Sin, Sex and Stigma

Anthropology Matters : Scholarship on Demand

A new series focusing on significant contributions that demonstrate the scholarship and depth of the traditional anthropological monograph, perhaps without wide commercial appeal, but with unquestionable academic merit. It will include important collections that open up new themes, and will publish research reports that deal with specific development or policy related issues, and are major interventions in current affairs and decision-making. All of these exemplify the way 'Anthropology Matters'.

Sin, Sex and Stigma

❖❖❖

A Pacific Response to HIV and AIDS

Lawrence James Hammar

Anthropology Matters, Volume 4

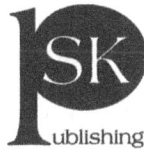

Sean Kingston Publishing

www.seankingston.co.uk

Wantage

First published in 2010 by

Sean Kingston Publishing
www.seankingston.co.uk
Wantage

British Library Cataloguing in Publication Data
A catalogue record for this book is available from the British Library.

Printed by Lightning Source

ISBN 978-0-9556400-4-9 hardback

Dedication

This book is dedicated to Olive, a girl who was traded by her father for three cartons of beer, some money and the promise of groom-service, a seldom used term now in anthropology but one that used to mean a man's support of his wife's parents. Olive was conned into marriage with an already twice-married provincial governor who soon infected her with STDs. He abandoned Olive due to her apparent infertility. This necessitated that she begin a short life of prostitution amidst the structural violence of gender relations, religious hypocrisy and increasing poverty. Officially, Olive died from cervical cancer, but if 'AIDS' means a systematic battering over time of skin, psyche, tissue and immune system in the process of living, well then, she died of AIDS. She had struggled unsuccessfully against a stubborn case of tuberculosis, and her vagina and cervix had been lacerated repeatedly by customer(s), boyfriend(s) and husband(s) alike, beginning with the then governor. Partly because Olive's church prohibited condom use, but partly also because she wanted to increase intimacy and avoid the stigmas that condom use would induce, she suffered several microbial STDs over the years, beginning but not ending with her husband's. Olive had been belted by her father (and then customers), raped (first by her husband) and robbed by father, boyfriend(s), customers, pimp and housemates. She was worn-out and miserable, and was carrying probably no more than ten *toea* in her skirt pocket when she died. Susan, Meke, Jackie, Kamaro, Agnes and countless others have died essentially the same way.

How many more Papua New Guineans must die before health bodies and officials, external donors and church leaders grasp that if there is an enemy, it is unprotected, infectious sex that is often as little consensual as it is pleasurable? I want to encourage responses to HIV and AIDS in Papua New Guinea to become less divisive and unrealistic and less slavishly devoted to acronyms and foreign concepts. I imagine a response built upon true Christian and secular norms of sociality, mutuality, multiplicity, compassion, desire and as much care for the Other as for Self.

This book is dedicated to Olive and to many more just like her. I hope that we may begin instead to embrace consensual, pleasurable expression of sexual desires on behalf of concern for healthy communities and relationships. Let us gain accurate knowledge of the only bodies we have in this world and use those bodies as we wish and at our pleasure in service of truly mutual goals, not because they are the tools of spouses, clans, churches or factories.

'God will lay his hand upon this nation', Taylor proclaimed in 1879. 'There will be more bloodshed, more ruin, more devastation than ever they have seen before ... We do not want them to force upon us that institution of monogamy called the social evil ... When they enact tyrannical laws, forbidding us the free exercise of our religion, we cannot submit. God is greater than the United States, and when the Government conflicts with heaven we will be ranged under the banner of heaven and against the Government. The United States says we cannot marry more than one wife. God says different ... Polygamy is a divine institution. It has been handed down direct from God. The United States cannot abolish it. No nation on earth can prevent it, nor all the nations of the earth combined; these are my sentiments and all of you who sympathize with me in this position will raise your right hands. I defy the United States; I will obey God.' (The third Prophet, Seer and Revelator of the Church of Jesus Christ of Latter-Day Saints, John Taylor, 1879–80, quoted in Jon Krakauer, *Under the Banner of Heaven*, 2003, p. 250)

The HIV virus [sic] is easy to spread because in the world there is not only a lack of medicines, but also a lack of education and awareness; there is poverty and unemployment, financial interests, uncontrolled risky sex behavior [and] polygamy. (Bishop Bonivento, *Do Condoms Stop or Spread AIDS?*, 2001, p. 5)

I plead on behalf of PNG, if an MP can stop the particular company producing condoms and also stop the awareness and advertisements on the media. People are happy when such awareness and advertisements occur knowing that it will save them from AIDS. But I [do] not agree on what you are doing. I believe the only way to stop AIDS is to accept Jesus Christ in to your life. He is the healer both physically and spiritually. (Lady Hennisha Paki, *Post Courier*, 31 January 2007)

Mr Hammer [sic] should not have been allowed into our country. I urge the government to carefully screen researchers coming into Papua New Guinea. (Paulias Matane, 'Research Tarnishes Our Image', *Post-Courier*, September 1992)

Contents

Foreword

We are fortunate to be reading Lawrence Hammar's *Sin, Sex and Stigma: a Pacific response to HIV and AIDS* because he was unfortunate. Just as he was about to take up a new position training young Papua New Guineans to assist in the fight against HIV and AIDS and just as his wife was about to join him in the Papua New Guinea town of Goroka, she fell seriously ill and he had to return to the United States to care for her. (Fortunately, she is recovering well from breast cancer.) When this occurred, he had finished his contract as Senior Research Fellow at the Papua New Guinea Institute of Medical Research and was about to begin working for the National Centre in HIV Social Research, based in Sydney, Australia. In this capacity, he was going to train 10 Papua New Guinean 'Research Cadets' in qualitative and quantitative research methods so that they could employ 'a multi-method, evidence-based approach to the rapidly expanding HIV and AIDS epidemic in Papua New Guinea' (Hammar, e-mail communication, 28 July 2006). Suitable and successful response to what was becoming a pandemic would demand, he believed, that Papua New Guineans, themselves, become appropriately trained researchers – able to collect the data necessary to argue persuasively for potentially successful interventions.

Unable to take up this position, he found himself back in Portland, Oregon with the time to ponder what he had learned over the years he had researched sexual violence in Papua New Guinea and its concomitant medical and psychological ills. As he tells us in Chapter 1, the Introduction to his book, many of his experiences have provoked the hot glow of anger and compelled him to speak Truth to Power. I will return to the truth he speaks in a minute, but first wish to say a bit more about the Research Cadets he wanted to train, focusing on the one with whom I, too, was privileged to work. I do this because it helps contextualize – it helps embody – the (productive) anger that hurt Lawrence into writing this book.

Rebecca Emori, the young Research Cadet in question, had already been trained in qualitative research methods at Papua New Guinea's Divine Word University by the anthropologist Nancy Sullivan. In addition to occasional teaching, Nancy runs a small research firm in the Papua New Guinea town of Madang and when Lawrence needed assistants to help with the work he was doing for the PNGIMR, he hired several members of Nancy's team. Rebecca proved a superb assistant (as I can personally attest since she helped me with my research project as well). And, so, it was natural that, when she applied for one of the Research Cadet positions, he signed her on. The job was to 'design research [about HIV and AIDS] and to analyze and write up data collected in the Highlands region' (Hammar, e-mail communication, 28 July 2006), and Rebecca was excited to take on the new position. Unfortunately, Lawrence left for home and, although things did not exactly fall apart, they became less structured than they might have been had he been able to remain. Rebecca wrote to me at this time, asking for help – as she did not know how to reach Lawrence. The problem was with writing an abstract. To apply for a scholarship which would allow her to travel to Sri Lanka to introduce the Research Cadet Program to delegates attending the International Congress on AIDS in the Asia and Pacific region, she needed advice as to how to write this abstract. I provided advice, but also contacted Lawrence for his assistance. Let me quote a bit from the message he sent. (I have translated the first paragraph from the Neo-Melanesian [Tok Pisin] in which it was written; the rest is presented as it was written, in English):

> Good morning, 'Last Born' [a term meaning a favoured dependent] ... do not worry: your family [literally, 'line,' or support network] is here and is in the 'same corner' as you. And I was once in the same shoes as you when I was in graduate school and I cried and cried and pulled out my hair. 'Ai, mama, please, not me, not me! How am I going to write this little paper [abstract]? Who will understand me? How come my teacher asked me to send this abstract to the big boss?'

> First of all, I want to congratulate you! It's a high honour even to be asked to do this and to travel to Sri Lanka to do so. I am absolutely and totally confident in your abilities ... Here are some general guidelines to follow... . First, make sure that your statement of ideas is well thought out and follows a logical, coherent direction. You will want to:

> ■ state the issue to be discussed (it sounds as if the ... practice of strengthening HIV Social Research in PNG is the 'big' issue here).

> ■ provide just enough 'background' ... to establish your knowledge-base and interest in [the subject so as] ... to compel further reading (when did this programme become important? ... why is it important now?) ...

> ■ provide a brief description of what you are doing as a Research Cadet ... (that is, where are you located? who is funding you? how many cadets are there? what are your activities?)

> ■ finally, discuss the implications and/or outcomes of this project (... when it's all over, how many cadets will be trained to do what? who is going to employ them?).

> When you have what you think is a good first draft, send it to us if you wish, or send it to another colleague, but do NOT send it to someone who is going to give it the once-over and just tell you that it is 'fine'. You want someone who has a critical mind and who will give you an honest opinion! When I give drafts of my writing to people to read, I always pick people who are going to be critical. I want the mistakes to be found and the strengths to be highlighted... . So, this is your chance to establish a career trait: don't be

afraid to solicit critical feed-back ... (e-mail communication from Hammar to Emori, 17 December 2006).

What is obvious about this e-mail communication is the degree to which Lawrence cares that Rebecca succeeds fully: he cares that she learns to do her best so that she can accomplish important personal and professional goals – and ones for the good of her countrymen and women. It is also obvious that he is not going to give Rebecca an easy time. He is not going to do the work for her, but he is going to provide her with skills and advice and be in her corner.

Over the course of his career, Lawrence has been in the corner of many Papua New Guineans from greatly varied backgrounds: those well-educated like Rebecca and those far less so, such as the *tu kina meri* (K2.00 women) with whom Lawrence worked at the island provincial capital town of Daru. These are the women in prostitution who used to sell sex for about US$.60 (now about triple that) and who are often coerced into doing so by kinsmen (who should be in their corner, but who are not). Lawrence has spoken with them at length about who they are, where they come from, to what they aspire and what they are prevented from doing. He has learned about the various political economies of sex that flourish throughout the country: about those derived from a patriarchal Christianity that demands fidelity on the part of wives, but not on the part of husbands; about those derived from other patriarchies which, for example, allow fathers and husbands to pimp their daughters and wives with impunity – sometimes to get by in the context of land alienation, sometimes just to buy a beer in the context of anomie. And, he has come to understand (as many HIV and AIDS researchers have also come to understand in Papua New Guinea and elsewhere) that many people, including variously located women, are becoming terribly, terribly sick – and not only those deemed at 'high risk'. Hence his anger: anger at certain pastors, with their ABC programmes (recommending **A**bstinence, **B**eing Faithful and – in Papua New Guinea – **C**hristian-Centred Values) who preach against condoms as being 'Satan's tools' which lead to immorality; anger at the husbands who bring diseases home to their good, Christian wives and then ostracize them when they become sick; anger at the NGOs that rely for their funding and access to the country upon a model of 'high risk' groups and settings which many know to be epidemiologically simplistic; anger at the politicians who siphon off funds, seduce whomever they choose and acquire their antiretroviral drugs with ease and efficiency; anger at the fear, silences, omissions and down-right lies.

And he has a right to his anger, I think – especially because, as I have said, it has proven a productive anger. It is not an 'ethnography of indignation' (Cassell 1991: xiv–xviii). It does not indulge in self-righteousness at the expense of understanding. It provides a detailed, rich, upsetting, perplexing, historically and culturally nuanced explication of why we all should be angrier – for the *tu kina meri*, for the good Christian wives, for Rebecca.

Dr Deborah Gewertz, Amherst, Massachusetts

Acknowledgments

This book has resulted from much collaboration and friendship shown and help given freely by many colleagues, friends and organisations. I want first to thank people in Goroka, capital of Papua New Guinea's Eastern Highlands Province. Having briefly visited Goroka in 1988 I never imagined that 15 years later I would be honoured by being able to spend three years there working for the Papua New Guinea Institute of Medical Research. I thank the (then) Deputy (now) Director of the IMR, Dr Peter Siba, and the former Director, Professor John Reeder (now of the Melbourne-based Burnet Institute) for their support of the nationwide project I was honoured to lead. Although I present no clinical data from that study here, my experiences in and out of the field (and literally bushes) could not help but influence much of what I have written. I worked closely with many fine technicians and colleagues at the IMR, among them Mition Yoannes, Lisol Luke, Tony Lupiwa, Martina Yambun, Tilda Wal, Gibson Winston, Mary Amos, Janet Gare, Matthew Omena, George Koki and Pamela Toliman. I cannot express in words how much I enjoyed working in the field with Herick Aeno (Sajen Swit-Gris), Mary (Moms) Aisa, Kim (Soupie) Papaso, Phili Manove (Gamo), Steven (Stiki) Yangi, James (Soge) Topo, Maggie Wagi (Sotpela) and Marynne Tom (Longpela). *Save i kilim yupela pinis. Wanbel i stap.*

I want to thank also officials and colleagues from the National AIDS Council Secretariat (NACS) and the National HIV and AIDS Support Project (NHASP), including Ms Sue Crockett, Ms Barbara Smith, Ms Cheryl Kelly, Mr Romanus Pakure and Drs John Millan, Joachim Pantumari and Ninkama Moiya. Dr Millan was a particularly interested and fine colleague. I have written this book in the hope that in the coming years their stated interest in the conduct of HIV social research will come to reflect so, wherever research findings lead them. Dr Greg Law was extremely supportive during conduct of our nationwide study. Ross Hutton (of Oil Search Limited), Cathy Reto (then of Porgera Joint Ventures), Jaime Carron, Patricia Bayly and Thomas Coombs (of JTA International, Brisbane) and David Masani (of Ok Tedi Mining Limited) provided friendship and logistical support and put kind and concerned human faces to resource extraction companies. Rose Uri stood out in Vanimo and Meredith Tutumang did the same in Lae as models of leadership against anti-condom nonsense in provincial AIDS committee settings. Sr Deli Wangama, Sr Primrose, Sr Frieda and Mr Mauri Nemantu also did so in their varied roles and settings of healthcare delivery. Each one of them is going to have to stand proxy for another 10 people at each of 11 field-sites who enriched my life and helped my crew. Mama Angela and Papa Jeff Bulage are my parents, fully and in every sense of the term. Papa Jeff has since passed away, of cerebral malaria, and I miss him so very much. In addition to being a great ethnographer and fine scholar, Richard Eves was gentlemanly in allowing me to use as my book cover the photo he snapped in Boroko, NCD: thanks! to him and to the poster's artist.

While I *could* say enough to thank my co-conspirators here for their labors here and friendship and support elsewhere – Deborah Gewertz, Mark Boyd, Alison Murray and Sarah Hewat – to do so would take way too many pages. But thank you! Anne Arthur and Michael French Smith provided good advice about one deadly dull and one too harshly pessimistic draft of Chapter 1 that has come in handy elsewhere. Phil Carr closely read and provided helpful commentary upon Chapter 2, as did Michael Wood in a prior version. Holly Wardlow read and commented upon Chapter 4 at a critical point and made many, many constructive suggestions: thank you! The friendship, works and writings of Leslie Butt, Kathy Lepani, Stuart Kirsch, Naomi McPherson, Nancy Sullivan and Deborah Gewertz continue to inspire me; they have been wonderful friends and e-mail colleagues over the years and have taught me the other Papua New Guineas they know. Sean Kingston and colleagues at his publishing house have been uncommonly helpful and supportive; frankly, this book would not have even been dreamt about had Sean not in 2004 expressed interest in it. I also thank greatly an anonymous reviewer of the first complete draft of the book, who made a number of extremely positive and helpful suggestions at an important time – in any event, I expected much worse. The penultimate draft was proof-read and commented upon by Amy Achor, Eli Hurwitz, Vick Mickunas, Mike Kelly, Michael Hall, Laurel Finch and Joel Smith. Crystal Bryson then improved the final draft with an extra-close reading. Glen Mola, Kim Benton, Jane Cousins, Tim Sladden, Philip Smith and Philip Gibbs deserve recognition, too, for the many newspaper reports and special insights they provided. Thank you, all!

My mother, Norma Garrison, and father, Les Hammar, gave me the best start in life one could ask for and have never left my side even when graduate school and fieldwork overseas separated us. My debt to my wife Urakume Mahala (neé Cassandra Lee) goes way beyond the words I know – she is worth every *toea* I paid for her in bride-price, that's for sure. She has enabled me to live freely, unapologetically standing up for what I think is right and for speaking out against what I think is not. I have persisted in being an anthropologist partly because she believes in me and in the worth of what we anthropologists do in the world.

Whether supportive or critical, good or bad, *sapos yu bel hat o yu bel isi*, I welcome your comments: gorokadubu@att.net.

Abbreviations and Acronyms

ABC   Abstain (from sex), Be faithful (to one's spouse), or (as a last resort) use Condoms, the major conceptual plank of more conservative HIV transmission prevention platforms worldwide; ABC remains the ideological fulcrum of the national response in Papua New Guinea.

AIDS   The Acquired Immune Deficiency Syndrome is a highly contested, often greatly misunderstood collection of signs (such as prolonged weight and hair loss), markers (lowered CD4 cell counts, HIVab seroreactivity) and symptoms (productive cough, persistent diarrhoea). 'AIDS diagnoses' in Papua New Guinea are highly correlated with these symptoms and especially persistent tuberculosis, but for complicated reasons do not require an HIVab+ blood-test result (e.g. Lavu *et al.* 2004)

ARV/ART/ HAART   Antiretrovirals, antiretroviral therapies and highly active antiretroviral therapies. Singly and in combination, these are the major pharmaceutical treatments for HIV infection.

AusAID   Australian Agency for International Development, based in Canberra, the primary external donor.

CBO   Community-Based Organisations, such as street theatre groups.

CSW/FSW   Commercial Sex Worker/Female Sex Worker, both being highly contentious terms favoured by NGOs and many epidemiologists but that tend to hide more than they reveal about sexual networking.

ELISA   Enzyme-linked Immunosorbent Assay, used here to screen for antibody to HIV.

FBO   Faith-Based Organisations, such as those that sponsor sites where HIVab testing and counselling occur.

HIV   Human Immunodeficiency Virus. 'HIV' is split into two main types (HIV-1 and HIV-2). The first is split further into three major Groups – M[ain], N and O-, Type C of the first of which is common in sub-Saharan Africa (and apparently Papua New Guinea).

HIVab   HIV antibody, what tests of our blood can register following sufficient exposure to HIV. 'HIV prevalence studies' seldom monitor HIV directly, but rather putative antibody to it. An 'HIVab+' test result can be 'false positive' in that current or recent pregnancy, infection with other viruses, recent experience of influenza shots and many other conditions and vaccinations can sometimes falsely register infection with HIV.

HIVab-	HIV antibody-negative, a test result suggesting non-exposure to HIV. Such can be 'false-negative', however, in the sense that exposure to HIV was so recent that the body had not yet produced antibody thereto, or because the integrity of the blood samples tested had been challenged (for example, by heat), or because of great differences in the ways in which individuals, laboratories and countries construct and carry out HIVab testing algorithms.
HIVab+	HIV antibody-positive, a blood test result that follows from application of a testing algorithm that finds 'Initial' and 'Repeat' Reactives ideally 'confirmed' by additional and/or different testing.
HRSS	High-Risk Settings Strategy, adopted at 30+ sites throughout the country, ideally to monitor and evaluate the efficacy of targeted interventions along the lines of communication, behaviour change, condom distribution, 'awareness' and street-based theatre, since 're-branded' as Tingim Laip.
NAC/S	National AIDS Council/Secretariat, located in Port Moresby, established in 1997 and revamped and revised and supported by the National HIV and AIDS Support Project (funded by AusAID).
NCD	National Capital District, where the nation's capital, Port Moresby, is located.
NDoH	National Department of Health, a government body located in the nation's capital of Port Moresby.
NGO/INGO	Non-Government, International Non-Government Organisations, both of which have greatly aided the national response.
NHASP	National HIV and AIDS Support Project, located in Port Moresby, which has supported and advocated the NACS since 2000.
PACs/DACs	Provincial AIDS Committees and District AIDS Committees. These were set up in each of Papua New Guinea's 20 provinces (including the NCD), each having a set number of paid staff and ideally supported by volunteers and other resources to promote HIV awareness and prevention.
PNGIMR	Papua New Guinea Institute of Medical Research, headquartered in Goroka.
STD/s	Sexually Transmitted Disease/s, such as gonorrhea and syphilis, including their symptoms.
VCT	Voluntary (HIVab) Counselling and Testing, increasingly promoted as an indirect method of prevention. As of this writing, there are 75 such sites of VCT throughout Papua New Guinea.

Part One

Sexual networking and sexually transmitted dis-ease in the Pacific

ABC: *Always Be Critical*

A MEMBER of Parliament says condoms are not always safe and has urged people to have sex with only person[s] they trusted. Unggai-Bena MP Benny Allen told a leadership program on HIV in Parliament on Thursday he had a case in his electorate where a woman got infected by her husband who said he was using condoms. But it was found later that he had actually torn it before using it, Mr Allen said. (*Post-Courier* 2007)

This book is about the cultural and religious politics in Papua New Guinea of sexuality, HIV, condoms, AIDS, mobility and marriage and other kinds of gender relations. In fact, this book is in many ways about the epigraph above: about why a man would tear a condom before using it – and without his wife knowing; about AIDS workshops that leave learned parliamentarians with yet opaque understandings of condom 'safety' and HIV transmission routes and risks; about why people think that 'trust' in a partner's fidelity (and non-infectiousness) helps to prevent transmission of HIV and sexually transmitted diseases (STDs) in the face of mountains of evidence that they do not; and about newspaper reportage that can fall down on the job. In discourses that I detail in middle chapters of the book, religious goals and aspirations seem to clash more than they mesh with those of the public health. In Chapters 4 and 5 I reveal considerable cognitive dissonance in both mainstream epidemiological models and anti-condom rhetoric in Papua New Guinea. I argue that the real focus is not and perhaps never has been as much about preventing sexual transmission of anything so much as about realigning sexual practice to fit certain Christian ideals of monogamous heterosexuality. I look closely at patterned condom disinformation, at misunderstandings of sexual networking dynamics and, above all, at debatable models of HIV epidemiology in the region. I argue that these have combined with nationalist and religious politics of sexual matters to blunt well intended efforts to stem the transmission of the STDs (and now HIV) that have historically devastated the bodies, health systems and social-structures of countries, cultures and territories in the Pacific.

I attribute many of the successes but also some of the challenges of the 'national response' in Papua New Guinea to HIV and AIDS to the fact that it is mostly externally funded and guided, mostly by the Australian Agency for International Development (AusAID). So much so, in fact, that sometimes even Papua New Guineans (such as Dr Ninkama Moiya, who now heads the Sanap Wantaim programme, after having been Director for three years of the National AIDS Council Secretariat, head-quartered in Port Moresby) are dubbed 'representatives from the Australian Government' (Gumuno 2008). Geoffrey Hayes has pointed out that 'the geographical variations within PNG in any case work against a "national" response'. Despite commonalities of health systems collapse, he says, Milne Bay and Southern Highlands provinces might as well be different countries (personal communication, 28 April 2008; see Hayes 2007). I argue that these geographic obstacles, alongside the imported nature of initiatives, messages and personnel often contradict otherwise well-intended efforts to slow the pace of the epidemic and at the same time fail to appreciate also the multiplicity of epidemics evolving and interacting with one another. By this I mean the types of HIV-I and HIV-II circulating about the region (e.g. Oelrichs 2004; Ryan *et al.* 2006; Lindenbaum 2008: vii–viii) that have different transmission dynamics, source points and even degrees of resistance to this or that highly active antiretroviral therapy (HAART). Added to these are ongoing regimes of resource extraction that make sexual networking more dangerous than it should be; continuing scandals of political and financial corruption that drub already struggling health services systems; seemingly unchecked sexual violence; and persistent shortfalls in matters of sexual health education.

In particular I show that the so-called 'ABC' approach to preventing transmission (where **A**bstinence and **B**eing faithful are enjoined, but where those don't work, **C**ondoms must be used) remains the ideological fulcrum of the national response despite the absence of any evidence that it works to prevent transmission. I argue that this borrowed, prescriptive model hasn't worked, that it isn't working and that it should not be expected to work, as many people hope, to prevent infection on a mass level. The ABC message functions mostly to placate the religious doctrines and leaders that drive the national response and who are not so inflamed by the presence of the 'C' that they feel a need to reconfigure it. The same dynamic has been found in Africa. The virologist-turned-intrepid-journalist, Helen Epstein, interviewed one Martin Ssempa, an Ugandan pastor who burned condoms in protest and who exclaimed thusly when encountering a condom promotion billboard: '"Look at this!" Ssempa yelled, pointing at the drawing of the condom billboard. "It's horrible. You can't promote condoms and abstinence at the same time! It would only confuse young people", he said, "and send the message that it was really OK to be promiscuous"' (Epstein 2007: 192). In Chapter 5 I show in great detail that in both religious and ostensibly secular settings 'C' now can mean 'Christian values', even 'Church doctrine' or 'Commitment' in some venues. One AusAID review team concluded that 'this misinformation (at worst) and ambivalence (at best) is undermining HIV prevention in PNG

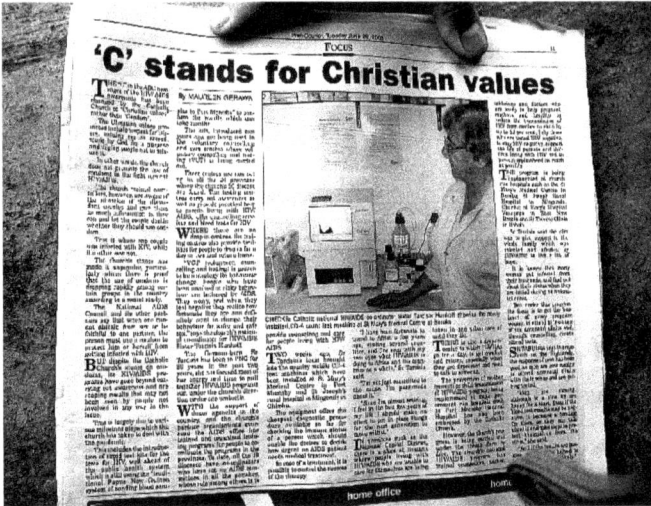

Changing the C in ABC

and denying people a full range of proven protective choices' (AusAID 2005a: 13). Another commentator, in this case upon the essays that make up the exciting new collection edited by Leslie Butt and Richard Eves, *Making Sense of AIDS: culture, sexuality, and power in Melanesia*, asked poignantly: 'How can adequate knowledge and protection be provided for communities in which conservative Christian beliefs, often aligned with preexisting cultural codes, adopt sin-based models of AIDS, and have a negative influence on the use of condoms?' (Lindenbaum 2008: ix). Eves and Butt rightfully credit the efforts made by mainline Christian churches and denominations in Papua New Guinea, but yet worryingly write that '[t]he fundamentalist moral agenda and worldview are increasingly dominant' (Eves and Butt 2008: 14). In a Pastoral Letter sent to his Sandaun Province faithful, Bishop Cesare Bonivento of the Vanimo Diocese reminded that 'lots' of people suffering from AIDS weren't at fault for having contracted HIV, so don't discriminate against them! As for the rest, well ... Like Eves, Butt, Lindenbaum and others, I call attention to the fact that Christian-based ideas and practices can also harm people – even when the desired purpose is not to do so. In doing so, they also dull the effects of HIV transmission prevention efforts. Attributions of 'innocent' infections invite contemplation of guilt; feelings of guilt alter perception of risk; and perceptions of risk have consequences for infection.

Eves and Butt remark in an endnote to their essay that '[n]o ethnography of AIDS in any part of the Pacific exists ... Neither are there any volumes detailing the failures and inadequacies of prevention campaigns' (Eves and Butt 2008: 269, n. 19). Having read these words for the first time on 6 June 2008, I have aimed to respond effectively to this critical deficit, and I hope that my readers and other researchers and activists will stand up and speak out. Debate has to this date been fleeting and too terribly polite, for example, in cyberspace on the Pacific islands-based discussion forum, AIDSTOK. For every point of contention raised, there must be 75 postings that advertise consultancies, report upon workshops, announce new organisations and re-post already published newspaper items. The rare flame is too often politely allowed to extinguish. Dr Sitaleki Finau, a prominent Tongan physician and current Director of Health in Niue, called recently for the erection of quarantines in the Pacific of those found to be HIVab+ and/or suffering from AIDS. Reaction was swift and negative. Nevertheless, this is the rare exception, and posters missed great opportunities to examine the sources of Dr Finau's misguided opinions – Christian doctrine-induced concepts of sin, promiscuity and social stigma – with which, I hate to say it, in other ways many more concur.

I will mention here briefly the seven 'big' points on which this book is founded. First, *both national* (Papua New Guinean) *and international public health and policy representatives have yet really to grasp the fundamental, root causes of HIV transmission dynamics or the burden of AIDS-related illness and suffering.* No fundamental shift in social-structure has been called for, for example, in political leadership, in the division of domestic labours or in the redistribution of land and its resources in a way that is gender-equitable. The focus for twenty years has been on individuals, often 'bad', socially despised people, and on individual behaviours, which have often been pathologised and stigmatised. The HIV and AIDS community in Papua New Guinea and Australia continues to 'target' dubiously constructed 'risk groups', for example 'FSW' or female sex workers, and 'MSM' or Men who have Sex with Men. This has both obscured the setting of the greatest bulk of infections (companionate relationships, plain-old marriage) and revealed the particular blindness of the national response to HIV and AIDS. The national response has been to refuse to question, much less intervene in heterosexual male privilege. It has utterly failed to recognise, much less to target the extraordinary transmissive risk that husbands, politicians and expatriate males often pose to others. It questions no Christian leaders or doctrines that mandate male dominance.

Second, *there are too few facts, too little empirical evidence on which the national response has been based.* This is not to say that empirical data have not been collected in abundance, for they surely have, but rather, to note that those of dubious character have been chosen over those of greater facticity. The ways that 'behavioural risk', 'identity', 'sex worker' and the like, have been framed

> '[I]t is also often assumed that the lessons learnt in the West will be instantly transferable to Asia. These kinds of assumptions are not infrequently found in papers presented at various international AIDS conferences, in which a successful "model" derived from projects in say Sydney or San Francisco is presented as being immediately relevant to the situation in Manila or Bangkok but rarely vice versa' (Borthwick 1999: 206, emphasis added).

show disrespect of the many dedicated social scientists whose data and models challenging them have been overlooked. Such cozy acronyms as ABC also ignore the tenor and motivations of sexual practice of most Papua New Guineans. I make this point especially in the remainder of this Introduction to Part One, but also in Chapter 4 and Chapter 5. In the Introduction to Part Two I also discuss patterns and motivations of male practices of genital cutting and manipulation. These issues have been generally overlooked by health authorities and bodies, even as they contemplate male circumcision en masse as a prevention strategy, as has been attempted from one hospital initiative in East Sepik Province. This may appeal to readers who have been following the extensive debates regarding HIV and male circumcision (see Aggleton 2007; Berer 2007a, b; Dowsett and Couch 2007). In any event, little breadth of analysis has been allowed by national health authorities and their expatriate sponsors to inform public health and human rights issues. The debate will surely heat up when men's sexuality and their genitals are 'put under a bright light for examination' (Berer 2007b: 8).

Third, the *overwhelmingly external nature of funding source, epidemiological model and surveillance system* has resulted in an epidemiological database that is too loose, opaque and insensitive to culture and mobility to guide the national response effectively. This will become evident in Chapters 3 and 4; there and elsewhere I critique the overwhelmingly urban-based nature of policy planning, awareness campaigns and resource-gobbling administrative overhead. The static, reifying nature of the leading categories in epidemiological modelling can be glimpsed in terms just of the facts that 'expatriate' is not 'heterosexual'; that noting the 'province of origin' of someone HIV antibody positive (HIVab+) says nothing about anything unless it helps to explain actual transmission; that 'bisexual' is only homosexual, not also heterosexual and can refer only to males, not also females; that 'MSM' (Men who have Sex with Men) has for some doctors turned itself into a 'transmissive mode' (not a sexual identity); and that anal intercourse is the suspected transmissive culprit when two men are involved but not when a man and a woman or child are involved. The national response in Papua New Guinea has borrowed from the West some of the language of HIV prevention but little of its nuance and without benefit of any of its gadflies.

Fourth, *national and international health bodies and authorities seem to be aiming for a 'fix' of some kind but that is too biomedical and technical in nature.* There are many unquestioned assumptions about HIVab testing and counselling, about the sustainability of the roll-out of highly active antiretroviral therapies (HAART) and about the benefits of male circumcision. In Chapter 4, in the Introduction to Part Two and in Chapter 9 I argue that too little attention has been paid to the level of social-structure. I mean this in terms of both the nature of bodily suffering and the rearrangements in sexual praxis that must be made so as to dampen HIV transmission. Additionally, my colleague Mark Boyd speaks perceptively in Chapter 8 to the complexities of technical, biomedical fixes. I cannot improve upon Marge Berer's comment recently that '[a]nyone who thinks that a technical solution to a sociosexual problem can work on its own, no matter how many millions of dollars they can throw at it is, I believe, deluding themselves' (Berer 2007b: 46).

Fifth, *the externalization of risk away from oneself, one's marriage and one's sexual partners is endemic,* being carried there by foreign consultants and sponsors, but also built-in to the national response on other grounds. This is hardly just a Papua New Guinean phenomenon, but nevertheless, it defines the national response there. In guides to implementation of the provisions of the President's Emergency Plan for AIDS Relief (PEPFAR), 'high-risk populations' are defined as sex workers, male homosexuals and IV drug injectors. Critics of the implementation of PEPFAR in Uganda note that 'US government-funded condom programmes are restricted to "high-risk" areas such as bars and discos and banned from locations, such as schools and universities, where they would serve the general population' (Cohen 2005: 24; see also Schoepf 2004a, b). Here, in the remainder of this chapter, and in Chapters 4, 5 and 6 I argue that health officials continue to refuse to look at where the bulk of transmissive risk lies: in companionate relations, in plain-old marriage. My colleague Alison Murray also deepens this critique in our conversation in Chapter 7. This externalisation is evident especially in newspaper reportage. It was recently reported that there were 'More Mothers, Students HIV Positive in Morobe [Province]'. The report included commentary from a spokesperson in Lae, the provincial capital, such that, while rates of HIV infection among 'sex workers' had 'stabilised', those of 'mothers in stable marriages and students in secondary and tertiary schools was rising at a very alarming rate' (*Post-Courier* 2008c). Excited to read further – *finally!* – my hopes were soon dashed: the article failed to show and explain what those rates were, how transmission had been established and what defined sex work or marriage stability. It explained that 'the men were usually in the mid 30s, had money and cars and they picked up women for sex and paid them' and then 'passed on the virus to their wives in their homes'. So, the infective source is girls and young women? How are *they* becoming infected? Why does 'student' mean female? Are not wives infecting husbands? Can people not be infected multiple times via many different routes?

Sixth, I show explicitly in Chapter 2 on historical and ethnographic grounds that this tendency to externalise risk and to blame the Other is related to the inability of programme managers and religious leaders to look squarely at broadly acceptable traditions and local expectations about sexuality and its products. Chapters 2, 6, 7 and 9 discuss male sexual prerogative most critically, but also discuss the place of sexual networking in the discharge of social obligations such as the transmission of names, the achievement of fertility goals and the furtherance of economic and social ties between groups. The fact that the discharge is often one-sided, that the obligations are often of and express sexual and other inequalities, hasn't yet really changed the approach that public health authorities, preachers and politicians take to sexual health and behaviour. This is most obviously so when it comes to contemporary debates around sexual pleasure and prostitution. By contrast, ethnographers such as Katherine Lepani have shown on various grounds what can be the benefits of more sex-positive, erotically playful attitudes (in her case, regarding Trobriand islander sexual praxis; see 2007b, 2008a). Holly Buchanan-Aruwafu and Rose Maebiru (2008) and Jack Morin (2008) have each but in different ways detailed the paradoxical nature of sexual desire

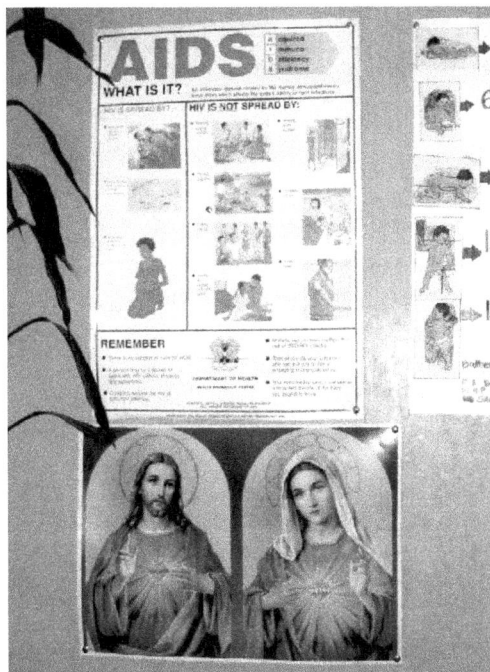

Likenesses of Jesus and Mary frame AIDS poster message

and categories of risk and identity elsewhere in Melanesia. Nevertheless, the rich ethnographic detail they provide and with such keen sociological insight has not been hitched to any wagon of epidemiological modelling or intervention. This is mostly because, in the first case, Abstinence is the only plank applicable in the Papua New Guinea platform, and in the second case, because male–male sexual contact remains illegal in Indonesia (and Papua New Guinea) and is thus made the more unsafe.

Seventh and finally, *I critique the ABC message in concept, motivation and implementation and lay particular responsibility at the doorstep of religious leaders and doctrine.* I argue that the ABC message has as little grounding in the realities of social-structure as in today's globalising political-economy, and that it is a gender-neutral message delivered in the most gender-saturated country one could imagine. Even ostensibly biomedical messages about the properties of viruses and their transmission dynamics are easily lost when situated in a context of religious icons and texts, such as those depicted here, which undercut rational public health information by encouraging viewers to interpret along lines of religious belief. The photo here, taken in a highlands STD Clinic, depicts a man said to have been a virgin (but who probably wasn't) and a woman said to have been a virgin (and who surely wasn't). In this argument I join a number of recent ethnographers. Lepani has written perceptively about the problems that ensue in the Trobriand islands, where local norms and understandings clank against ABC:

> communication about HIV and AIDS is based persistently on biomedical and epidemiological constructions of meaning, with little consideration for how such information interacts dynamically with diverse and changing cultural

beliefs and practices. These models infuse the language of HIV prevention with predominantly Western assumptions and moralities about human sexuality, gender relations, and individual behavior. (Lepani 2008a: 246)

* * *

Taking these seven points together, and especially in view of ABC, I argue that Christian churches in the Pacific *more than any other institution* have encouraged unsafe sex and disabled the more accurate risk assessments needed to guide safer, more pleasurable and less infectious sexual behaviour (Hammar 2006b). By this I don't just mean prohibitions of demonstrably safer sexual practices, for example, missionary musings about the adverse psychological consequences of masturbation, the exaggerated dangers of oral sex or even the specific banning by Christian missionaries of 'thigh sex' (*ukusoma*) in rural South Africa (Harrison 2008: 177). Naomi McPherson has pointed out that 'the church is responsible for exacerbating the problem in another way as well, for in laying such stress on the sinful nature of promiscuous sex, it makes condom use even more out of the question' (McPherson 2008: 244). Richard Eves has suggested that '[f]aith healing and miraculous cures license unsafe sex because repentance and conversion are such readily available means of saving sinners from both the ravages of AIDS and the fires of hell' (Eves 2008: 223). The head Pastor of Papua New Guinea's Revival Fellowship Church claims to have cured 40 people of their HIV infections through prayer alone and has argued that condom promotion campaigns are sinful, verily anti-Christ (Bennett 2008; see the photo and accompanying story in Chapter 8). How many of those 40 still-infected people, do you think, will *now* start using condoms, assuming that any of them had previously? Holly Wardlow writes on the basis of her long-term involvement with the Huli-speaking people of Southern Highlands Province that 'some community leaders asserted that the arrival of AIDS in Tari was a good thing, since the threat of death and stigma might spur people to finally become good Christians' (2008: 187). AIDS showed Huli villagers that 'Christianity was nevertheless the right path' (2008: 188). Such moralistic attitudes can drub treatment initiatives. Like Eves in New Ireland Province, Daniel Smith has shown that, for the mainline and Pentecostal denominations of Christian Igbo in Nigeria, 'testimonies included stories of cure through religious healing, which is arguably one of the most dangerous religious messages proffered in relation to HIV/AIDS'. '[T]he larger religious message that HIV/AIDS is the result of immorality and can be prevented by being a good, moral Christian', he notes, 'contributes to a social environment in which the disease is highly stigmatized' (Smith 2004: 429).

I argue in Chapters 1, 4 and 5 that missions throughout Papua New Guinea and the Pacific have monopolised not just the content of sexual health educational materials but also the means by which and social spaces within which they may be disseminated. At the South Pacific Games held recently in Samoa the sporting bodies of Samoa and Fiji convinced games organisers on Christian grounds to remove female condoms from the gift bags given to all athletes so that they could enjoy Safe Games, though they left in the male condoms (postings made to AIDSTOK, September, 2007). Being often influenced by variously understood Christian doctrines, behaviours and ideals, public health programmes and personnel have in Papua New Guinea contributed also to massive cognitive dissonance about HIV transmission risks. By externalising risk away from 'husband' and 'marriage' toward 'sex worker' and 'prostitution' (each being also extremely contentious terms), and whether or not churches and church leaders have always meant consciously to do so, they have increased stigma and fuelled misogyny. To their credit, several mainline churches and their representatives have owned up to the stigma they have fuelled, and to make amends they are now to be counted among the most vociferous opponents of sexual violence (though not of male domination *per se*). Just like in Hollywood film codes, straight men are both villain and hero.

Gendering groups and others

Of these seven points I've mentioned above, there are three kinds of examples that I present in greater detail in Chapters 3, 4, 5 and 6. First, public health, political and Christian authorities blame not just sex or social change *per se* for the spread of HIV, but prostitution and particular kinds of women and girls. By aggressively marketing conservative gender ideals they tell people with whom *not* to have sex and exhort them to have less sex, as opposed to showing them how to have sex more safely, pleasurably and consensually. As well, by promoting individualising messages and initiatives they have blurred the social nature of HIV epidemics. Bettina Beer has been conducting field research alongside the Wampar, who live in the Markham Valley of Papua New Guinea's Morobe Province. She reports on the basis of her recent fieldwork that a locally made AIDS video, featuring Wampar themselves, 'in common with other early campaign materials, presented promiscuity as the main reason for the spread of HIV, showing married village men drinking with city prostitutes and subsequently infecting their wives' (Beer 2008: 97). The 'HIV/AIDS Action Drama' presented to Kaliai villagers in West New Britain Province featured 'the Husband, the Wife, two Sex Workers and the Narrator' (McPherson 2008: 227). In like manner, a South African AIDS drama featured the protagonist and his wife and two bar girls; the American development agency representative asked the sparse audience 'what was the message here?', and the reply was '[d]on't go out with bar girls. Stick to one partner' (Epstein 2007: 253). It is not completely clear to what extent the play's content (Western-dressing sex workers transmit HIV to hapless village men) and its implicit moral (Christian, village-based lifestyles will prevent HIV infection) had been endorsed by the NAC. Nevertheless, the drama troupe members had recently attended a workshop sponsored by the Provincial AIDS Committee, and I have seen other plays produced and performed with similar intent and effect and also underwritten by NAC and PAC (Provincial AIDS Committee) materials and direction. Some fail altogether to mention condoms, and others conflate HIV and AIDS and thus confuse listeners. Yet others imply religious cures and means of prevention, as when the touch of Jesus is presumed to remove both HIV infection and its associated stigma, as I witnessed being performed by health workers and women's group representatives in Mendi, capital of Southern Highlands Province. Promoting condom use or critiquing male sexual prerogative are not yet part of the script. Bashing 'sex workers' goes over a lot better.

Contradictory models of gender comportment in the face of *kastom*, the nation and especially the Church are evident in other Pacific island countries and cultures. Maggie Cummings wrote in her recent essay, 'The Trouble With Trousers' (Cummings 2008) that '[t]oday, despite its "foreign" roots, the Mother Hubbard (or island dress) is lauded as the "national" and *kastom* dress for ni-Vanuatu women. Trousers, on the other hand, are understood to be for men or for foreign, white women. When worn by ni-Vanuatu women', she notes, 'they are considered indicative of sexual availability, promiscuity, and *rabis* behavior' (2008: 142). The Bariai-produced play and its performance mentioned above did not mention condom use; neither were they handed out at the play's conclusion, nor did instruction as to their use occur. Not surprisingly, the narrator seemed puzzled at the ethnographer's commentary that men posed a transmissive threat to wives and mothers, to foetuses and infants. I have sat through entire AIDS-related programmes without any mention whatsoever of condoms, unless it was to disparage them as 'only 50/50', 'not proper for Papua New Guinea' and the like (see also Eves and Butt 2008: 3). The words and terms 'consensual', 'condoms' and 'safe sex' appear in workshops and seminars sponsored by national health authorities and their expatriate supporters, but I have never seen them discussed or demonstrated in any depth. Who is responsible for this?

Second, the heading 'Sentinel Surveillance' was defined in the Papua New Guinea government's most recent National Strategic Plan as relating to 'a particular group (such as men who have sex with men) or activity (such as sex work) that acts as an indicator of the presence of a disease' (NAC 2007: viii). The review commissioned by the National HIV and AIDS Support Project (NHASP) of one of the major components of the national response, the so-called High-Risk Settings Strategy (HRSS), suggested that there be an '[e]xpansion of a broad range of approaches, including behaviour change programmes targeted at high-risk groups, such as sex workers and men who have sex with men' (NHASP 2006e: 2; see also Jenkins 2007: 5). There can be no way forward when groups are identified with disease and insofar as sex is seen and condemned in such negative terms. I detail these problems especially in Chapters 1 and 4.

Third, frank sex education curricula for youth have also been opposed by community leaders and church bodies because sex is not *for* them. Joe Egu, an 'anti-HIV/AIDS campaigner', lectured fourth-year Divine Word University students in a health management course that 'sex is not something to experiment by young people ... It is a blessed and sanctified activity of God to be enjoyed only in marriage' ... but also after completing a college education and finding a job (see Pamba 2008). To that end the new *HIV & AIDS and Reproductive Health* course for student teachers and lecturers is a welcome substitution of education for ignorance, as its Introduction states (Department of Education 2006b: 4). Unfortunately, this exciting new resource is one that Bishop Bonivento of the Vanimo Diocese thinks is so dangerous that he released a Pastoral Letter (Bonivento 2008) requesting that the government withdraw it and that parents send their children to Catholic schools forthwith (see also Agenzia Fides 2008). Religious instruction has long prevented and community attitudes have shied away from the clear presentation of factual information to youth. This has further blunted the accuracy of personal risk assessments.

> '*I experienced stigma and discrimination for three years. From my family – my brothers' wives didn't want me to talk to or hold their children and it was something that I was so sad about. And they got over it and I educated them on HIV and now we are friends. And around the community people were so, kind of, scared about me. Scared of me and they were always gossiping, but then it took me a couple of years to work with my community to break that stigma down and my whole community is very supportive of me*' (Maura Mea, in AIDSmeds & Poz, see Hofman 2007).

These three developments have greatly blunted the national response to HIV and AIDS. At the level of policy, debatable assumptions were made in the early 1990s about what constituted 'high-risk' and 'low-risk' that continue to (mis)inform policy and activities today. In Chapter 4 I discuss several examples of the formal model, such as Caldwell and Isaac-Toua's 'AIDS in Papua New Guinea: situation in the Pacific' (2002). This model hinges on the assumption that, as they put it, '"[l]ow-risk" means general population and "high-risk" refers to persons attending STI clinics or employed in commercial sex' (2002: 105). I show why 'general population' is an ill-chosen term to use in such a diverse country and why targeting STD clinic patients or 'MSM' (Men who have Sex with Men) and 'FSW' (Female Sex Workers) may make policy-makers feel good but does not very well enable them to understand sexual practice and transmissive risk. Moreover, because prostitution remains illegal in Papua New Guinea the idea that persons are 'employed' in it (as they might be in legal brothels in Nevada, Bangkok, or Jayapura) is misleading. More positively, I show that religious leaders and followers from Anglican, Adventist and Catholic churches in Papua New Guinea have contributed in profound ways to developing home-based care (HBC) for those suffering from AIDS and for those taking care of them, to sponsoring HIV-antibody (HIVab) testing and counselling initiatives and to assisting in community mobilisation.

Nevertheless, little critical attention has been paid to what kinds of effects these efforts have had, progressive and untoward, helpful and less so. Usually, that has been for fear of offending hosts and colleagues, of muddying the funding streams or of appearing to threaten the ties of collaboration. In ways little and big, at workshop presentations no less than in cyberspace, this has led over the years to a sort of rhetorical, public stalemate about what should (and shouldn't) be 'Christian Church' responses to HIV and AIDS and what one can say about them. Foreign observers have noted that condoms or brothels or masturbation 'work' in their home countries in preventing infection, but that we can't have that in Papua New Guinea, for it is 'is a Christian country'. A visiting parliamentary delegation from New Zealand remarked that Church-sponsored 'stigma and ignorance' were everywhere in Papua New Guinea and that Christian churches were both 'cause and the remedy to so many of PNG's woes' (Flaws 2006: 2). As the examples in these two text boxes indicate, such stigma is not peculiar to Papua New Guinea, where the first is situated; the second one comes from Fiji and assumes that someone who is only HIVab+ is already 'an AIDS victim'. Stigma has to do with more than just religious forms of discrimination, too, for example, with the visual spectre of AIDS, with lacking or absent health services and with the moral questions raised by human sexuality, illness and suffering. Sarah Hewat and I show in Chapter 6 what are the key similarities and differences in Indonesian Papuan (instead of Papua New Guinean) responses along these lines.

'An AIDS victim says she was arrested by police and kept in a cell overnight after they accused her of having sex with a villager. Joana Cagivinaka said she was taken in by police at Savusavu on Sunday, questioned over the incident – which she denied – and told to sleep overnight in the cell. "I have never been so humiliated all my life ever since the time I came out publicly about being HIV positive," she said. "What I experienced with the police officers was total discrimination. They questioned me whether I had sex with the villager and what happened after we slept together. After they questioned me, the officers went outside and made fun of me. I could hear them joking about my sex life. I slept in the cell on Sunday night." ...Police Media Liaison Officer Sergeant Ajay Nand said last night he did not have enough information on the matter. But a police source ...said no charges were laid against Ms Cagivinaka and police only wanted to know whether she had slept with a villager' (Fiji Times Online, see Qalo 2007).

Although I focus in this book mostly on Papua New Guinea, I draw also on examples, approaches and data from other countries in the insular Pacific, especially just across the border in Indonesian Papua. Contrary to popular belief, 'the insular Pacific' is not a homogeneous unit that is in some simple way comparable to other regions of the world. Its 21 different nation-states differ greatly in terms of their political affiliations and evolution. They differ in geographic breadth and cultural depth. They have taken part in and have been absorbed by globalizing forces differently, too. Their health profiles, not least of which is the state of their HIV and AIDS epidemics and what kinds of donor agencies are helping to manage them, can appear as different as night is to day. All too often, notes the renowned demographer Peter Pirie, 'the Pacific islands are lumped together in ways that outrage fact' (2000: 8). For this reason I tread with care upon those Pacific island peoples and culture I do not yet know very well.

I argue in this book that an over-focus upon microscopic entities and individual behaviours, combined with a fetishizing of often dubious quantitative data, has obscured both the social-structure of the epidemics and the cognitive and social contexts of infection. I suggest that AIDS is a problem not just of viral sources and biomedical proportions but also of and with social-structures and interpersonal relations. Women and girls in the Pacific are at special disadvantage in trying to prevent infection by negotiating safer sexual practices with their various kinds of partners and in trying to avoid the stigmas of real or imputed promiscuity. Their already significant burden in terms of domestic and other caring labours has increased in terms of caring for those sick from and dying of AIDS. The problem is not just with divisions of labour, however. Disparities in land tenure and behavioural norms have combined with male-dominated resource extraction companies and local communities to put royalties, salaries, employment and 'compo' (compensation for environmental and other forms of degradation) in the hands of individual men and male corporate groups. That they don't tend to spend the bulk thereof on their wives is seldom addressed forthrightly and denounced in a way that implicates anything other than individual prerogative. Male prerogative in Culture, Capital and Christianity is thus protected and strengthened.

There has recently occurred increased attention to disparities in gender relations and the gendered aspects of the epidemiology of HIV. That is all to the good. I argue, however, that it has been too long in coming and that the fact that too many have hopped onto the gender bandwagon too easily and sometimes for untoward purposes is telling of yet conservative ideas. For example, it is virtually a truism nowadays to say that girls are 'biologically' more vulnerable than boys owing to brittle cervixes and underdeveloped vaginas. I hasten to point out that this represents extraordinary effort by women's health advocates and feminist theorists over the years to change the mind-set of policy-makers and programme managers around more specifically sexed and gendered understandings of sexual physiology. Nevertheless, girls who aren't sexually assaulted by male relatives, preachers or teachers, who aren't poked and prodded by early boyfriends, and who aren't harmed by medical techniques and technologies seem to do just fine, so it can't be *just* 'biology'. The quick leap to positions of women-are-especially-vulnerable-because-they're-female is conservative in its understanding of sexual matters since it avoids men and the social-structure.

The limited grasp of gender relations can be seen in the frequency of calls made to keep girls and women home, where they belong, and off the streets. This mistakes not just the location of much sexual molestation and violence (the home and its institutional proxies) but also the real culprits, the sexual predators to whom 'the street' and other public spaces have been ceded and the unhappiness in many homes and within many marriages. No clear-thinking person can fail to grieve when reading of a description of sexual practice such as the following about the Gumine of Simbu Province: 'A wife is expected to give birth and nurture children for her husband, and sexual intercourse is necessary for this; but it is a relationship fraught with tension, and may not be very pleasurable … Sexual and emotional satisfaction seem to be of little importance in the marriage relationship' (Whiteman 1973: 30, 37). A 16-year-old girl interviewed by Carol Jenkins' team in the mid-1990s said 'I don't want to get married. I want to be a prostitute and get feelings. Get feelings like happiness' (quoted in Jenkins 2007: 45). I am not suggesting that in no marriage can be found pleasurable sexual expression or even that sexual enjoyment must be experienced inside marriage, but only that marriage is no more inherently protective than the sex in it is inherently pleasurable. No one would deny that this is true of a large proportion of heterosexual marriages in Papua New Guinea, elsewhere in the Pacific, or throughout the world, but this fact features prominently in no public health initiatives or messages about HIV and STD prevention. The conclusion to which Ruta Fiti-Sinclair came regarding the marriage:prostitution dialectic (see below) was that

> Most of the women stated that they hoped to be a *pasinja meri* [newly independent, highly mobile single women], although three women who had had a violent relationship said they did not want steady relationships ... and that they liked the fact that these men [their clients] do not treat them as their property. They reported enjoying the freedom they have which their married sisters do not have. (Fiti-Sinclair 1996: 121)

Thus there are many reasons beyond the mere 'promiscuity' of women or a somehow different 'nature' of the sexuality of men that explains the existence of prostitution and normative male infidelity. Mainstream HIV and STD prevention programmes have tended to opt for gender-neutral messages, however, and in doing so, badly misrepresent transmissive risk. I do not believe that 'prevention' lies in greater 'awareness' – or even that 'awareness' is really the problem. Instead, patterned unprotected intercourse is the problem because it occurs between infected and uninfected people who so frequently hold such different degrees of physical, economic and social power. Curbing HIV transmission and preventing AIDS demands that gender and other harmful social relations be healed. Neither health bodies nor most external donors yet 'get' gender relations very deeply, because they see gender as a variable, not a social relation, and because they don't see themselves in it.

In the next two chapters I lay out some of the behavioural dynamics, historical forces and ethnographic data and insights that are relevant to today's HIV and AIDS epidemics. These two chapters become something of a conceptual backdrop for three more chapters that examine the problems of and in HIV serosurveillance and intervention programmes in Papua New Guinea. I show that some messages from certain religious leaders and particular public health initiatives have induced massive cognitive dissonance in Papua New Guineans regarding the properties of condoms, their real and alleged failure rates and the nature and dynamics of transmissive risk. Such campaigns have not much informed people of the signs and symptoms of STDs, have instructed little about safer and less safe kinds of sexual acts and have opened up few possibilities for transmission prevention in a more sex-positive way. Instead, they have enjoined people to have less sex but with people in situations *more* likely to be infectious to them: with their 'intimate' partners. Many of them, of course, do not know they are infected and they have been told in various ways, for God's sake, not to use condoms. Messages and programmes are thus not so much about preventing transmission as about maintaining some and realigning other gender roles to fit conservative ideals. Henry Ivarature, a Papua New Guinean researcher who has conducted research in Tonga, found that the Tongan government, too, 'used the media to restructure reproductive behaviour and perceptions of family size. Indirectly, such campaigns promoted the restraint of desire, such as the need to discipline and channel sexual energies' (2000: 49).

In brief, I demonstrate in the five chapters comprising this first Part that by demonising the sexual Other and by promoting sex-negativity, public health campaigns in Papua New Guinea have over two decades externalised the nature of risk and disabled more accurate Self assessments. 'Male immigrants are ideologically represented as dangerous', says Bettina Beer about her work in the Markham Valley of Morobe Province, 'and female immigrants as given to prostitution as well as being transmitters of HIV'. 'Interestingly', she notes, 'another possible threat is not discussed – unprotected sex that Wampar women may have with men from other parts of the country' (Beer 2008: 112). Not surprisingly, condom usage goes out the window – when condoms can be found. I argue that, owing to the logic and tenor of such messages, less effective means of avoiding HIV and STD transmission have been implemented, such as renewed dedication to Christian beliefs, (male) genital cutting, the ingestion of 'bush medicines' (depicted here), the

Local herbal preparation said to cure AIDS

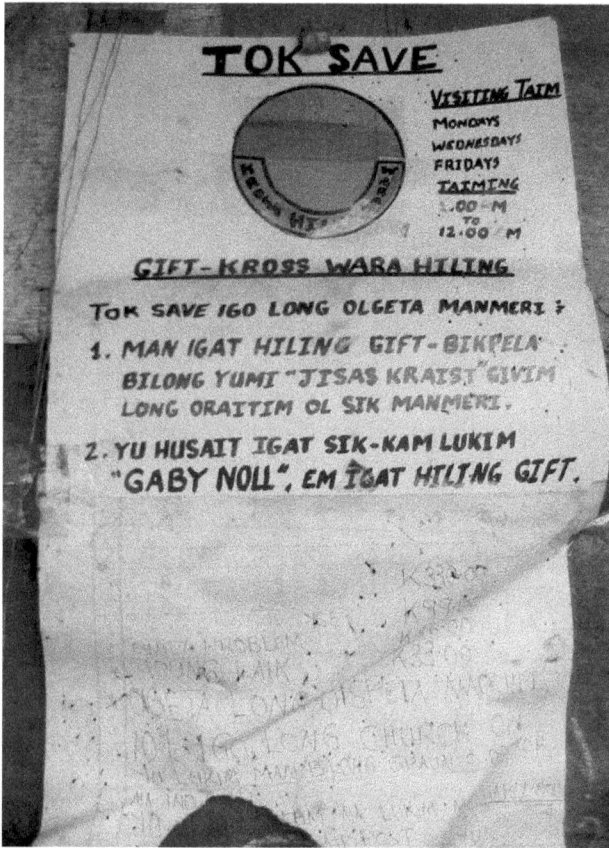

Alleged AIDS cure via wooden cross dipped in water

drinking of 'healing waters' said to be given as a gift from Jisas Kraist, in the next photograph, and renewed faith in one's partner's fidelity. Each of these 'methods' has further dissuaded people from realising the true transmissive risks right there in front of them. In Chapters 3, 4, 5 and 6 I show that the tendency to blame instead of explain is just as common in high places as low in Papua New Guinea, as elsewhere. Leslie Butt and colleagues (Butt, Numbery and Morin 2002a, b) provide many examples across the border in Indonesian Papua of similar displacement of risk. So-called 'experts' in *The Jakarta Post*, for example, 'blamed the spread of the epidemic on Papuan lifestyles: Papuans have multiple sex partners,[the newspaper claimed they] freely exchange wives, and do not engage in sexual foreplay' (Butt, Numbery and Morin 2002b: 8; see also *Jakarta Post* 2007a, b). Such sentiments are carbon-copies of the fantasies that began to circulate two decades ago in the US regarding 'Africans' and Haitians.

Some of these ideas are taken up also in the four chapters that make up Part Two, which focuses upon other countries in the Asia-Pacific region such as Indonesia, Thailand and Australia. I and my three co-collaborators discuss questions of state legitimacy, public health discourse, courtship and secrecy, religious attitudes to sex and legal prohibitions on prostitution and homosexuality. In Fiji, Christian churches and other institutions organised massive marches in protest of homosexuality and urged that homosexuals be stoned to death (Eves and Butt 2008: 18). Because heterosexual marriage is *the* culturally and theologically sanctioned form of sex, critique of it doesn't yet dine at the policy table. 'Single in town, married in the village', say the scooter-driving *bodabodamen* of Southwest Uganda (Nyanzi *et al.* 2007[2004]). Of course, they also get married in town, often multiply so, and they have other kinds of sexual relationships, too, each of which strains the marriages back home in the village. Would that surveillance and monitoring experts were capturing this cognitive and behavioural dynamic.

✳ ✳ ✳

Indeed, if there is a single thread running through the following five chapters, it is that there is a dialectical relationship between prostitution and marriage but that is hidden in policy discussions in ways that harm the national response to HIV and AIDS. Any field-based researcher in New Guinea during the past couple of decades who has conducted research about sexuality and gender relations can verify the rule of thumb that women will frequently use condoms with those men who pay for their sexual services but tend not to use them with their boyfriends, pimps and husbands. (These three kinds of men can be one and the same man developmentally or even simultaneously, of course, depending on what and how the questions are asked and on the context of research.) I examine this dialectic explicitly in Chapter 2 with regards to a particular 'culture area', south coast New Guinea, and the growth and development there during and following the colonial era of one of the many 'labour forms' of prostitution now existing (see also Hammar n.d.). *Tu kina bus* is an often brutalising form of cheap ($2), largely anonymous sexual toil that takes place outdoors (in the bush) and that is now a common feature of enclaves of resource extraction. I examine the dialectic also in Chapters 3, 4 and 5 regarding policy assumptions, public discussions and models of HIV epidemiology that ignore it. This can be seen on the web-site maintained by the head of AIDS Holistics, Mr Bruce Copeland (http://www.geocities. com/aids_holisticspng/), and in the many letters to the editor that he writes. 'Condoms', he writes, 'belong to Caesar', whereas 'Family belongs to God'. It is encountered daily in newspaper articles, letters to the editor and press releases, too. The influential editorialist for *The National*, for example, wrote that were Christian families to test their children for HIVab prior to marriage, 'HIV/AIDS would be an isolated issue, associated with prostitutes' (Pamba 2005). Sex industries, though they are often excoriated by civil, ecclesiastical and especially 'disciplinary' authorities, have nevertheless had cozy relationships with them. They have played a significant role in fulfilling sexual desires going apparently otherwise unfulfilled in often sex-negative marriages, communities and cultures. These facts, however, still inform remarkably few policy positions or intervention strategies. The NHASP document cited above, for example, mentions the word 'sex' 371 times, but 'prostitution' only twice, and not at all in the text. Those policy documents that most mention prostitution, however, present it in the flattest terms possible, just as 'sex workers' emerge as faceless, storyless, historyless reservoirs of infection to foreign sponsors and to national politicians. Papua New Guineans thus link HIV and other epidemics more to categories such as 'prostitution' and 'outsiders' than to their own selves and marriages or to intimate relationships and unprotected sex *per se*. This is killing HIV prevention efforts.

What I meant above by 'dialectical' is that the *Thesis* produces an *Antithesis* whose temporary resolution constitutes a *Synthesis* but because of whose persistent internal contradictions that need working out becomes the germ of another *Thesis*. Readers may refer to the works of Fichte, Hegel and marxians (but not Marx himself). My use of 'dialectic' underscores the social consequences (marital dissolution, stigma, sexism, etc.) of material differences (in access to land and other resources, political power, and so on). Here's how it works, conceptually and behaviourally, in ways that are relevant to chapters that follow: the Thesis consists of the norms and behaviours and ideals that move people toward marriage, whether putatively lifelong monogamous or serially so or casually so or frankly polygynously so. Despite that the elements may spring from different sources, both pre-contact and introduced Christian norms and ideals move differently gendered and sexed bodies toward a form of union that is heavily gendered in its rights, obligations, duties and outcomes. *Many tens of thousands of times annually,* girls and women (and sometimes boys and men, for different reasons) are forced into marriages they don't want. Girls in particular experience coitarche (first vaginal intercourse) in ways that are often traumatic and that involve male relatives, 'family friends' and sometimes even a particularly brutalising form of serial intercourse akin to pack- or gang-rape. Even when the sex is consensual, rates of condom use at first intercourse are often quite low, for example, 6% in Tokelau (Peseta 2007: 27). It may be difficult for those ill-attuned to the study and frequency of rape to appreciate fully the scope of the problem, but think on this: police statistics from 1992–95, when rape was by all accounts occurring far less frequently than it is now, showed that there were 'an average of 2.5 offenders recorded per victim' and that half of all victims reporting sexual assault between 1991–1996 were 15 years old or younger (Department for Community Development 2004: 3). That was the *average*. This is a developmental precursor to well known trajectories in terms of poor health and later engagement in prostitution (Hammar 1996a, b, 2006b). Many of the ideas about and obligations of fertility and reproduction are sexist in that females are not considered persons in their own right unless and until they can bear children, produce agricultural value and gain social worth. Penelope Schoeffel rightly points out that, regarding the introduction in the Pacific of Christian ideals of womanhood and marriage, they have tended to be of the St. Paulian variety, that 'a man should have one wife over whom he had the right of command but the duty to care for and protect' (Schoeffel 1994: 365). Family planning is considered 'women's business', just as STD is often gendered female and infertility is assumed to be women's fault. There are many gendered contradictions in religious doctrine and practice, too: the husband rules the wife, the father heads the family, and the man speaks for the family, community, church and culture.

There are multiple contradictions in the rules and exceptions of Melanesian social-structures, too, or what Eves and Butt have called 'a lack of reciprocity in regard for the other' (2008: 18). Buchanan-Aruwafu and Maebiru (2008), for example, write of the Auki of Malaita that '[t]he expectation to have sex only with regular partners also differed significantly with regard to gender'; while 70% of young women surveyed felt that infidelity was wrong, only 15% of their male counterparts felt so (2008: 172). Christine Salomon and Christine Hamelin inform us that for the Kanak women of New Caledonia, '[r]ape at first intercourse appears relatively ordinary, especially since there is no norm of premarital virginity' (2008: 90). Not surprisingly, there is an extraordinarily high frequency of rape, especially in marriage – 14% of Kanak women studied – and the perpetrators prior to marriage were most often male relatives (2008: 93). Land tenure, education, employment and sexuality are also male-dominated.

> 'Two-thirds of sex workers had been married; most sex workers who were married became separated or divorced, and started selling sex after their marriage ended between the ages of seventeen and twenty. The majority of women interviewed reported being victims of sexual and physical violence over the past year, and that they had experienced stigma and discrimination' (NACS 2007: 17).

Such unions therefore frequently produce an Antithesis in the form of sexual networking, often frank prostitution. Sexual prerogative begets coercion begets sexual refusal begets sexual violence begets women voting with their feet against a bad marriage. Wherever sex industries flourish, those can occur quite directly in marriage and family, insofar as husbands, boyfriends, family friends and male relatives act as pimp (see Chapter 2) or more passively support female choice in prostitution. This has been the case in Papua New Guinea for at least four decades. Ruta Fiti-Sinclair's study conducted in Port Moresby found that nearly two-thirds of the women in prostitution with whom she worked were married, and that the remaining seven were either divorced or separated. 'Five women said their husbands know what they are doing', she noted, 'and make no effort to stop their activities, and two others said their husbands encourage them to prostitute, providing they bring the money home' (1996: 121). Females can come to engage in prostitution also out of economic desperation that is borne of long-term male absenteeism and the social and economic costs to women of divorce, their seeming infertility and widowhood. As well, they can be forced or coerced into it, as is made plain with reference to periodic upswells in concern over the importation of Asian females by 'the Chinese mafia' into Papua New Guinea's seaports and provincial capitals or the use of provincial government-owned ships as 'floating brothels' (e.g. *Post-Courier* 2008a, 2008d).

When these antitheses (sexist beliefs, expectations and elements of the social-structure) are resolved in forms of companionate relationship (that is, the forging of new marriages), they constitute a Synthesis of sorts (that is, paying bride-wealth, becoming married, attempting to become pregnant, creating trade partners), but it is often only temporarily so. These new syntheses (formal marriages and other recognised unions) are still riddled by the same gendered double-standards, for example, that second and third wives enjoy fewer rights than do first wives, that subsequent wives get younger as husbands age, that men can openly have multiple wives and that they can get away with infidelity in ways women generally can't. Second and third wives are now also increasing the pressure they put on husbands to disown first or prior wives and displace their affections, especially if they haven't borne children or not recently. For women in polygynous settings, marriage causes divorce, a sociological point that many ethnographers have established (e.g. Clark and Hughes 1995: 322; Hammar 1996a, b, 1999a; Wardlow 2006a).[1] Dragging feet at, protesting or leaving those marriages and the new slings and arrows they attempt to dodge in the form of co-wife jealousies, male drinking, continued infidelities and repeated STDs become the germ of another Thesis, that is, women's attempts to marry again by engaging a series of male sexual partners and admirers in would-be marriages but that soon enough become frank prostitution, just as the text box case-study of Mary Andrews indicates. Unlike what the international 'best-practices' manuals (or rather, dictionaries) mandate regarding 'sex work' and 'FSW', the notion of regular, routinised and rationalized sex work is often missing in Papua New Guinea. 'Only when money is needed do they go looking for clients', said Fiti-Sinclair of the participants in the study she conducted in Port Moresby in 1993. Because payment is seldom sought immediately, such sexual networking 'makes it more like a Melanesian exchange relationship, rather than a modern economic transaction' (Fiti-Sinclair 1996: 122), money being collected on their boyfriends' and steady clients' pay-days, just as many wives do.

Marriage can thus for women be a dangerous 'total institution', a 'total social fact', in the words of Erving Goffman and Marcel Mauss, respectively, when they come to it, suffer it and leave it under great duress. Anna-Karina Hermkens pursued research among Catholic women in Papua New Guinea's Madang Province capital town of Madang and also in the nation's capital of Port Moresby. She found that 16 of 19 members of the Catholic Women's Association she interviewed in Madang had been beaten by their husbands, some of them many times. Another six of the 23 members of the Legion of Mary she interviewed in Madang and Port Moresby had also been beaten by husbands (Hermkens 2007: 5, n. 5). The ability and propensity of men *qua* husbands to do so is of course buttressed or at least not opposed by a number of sources, including Christian doctrine itself. Christine Bradley has noted that 'Christian missionary activity, for the most part critical of bride-price, has nevertheless tended (with recent exceptions) to reinforce the traditional dominance of the husband in the family' (1998: 352). The works of Ian Malins, especially *Christian Marriage and Family Life* (1987), are especially popular in Papua New Guinea and are used to explain away husbandly abuse.

The case in the text box is a good example of the behavioural outcome of Christian-based 'submission' of women. Mary Andrew is now a well-respected advocate for suffering women and in fact gave testimony to the Special Parliamentary Committee on HIV/AIDS (see Chapter 4). Women can initiate divorce, 'but as Christians they come under considerable pressure to maintain the marriage' (Clark and Hughes 1995: 322; cf. Malins 1987; Hermkens 2007).

> 'Every time Mary Andrew's husband drank, she got a hiding. A policeman, he used his work boots to kick her in the face. "He told me not to tell my family," recalls Mary, a petite, care-worn woman who looks far older than her 36 years. "He threatened to kill me and chop me up. I was a punching bag. I was his slave." During an 11-year marriage, she had to turn a blind eye to his drink-fuelled womanising, an accepted part of male culture in Papua New Guinea. Mary, a mother of two, drops her gaze as she recalls, with embarrassment, how he forced her into a threesome with another woman. When Mary's husband announced he wanted a second wife, she objected, telling him that while polygamy might be acceptable in many parts of PNG, it was against her Catholic beliefs. After delivering another fierce beating, he threw her out of their Port Moresby home. Without a welfare system to draw on, Mary was forced to leave her two boys with their father and resort to prostitution: 20 kina ($11) for sex – maybe 50 kina ($27) if she was lucky. Some sex workers will accept bags of rice. When her husband heard, he ensured Mary was ostracised from her children' (Middleton 2006a).

I show in chapters to follow that this dialectic is hidden because it is too revealing of the contradictions of culture and religious faith to be spoken of openly. Chapter 2 is titled 'The Women in Traffic: *tu kina bus* in town and country', and it analyses the growth and development of the kinds of sex industries that now flourish throughout Papua New Guinea as throughout the remainder of the world. 'Prostitution' and 'prostitutes' (variably defined) are usually the first – and marriage and husbands the last – to be singled out as the cause of disease outbreaks and moral decline. Dr Thomas Vinit called in 2008, for example, for a much tougher Adultery Act and specifically criticised women's groups for not heretofore taking a sufficiently strong stand! Passage of a tougher Act, he argued, would result in the wife being 'on guard to ensure the husband is faithful, hence it is a win-win situation in the fight to stop the spread of HIV and the restoration of moral fabric in the family and society' (Vinit 2008). Dr Vinit did not say where else these wives would stand guard, since they're instructed by Christian edict to stay home.

Political, public health and community leaders, especially religious officials, remain unwilling to realise this dialectical relationship. Few can admit that regular-old marriage is also a form of sexual networking, that such exists on a continuum with other forms and that marriages are social processes (not events) that as often as not require or at least lead to sex ahead of time. This renders rotten the A plank in the ABC platform that undergirds the national response. Holly Wardlow writes that 'premarital sex, either consensual or forced, is a common tactic young people employ to obtain their desired marriage partners' and that sixteen of 50 of the women in one of her fieldwork samples 'were made to marry because of premarital sexual activity' (2006b: 52, 60). Needless to say, that Huli girls and young women have to 'choose' something sometimes forced on them crimps their life opportunities as it structures their STD and HIV transmissive risks; she notes further that three in her sample stated forthrightly that they had been raped 'and then forced to marry their rapists', and another seven claimed that they had been '"sort of raped"' despite knowing their assailants and wanting anyway to marry them (2006b: 60, 61). Despite the tenets of ABC and the public health and religious authorities who preach them, sex is seldom something that can, in a sense, be *saved* for marriage. Rewards in the form of names, favours, land claims, social status, money, heirs and not being beaten (or suffering a worse fate) are far more important than ideal chastity.

'Condoms with spermicides are spreading rather [than] stopping AIDS' (Bonivento 2001a: 16).

'In fact by advertising condoms in this way, an ever-greater number of people will be encouraged in using condoms, increasing the number of those already having risky sex. These people are very confident that condoms can protect them, because of what they have heard from the propaganda. But they are not informed of the limitations of condoms, and they do not realize how they are dangerously exposing themselves to AIDS' (Bonivento 2001a: 29).

'100% of those having risky sex behavior and using condoms for more than four or more years can be predicted to get AIDS' (Bonivento 2001a: 25).

Chapter 3 is titled and discusses 'HIV in history: serosurveillance and other studies, 1987–2007'. Chapter 4, 'HIV in discourse: problems and prospects of the national response, 1987–2007', discusses what the anthropologist Graham Fordham has called with reference to Thailand, the 'normative AIDS paradigm'. I examine the structure and function of the national response in terms of numbers that are seldom conceptualised clearly in a system of case reporting that by even national health official estimates are inconsistent and noncomparable across time and space. I argue that we need a nose-down, tail-up grappling with the existing knowledge base, with the breakdown of health services delivery systems and with the high costs of sex-negativity. Chapter 5 looks at the facts and fantasies of condom usage, three examples of which appear in the text box. I show that the positioning of condoms culturally, religiously and in terms of public health interventions has had more to do with tropes of good and evil (things and people) and with sex-negative attitudes than with their potentials to prevent unwanted pregnancies and STDs. Mainstream constructions of condoms as being inherently wrong, or being only for morally 'bad' or 'high-risk' people, show how blurry are the lines between religious and ostensibly 'secular' policies and settings. By analysing in some detail the anti-condom discourse of Bishop Bonivento from the Vanimo Diocese I show how much this has damaged the national response. The differences between one church and another on this issue can get blurry, and there are often significant disjunctures between stated policies and on-the-ground realities. A journalist travelling about in the highlands on behalf of the Asian Development Bank (ADB) quoted Banz-based Sister Rose Bernard as saying that '[a]s a Catholic, I do not promote condoms for birth control, but the Church recognizes the right of an individual to protect himself or herself from life threatening danger. As counsellors, we used to have difficulty teaching pastors and priests, who wholly disapproved of condoms, but many are now beginning to recognize them as a means of preventing the disease' (quoted in Gill 2007). I show in Chapter 5 that she has a long way to go, that anti-condom forces have dug themselves in more deeply.

In these first five chapters I present a lot of ideas and data about stigma, beatings and cultural dislocation that, alongside the potential of protozoa, viruses, funguses and bacteria to sicken and kill, are greatly immiserating people, families and communities. This 'STD', this form of sexually transmitted dis-ease, I conclude in Chapter 9, is the mass effect of the embodied experience of sexual intercourse insofar as it occurs between unequal persons. The fact that condom usage is difficult, however, since it has been constructed as pertaining to illicit sex, to 'bad' people and to 'high-risk' settings, has led young females to forego condom use in favour of hopes of love and has led young males to seek other means of 'protection' in the form of genital cuttings. The epidemiology of HIV in Papua New Guinea shows that the Body Politic has been made sick in its inequalities. Younger females are bearing the brunt of HIV infection among all females, whereas for males, the older ones are exhibiting higher HIVab seroprevalence. Females, whether young or old, are bearing the burden of caring, whether for anxious HIVab test candidates or those sick and dying in their huts. Females have been told to worship God in church more regularly, not to go out at night, to stay close to home and to protect their virginity (Bonivento 2001a, b; Malins 1987; cf. Cummings 2008; Hammar 2008; Harrison 2008). Over Independence weekend in Madang town in 2007, a 13-year-old girl and a 4-year-old toddler were raped, but a 'police source' said that '[c]hildren must be told who to talk to and not at a young age so that this vital message will stick in their minds to avoid such nasty incidences' (*Post-Courier*, 18 September 2007). I guess that messages that don't stick are the causes of such sexual violence ... Males, on the other hand, especially younger ones, have been subject to and have responded to awkward discourses of risk by means of engagement in supercision, circumcision and other forms of genital surgery or embellishment. These conservative sexual ideals are multiplied by the right of men to and the need often for women to engage in multi-partner, concurrent sexual networking. In a recent, sterling essay, Martha Macintyre writes that the 'high incidence of violent crime in Papua New Guinea (PNG) means that, for many people, violence has become a part of mundane social life [reference omitted]. Women fear violence at home and in the street; people fear theft and violence' (2008: 180). Papua New Guineans are not alone in this, of course. Salomon and Hamelin (2008: 90) report upon their research in New Caledonia by saying that '[v]iolence is still used to force women into nonconsensual sex, particularly when the man who forces her is classified as allowed to do so, because he is her actual or potential husband'. The similar rottenness of the B plank in the ABC platform will be detailed throughout the entire book.

From this perspective AIDS really *is* a rent in the social fabric, not just a metaphoric one. I think that lesions, pains, discharges and sores that occur in or to or on human bodies are signalling and mediating relations *between* those same and other bodies. Those relations are, in addition to viruses and bacteria, also sickening and killing. From my perspective the 'cure' for AIDS doesn't lie therefore so much in a vaccine, and it certainly doesn't lie in more prayer or ingestion of bush medicines and miracle healing waters – those have been tried already and they don't work. I suggest that we try something new and different that we already hold in our hands: healthier sexuality, a dedication to protect human rights, the valorisation of qualitative ways of knowing about ill health and the agreement not to stigmatise anyone. Inducing fear when discussing bodies and pleasures, consent and community, is a big part of the problem facing Papua New Guineans. Repeat after me: sex is good, consent is hot, pleasure induces good health and condoms are our friends ...

An awkward fit

The major aim of this book is thus to pay critical attention to several aspects of Papua New Guinea's national response to HIV and AIDS and hopefully thereby to strengthen it. I will mention several briefly here that will be unpacked in chapters below. First, there are urban biases of programme location, medium, ideology and epidemiology that don't translate well to the rural realities of the remainder of the country. Though it is by international comparison a rather small cosmopole, having fewer than 500,000 inhabitants, Port Moresby absorbs a disproportionately large amount of resources and attention, partly because it is where donor country and programme representatives live. The review commissioned by Oxfam Australia of the progress made in involving people living with HIV and/or AIDS in the national response was helpful and much needed, but it noted that '[t]he review budget provided for fifteen days of external consultancy work plus five days from the in-country consultant. The budget did not allow for travel to parts of PNG other than Port Moresby' (Leach *et al.* 2006: 13). Of course, were they to have avoided Port Moresby altogether, they would have saved money and been able to visit provincial capitals or rural enclaves or care centres instead, which might have provided for a more realistic assessment of the situation. The review did note that 'the experience for PLHA outside of Port Moresby has not been captured as part of this limited review' (2006: 13). The review commissioned by the NHASP of the social marketing campaign noted that only 25% of the respondents had been interviewed in rural settings, despite that 85% of all Papua New Guineans live there (NHASP 2006h: 14). The National AIDS Council Secretariat (NACS) reported that, while 2004 financial outlays from the government amounted to only US$180,000, most of that 'was used to provide salaries for the staff of NACS at the national capital' and that even when expenditures had more than quadrupled by 2005, '[i]n all cases salaries and administrative cost used up the bulk of money and not much was left to carry out activities' (NACS 2006a: 11).

The extremely valuable work that NGOs headquartered elsewhere do, such as the Goroka-based Save the Children (in Papua New Guinea), Help Resources (located in Wewak), Tokaut AIDS (based in Madang) or ATProjects (based outside Goroka) often gets lost in the shuffle. Already debatable assumptions about transmissive 'hot-spots' and the sexual behaviours said to be linking them that are driven by desk-bound, not field-based programme managers are made more dubious by neglecting the multiplicity of transmissive modes and routes and the fact of multiple infections and viral or bacterial strains. The problems facing voluntary counselling and testing (VCT) or prevention of mother-to-child transmission (PMTCT) or other initiatives based in rural areas, where there might not be running water or a trained doctor, much less an Internet Service Provider, can be of a different kind altogether. Moreover, the divide between religious and ostensibly secular healthcare settings is in rural areas often even blurrier than in provincial capitals. The rural realities of language diversity, geographic access to health centres and ideological interest in epidemics seemingly originating elsewhere can be lost in urban-conceived programmes that rely upon television, newspapers or even radio for conveyance. Case reporting systems that are formulated in and for the realities of city life remain stuck on categories such as 'province of origin' and 'province of detection' that few field researchers would ever use and that are not guided by qualitative approaches to sexual behaviour. Such dubious categories fail even to appreciate normal mobility, much less capture transmission dynamics. While there is much attention paid to collecting *more* data, few seem worried about their quality or veracity. I show this in Chapters 3, 4, 6, 7 and 8.

Second, the ABC approach has not a chance in the world to work on a mass level. Attitudes to sex are already negative and made the more so by it. Sexual cultures are in many places too misogynous to take seriously other well intended calls to 'empower women' and 'put an end to violence'. Holly Wardlow tells an extremely poignant story of one 'Yalime', a young Huli woman from the Tari Basin, who in 1997 wished only eventually to marry her boyfriend, get a job in Port Moresby as a secretary and live a modern, Christian existence. Unfortunately, senior members of a Huli women's group conspired to expel her from school and compel her to return home and marry a much older and prominent Huli politician; 'in return, the politician would channel funds to the women's group for development projects' (Wardlow 2006b: 51). What are the chances that her abstinence and fidelity would be matched by his?

Most obviously, attitudes to condoms are deeply entrenched and mostly, although not wholly negative. An 'educated single woman' complained to a newspaper reporter that 'she will not wear a condom because she is not a "rubbish dump"' (Tonny 2008). (In Tok Pisin, semen is rendered *rabis*, 'rubbish'.) When he was Minister of Inter Governmental Relations, Sir Peter Barter, who had to that point not been 'engaged in, or supportive of, the national HIV program ... ripped down a "Protect yourself from AIDS" billboard' (NHASP 2005h: 5) that featured condoms. In another well-known case a peer educator for Hope Worldwide (an INGO) disfigured a condom dispenser, so disgruntled was he at the promotion of condoms (NHASP 2006g: 22). I have been on the receiving end of moral diatribes from Diocesan Health Services officials in context even just of STD treatment, much less of condom promotion. Several other provincial AIDS committees (PACs) have been thwarted by religious organisations or have themselves more actively opposed condom promotion despite the fact that such is expressly against the policies of the National AIDS Council (NAC). This has occurred even in the PAC that represents the National Capital District (NCD). In the face of such opposition to frank talk about sexual matters and condom promotion the sheer number of condoms sent to Papua New Guinea is not really the issue, although the disruption of supply and distribution chains is a constant problem. The larger problem is that many politicians, peer educators, health officials, church leaders and community activists disinform people about condom efficacy. They ignore or misunderstand the multiple-partner, concurrent nature of sexual networking in Papua New Guinea. Instead of trying to work with cultural norms of sexuality that are multiple to make it safer by promoting masturbation, consensual sex and condom use, they promote the ideals of abstinence and fidelity that work against them. A and B have as little support in social-structure as they have in political-economy.

Third, the fact that funding is external in source and priority makes for an awkward fit between otherwise laudable goals and often untidy realities. One of the many perceptive points that John Ballard and Clement Malau make in their essay, 'Policy-Making on AIDS in PNG to 2000', is that 'the international process of defining AIDS and of establishing a repertoire of policy responses has ensured that external precedents have been unusually forceful for national AIDS policy in PNG and elsewhere' (2002: 1). Some external precedents result in unreasonable expectations, such as that the government of Papua New Guinea will increase its annual AIDS-related budget by 20% per year throughout the life of a proposed joint project and that *thousands* of condom distribution points and *hundreds* of VCT sites will be erected and maintained (WB-ADB-AusAID 2006). This sets up people to fail at projects they didn't design or fund, just as do expectations that females can remain abstinent until they marry or that male fidelity and uninfectedness thereafter will protect them. Much criticism was aired in cyberspace and elsewhere when it was reported in September of 2008 that Papua New Guinea would be unlikely to meet the Millennium Development

Goals set forth by the United Nations such that there would occur by 2015 a reversal of the increase in HIV transmissions and people suffering from AIDS. 'This was because', said a reporter for *The National*, 'the country still had a long way to go in meeting its 2010 goal of scaling towards universal access to HIV prevention, treatment, care and support set two years ago at the UN General Assembly' (Arek 2008). Significant challenges to even HAART roll-out, much less those posed by people's attitudes to those who declare HIVab+ status or the parlous state of health care delivery systems, were aired in a 2006 article by Raynes and Maibani (2006), which showed a great willingness of health care professionals to take up the challenge of scaling up antiretroviral therapies but significant realism in terms of what's actually possible, given the high costs and considerable technical and technological requirements. For reasons of cost, security and sometimes of ethnocentrism, external donors have tended to the more impersonal dependence upon distribution of 'awareness' materials instead of close-in, painstaking observation of and participation in social process and behavioural flow. Consultants have seldom been hired to study the systems, the messages and the players that aren't working – in other words, to contribute to a sociology-of-knowledge approach. Seldom have they been encouraged to help consolidate and disseminate that which has already been achieved or jettison that which has demonstrably failed, such as ABC and HRSS (see Chapter 4 especially). The assistance of NGOs and INGOs has been invaluable and their intentions are usually good, but their relevance has been contentious. Their presence has sometimes been resented owing to salary and housing provisions. Papua New Guinea's current Prime Minister has referred to NGOs as 'enemies of the government' (NZPGPD 2006: 34). Carol Jenkins noted in a 2000 review of three different sex worker intervention projects that '[p]oor coordination between national and provincial health departments as well as mutual distrust between government and NGOs has hampered a solid national response to the epidemic' (2000: 21). Internal precedents can also stymie work, for example, by protecting Christian sensibilities and seldom urging modesty and caution in setting goals. I have sat in on workshops during which were presented plans for 'universal' access to antiretroviral therapies even in the face of reports of absent medical workers, of supplies languishing in storehouses, and of counselling and testing sites that are inaccessible to many Papua New Guineans. The same can be seen in press releases and bulletins from elsewhere throughout the Pacific.[2] Sitting political leaders can only be praised for what they *may* have said about HIV and AIDS, not held accountable for what they had multiple opportunities to do previously and didn't. The tourism industry cannot be implicated by legislation of more sensible HIVab testing requirements. However sexually active *tourists* may be – sexological research shows that they normally are – they need not show proof of HIVab negativity, but researchers and aid workers do. Papua New Guinea is not alone: the policy announced in September, 2006 on Niue mandated HIVab testing for visitors planning to stay more than 60 days, but not for those staying 59 days or fewer.

Fourth, the trend seems toward largely technical and/or biomedical solutions for what are problems rooted greatly in social structure. What I mean is that the burden of suffering and of taking care of those suffering from AIDS is just as heavily gendered as we might expect – women doing most of it. They are not the ones guiding the national response, however. The burden of blame and stigma is borne also in sociologically predictable fashion – with the more powerful and wealthy being able to insulate themselves from broken confidentiality, community scorn and substandard living conditions. Compare the rumoured seroprevalence of HIVab among politicians with that in the country overall. In the same way, Stuart Kirsch has rooted his sensitive argument about the situation facing those living downstream from the Ok Tedi mine in Western Province just where it belongs: firmly in social structure. In *Reverse Anthropology* he has argued that

> The resulting compensation claims show how pollution should be seen as a social relationship rather than an environmental problem that can only be addressed by technical means. These analyses also formed the basis of political action against the mine. (Kirsch 2006: 106)

In the context of problems raised by HIV and AIDS, antiretroviral therapies will undoubtedly help many Papua New Guineans, but their sourcing, distribution, prescription, usage, adherence and monitoring are wildly more complicated than most allow. They can't help but reveal more fundamental, underlying problems of the health services delivery system itself, of its weak position in the social-structure, so to speak, and of people's differential access to and deeply ambivalent feelings about medical care (see Amstel and van der Geest 2004; Eves 2008; Hauquitz 2004). Much has been made of the shortfalls in supplies, logistics and timeliness of health care services in the country's flagship healthcare centre, the Port Moresby General Hospital (e.g. Curry *et al.* 2005; McBride 2005), much less at the flagging nature of services throughout the country; half of the country's aid posts that were operating at Independence have in the past decade closed down permanently, and the government estimates that 27% of the population is undernourished (Pincock 2006). With regards specifically to the roll-out of antiretrovirals, consulting physicians and epidemiologists have written consistently about the problems in and of the clinic, not just of and with the patients. For example,

It is painful to write forthrightly about social and medical ills in a country that one loves. Although I do not want my words to harm anyone, least of all those who are already being harmed, and despite the fact that I hope my analyses will be put to good use, I know that Papua New Guinea has already a dicey and in some ways undeserved reputation among journalists, foreign donors and tourists regarding sexual and public health matters.

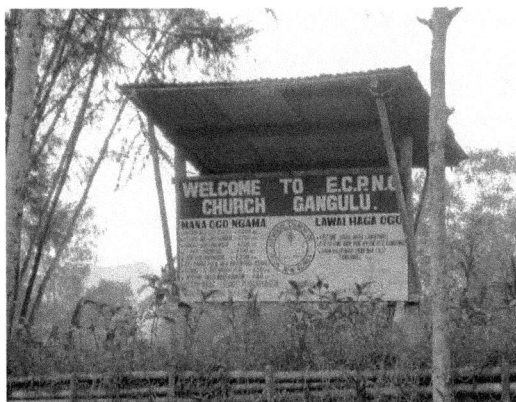

Village signboard warns against outsiders

The detail information about HIV/AIDS cases and treatment were written by physicians. There is no systematic recording form, to be filled in. The physicians and nurses in the clinic will extract the information from the patient's charts and fill information into the computer ... However the computer data recording form was quite weak and did not contain some important information. There were many open questions that was very difficult to be analyzed ... The consent form is still not in practice. (Pathanapornpandh 2005: 13, 14)

These observations do not bode well for the roll-out of antiretroviral therapies. Given their cost, technical requirements, extreme toxicity, spotty distribution (so far anyway) and the resistance they can induce, some have worried (but mostly privately) that prevention efforts will be compromised. Papua New Guineans cannot afford this. Because so few results of the antiretroviral therapy roll-out have been published (e.g. NACS 2007; NHASP 2005a; Tau 2007), I take up these issues in Chapter 4 and in Chapter 8 with my colleague Mark Boyd.

Fifth, the national response is plagued by the externalisation of risk. This innocuous-looking village sign-board erected by the Evangelical Church of Papua New Guinea, for example, instructs villagers of the high costs of adultery, of allowing one's pigs to mess about in the pastor's garden, and worst of all, of having sex with 'outside' women and girls. Many such signboards now dot the countryside. People seem convinced ever more that AIDS comes necessarily from somewhere else and from qualitatively Other kinds of people. 'It is still a popular belief', said a community research team over a decade ago, 'in some parts of the Eastern Highlands and other societies of the highlands provinces that *getos* [usually divorced or widowed women dubbed sexually promiscuous who may or may not sell sexual services] are the main ones at risk and are thought to be primarily responsible for the spread of STDs' (Lemeki *et al.* 1996: 240). Gulf Christian Services, a faith-based organisation (FBO) based in Gulf Province that takes admirable care of a teaching centre at Kapuna and a hospital in Kikori, promotes a Tribal Protection Concept. This 'requires a Chief of a particular village to sign a declaration prepared by the Gulf Christian Health Services to make an obligation to protect the village community from any harm *from outside'* (NHASP 2006g: 25, emphasis added). The former Secretary for Health, Dr Nicholas Mann, took extreme exception at reports (by his own Minister of Health, Sir Peter Barter) of double-digit HIVab seroprevalence at the Porgera mine-site in Enga Province by remarking, 'This is an isolated town where there is economic activity and many males, who take sex workers' (People and Planet 2006). All towns, of course, have many males and economic activities. Moreover, no HIVab seroprevalence figures for females were provided, no evidence of 'sex workers' was presented and transmission seems to run only one-way. Dr Thomas Vinit, who is neither a highlander nor a Papuan, argued that being one put one at greater risk (Vinit 2004). A NHASP representative based on Daru returned from a trip he took in 2002 to Western Province outstations and reported that '[a]n Irian Jayan was detected to be carrying the HIV virus at Bula from Wambi in the Republic of Indonesia. The Police authorities and Foreign Affairs are to be told to force these people back to where they came from because of rebel incursions. The person carrying the virus is sexually active' (Paradi 2002: 2). The grounds on which his or her HIVab status and prior sexual activity had been 'detected' were not given, but Members for Parliament, expatriate logging barons and housewives are also known to be HIVab+ and sexually active, but yet they are not targeted. Slogan after acronym, programme after policy document, poster after press release continue to promote this externalisation.

> The most liberal of Papua New Guinea's national religious leaders, the Anglican Church Bishop of Port Moresby, Peter Fox, in a letter he sent to the editor of The National, yet externalized risk away from marriage: '[i]f you insist on having sex with people you do not know, then for God's sake I beg you please use a condom' (Fox 2006, emphasis added), as if people one knows – i.e., spouses – are less likely to be infected.

Sixth, Papua New Guineans believe just as strongly as anyone else in the ability of sexual intercourse and its outcomes to forge and to maintain social relations. Like many people they believe also in the ability of and practice in sorcery to deal with perceived affronts thereto. On both counts Papua New Guineans are pronounced in Australian newspapers and policy documents as 'ignorant', 'promiscuous', 'backwards', 'dangerous' and 'immoral'. Their culture is said likely to make the problem worse and to lead to further stigma and isolation (e.g. Casey 2006; Fink 2006; Gibson 2006; *Sydney Morning Herald* 2007a; Tobias 2007). Nevertheless, the most palpable nonsense about condoms, say, from an Australian Cardinal or Italian Bishop can pass without comment. I show this in detail in Chapter 5. The larger point is that the very language of international public health, Australian journalism and Western NGOs that most trades in acronyms and slogans that muddle cause and effect, that criticises technical capacity and that produces and essentialises

TAMBU TRU LONG
PASINDIA MAN/MERI NR

PUBLIC TOKSAVE
SAPOS YU KAM LONG DISPELA PLES KAIPU 1 NA 2 BIHANIM DISPELA LO:
TAMBU TRU LONG:
1. DRINK BIA   3. PILAI DAT BOT   5. SIMOK   7. PASINDIA MAN/MERI
2. PILAI KAS   4. KAIKAI BUAI   6. PASIN STIL   8. SIMOK MARIWANA
AUTHORISED BY COMMUNITY LEADERS
1. AFAYA SIRI   3. NATO EWAE   5. PASTOR I. SIRI
2. DOUGLAS FAIYABE   4. GIBSON SASUE

Jeremaia 29:7   1 Korin 5:11

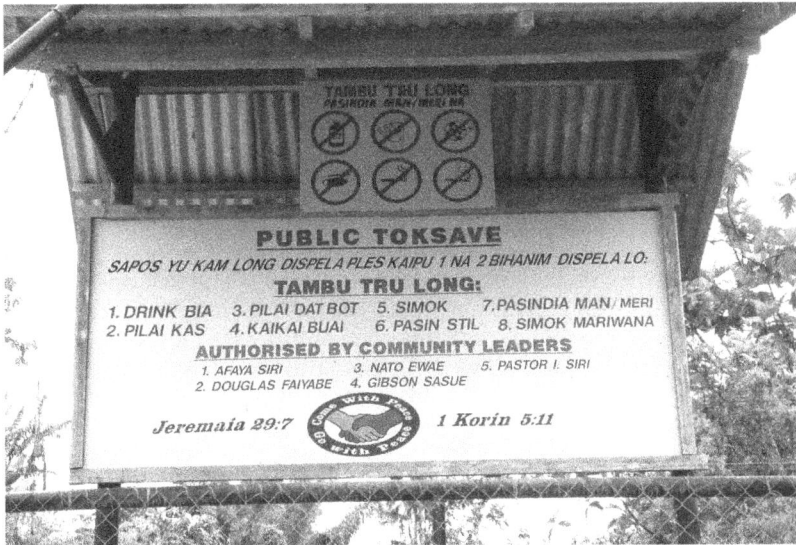

Village signboard warns against vices and outsiders

sexual identity and then relentlessly 'targets' already stigmatised people remains immune to criticism. Miranda Tobias (2007: 4) from the Centre for Independent Studies, denigrates Papua New Guineans for their educational deficits but she uses such unfortunate phrases as 'HIV takes time to develop into AIDS' and 'HIV/AIDS infection' in doing so. Many times conflating cause and effect, she even confuses syphilis seroprevalence with that of HIVab, which made for even more alarmist press coverage! In this she shares with other policy-writers and journalists the tendency to promote sensational leads over verified facts and to hold Australians to standards that are different than those to which Papua New Guineans and other Pacific islanders are held. Her right to pronounce about things about which she knows not is guaranteed in a way that an average Pacific island villager's is not. In terms of media play and policy weight her misinformation tramples over the embodied experience of a wife who is beaten by a husband into not using a condom and who, by doing so, appeals to the authority granted him by Church, State, Culture and Capitalism.

Seventh, the 'national response' in Papua New Guinea has for two decades, despite many good intentions, been based very little on the empirical facts of infection and transmissive risk. Person for person, mission by mission, the ones in Papua New Guinea whose work is most responsible for the way I craft my argument here are good, hard-working people and for the most part well-meaning. Beyond personal idiosyncrasies, however, there is a darker side to intervention programmes to which an increasing number of social scientists has called attention. 'While legitimating the increase in their power and influence by recourse to humanitarian sentiment', says Graham Fordham, 'these groups and individuals seek the domination of the AIDS sphere in the South East Asian region through defining the nature of the HIV/AIDS epidemic(s) as a social and medical problem relevant to their own spheres of interest and control'. He continues:

In the case of large international organisations, their manipulation of AIDS research agendas due to the control they exercise over research funding gives them a high degree of influence over the direction of most AIDS related research, and a near total domination of the social and behavioural interventions indicated by that research. (Fordham 2005: xv)

In like manner, Stacy Pigg has documented in a number of provocative essays that public knowledge in Nepali communities about STDs, HIV and AIDS was formed largely

out of an already formed template of accepted facts about HIV, and the public health wisdom of AIDS prevention that accompanied that information, as set out by powerful international organizations. This means that Nepali health planners and activists, together with the public at large, encounter AIDS – as an idea, and for some, a physical reality – through the mediation of an AIDS expertise that is already firmly consolidated. (Pigg 2001: 481)

Leslie Butt and her colleagues (Butt, Numbery and Morin 2002a: 283) have contributed a similar point about their fieldwork across the border from Papua New Guinea:

[T]he failure of programs to reach Papuans is due to a combination of cultural and structural aspects of Indonesian rule in Papua. Most program managers and state bureaucrats are Indonesian migrants who bring with them specific and explicit ideas about appropriate sexuality. These Indonesian bureaucrats generally hold an implicit but widespread, belief about the role of 'Papuan' culture in increasing sexual risk by promoting risky sexual behavior.

Papua New Guinea therefore differs from Central and East African countries, Australia, and even Haiti in the early–mid 1980s, where *rapidly evolving knowledge bases* reflected *rapidly evolving research agendas and output*. I show particularly in Chapters 3, 4, 6 and 7 that Papua New Guinea's AIDS paradigm remains stuck, despite re-branded campaigns such as Tingim Laip (Think Life), which replaced the High-Risk Settings Strategy.

I aim therefore to help dig it out. The patent gobbledy-gook that was the notion of 'Pattern I/II/III' countries in early Western HIV epidemiology was effectively outed by concerned social scientists and critical theorists, and it did eventually die. By contrast, ABC has new life breathed into it daily by crusading evangelicals, by politicians and by donor country programme managers who are anxious to increase the size of their toehold in the country. In Papua New Guinea no amount of empirical evidence to the contrary has been able to shake the foundations of a model of HIV epidemiology and a plan for intervention that were laid down much earlier and with almost no input from concerned social scientists or men and women in the towns and villages of Papua New Guinea. No matter the voluminous sociological insight and ethnographic data to the contrary, the 'normative AIDS paradigm', as Fordham calls it, is not in Papua New Guinea and has never been focused where the great bulk of infections lie: in companionate relationships, especially in marriage, whether frankly polygynous or putatively monogamous. These are the hopefully intimate settings where belief in the safety of companionate relationships and Christian faith rule. For this reason, and although it is empirically false, as I show in middle chapters, the following statement makes certain perverse sociological sense: 'Understanding what is actually driving the HIV epidemic in PNG is quite unknown in most at risk groups and the general population' (NACS 2008: 23). Well, we'll see.

Notes

1. In Chapter 2 I will discuss in some detail ethnographic accounts of the dialectic relationship between marriage and prostitution. Christian missionaries inadvertently enabled the prostitution of women who had been the second, third or fourth wives of polygynous men; when they prohibited polygyny they introduced the idea of divorce. Such outcomes are not uncommon to other religious faiths, too. Jon Krakauer's social history of Mormonism, for example, *Under the Banner of Heaven*, includes the following example: 'Apostles John Taylor, Willard Richards, Brigham Young, and their brethren in the pro-polygamy camp wanted just as desperately to install a prophet who would uphold the doctrine, lest the plural wives these men had covertly married be branded as whores' (Krakauer 2003: 193).

2. The recent publication from WHO/UNAID/UNICEF (2008: 50), for example, would appear to urge modesty even while recognising Papua New Guinea's significant accomplishments. Comparing 'generalised epidemic' countries of low, low-to-middle, middle and high income countries, the study found 'large disparities in the availability of testing and counselling facilities in relation to population size'. Botswana, for example, has one facility for each 1,900 people, whereas Papua New Guinea has one for each 120,000 people. In any event, only 5% of Papua New Guinea's health facilities to date had HIVab testing and counselling sites attached to them (2008: 51, Table 3.1). The November 2007 issue of PASA, the *Pacific AIDS Alert Bulletin*, blurted out in headline that 'Universal Access to HIV Treatment Achieved in Pacific Small Island Countries'. A consulting doctor interviewed, Gary Rogers, was said to have asserted that 'small Pacific islands now have universal access to treatment' (PAAB 2007: 8, 9). Nevertheless, such centres of testing and treatment are located in capital cities only of French Polynesia, Kiribati, New Caledonia, Palau, Samoa, Solomon Islands, Tuvulu and Vanuatu. As well, the claims of religious groups have restricted access to treatment in other ways (Eves and Butt 2008: 14), distribution of antiretrovirals has been spotty according to newspaper stories and the stigma and possibility of breaking confidentiality has held yet others back. It is simply counterfactual to claim 'universal access'.

Chapter 1

Introduction

HIV, human rights and the hot glow of anger

Managing impressions

Certain secrets remained too dark to be told even by those who trusted us most. The village remained a team, united in its performance, with regard to some practices or beliefs which were too damaging to all (or to certain powerful high-caste people) to permit their revelation to an outsider. (Gerald Berreman, *Behind Many Masks*, 1962, p. 19)

If men speak to hide their thoughts, they write to hide their society. (Ernest Gellner, 'Original Sin', 1986, p. 13)

Sir Peter [Barter, the then Minister for Health for Papua New Guinea] said while there was a 'levelling-off' in the urban areas due to establishments of Volunteer Counselling and Testing (VCT) sites or projections from the estimation report showed the epidemic was increasing in the rural areas where majority of the people live. 'The HIV prevalence of 1.28 percent which was less than previously documented does not mean that the HIV epidemic was decreasing. Rather all projected HIV indicators show an increase', he said...
. 'Papua New Guineans should continue prevention methods like abstaining from sex, being faithful or using a condom every time to prevent infection, and also go for testing to know their HIV status', Sir Peter said. (*The National*, 9 August 2007)

Social scientific debates have for two decades revealed impression management to feature in ethnographic writing not less than in other forms of social intercourse. Perhaps it is even more so because of the rapt attention ethnographers pay to time and context and the usual cross-cultural nature of their inquiry. Anthropologists have often and in different ways hidden themselves in the texts they produce; think of E.E. Evans-Pritchard in *The Nuer* or Laud Humphreys in *The Tearoom Trade*. Sometimes they bracket off the societies to which they belong in trying to understand the ones to which they don't. Gerald Berreman concluded his provocative essay from nearly half a century ago by reminding would-be ethnographers that competence in the field and out of it is measured partly by understanding the structure and function of impression management. That includes verbal performances, memories, enacted dramas, gossip and written history. Methodological approaches must even be taken in earnest, he said, so as to reveal and explain it. He notes that special care must be taken to reveal in the field not just the performance of impression management but also and perhaps more importantly, 'the nature of the efforts which go into producing it and the backstage situation it conceals' (1962: 24).

This book is also about impression management. The third epigraph above is drawn from a story published in one of Papua New Guinea's two daily English newspapers, *The National*, the Papua New Guinea *Post-Courier* being the second and both being significant sources of news and perspective on the HIV and AIDS epidemics. The upbeat, congratulatory tone of the remainder of the story conceals (but not very well) a backstage situation requiring much impression management along the lines suggested by Berreman. There appears to be a Rural–Urban divide in programme location and transmission dynamics such that figures from the one are difficult to square with those from the other. There are significant gaps in case reporting of HIV antibody-positive (HIVab+) blood-samples that are grounds for concern. As of 2006, HIVab seroprevalence from only 20 of the 75 VCT sites throughout the country were being reported (NACS 2006b; NHASP 2006b: 11, Table 1.11). The epigraph shows difficulties with issues of statistical significance and confusion in conceptualising epidemic increase, decrease and levelling-off. Sir Peter Barter, a naturalised Papua New Guinea citizen who has for four decades had an admirable life in business and politics, seems to be assuming that more HIVab testing has resulted in lower overall seroprevalence, when just two years ago the opposite was being said, when absolute numbers of those seeking and receiving counselling and testing were blamed for an apparent steep increase in seroprevalence. In any event, it's difficult to warn the populace of the coming menace ('all projected HIV indicators show an increase') ... when simultaneously claiming an annual decrease. How does an organisation seek funding from donors to mount an 'emergency response' ... but that needs to be sustained indefinitely?

I show throughout the middle chapters of this book that impression management is also evident in a national response to HIV and AIDS that has been informed by as little theory about sexual behaviour as about its own structure and function. To take one set of figures for example, HIVab seroprevalence among females attending antenatal clinics (ANC) in Papua New Guinea is higher (1.6%–NACS 2007) than the 1.28% figure of countrywide seroprevalence. It is way, way higher for VCT sites (11.3%), STD clinic attendees (12.7%) and tuberculosis patients (16%–see NACS 2007: 12). As well, rural enclaves and health centres in highlands provinces have been reporting double-digit seroprevalence. For two decades, however, ANC attendees have been used rhetorically as a 'low-risk' proxy for 'the general population', an epidemiological model into which the 'good' fit (Us?) but into which 'sex workers' don't (definitely Them). Family Health International, for example, concluded that '[s]ince 2003 ... HIV prevalence among pregnant women attending antenatal clinics has consistently been above 1 percent, *which indicates a generalized epidemic in the country* (FHI 2007: 9, emphasis added). For years social scientists have been ignored when they pointed out or criticised when they persisted in challenging on intuitive, sociological and empirical grounds the dogma that ANC attendees necessarily represented 'low-risk' transmission dynamics. Now, however, pregnant females have finally been accepted to be a 'higher-risk' group (NACS 2007: 11–2). Even this conclusion is difficult to accept uncritically, however, in that ANC figures aren't adjusted for age or gender, and probably half of all pregnant women in Papua New Guinea don't attend them anyway. The degree to which ANC attendees stand proxy even for other women, much less the remainder of 'the general population' is therefore debatable. By the same token, it has for a long time been assumed that an STD clinic attendee was at necessarily higher risk of HIV infection. This book, however, implicitly asks: higher risk than who? Official estimates have it that 1,000,000 STDs each year go untreated. At least those patients attending STD clinics are getting them treated, closing the wounds and staunching the flow of discharge, obtaining condoms (hopefully) and counselling advice. STD clinic patients are thus at lower risk than STD sufferers *per se*.

The newspaper story also appears to fetishize numbers, since the percentage isn't questioned and since nothing is offered along the lines of transmission routes and risks or any relevant cultural or sexual practices. No structural factors are cited to help explain why HIV epidemiology is so starkly patterned by age and gender. Despite there being social scientific evidence in abundance around these issues, no attention is paid here and little is paid elsewhere to changes that need to be made in social-structure around land tenure, kinship obligations, divisions of labour, health services, resource extraction, reproduction and especially male sexual prerogative. No evidence is presented that clarifies the advantages of knowing one's HIVab status, either. Sir Peter also doesn't hint at the many disadvantages of such, which in Papua New Guinea can mean court cases, spousal retribution, community scorn and far worse – including isolation, torture and being buried alive.

Above all else, the impression is communicated in the story that faith in ABC has been well placed. Keep on usin' those prevention methods! How many people, however, actually *use* abstinence – or fidelity, for that matter? Despite this continuing faith in the efficacy of ABC, a small army of social scientists has showed that the **A** isn't currently in the power of many Papua New Guinean women and girls to negotiate. Similar degrees of doubt have been expressed by the same sources about the **B**. The anthropologist Holly Wardlow reported recently the estimates made by a head nurse in just one health centre regarding the 72 cases of HIVab seropositivity it had reported. She knew well enough of the 72 to say with confidence that 'at least 19 of the 31 women who were HIV-positive or who had died of AIDS had been infected by husband-to-wife transmission' (Wardlow 2007: 1007). Lots of evidence shows that the situation Wardlow describes for the Tari Basin of Southern Highlands Province is common throughout the country. The nurse's phrasing, 'husband-to-wife transmission', also tantalizes, since relationship is not a usual epidemiological category. In another context, 'MSM' and 'gay' have become transmission routes (Tau 2007), not just sexual identities.

As for the **C** in ABC, the huge disconnect between rhetoric and reality requires massive impression management. About the same time as this newspaper article was published it was also being claimed that the Australian Agency for International Development (AusAID) had distributed 700,000,000 condoms through the National HIV and AIDS Support Project (NHASP). *Seven hundred million.* The National AIDS Council Secretariat (NACS) had claimed at the same time on its web-site that 19,000,000 condoms were to be distributed in 2007. *Nineteen million.* Several of the six Area Medical Stores that manage their distribution and dissemination, however, had at the time only a few tens of thousands on hand, and others had even fewer. The AMS in Badili in the nation's capital of Port Moresby, for example, had only 1,584. This dashed the hopes of a leading physician who told me (in a personal communication, 26 July 2007) that he had wanted to lead his medical students in HIV and AIDS awareness campaigns but now couldn't.

Lengthy e-mail logs he showed me about this issue, carried out between NACS, NHASP and the National Department of Health (NDoH) officials, combined with my own experience over the years, tell me that impressions are managed by iterating and reiterating numbers, slogans and acronyms (and not so much by worrying about their truth content). Someone brought the ABC mantra to Pacific island countries, and many seem to believe that, by repeating it, transmission is somehow averted, even when the 'C' is changed to mean 'Christ-centred', 'Christian doctrine', 'Christian values' or even 'Commitment' (Gerawa 2006). Worse, it has been extended alphabetically to 'ABCD' and 'ABCDE' where 'D' and 'E' stand, respectively, for 'Delay sex' or (again) 'Don't have sex outside marriage' and 'Early testing'. Hellena Tomasi, head of the STI/HIV/AIDS Unit of the Ministry of Health in Solomon Islands, has proposed an 'ABCDEFG' such that 'C' doesn't even mean 'Christian', much less 'Condom', but rather 'Changing behaviour', since condoms are only for sex workers. 'F' stands for being a Family man and 'G' for fearing God (Mamu 2006).

ABC has stuck in Papua New Guinea for all manner of reasons. First and foremost is the fact that the social field is already sticky now with movements of Christian crusade. Mainline churches are attempting to revivify their congregation in one crusade after another activity. Pentecostal and Charismatic reform movements are sweeping especially throughout the rural countryside, instructing in sin, counting the sins and exhorting the sinners not to do so. American televangelists such as Joyce Meyer, James Hagee and Charles Copeland blitz the airwaves and Benny Hinn and others who claim faith-healings – though whose black and grey comb-overs do not also feature mullets – drop in from time to time to John Guise Stadium for week-long crusades that enmesh government workers and siphon monies (Sullivan 2006). Excellent studies such as that by Joel Robbins, *Becoming Sinners* (2004), Richard Eves' several fine essays, especially 'AIDS and Apocalypticism' (2003a, b) and Dan Jorgensen's 'Hinterland History' (2006) each show the great fervor and also social and public health consequences of Christian movements.

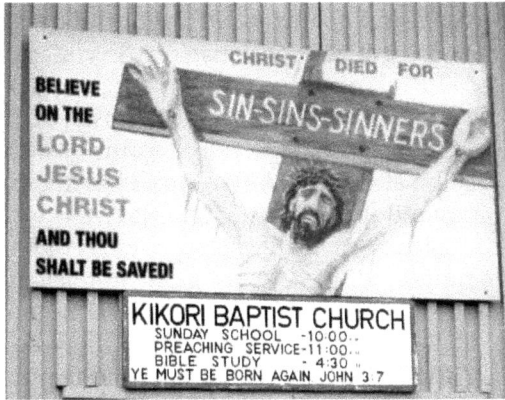

Gulf Province church signboard

Acronyms flow in funding streams, too, and donors don't look kindly upon those who question their meaning or challenge their efficacy. Thinking in terms of such packaged phrases and snappy acronyms as 'self-described FSW', 'the general population', or 'high-risk groups such as MSM' is certainly easier than critiquing them and thinking through their untoward consequences. Conducting fine-grained, empirical field research that builds up from the community level is more difficult than applying well-funded foreign-inspired templates upon it. Because taking evidence-based approaches is theoretically open to the very contrary evidence and counter-intuitive insights that require cultures of debate and critique to sustain them, such have come late and haltingly so.

✳ ✳ ✳

The fact that I have registered these developments suggests that I have engaged in a little impression management myself, so let me explain. It may appear, for example, that I am anti-religion or anti-Christian, but I am not, even though I am agnostic. No, I don't think that Christian faith *per se* makes a good platform on which to base an entire nation's response to the challenge of preventing sexually transmitted disease or reducing fear and stigma around HIV. Neither would I expect Muslim or Hindu or Confucian faith *per se* to be effective on those grounds. It may appear that I am opposed to quantitative forms of reasoning, in this case to estimates of HIVab sero-prevalence, but neither is that so. What I am against is the uncritical ways in which they are bandied about and the blunt force trauma they exert against critical faculties when it comes to monitoring and surveillance. Chapter 4 shows in detail that even though admirable responses have been mounted, official estimates can yet go off the rails and so need to be challenged and put aright. Interestingly, it was the same Minister of Health above who pre-viously announced 30% HIVab+ seroprevalence at the Porgera mine-site in Enga Province and that 'youth' in an adjacent province were testing HIVab+ to the tune of 40% or more. It may appear that I am merely poaching from the sidelines or that I don't support the national response, when nothing could be further from the truth. I have myself lived and worked in Papua New

Guinea for over five years and I care deeply about the near and distant future of Papua New Guineans. I grieve especially for the collapse of health service delivery systems, for the rising tide of all manner of sexually transmitted infections and for the likely devastation that will ensue on systems of kinship, patterns of residence, levels of production and forms of sociality. I know that I am not alone in worrying about the downside of having external donors and countries manage more and more of the 'national' response and at how little room there seems to be for registering one's dissent. For example, there is no real consumer movement afoot that would guide in relevant issues of medical licensure, bush medicine promotion or financial accountability. I sympathize with the many doctors who privately worry about the wisdom of the way the antiretroviral therapy roll-out has occurred but who cannot say so in public. Critical dissent is stifled in high places as in low. Simplistic models of HIV epidemiology and the silencing of viable alternatives to them help no one.

In terms of these difficult issues of sovereignty, medicine, religious doctrine and sexual matters, social capital is gained in Papua New Guinea only with great difficulty but is lost with comparative ease. I want to help strengthen the national response, but I recognise that I do so from an extremely marginal position. I want social scientific perspectives, data and approaches to become more central to the national response, but political leaders and policy-makers have shown little interest in them and in fact have often been quite hostile to them. This is mostly because their findings tend to run against the grain of public health campaigns and foreign donor assumptions about what's really driving the epidemic. I want the national response to be bolstered by a sex-positive attitude and to expand sexual options and gender identities, but such is not possible in the current climate of risk externalisation and Christian fervor. I want to support the national response by addressing its persistent weaknesses, even though that doesn't sound very supportive. I expect fallout from predictable sources for predictable reasons, but yet I feel I must persist because the very future of Papua New Guinea hangs in the balance.

Out from behind many masks

Ethnographers often begin writing by searching for the right words to explain their work to the people with whom they have lived and studied and about whom they have written. This is so even when they know that those about whom they write may not ever be among their readers. Papua New Guinea first became my home-away-from-home from 1990 to 1992 on Daru island, the capital of Western Province, where I studied sexual networking, sexually transmitted disease (STD) and sexual violence. The study of Melanesian gender relations and especially those in highlands Papua New Guinea had to that point greatly fascinated me (e.g. Hammar 1989), and they still do. Several articles I published upon completion of Ph.D. dissertation-related research (e.g. Hammar 1992, 1993a, b, 1996a, b, 1998a) warned of precisely what is happening now, just as did those of other concerned social scientists (e.g. Hughes 1991, 1997; Jenkins 1996, 1997; NSRRT and Jenkins 1994; Wardlow 2002a, b, 2008b). From 2003 to 2006 I had the good fortune to live in Goroka, the capital of Eastern Highlands Province and where is headquartered the Papua New Guinea Institute of Medical Research. The IMR made me a Senior

Research Fellow in their Operational Research Unit and I was privileged to work alongside Papua New Guinean colleagues as we studied HIV, AIDS, STDs and sexual health and behaviour.

> *I take a critical and reflexive approach to HIV- and AIDS-related policies, numbers, behaviours and activities. I lament that sex toys, being gay and abortion are illegal anywhere and that prostitution has not been decriminalized in Papua New Guinea. I am resolutely pro-sex, decidedly agnostic, and far more respectful of other people's religious beliefs about these topics than by and large they have been of more secular ones. I am convinced that serosurveillance findings are not up to the demands made upon them and that what have been asserted to be 'high-risk settings' have not been demonstrated to be so. Some public health officials and NGO reps will say that, but only in private.*

The study proper and its internal politics regarding sex and ethics, method and personnel, condoms and Christianity were extremely complicated. The periodic dissemination of its results to the NACS, to the NHASP and to local- and provincial-level stakeholders was even more complicated in that we conducted our study amidst collapsing health systems, absent health workers and considerable rumour. What we found in the field was broken confidentiality, large numbers of infected housewives, absent HIVab test counsellors who had been trained to be at the ready, anti-condom discourse, low levels of knowledge about sexual function and physiology, sexually predatory male health workers and misogynous AIDS theatre dramas. Our publicising of such didn't sit well with authorities. Although it makes perfect intuitive sense from a social scientific perspective, the finding of lower risk in 'high-risk' settings and correspondingly high risk in 'low-risk' settings (see especially Chapter 4) won us few friends. Results often sailed into one ear, for example, about the inappropriateness of ABC or the sexual shenanigans of medical workers, and out the other, sometimes in the space of a single presentation. The study and its personnel were frequently queried about issues of method and instrument in ways that quantitative researchers generally aren't and regardless of the dubiousness of the quantitative data often collected about topics (for example, sexuality, fertility, blood and marital strife) that demand slower, often more inductive approaches. Thankfully, others have experienced similarly rocky times in the field and have had to make adjustments in their methodology accordingly and report upon them. The NHASP-sponsored Social Marketing Evaluation Review, for instance, noted that while a randomising probability sample would have been ideal, the census data available from 1997 were 'unreliable', few Papua New Guineans are home during the day, strangers are not welcomed into the home at night, and there were issues of researcher safety to consider (NHASP 2006h: 6–7). Things were complicated further insofar as the field component of our study was conducted in the shadow of much physical violence and many dead and dying people. This heightened emotions and sparked defensive reactions. There were extremely complicated local politics between the local provincial AIDS committee (PAC), the provincial health office, the hospital, churches and NGOs, even though the image promoted is usually of a cooperative, uniform national response. The NACS did not in a timely fashion vet the site reports I wrote, although I kept my promises not to release them to other than our sponsors. Consequently, health officials, PAC members and activists at each field-site came away with a poor impression of 'research' – since they weren't benefiting from the data we collected – and said many unkind things about me that still rankle. At least 20 people asked me in the ensuing two years to share with them the Final Report I wrote, '"It's in Every Corner Now"' (Hammar 2006b), based upon the hard work of the entire IMR team, and when I had of necessity to reroute them back to NACS and NHASP and other officials, they wrote back to me detailing the many ways they'd been ignored and rebuffed. The report did eventually surface, although neither the data in their staggering negativity, for example, about overall STD prevalence, nor the radical nature of the sociological insights – marriage increases risk, churches more than any other institution enable unsafe sex – have dented the sunny attitudes and comfortable assumptions in Port Moresby among the national and expatriate leadership.

Nevertheless, the work was life-affirming, we did our best to make our mark, and we brought to the light many issues and problems that leaders and led want to this day not to air. Nothing of what we found can in any way be read as supporting the 1.28% that stood as the 'official' figure of HIVab seroprevalence countrywide. I say this not as a personal slight, but rather, to indicate that empirical evidence and sociological insight are not where it's at – nor are they where they should be.

Many of the things I couldn't say then, I say here, although it remains to my former IMR colleagues to publish the results of our study. To some of them and to many other colleagues my analyses may appear strange and my conclusions unfair, even though they witnessed the events that inform the stories I tell and have themselves in many cases experienced similar things. For example, as many times as they heard me rail about clinics around the country that didn't provide condoms and whose personnel blamed AIDS on *pamuk meri* ('prostitutes') or on *pamuk pasin* (promiscuity), I came to find from experience and from disgruntled clients that these problems were also evident in our local clinics and at our local PAC office. Many quantitative-inclined colleagues rolled their eyes good-naturedly at my worrying about the methodological complexities of establishing 'marital status' in the context of formal interview, even though many of their relationships were similarly multiple and just as disputed by spouses and community members. Visiting scholars and researchers many times showed with ideas, data and sociological insight why the assumption that marriage was a safe institution and that there was a 'general population' to worry about was false and dangerous. Neither their presentations nor mine, however, made an appreciable dent in faith in variously Christian solutions to HIV and AIDS in abstinence and marriage. Although 'Christian' approaches to everyday behaviour and to an emergency national response are called for daily, most infections with HIV and STD are transmitted and suffered by Christians. Christian belief in the preventive properties of prayer, that 'two bodies must become one', that only the immoral get infected and that God wishes us to eschew condoms is clearly a problem on a number of levels, moral as well as public health, but to say so is to appear to slander Papua New Guinea's 300 or so Christian churches, denominations and sects. To this agnostic, moreover, it surely seems obvious that one sect trashes another, that one denomination slanders another. It is a sad indictment of the tendency to externalise risk to note that it 'was only in 2006 that there was any acknowledgement that HIV was infecting church members and clergy' (NHASP 2006c: 15), when that has been occurring all along. Such recognition, though it has come late, is structurally similar to the externalisation of public health messages and campaigns of 15 years ago. One booklet published by the then STD/AIDS Unit of the Department of Health in 1990 pronounced that 'You are especially at risk if you have more than one partner' (which ought to have alarmed all polygynous men and the wives thereof) and implied that condom use was for extra-marital sex: 'If you have more than one sexual partner, the proper use of condoms … '.

'You asked if I had any more insights/recollections of my stint in the hospital. There were about 60 beds in the pediatric ward, and as I recollect, there were usually four or five kids that we suspected as suffering from AIDS, but confirming it with serology was a lot more challenging. My instinct was simply to talk to the mother about our concerns and draw blood and send it to the lab, but it wasn't as easy as that. I didn't realise how much talking needed to happen before the test could be carried out. Staff knew that a 'positive' HIVab test result given to the wrong person could and does result in the beating and murder of mothers, since the man will assume that she has been unfaithful, so this threat of violence and negative family reaction was a direct obstacle to testing and few children were actually tested. The counselling seemed highly opaque, carried out by nurse, social worker and doctor. When I think back to that time I think of a constant stream of warm, small, dead, bundled up babies accompanied by wailing mothers, burnt out nurses and squalor. Drug shortages, bed shortages, reused needles, preventable disease, and a population of warm, friendly, welcoming, generous people that I think about every day' (Personal communication, medical doctor posted to a provincial hospital, September, 2007).

I hope therefore that this book nudges my colleagues in that direction even half as much as I have come to appreciate how crucial is the work they do in bettering community health. Those dedicated professionals and their counterparts in the NHASP, the NACS and the National Department of Health (hereafter NDoH) will find in Chapter 3 a detailed and healthily critical appreciation of the work they do and that opposes the criticisms made by many Australian journalists and policy-makers. I was honoured to work with many colleagues from government, business, academic research and faith communities, too. I admire those who from within private companies such as Oil Search Limited and Ok Tedi Mining Limited advocate for the communities whose health has been negatively affected by the logistics and economics of resource extraction. They, the NACS, AusAID, the NDoH and the NHASP have guided the national response to HIV and AIDS despite great political turmoil, fiscal downturns, a smoldering civil war along the border with Indonesia and contentious evangelism. International non-governmental organisations (INGOs) such as Save the Children (in Papua New Guinea), the European Union (EU), which is headquartered in the nation's capital of Port Moresby, and the Adventist Development and Relief Agency (ADRA), which is located in Lae on the north coast, are three more of the many examples that could be cited. They have bravely voiced the rights and sometimes special needs of sexual minorities who have been stigmatised in terms of sin, sex and HIV. Help Resources, Family Voice (Goroka-based) and AT Projects also do great work in peer education, victim advocacy, condom promotion and home-based care (HBC).

Programmes and initiatives sponsored by faith-based organisations (FBO) such as Anglicare-StopAIDS and the Catholic Church-funded Diocesan Health Services have also done much good around issues of VCT and HBC for those suffering from AIDS and for those trying to take care of them. One can disagree – okay, I disagree strongly – with the conservative, misogynous and homophobic attitudes that some FBO representatives take to sex, condoms and gender relations. Nevertheless, many FBOs are taking Christian exemplary care of the bodies (and if they exist, souls) of suffering people. The Franciscan Father Jude Ronayne-Ford runs an AIDS hospice in Port Moresby under extremely trying conditions; the weekly radio programme he directs never fails to defend the downtrodden and misunderstood. The Anglican Church Bishop from Port Moresby, Peter Fox, has made faith-based and interdenominational dialogues about gender relations and condom usage more progressive. Sister Rose Bernard is an American nun who manages the Shalom Care Centre in Banz, Western Highlands Province. She provides HBC training and HIVab testing services and also ministers to the sick and dying. Her skills and compassion are trained especially on the serodiscordant couples (in which only one spouse is HIVab+) who then have to navigate the waters of likely infection in the face of male sexual prerogative and community and church advice to stay married but not to use condoms. Bishop Cesare Bonivento of the Vanimo Diocese (see Chapter 5) is controversial for opposing condoms, non-Catholics, homosexuality, population control, masturbation and safer-sex initiatives. Nevertheless, he is doing what he thinks is right, and no one can blame him for not caring. Bishop Bonivento also defends the rights of West Papuans to their homeland and opposes Indonesian incursions. He doesn't like sexual violence any more than I do. Religious doctrines undoubtedly crimp frank discussions of sex, disease, risk and condoms, but yet many devout Christians deserve credit (alongside a long list of agnostic social scientists) for doing what they have to crack open this difficult nut.

Albeit from quite different vantage points, these individuals and organisations have had to deal with the public health fallout of largely unanticipated social change and medical disasters that have affected Papua New Guineans, just as they have others in the Pacific. Fijians and Tuvaluans, New Caledonians and their counterparts in the Solomon Islands, Pohnpei, the Cook Islands and Tonga are beginning also to register now what Papua New Guinean authorities began registering a decade ago, and the rates of STD infection are everywhere worrying. If at times it seems to American or Australian observers that the response to HIV and AIDS has been too slow, just imagine how fast all of this has hit Pacific islanders. A 65-year-old woman in the 'developed' US would have been born prior to the advent of birth control pills, television, mammograms and penicillin. Her male counterpart didn't have iPods and photocopy machines growing up, and his shaving razor was neither quadruplicate nor powered by an on-board computer. None of their age-mates had access to the Internet, HIVab tests, global positioning systems or many other medical and technological marvels. None of their children attended school wearing bullet-proof back-packs or entered the classroom through metal detectors, either.

> 'Another centre …had run out of condoms and said that they had stopped advocating the use of them because they could not supply them. The same centre stated that some time ago they had had rapid test kits but the supply had run out so they had stopped doing rapid tests and now sent the clients to the nearby town. Some centres had not received a supply of test kits recently so were using expired test kits. Another centre had none of the cardboard sharps containers and was using a recycled plastic detergent bottle which had congealed and old blood around its opening' (NHASP 2006a: 20).

Just imagine what the late-twentieth and early-twenty-first centuries have meant to Papua New Guineans, many of whom travelled their first road, ate their first fast-food, saw their first television programme and cooked with electricity for the first time in the 1980s. Suddenly, their country has been pronounced by Australians as being 'a catastrophe on our doorstep' (Carney 2006; Cronau 2006) and 'a national catastrophe' (Alexander Downer, in *The Economist* 2006: 56). How unfair. Papua New Guinea is seen as being 'at the epicentre of' the regional HIV epidemic (Casey 2007), responsible for 85–90% of the entire burden of HIV in the Pacific. This, too, is unfair and makes no sense in terms of epidemiology. The geographic, sexual, diplomatic and financial links that Papua New Guinea has to its neighbour Indonesia should by rights move it from epicentre to opposite end of the spectrum from the west or at least make 'New Guinea' (not Papua New Guinea) the epicentre of the Asia-Pacific region, but that has not happened. Indonesia's viral threat to Papua New Guinea is not registered. Strange, but Indonesia thinks about its Papua in about the same way as Australia deals with Papua New Guinea.

This book is therefore greatly about the discourse of AIDS, too, about the models and metaphors by which HIV has come to be known. Some evidence suggests that epicentre motifs are being ditched in favour of linear ones even though the metaphors are still of disaster. For example, Tuvalu is to two observers in danger of 'extinction' from AIDS, even though very few cases have been reported. Major changes need to be made, they say, if it and the rest of the Pacific are not to 'follow in the wake of Africa and Papua New Guinea' (Gross and Manning 2005). Tim Rwabuhemba, not himself Papua New Guinean but who is the Country Coordinator for the UNAIDS mission in Papua New Guinea, warned that if political leaders didn't sufficiently deal with things now, 'it could very much become an Africa-type situation' (O'Brien 2007). While other Pacific island countries excluding Papua New Guinea are 'believed to be where PNG was between five and ten years ago', according to a Fijian journalist, 'PNG itself is today surmised to be where Africa was ten years ago' (Islands Business International 2007).

This just antes up the rhetorical stakes. For three years I sat in innumerable workshops and seminars and listened to one speaker after another health official warn about an 'African-style epidemic' washing ashore ... and now other Pacific islanders are worried about the behemoth of Papua New Guinea. Treat Asia Network opined that Papua New Guinea's generalised epidemic 'threatens to become one of the most severe in Asia [sic]'. 'Men often have multiple partners', says Neil Brenden, head of an ADB-funded project, 'but the HIV/AIDS situation here has the makings of an Africa-style epidemic mainly because of the risk behavior of the women' (Brenden, quoted in Gill 2007).

In addition to mislocating Papua New Guinea geographically, it claimed that Papua New Guinea had been 'largely untouched by the currents of globalization' (Treat Asia 2006)! Its outgoing Minister of Health was quoted in the *New Zealand Herald* (12 April 2007) as saying that it was 'up to leaders to fight the disease' and that Papua New Guinea had done more on the issue than its Pacific neighbours: 'The rest of the Pacific is in a state of denial', he asserted. Hmmm. Internet postings and press releases have favourably compared other insular Pacific countries (especially Fiji and Tonga) to Papua New Guinea, which is being compared increasingly with 'Africa' (Gross and Manning 2005; Nalu 2004; O'Brien 2007), a continent many of whose countries have been accused of just such denial.

Why are Papua New Guineans even looking to the continent of Africa when there is plenty to look at in their own back-yard? Why are other Pacific islanders worried about Papua New Guinea? Why isn't Papua New Guinea more worried about Indonesia or an 'Asia-type' epidemic? What does the situation in Indonesian Papua have to teach us about the place of governance in managing crises of the public health in Pacific island states and cultures? Looked at over the span of several years, the pendulum of recognition of a serious problem seems to be swinging ever harder from one end to the other. Part of the Pacific ... but not really. Doesn't yet have a big problem ... but is now the epicentre of one. Doing the most of any Pacific country ... but nowhere near enough. AIDS is a huge problem somewhere ... but not here, because we're a Christian nation. Okay, yeah, we've got a problem ... but it's affecting only sex workers and a few gay expatriates. Yeah, okay, our HIV epidemic has 'generalised' ... but we're effectively 'targeting' those 'high-risk' people who represent the 'bridging' groups. Yeah, I know, way more of us housewives than sex workers are infected ... but it all started with them chasing after our husbands anyway. They'll get theirs. In addition to disabling more accurate risk assessments, these kinds of denial and this extent of externalisation feed inter-country name-calling and one-upmanship, which are distinctly not valued Pacific island traits. If in the Pacific HIV constitutes a regional security threat, what kind of a threat is that? If Papua New Guinea is all of a sudden so threatening to others, then why is the HIVab seroprevalence so low? If the officially accepted figure is so obviously a sham, why hasn't anyone said so? If only 'a handful of [Australian] expatriates' in Port Moresby are at risk, then why the big fuss; why is it that already infected Australian businessmen are said to be *at risk* when they have sex with Papua New Guineans instead of *to pose a risk* to them (*The Australian 2008*)?

The hot glow of anger

My experience in Western Province during 1990–92 when AIDS was a distant rumour and then again more recently throughout 11 provinces as the national response was finally kicking into gear has led to new heights of clarity about these topics, but also to new lows of depression. Maybe even to a little 'hot glow of anger' at discovering a wrong, as Jules Henry confessed in *Pathways to Madness* (Henry 1965). This resulted, he wrote, from engagement in deep thought about social injustice, but he warned that it can still choke off constructive ways forward if allowed to take over one's work. I don't want that to happen here. Joan Cassell also warned in her fine study of US surgeons, *Expected Miracles: surgeons at work*, that what fuels 'the ethnography of indignation' (Cassell 1991: xiv–xviii) is precisely what allows this hot glow of anger, this indulgent self-righteousness, to compromise the search for understanding. The ethnography of indignation, she says, leads to a certain coarseness of analysis and enables the tendency to blame instead of explain. 'Those who practice the ethnography of indignation', she says, 'may be able to expose the misbehavior of the powerful, but exposure, although valuable, cannot help us understand why they behave this way' (1991: xvii). An editorial published in *BMJ* (Sims 2003: 165) called for law-and-order-type remedies for a social milieu in which, the author claimed, community caring was no longer evident. The author's further claim that health workers 'are not prepared to go into the settlements to provide a home nursing or palliative care service', being too frequently 'attacked or murdered [or] raped', led to his vilification. Notable politicians, journalists, consultants and health professionals such as Alexander Downer, Bonnie Flaws, Matthew Carney, Miranda Tobias, Sean Dorney, Carol Jenkins, David Gordon-Macleod, Peter Cronau, Bill Bowtell, Scarlett Epstein and Peter Piot have received the same kind of treatment from some quarters. Saying publicly that HIV epidemics are largely home-grown (Dundon and Wilde 2007; Hammar 2007b; Keck

2007) is just as unpopular as is questioning the intelligence of promoting abstinence as a viable safe-*sex* method. In like manner the alarmist reporting of 'boys' and 'innocent men' being pack-raped by women, typically said to be 'from the highlands', detracts from the very real and really high rates of such suffered sometimes by boys but more often by girls at the hands of males, individually and in groups. It was reported in early April of 2004, for example, that a 16-year-old boy from Madang had been raped repeatedly at knife-point by three women at the old Lae airport. The boy reported his 'ordeal' to police, who said that the women 'alleged to have committed the offence were from the highlands' (*Post-Courier* 2008b).

✳ ✳ ✳

This book, therefore, looks critically at discourses of HIV and AIDS in public discussion as much as in epidemiological modelling. It asks why ABC remains the ideological fulcrum of the national response to HIV and AIDS despite the absence of any evidence that it works. The book explores which attitudes in public health (now and in the past) help explain why so many people are afraid to be treated for an STD. It looks at why so many so quickly become reinfected. Regarding the question as to why so many health officials – not just religious leaders – repudiate condom usage, I'll say here what I explore more fully in Chapter 5: there is a Pope somewhere, the Pope is Catholic and the Catholic Church is the biggest donor among the FBOs to the AIDS fight in Papua New Guinea. Australia's Cardinal George Pell believes that usage of a 'rubber contraption' (quoted in Cronau 2006) causes sexual irresponsibility, too. Bishop Bonivento claims that condoms 'accelerate the spread of AIDS' (2006–and in other publications [2001a, 2001b, 2005a, b], actually *cause* AIDS). George Bush's administration had progressive family planning and HIV prevention programmes in a stranglehold over condoms and abstinence. Speaking forthrightly about these issues is not really allowed, however; the national response welcomes little frank talk or dissent and that which appears to speak ill of churches.

Well-meaning journalists, consultants and researchers are trapped thus in a paradox: working for an NGO, a prominent newspaper or a national research institution provides an institutional backing but that handcuffs them in what they can say and how they can say it. Noting the routine absence of condoms in religious and ostensibly secular health care settings and writing about the sex-negative attitudes that dampened women's clinic attendance there wins no one new friends. Questioning the beliefs of one's colleagues that God produces drug-resistant forms of STD, instead of the forces of natural selection working against often over-prescribed antibiotics, only makes them look at one sideways. Asking for proof of their claims that God can cure the HIV that is the wages of their sin leads them to point to people who are still alive. And when they die? Well, such people clearly didn't sufficiently believe in the Lord, and so provide a handy object lesson in abject suffering. Solo-flying researchers, however, while not perhaps shackled so, are the more easily ignored for lack of institutional backing and the often isolated ways in which they work, often in cahoots with the very marginalised people to whom they hope to give voice and provide support. Helen Epstein commented recently that '[h]itchhikers live cynical, parasitical existences, but sometimes they see the landscape more clearly than the driver' (Epstein 2007: 27). The anthropologist Graham Fordham has written painfully and insightfully about this dynamic in Thailand where, he argues, from the perspective of donor organisations, the 'kind of in-depth ethnographic AIDS research social scientists conduct' becomes in the eyes of NGOs 'totally irrelevant. Most were unaware of the existence of such work ...' (2005: xv). He continues:

> The insights that long-term field research and laboriously crafted analyses of the Thai AIDS epidemic may contain, the fruits of finely nuanced and critically reflexive analyses, spoke neither to their AIDS epidemic, nor to their AIDS epidemic agendas. (2005: xvi)[1]

> *Nun: I asked if you know anything about AIDS and you said you don't know ...How can you get this sickness? Do you know how you get this sickness?*
>
> *Man: I don't know.*
>
> *Nun: Of course you know.*
>
> *Man: Sinful acts?*
>
> *Nun: That's it.*

Either way, health workers, NGO heads and government officials who feel threatened by 'negative' publicity (say, regarding a wandering speculum in an STD clinic, dubious statistics or a project manager who has falsely claimed medical credentials) can easily block otherwise good work, quell constructive criticism and preclude the airing of sound research findings (see also Cullen 2006; Dorney 2005; Gibson 2006). Many times have social scientists been discouraged even from asking questions. Muck-raking journalism can make things worse. The producers, camera-people and reporters of 'Sick No Good', a sensational documentary produced by the Australian Broadcasting Corporation (see Carney 2006; Cronau 2006), used a hidden camera in a prominent Port Moresby night-club setting to observe sweating dancers and to conduct boozy interviews. The day following the airing of the documentary the young females residing in the night-club were punished by the club's expatriate manager for what he and the owners and the patrons openly condone and/or engage in: having sex (author's fieldnotes, 28 August 2006). The producer took another cheap shot by going after a very nervous-looking Minister of Health. Papua New Guineans and those who live and work in Papua New Guinea know that Members with Portfolio regularly shuffle horizontally between appointments, and so this Minister's mishandling of questions regarding the distribution of antiretrovirals was unsurprising.

Sad, but unsurprising. Less forgivable were his blaming of hospital capacity ahead of government inaction and prior lack of financial accountability to INGOs such as UNAIDS and WHO and his misstatements regarding HIVab seroprevalence in miners in Enga Province and among youth in Southern Highlands Province. In the documentary softball-sized questions were served up to a passionately dedicated nun who cares for the infected, but the reporter skirted tougher questions regarding her church's stance toward sex, the extent of the untreated STDs in her congregation, their access to condoms, the specific content of HIVab counselling sessions and what might be her feelings about having to hide what condoms she dispenses. The text box translation from the Tok Pisin of a portion of the broadcast shows that there is room for critique of the content of the components of the national response. None of this should in any way be taken as lessening appreciation for the impressive effort expended in the national response or of the enormity of the obstacles to its mounting. I only want that other kinds of labours be allowed to inform the national response and that self-critique be allowed to take its rightful, healthy place.

The documentary generated little negative commentary by Australians because, just as with the national response, it blamed AIDS on easy targets: their former colonial charges, disaffected youth, night-clubs and women in prostitution. It ignored the high transmissive risks in a statistically average marriage. It touched not on the constraints of evangelical Christian discourse regarding sexual ethics. It probed no misconstrual of transmission risks by mainstream public health messages and officials. It omitted scrutiny of the sexual behaviour of elite males, both national and expatriate. It neglected also to mention the many more progressive moments and opportunities of the national response, for example, the training of physicians in the principles of syndromic management of STDs, of youth in the methods of street theatre and of female peer educators in condom distribution and promotion. The massive disconnect between 'knowledge' of HIV transmission risks (as measured following distribution of posters and pamphlets and other materials) and their self-perception (as somehow monitored in behaviour) took a back seat to the fact of spotty distribution of medicine. Moreover, how antiretroviral therapies will be expected to work in the shadow of faltering health systems and of endemic corruption of accountability was elided. A story published in the *Post-Courier*, 'Drugs Go Bad at Port' (11 September 2007), mentioned that four containers of vitally needed medicines that had been donated by Rotary service organisations overseas had languished on the docks in Lae, Morobe Province, since March of 2007 and had expired, needing thus to be dumped or destroyed. The sociologist Maxine Pitts remarked in 2001 that '[y]ears of junketing, greed, sloth, sheer incompetence and outright corruption is sending Papua New Guinea into an economic tailspin, exacerbated by the accompanying increase in crime' (Pitts 2001: 127).

Conservative religious ethics and movements are clanking the more loudly against rising STD and HIV transmission rates. Papua New Guineans have in recent years promoted and been exposed to conservative realignments in gender relations by civic and religious leaders alike. The scorn meted out not long ago in newspaper stories and letters to the editor to *tu kina meri* in

> *The embodied experience of a woman in Papua New Guinea*
> *tells her to fear her husband, but her priest, papa, politician and*
> *public health official each tell her to have sex with him and him*
> *only – and for God's sake, not to use a condom. The general tenor*
> *and specific content of mainstream public health messages and*
> *programmes betray women's embodied experiences and continue*
> *to privilege male sexual prerogative. They are precisely the 'good*
> *ideas' that imperil a struggling country filled with wonderful*
> *people and fascinating cultures but that are already under siege*
> *of ill sexual and reproductive health that is becoming worse.*

prostitution is now apportioned also to the *New Age Woman* of newspaper pullouts and hallway talk. Both kinds of femininity are under pressure to conform to models of gender comportment that put men and their needs at the centre. Mobile, carousing males are generally let off the hook, but females are expected to be sexually naïve and submissive to their husbands. Both men and women, however, are expected to select and groom sexual partners according to moral attributes of decency, fertility obligations and religious faith, not the olfactory and dermal signs of STDs, not the serological markers suggesting HIV infection and not by questioning anything. As with other related issues, there has been neglect at the level of policy-making and programme directives of the admirable corpus of qualitative literature regarding sexuality, health services, gender relations and risk-assessment that has amassed since the 1980s. The ground-breaking nationwide study conducted in the early 1990s (NSRRT and Jenkins 1994) is mentioned frequently but yet its signal findings are ignored in substance. This is a shame since it and other more focused, geographically specific qualitative studies (e.g. Clark 1997; Clark and Hughes 1995; Eves 2003a, b; Hammar 1996a, b; Hughes, 1991, 2002; Wardlow 2002a, b, 2006, 2008a, b) are so relevant to today's crises.

A little background

Before I lay out the specific contents of the book I want briefly to mention important issues of context and perspective that will be unpacked in chapters below. These cross-cut and add a dimension to those mentioned above. First, the cultural and religious politics of sexuality, gender relations and fertility mandate that 'good', 'proper' sex be unprotected. That fact, however, is the subject of remarkably superficial and non-reflexive thought. Based upon injunctions to 'Just Say "No"', transmissive vulnerability and reinfection are chalked up to deviance and ignorance more than to the normative ideals of trust, reproduction and faith. Explanations of the current crisis tend to the too easy and too quick: 'STDs are new', 'condoms are foreign introductions' and 'it is taboo in many Pacific cultures to talk about sex'. In fact, STDs are three times older than the oldest commentator's lifetime, no more foreign than Pentecostal and Charismatic revivals, and such taboos are made to be broken, especially in times of such great stress. There is consensus among health officials that STD has vaguely to do with social change and rural-to-urban migration and that a 'breakdown in values' and compromising of 'tradition' has occurred (read: women, gays and youth are getting uppity). There is little attention paid to male sexual prerogative *per se*, however, or to the good health-inducing effects of sex-positive ethics that include condoms, bodily knowledge, pleasure and consent (see Lepani 2007b, 2008a). Works by Holly Wardlow, Adam Reed, Holly Aruwafu-Buchanan, Martha Macintyre, Carol Jenkins, Charles Wilde, Jeffrey Clark, Michael Wood and Anou Borrey among others show the contingent nature of men's sexualities in specific and sometimes historically unique settings. This means that things can get better, if only because they have so obviously changed for the worse.

> '*Female Patient: Oh, but doctor, you told me to undress and lie down on the couch for an examination. But I only came for advice about getting married and bringing my boyfriend for a blood test, so why are you undressing too?*
>
> *Male Doctor: Well! It's only right that you should get both a doctor's advice and a demonstration of safe sex too!'*
> ('Safe Sex' cartoon, Thailand; Borthwick 1999: 215).

Second, few see anything wrong in and with the Clinic itself, preferring to blame the patient's hygiene, not that of the health centre; to suspect the climate, not the historical influence of colonialism upon sexuality; to lament geographical access, not the legacy of medical experimentation; to finger the culture of the native, not that of the health-care setting; and to blame the sexual behaviour of the patient, not the genitophobia and sexual anxieties induced by church doctrines.

The photo here was snapped in an urban clinic that was still serving clients (April 2006), and no, there was no toilet paper or running water. Both nurses and patients must use it. STD clinic (non-) attendance is blamed on the tendency of patients to abscond, not on the fact that health workers are thought or known to be sexually predatory or that such clinics are located in full view of others. Street-sellers of Amoxicillin and purveyors of 'bush medicines' are blamed for blunting antibiotic and health worker efficacy, but it is from health workers that they get their supplies and who sometimes endorse their products.[2] People who become HIV-infected and then ultimately die of AIDS are sometimes blamed for their own demise insofar as they were short on or not sufficiently persistent in the faith in God that allegedly kept them alive. 'The charismatics therefore do not always encourage people to seek medical care, as this is an indication of lack of belief in God's healing power' (McPherson 2008: 241). Not surprisingly, claims abound by charismatic movement representatives of the AIDS cure that their faith offers (2008: 243). Proponents of 'faith healings' get a free

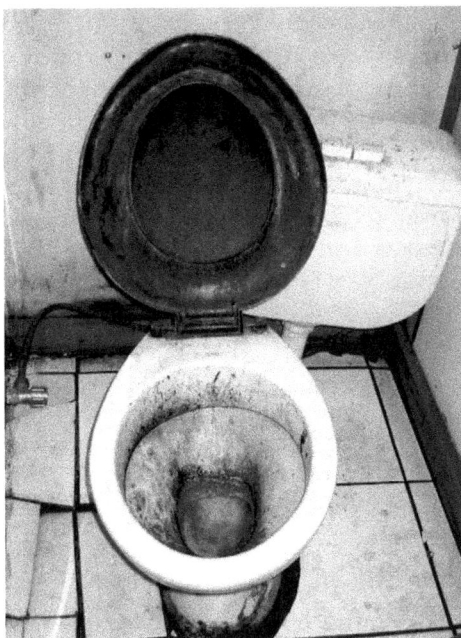

Health Clinic toilet

pass in the newspaper and in the countryside because they are endorsed formally and less so and because they seem to fit Christian ideals. This is unfair and unhealthy. One NHASP review (2006a: 19) noted 'misconceptions' among focus group interview members insofar as two who were HIVab+ were convinced that it constituted a death sentence but also believed that the herbal concoctions they were taking would cure them within the year. The problem is that many health officials have formally and informally endorsed such products, although *their* misconceptions have gone unreported. The language, geography and culture of the Other are routinely cited as 'barriers' to swifter and to more effective treatment of STDs (see Butt, Numbery and Morin 2002a), but long waits on a bench in view of judgmental relatives are not. Posters of Jesus and Mary in an STD clinic and images of bright-red emblazoned coffins awaiting the descent of uncomprehending AIDS victims (see the posters in Chapter 5) can't help but induce fear and shame. Few seem concerned about the confidence sometimes broken there or about the penal attitude taken toward STD sufferers in decades past, which is one source of iatrophobia. Encouraged by external donors whose monies need acquitting, this has underwritten the conceit that problems of serosurveillance or of antiretroviral distribution and treatment are relatively new, when they aren't. Problems of the past have not been allowed to inform those of the present.

A third important contextual factor is the overwhelmingly sexual nature of Papua New Guinea's HIV epidemics. Unlike, say, in the People's Republic of China, Thailand, Peru, Romania, France, the US or Indonesia, there seem to be few infections due to sharing of contaminated medical or drug-injecting equipment or to blood supplies or to nosocomial sources. Not surprisingly, conservative sexual ethics have been promoted that are often 'confounded with public health matters' (NZPGPD 2006: 20). Verena Keck tells in a recent essay just how difficult it is for Yupno youth (especially male) in the mountainous regions of Madang Province to obtain condoms from scattered health centres. One teen's comment, she says, well represents: '"the health workers ... have taken a new course and that is why they now say: 'All married men may come and get condoms. But all the young men and teenagers are not allowed to come and get any'. That is what they say"' (Keck 2007: 50). Alison Dundon and Charles Wilde remarked that in a Gogodala (Western Province, Papua New Guinea) women's Christian Fellowship group,

> many agreed vigorously when one woman argued against the use of condoms as the platform for prevention of the spread of HIV, stating that 'when God created man, he gave them [sexual] organs, and [told them] not to put other things [like condoms] on them'. Another noted that 'our mothers didn't know this sickness [AIDS]. When the sickness came, they introduced the condom: so all the ladies are living in fear of their husbands going away [to work] and coming back wanting to wear condoms'. (2007: 1)

These kinds of behavioural and cognitive paradoxes are a fourth contextual factor and are woven throughout later chapters. The snippet above suggests that while women are embracing infection and fearing protection, which is precisely the opposite of what we would want them to do, men are disavowing responsibility and engaging in sexual experimentation. Additionally, while Christian churches and church leaders have in many ways modelled proper care and compassion of the suffering and dying, they have done this so well that they have become in effect impervious to commentary upon the specific content of their HIV and AIDS programmes or to their policies and individual attitudes about gender relations and sexuality more broadly. They had so constrained discussion of sexual matters in one Papua New Guinean community, writes Holly Wardlow, who and whose team wished to show AIDS-related videos, that returning university students were reduced to saying that AIDS was caused by 'young girls writing love letters to high school boys' (Wardlow 2008: 194). The 'Faith Community Leaders Covenant on HIV/AIDS', a document that was formulated and approved in remarkably quick fashion (see Chapter 4), does not mention the word 'condom', and neither does the Catholic Church's equivalent document. The so-called 'Nadi Declaration' made in 2004 at least claimed not to want to engage actively in opposing condom distribution and usage and allowed that, yes, there was scientific evidence showing how effective condoms were in preventing STD and HIV transmission (World Council of Churches 2004: 4). In response to the proclamation that followed from the first-ever HIV Prevention Summit in 2006 such that the government would encourage '100% condom use', several church leaders said that they 'would not be threatened' by the increasing suffering of and dying from AIDS and end up promoting or distributing condoms. Pastor Daniel Hewali, who holds a prominent position in the National Capital District PAC, added that Papua New Guineans did not have to 'adopt ungodly ways to win this battle', and that condom promotion would have long-term, devastating effects (Gerawa 2006). As I show in Chapter 5, it remains difficult to voice such concerns, however, for fear of appearing anti-church and immoral. I recognise that this must be difficult for devout Christians (e.g. Bouten 1996; Farmer 1996). No document, programme or pronouncement about HIV and AIDS should be considered immune from criticism, however, least of all this one.

Fifth, by most accounts, politicians and health officials came late to the table. 'The major driver of the spread of HIV', concluded a recent Policy Brief (Bowtell 2007: 3), 'was the failure of political will to translate scientific evidence into good policy in time to cap and control the spread of the virus'. The 1st National Surveillance Plan wasn't announced until two decades following report of the first HIV infection, and to date there remains no formal notification system for AIDS diagnoses or suspected HIV infection (NACS 2007: 1). Depending on one's preference for metaphor, Papua New Guinea is either 'on the brink' or 'under siege' or 'at the crossroads' or 'at the frontline' of, 'cursed' by God in the form of, engaged in 'war' on in a 'national fight' against, sitting atop a 'ticking time bomb' of, caught in a 'snowball' of gathering infections of, fighting multiple 'bushfires' in the form of or staring at the Apocalypse or the End Time that is now taking the shape of HIV and AIDS epidemics that are racing, galloping and burning (Bowtell 2007; Cullen 2000, 2003a, b, 2006; Dorney 2005; Eves 2003a, 2003b; Gross and Manning 2005; Hammar n.d., 2004a, 2004b, 2008a, 2007b; Middleton 2006b; Ostroff 1998; Tobias 2007; Windybank and Manning 2003). Differences of scale, religion and social milieu aside, the metaphor in Thailand of AIDS victims placidly 'falling like leaves' from a tree (Fordham 2005) doesn't well capture the sense in Papua New Guinea that things are spiraling wildly out of control or, as in other Pacific countries, are poised for take-off. Sticking with the climatic metaphor, if Papua New Guinea is yet in the eye of the storm, the weather is quickly becoming very, very nasty. It is a pity, how long ago this storm blipped on the radar.

Contents of the book

I argue throughout the book that, despite massive effort and good intentions, the national response to HIV and AIDS has in Papua New Guinea gone wrong in some of the same ways it has gone wrong in Indonesia (Butt 2005, 2008; Butt, Numbery and Morin 2002a, b; Butt, Munro and Wong 2004; Murray 2001), Thailand (Fordham 2005), Uganda (Schoepf 2003), South Africa (Epstein 2007; Gauri and Lieberman 2006) and elsewhere (Bowtell 2007), especially in several countries and territories of the insular Pacific (Butt and Eves 2008). Brooke Schoepf in the case of Uganda (2003), Alison Murray in view of Indonesia (2001), and Graham Fordham in context of Thailand (2005) have argued that the cultural politics of sexuality and intervention and the foreign donor-nature of funding sources have in effect sped up the pace of epidemics instead of slowed them down.

Why and in what ways this might also be the case in Papua New Guinea will be unpacked and discussed in the several chapters to follow. This Part One is titled *Sexual Networking and Dis-ease in the Pacific* and contains in its several chapters some of the historical, behavioural, conceptual, ethnographic and policy-implementation backdrop of especially Papua New Guinea's response to HIV and AIDS. Part Two, *What the Experts (Still) Don't Get*, extends my analysis to other countries, cultures and topics but by handing over the analytical and editorial reins to three colleagues. Drawing upon their personal experiences and disciplinary perspectives, we discuss points of comparison and contrast between Papua New Guinea, Australia, island Indonesia, Thailand and Indonesian Papua.

The second chapter in Part One, 'The Women in Traffic: *tu kina bus* in town and country', reverses the direction and title of three variably famous essays each titled 'The Traffic in Women': Goldman (1970[1917]), Rubin (1975) and Skrobonok, Boonpakdi and Janthakeero (1997). I explain the slow transition in one culture area in the meaning, frequency and monetary value of women's bodies and the sexual services they provided. Just as soon as they began to arrive in what became the territories of New Guinea and Papua, Christian missionaries began to denounce, colonial authorities became concerned by, and ethnologists tried to record and explain what were perceived to be 'traditional' behavioural excesses. 'All missionaries opposed "licentiousness" in any form, their main concerns being "fornication" and adultery', according to Diane Langmore, in *Missionary Lives* (1989: 125). They were particularly concerned by serial and transactional forms of sexual intercourse, both 'homosexual' and 'heterosexual', though those were of course not the terms then used. Colonial administrative discourses of racial defects and promiscuity denigrated a particular tribe, the Bamu, for literally stagnating in the mud and metaphorically stagnating by taint of participation in certain sexual transactions. Their engagement since the mid-1960s on the nearby island capital of Daru in *tu kina bus*, or $2 bush prostitution, has long made them vulnerable to social scorn and to STDs. Now it exposes them to HIV. Once considered the 'backwater of the backwater' of colonial reach, Western Province has become for external donors a 'high-priority province' in terms of AIDS and HIV and their seeming migration southward across the Torres Straits into North Queensland, into Australia. This chapter suggests that norms of sociality and regional trade imbalances better explain transitions to contemporary prostitution than do the tropes of backwardness and promiscuity common to colonial administrative, public health and mission-inspired works of the period. In a sense, the 'traffic in women' is about heathenness, backwardness and vulnerability, whereas the 'women in traffic' is about gender relations, male sexual prerogative and social-structure.

In the Introduction to Part Two I argue that Papua New Guinean males seem to be responding behaviourally (by not using condoms) not just to anti-condom discourse, but also to misunderstood, ambiguous and misconstrued messages about 'circumcision' that only rarely result in an actual circumcision. These four text box quotes, each from Bishop Bonivento of the Vanimo Diocese, suggest something of the discursive context of today's 'Rubber Wars' in Papua New Guinea (Gamson 1990). Into the breach, as it were, a dermal gap has been opened by Self and by Other, using home-made and clinic-purloined scalpels, dressings and antibiotics. The increasing prominence of 'the invisible condom' shows that Papua New Guinean and other Pacific island men are struggling to appear modern and gain in their masculinity, but without parting with or opposing Christian teachings. A prominent newspaper editor in Papua New Guinea commented to Trevor Cullen in 1999 that 'not using condoms has become among many PNG men a mark of masculinity, a macho rite of passage. Using condoms is totally uncool' (Cullen 2000: 192). Other sources related that '[s]ome men refuse to wear condoms because they believe it lessens their manhood' (ESCAP 2005: 9). It may seem counter-intuitive to point out, but many men believe the need for using two, three or even four condoms at a time or using a condom with another device, for example, a plastic sack or even rice packet (part of what has been dubbed in the US 'redneck contraception').

> *Bishop Bonivento, Do Condoms Stop or Spread AIDS? (2001a):*
>
> *'It is a joke to say that condoms are safe or safer' (p. 25).*
>
> *'If we consider all the factors present in the use of condoms as prevention from AIDS, we can state that the risk of getting infected in the first year is as high as 100%' (p. 33).*
>
> *'100% of those following abstinence before marriage will never get infected' (p. 31).*
>
> *'spermicides increase the risk of catching ...HIV' (back-flap).*

Chapter 3 is titled and discusses 'HIV in history: serosurveillance and other studies, 1987–2007'. The first few editorials and case reports that appeared in Papua New Guinean and Australian medical journals and newspapers laid the foundation for policies initially formulated and implemented and that still inform policy today. Chapter 4, 'HIV in Discourse: problems and prospects of the national response, 1987–2007', critiques the unreliability of numbers, which has led to the false construction of risk groups and misled people about the nature of and reasons behind sexual networking. Chapter 5 is titled 'Foreign Objects and Cognitive Dissonance: the strange waters of anti-condom discourse' and examines the 'rubber wars' (Gamson 1990) in Papua New Guinea. The quotes in the text box are from one of the writings of Bishop Bonivento, who argues that condoms and their usage are variously correlated with, cause, or spread AIDS and promiscuity. I show that debates about condoms are seldom about their tensile strength or STD and HIV preventing properties so much as about sex-positive and -negative attitudes. Indeed, the rubber wars are in Papua New Guinea about Good and Evil, almost always about God, sometimes even about Satan.

The four chapters that comprise Part Two, *What the Experts (Still) Don't Get*, are designed to stir up discussion amongst interested health professionals, policy-makers, donor country representatives and researchers. I have invited in Chapter 6 my friend Sarah Hewat to compare and contrast HIV- and AIDS-related numbers, behaviours and policies in Papua New Guinea with those across the border in the Indonesian province of Papua, where she has for a long time worked. Sarah's intimate grounding in the social poetics of daily life (a life enhanced by having lived also in Bougainville for a year) have attuned her to the special risks of companionate relationships, of intimate love and of underground romance (see Hewat 2008) that bear obviously on the situation in Papua New Guinea. Just as do Abigail Harrison in context of rural South African youth (2008) and a host of other ethnographers worldwide, Hewat shows that specifically gendered vulnerabilities relate to age differences in sexual 'partners', coercion in sexual matters and the purposeful forgoing of condom use. Harrison in context of South Africa, Schoepf in terms of Uganda and other African countries (2004a, b), Alison Murray with respect to Indonesia (2001), Leslie Butt and Hewat in terms of Indonesian Papua (Butt 2008; Butt and Munro 2007; Hewat 2008) and myself and others in reference to Papua New Guinea (Dundon 2007; Wardlow 2006a, b, 2007; Wilde 2007) have shown the ill effects upon STD and HIV transmission of gender ideals and practices that encourage unsafe sex.

Chapter 7 enlists another friend and colleague, Alison Murray, who has conducted ethnographic research and engaged in activism throughout the Asia-Pacific region. Some of the ideas and commentaries of these two chapters alongside many others from Chapters 4 and 5 are then discussed with another friend and colleague, Mark Boyd, in Chapter 8. Mark has a wealth of experience to share regarding his work in Thailand, the US and Australia on the management, efficacy and suffering of antiretroviral therapies. Conducting surveillance activities and thinking critically about disease causation in less microscopically small terms are each tasks that, however gargantuan they may be, have never been needed more. Aly's and Sarah's contributions have direct application to work that touches on community mobilisation, advocacy and risk assessment and prevention methods. Mark's comments, by contrast, have direct application to the ongoing antiretroviral roll-out, questions of ethics in clinical research and the need to develop indigenous research protocol. I draw upon earlier arguments to urge in Chapter 9, the Epilogue, for an understanding of disease that is rooted in social-structure, too, not just concerned with the level of microscopically small pathogens.

This book aims thus to lay out what has already been learned about HIV and AIDS in the insular Pacific and to insist that social scientific findings and analyses also guide policy. I show that the social construction of HIV and AIDS epidemics in policy and political discourse are significant problems in their own right. They misconstrue risk, target already vulnerable people, remain uncritical about male sexual prerogative and deny the pleasure and good health-inducing potential of consensual sex. HIV and AIDS are rooted firmly in social-structure and in social relations that, just like in the US, Thailand and Australia, must, can and in some ways and places have already changed.

NOTES

1. Fordham's candor resonates with me. No more than a couple of months had elapsed from the time I left Papua New Guinea in 1992 when an evangelical parliamentarian (now the Governor-General) who had misread a draft manuscript of mine excoriated me in the pages of one of the two national daily English newspapers, the *Post-Courier*, for allegedly having done a 'sex survey' and having sought to demonstrate that Daruans are all 'sex-crazed

maniacs' (Hammar 1993a, b). I hadn't – and they aren't – but that's what can happen when They read what We write, or rather, when they hear what someone says she thinks we meant when we wrote what she says someone told her we wrote. Without casting doubts of veracity upon public presentations that social scientists have given and reports they've submitted or on-line discussions into which they've entered, health officials nevertheless can slow their dissemination and preclude frank discussions of sexual health, HIV prevention programmes and sexual violence. This is pulling the card of nationalism or of Christian chauvinism when it suits them, but not, when it doesn't, for example, in the face of funding streams that attempt to initiate programmes that work against instead of with Papua New Guinean norms and forms of sociality.

2. It was reported in the pages of *The National*, for example, that Health Department workers in Buka were caught redirecting shipments of medicine to at least one private company, having sold about K80,000 worth of drugs and supplies for 'a substantial amount of money' (Philip 2008). Director of the Health Department, Igo Baru, said that 'there is a syndicate operating from Badili [in Port Moresby, where is located the Department of Health]' (quoted in Philip 2008).

Chapter 2

The women in traffic

Tu kina bus in town and country

The traffic in women

[Resident Europeans in the 1920s] planted crotons whose many-coloured leaves shone in the sunlight, and hibiscus shrubs with glorious blossoms, and the frangipani with its sweet-scented clusters. Poinciana trees in flaming red fringed the shore and made a wonderful splash of colour against the dark green of the mangoes that lined the main street. (Benjamin Butcher, *My Friends, the New Guinea Headhunters*, 1964, p. 37, writing of Daru in the nineteen teens and early twenties)

Is this place real? (Papua New Guinean colleague, after four days spent on Daru, November, 2003)

Now I see what you mean! She asked to come to our room, and she was holding onto a little girl! (same Papua New Guinean colleague, February, 2004, after two field-trips to Daru)

When I visited Daru for the first time in the 1960s, it was one of the most beautiful places in our country. The roads were good, houses were well looked after with flowers around them while the cemetery was kept clean ... Life there [now] appears dull, and, progress had stopped a long time ago. One wonders why this is so when Ok Tedi Mine is in the Province; the Province also has a lot of sea cucumbers, prawns, barramundi and timber ... (Paulias Matane, 'Research Tarnishes Our Image', *Post-Courier*, September, 1992)

This chapter reverses in title the direction of three variably well known works but of the same name. Gayle Rubin's 'The Traffic in Women' (Rubin 1975) enjoyed underground popularity even before it was published in 1975 in the second anthology of writings in feminist anthropology. *The Traffic in Women*, written by Skrobanok, Boonpakdi and Janthakeero (1997), documented the systematic human rights abuses of and in sexual slavery in south and south-east Asian countries and cultures. 'The Traffic in Women' is the name also of an essay penned, published and delivered many decades ago to not particularly admiring audiences by the feisty American feminist-anarchist, Emma Goldman (1970 [1917]).

Rubin's exegesis of the works of Marx and Engels, Freud, Lacan and Levi-Strauss was successful partly because of the deft usage she made of ethnographic data and theory from New Guinea. It doesn't delve deeply into the origins of or contemporary systems of prostitution, but yet her argument is greatly relevant regarding the scope and scale of trade in female sexual services. She notes that, in specific reference to Levi-Strauss, '[t]he "exchange of women" is a seductive and powerful concept ... [suggesting] that we look for the ultimate locus of women's oppression within the traffic in women, *rather than the traffic in merchandise* ... Women are given in marriage, taken in battle, exchanged for favours, sent as tribute, traded, bought, and sold' (1975: 175, emphasis added). This chapter, too, presents ethnological data that challenge his formulation in showing that 'women' and 'merchandise' cannot so easily be separated in the early development of sex industries. These data and this chapter more generally are designed to focus the argument in Chapters 3, 4 and 9 on the inequalities in contemporary Papua New Guinea social-structure that are so intimately linked to the HIV and AIDS epidemics.

Skrobanok, Boonpakdi and Janthakeero's survey of systems of sexual networking is valuable, but also contentious in concluding that 'the trade in human beings is an outcrop of international labour migration' (1997: 98). Nevertheless, they acknowledge the intimate, largely domestic forces of gender and expectations of filial piety that push girls and young women out of their families and villages into the hands of brokers, pimps and legal authorities. Just as I do in this and other chapters regarding contemporary Papua New Guinea, these three authors reveal normative male prerogative in all the regimes of classic anthropological interest: sexuality, residence, reproduction, marriage and kinship. That they do this despite there being a lot of 'female choice' and exhibition of sexual agency is an important lesson that seems to have been lost in the past several years' worth of debates in and over prostitution and sex work. (The two-volume *Encyclopedia of Prostitution and Sex Work*, edited by Melissa Hope Ditmore [2006], makes in this regard an extremely valuable contribution to these debates.) Perhaps springing from Levi-Strauss's famous caveat that women could never be merely objects, Rubin also highlighted ways in which female agency was expressed even in otherwise constraining ideas and practices of social-structure.

Goldman's fiery essay also recognised the enduring but punishing ties of intimacy in asking a still pregnant question: 'What is really the cause of the trade in women'? 'Exploitation, of course', was her answer, 'the merciless Moloch of capitalism that fattens on underpaid labour, thus driving thousands of women and girls into prostitution'. For Goldman, prostitution's origin was to be found less in international labour migration than in the local conditions and relations of work and production. This approach is amenable to mine and to Holly Wardlow's in her *Wayward Women: sexuality and agency in a New Guinea society* (Wardlow 2006a). Also relevant here to Papua New Guinea is the way in which Goldman fingers the hypocrisies of Christian doctrines and Catholic popes. Many thousands of clergy worldwide and for many centuries have committed sexual offenses against parishioners, especially youth. Nevertheless, they have excoriated women qua women and the non-heterosexual for sexual offences. Goldman also highlights, as I do here in other ways, the profound dialectic between marriage and prostitution. In reference to the large proportion of the 2,000-woman sample comprising William Sanger's massive study of prostitution in the US who were married, she noted that there didn't appear quite the guarantee of their 'safety and purity' in the sanctity of marriage as people might assume (1970 [1917]). Indeed. Whether we're talking about the US or Papua New Guinea, Fiji or Indonesia, marriage is often considered the solution to HIV transmission, even though public health and social scientific studies have demonstrated that marriage is as often as not the problem.

This chapter is designed to address some of these pressing questions of agency and exploitation and to push for a historical analysis of sex industries in Papua New Guinea. In doing so, I hope to introduce the social history of HIV and AIDS in the following two chapters. I look closely at one particular people – the Bamu of Western Province – in terms of the emergence of a particular 'labour form' of prostitution. *Tu kina bus*, as it is known throughout the country, was a $2 outdoor, bush form of prostitution that emerged in pre- and post-colonial settings. I sketch out the emergence on Daru at *sagapari* – 'small mangrove garden' – an ethnographically unique form of *tu kina bus*. I draw upon missionary memoirs, patrol officer reports and ethnological literature in highlighting four proximate reasons why *sagapari* developed and why the Bamu seem to have been predisposed to predominate in it. I don't argue that there is anything particularly exceptional about the Bamu case, despite there being all manner of ethnographic uniqueness. Adult female and child prostitution was 'common in colonial times, when many girls were trafficked among the colonial administrators and business personnel, even in the remote rural areas' (Department for Community Development 2004: 3).

First, there were a number of migratory pushes and pulls at work. As to the former, 'development' opportunities are in Bamu-land few and far between, despite there having been natural gas, logging and other activities in Gulf and elsewhere in Western Province. Consequently, Bamu were pulled to Daru, to Balimo, to the Ok Tedi mine wharf up the Fly river at Kiunga and to other centres of administration and commerce so as to participate in the cash economy. Kamusi, for instance, as pointed out to me by Phil Carr (in a personal communication, 24 June 2007),

> is well beyond Bamu territory. The veneer factory at Panakawa was only established in the late 1990s, and is at the very extreme of the northern-most Bamu village (Gagoro). Except for a *wokabaut* sawmill at Kuria village in the Aramia mouth since 2004, no milling has taken place on Bamu land since the Bamu River Mission operated a mill at their station next to Iowa village in the 1950s and 1960s. Of course, the tug boat and barge traffic has all been through the Bamu area. Nevertheless, Bamu people have had to find ways to travel to these places, and … they own no land there.

Second, their 'traditional' styles of sexual networking were already heavily transactional, just as they appear to have been in the Trobriand islands and among the Lesu (Powdermaker 1971[1933]), although it would appear that female agency then was greater. Just as with several other south coastal tribes, shell valuables were once given to new brides to recognise their beauty and sexual prowess, but now hard currency goes mostly to husbands in recognition of wifely subservience, the needs of a cash economy and a man's right to beer.

Third, the Bamu lived an extremely muddy, riverine existence but in which fishing was relatively marginal to their diet and culture when compared with the importance accorded it among neighbours. Because the Bamu pursued gardening less intensively, lived more nomadically and produced few surpluses, they were more dependent upon trade to maintain themselves. In keeping with regionally accepted practice, this interpersonal pot was sweetened often by the sale and barter of female sexual services. During this period, roughly the 1890s to the 1940s, the Bamu linked more tenuously to the regional political-economy than Kiwai and others, and they still do.

Fourth, Bamu once provided products and services that were valuable to themselves and others but that were later replaced by steel, plastic and other European goods and practices. The things they made from a precious black-palm species; the bows, arrows and other decorative finery, drums, belts and masks in whose making they specialised; the canoes and canoe hulls they provided to trading partners throughout the south coastal area into the Torres Straits – the manufacture and provision of each of these enabled Bamu to reproduce themselves as a people. Bamu predominated once in the provision of sexual services and of completely manufactured canoes and canoe hulls, just as they now predominate in the provision of different kinds of sexual services. The reasons then as now have less to do with moral taint – either theirs or of their European oppressors, which is how missionaries, non-Bamu Daruans, some academics and colonial officials saw it – than with political-economy.

The relevance of the Bamu case and that generally of *tu kina bus* is not perhaps crystal-clear, but today's struggles over HIV transmission prevention involve the potential of legalising prostitution and having the state sponsor and regulate brothels. Prostitution, not companionate relationships, has been blamed for the bulk of STD and HIV transmission. In this chapter I ask: on what does one blame prostitution? In this and in other chapters I answer: marriage.

Tu kina and other bushes

If, as the old adage has it, civilisations are founded atop middens, the polite term in archaeology for garbage heaps, what might future archaeologists say about Daru island, Western Province, 'the world's smallest capital' (Clune 1943), located just off the mainland of New Guinea near the mouth of the Fly river?[1] In such a hot and humid environment as this, one that is for two months each year rained on torrentially and also swept clear periodically by high tides, few material remains will ever be dug up beyond bottle tops and broken glass. Daru's original inhabitants – the Hiamu, said by one writer to have been a 'guileless, inoffensive group' (Singe 1989: 76) – were forced out around 1840 by the more numerous, coastal Kiwai peoples migrating from the east and who wished only to use it overnight in transit up the Fly (Landtman 1927: 293). A small sea cucumber-collecting station was established in 1863 at nearby Somerset on Cape York (Shnukal 2004: 327). The London Missionary Society established itself in 1871, and a British Protectorate was proclaimed by 1884, which consolidated into British New Guinea by 1888. Pearling luggers began to arrive in the area by the 1870s and were joined later by additional England-based missionaries. Japanese females were brought in the early 1880s to brothels erected on Thursday island, the first one being a 12-year-old girl sold by parents to a trafficker who smuggled her in (Sissons 1977: 478). They, their male handlers and their customers each introduced syphilis and other STDs to this region, as did escaped convicts and black-birded labourers. An 1879 report from the HMS *Beagle* noted a huge prevalence of STDs among pearl-divers, and attributed it to 'native women, there being camps of natives along the Australian coast where regular prostitutes are kept who are badly diseased' (quoted in Singe 1989: 53). Within two decades officials on Thursday island called for application of the 1868 Contagious Diseases Act to the Torres Straits, so staggering to the fishing and diving industries had been the losses of labour productivity owing to syphilis and gonorrhea. In 1883 the Australian Pearl Company brought 37 Japanese men to Thursday island to work aboard luggers, but there were already nearly one hundred Japanese labourers in the region. Not much longer thereafter the Japanese male:female ratio was along the lines of 17:1 (Nagata 2004). Having previously been established on Thursday island, the British New Guinea administrative apparatus for this area was headquartered by 1890 down-coast in Mabuduwan village at the mouth of the Pahoturi river. Three years later, on 18 April, but then being otherwise uninhabited, Daru became the new capital of Western Division, which became a District and eventually Province in 1975, at Independence. The first building erected on Daru was the jail, built *from* logs and *bili*-leaf roofing sufficient to house 25 prisoners (Clune 1943: 65–6) but built *by* convicts whose only 'crime' had been refusing to construct the jail. I and others have written about colonial and immediate post-colonial developments in the Papuan Gulf region in industry, missionary activity, plantation economy, resource extraction and administrative patrolling (Hammar 1998b; Knauft 1993: 25–41; Lawrence 1995; Maher 1961).

By 1988, when I first visited Daru, and certainly by celebration in 1993 of the centenary of its founding, it had become densely populated and mired in relations of dependency. It was characterised by admirable heteroglossia and was actively engaged in nation-making and pluralistic Christianity. Based upon ethnographic research I conducted there from 1990 to 1992, I detailed the slow decline in living conditions and recent upsurge in crime, corruption and public health crises, including of STD (Hammar 1996a, b, 1998a, b, c, 1999a, 2004b). When David King (1994: 2) returned to Daru as part of the social monitoring project related to the Ok Tedi mine, he found that 'morale in Daru was not high, as government officers alleged that corruption was widespread and admitted the failure of the provincial government to bring about development'. Since then, newspaper articles about Daru most often report upon alcohol and other drug consumption, gun- and drug-smuggling, communicable disease and the political and economic fallout from the Ok Tedi mine. It was reported on 8 August 2007 that authorities in Port Moresby had tracked a shipment of marijuana flown from the Eastern Highlands eventually to Daru, where was arrested a woman thought to be involved in the drugs-for-guns smuggling ring between Papua New Guinea, Australia and Indonesia (Couriermail 2007). In 2006, Daru's policemen living in condemned barracks carried buckets-full of their own excrement to and locked them inside the provincial health office to protest unhealthy living conditions and unpaid wages. The drugs-and-small-guns survey of Papua New Guinea had this to say about some of the circuits involved:

> The demand for firearms in PNG is increasing, particularly in the Highlands which is also the centre for the production of most of the 'Niugini gold,' that is high quality PNG cannabis, and Daru appears to have emerged as a centre for the purchase of illicit firearms ... By walking another 80 km south from S[a]mberigi [Southern Highlands Province], traffickers can reach the Gulf of Papua at the Kikori River delta, then move by land or by sea to PNG's closest settlement to Australia – Daru Island, on the Torres Strait. According to Southern Highlands provincial police commander Simon Nigi, this is the province's major 'guns for drugs' route. Gerry Kela, a senior detective with experience in undercover narcotics work, remembers Daru as the entry point for guns. (Alpers 2005: 60, 68)

By written and oral historical accounts such as that of Benjamin Butcher and reminiscences of the current Governor-General, Paulias Matane, Daru was a clean, well-organised, sweet-smelling place well into and through the 1960s. Its population had been limited once by colonial decree to 3,000. When villagers from down-coastal and inland villages arrived periodically to Daru in large canoe fleets and began pressing too hard on available resources they were rounded up and sent back home. When restrictions on movement were lifted in 1975, however, Daruans began to experience an upsurge in poverty, malnutrition, social strife, binge-style drinking and new forms and frequencies of sexual networking. An article published in the *Pacific Islands Monthly* noted that two men had died, that another six had been hospitalized after drinking methylated spirits at a party held on Daru and that a ninth man had been blinded (PIM 1975: 22). On my third day of fieldwork, in September of 1990, I watched a young Kiwai man begin to turn yellow and die of the same fate, two days after consuming a combination of cordial and both methylated and ethylated spirits. I later met a Christian string-band group of seven young Kiwai men who had celebrated a successful rugby match by blinding themselves by alcohol poisoning. Eleven men were hospitalized in June of 2002 and two died after drinking methylated spirits mixed with fermented coconut shoot sap and turpentine.

Those living in villages along the Fly and its tributaries have been harmed by the ecological devastation unleashed for two decades from the Ok Tedi mine, but whose environmental, social and political fallout has been felt on Daru, too. Having been to the Ok Tedi mine and seen the headwaters, I can more easily grasp Stuart Kirsch's poignant comments on some of the human costs involved, even for an expatriate:

When I walk beside the Ok Tedi River with a friend, it is difficult to identify the places where we once shared a meal or went swimming. Where towering trees stood, only ghostly tree trunks remain. The creeks are all buried by sand. Not only are these changes to the landscape physically disorienting, but they displace memories of the past ... Memories previously anchored to the landscape have lost their mooring. (Kirsch 2006: 189; see also Kirsch 2001)

Those living alongside or near many of the majestic rivers of Western and Gulf Province have also suffered from the effects of timber and oil exploration camps that now dot the countryside. Rampant deforestation and attendant environmental ills, communicable diseases, prostitution, alcohol abuse, cultural loss and police brutality have worsened the lives of families and communities. 'Our life in the past was better than today', says an old Bamu woman. 'Our creeks and rivers', she continued, 'were deep and clean. The river was our main water tank. We drank and cooked food with water from the river ... Making sago was easy for us. Our husbands cut the sago trees in the bush and floated them in at the village creek at high tide' (Lennox 2000). (Phil Carr pointed out in a personal communication [24 June 2007] that this old woman must have been speaking of the Gama river, and more likely, creeks, because the Bamu river has always been too sedimented to drink: the Bamu of Bladon's *Tidal Waves on the Bamu* and *Song of the Bamu* drink the water when it's not too salty or muddy.) 'Development' has for Bamu and others in their ancestral homeland and on Daru meant interpersonal violence, political corruption, public servant apathy, growing expectations of 'compensation' and changing gender relations that have perverted and distorted relationships and compromised the public health.

Industrial sex

We explore 'sites of desire' formed by confluences of cultures, be they the tidal waves of European colonialism or the smaller eddies of sexual contacts and erotic imaginings created between cultures. (Margaret Jolly and Lenore Manderson, 'Sites of Desire/Economies of Pleasure in Asia and the Pacific', 1997, p. 1)

The place of sexual servicing in regional trading systems has not featured much in ethnological accounts. McNiven, von Gnielinski and Quinell (2004) have presented compelling new evidence for a Torres Straits (not, that is, New Guinea Highland) origin of the 'Kiwai type' stone axes and clubs that so puzzled early colonial officials and ethnologists. 'Papuans', they say, 'required Islander axes to manufacture canoes for Islanders (and themselves), while Islanders required Papuan canoes to support their specialised maritime lifeway' (2004: 283). Nevertheless, they make little of the presence and provision of female bodies and sexual services in this widespread trade. Neither does Grimwade (2004), despite the topic of his fine essay being the archaeology of Japanese bath-houses on Thursday island, nor Vanderwal (2004), whose fascinating treatise on early contact narratives and sources doesn't even mention sexual networking. Yet and still, as canoe-loads of men handed over one item for another, as one village entertained another, as one husband received another man's wife for the night (just as he provided his own for his trading partner's enjoyment), existing ties were maintained and new ones forged. Such trade wasn't strictly utilitarian, that is, sago bundles for turtle meat, A providing B with what B has not, in exchange for what A has not. David Lawrence (1989a: 62) points out that two men from different areas, having exchanged names, 'maintained a preferential position in all bartering transactions and formed a close personal relationship which required the giving of presents and attention'. In another publication Lawrence has aptly summarised his own research and that of others regarding the necessity of local and regional trading systems:

> External contacts with the Papuan people to the north and the Australian Aboriginal people to the south were maintained. The creation of artificial dependencies through patterns of customary exchange, ritual, and marriage bound the people of the Torres Strait into small self-contained groups. The patterns of customary exchange which linked Islanders to Papuans and Aboriginal groups provided a means for the circulation of such garden-foods and fresh and dried seafoods. This exchange enabled the small, acephalous groups to survive during periods of drought and famine and permitted reciprocal exchange and distribution of surplus during periods of plenty. (Lawrence 1990b: 482)

Nevertheless, the fact that many of the presents were females and that much of the attention was of a sexual nature is rarely analysed with sensitivity or in terms of political-economy. None of the 41 essays of which the publication above was a part, for example, considered sexuality at all. Perhaps this is more evident under changed circumstances. The replacement of the products that Bamu made by guns and dinghies, laplaps and t-shirts, sauce-pans and hoes, bush-knives and lanterns dampened the pride Bamu once felt in carving, making pottery and wood-working (e.g. Butcher 1964: 91), but worse, it left them bereft of much else to sell, save sexual services. Landtman noted that by 1910–12 the 'canoe traffic' had already decreased, due mostly to colonial decrees about the movements of individuals and the substitution of steel and iron for wood (1927: 216, 64). Later, the manufacture of plastic buttons spelled the end of those made from pearlshell. This time period coincided with reports made by colonial and mission officials regarding the trafficking in women, but which wasn't possible without there already being women (sexual services) in traffic (regional trade systems) and already extremely dense and contingent social relations. The work of Yuriko Nagata (2004) is relevant here in showing the importance of (the colloquial) 'Yokohama' on Thursday island in the introduction of brothels where they hadn't previously existed. Nagata remarks upon the mollifying effect upon Caucasian men of the presence of Japanese women and girls available for sexual servicing in a time and at a place when cross-racial sexual boundaries were crossed at great peril. Quite unlike Bamu women, and despite being confined to brothels, many Japanese women during and following their confinement invested wisely in shares in fishing and pearling luggers and amassed significant income with the help of Australian and Japanese boyfriends, backers and states.

It is difficult to state with any precision, but these processes are likely in at least general terms to have introduced in the minds of lowland Papuan males, highly mobile and newly flush with cash, the idea of easily available, sexually pliable females. Such processes may have put ideas in the heads of Papuan females, too, that sexual servicing could bring them much needed cash. The Wabuda live in the north-eastern corner of the mouth of the Fly river near the Kiwai Island Kiwai, and they were from the 1890s associated with sexual networking in the pearling industry. The Gogodala live in scattered villages surrounding the swampy lagoon near Balimo, but stretching from the north bank of the Fly river, to the west, to the western bank of the Aramia river, to the east. Their renunciation in the 1930s and 1940s of 'pagan' lifestyles required confession on their part of the sexual nature of canoe-racing and licentiousness of longhouse-style living. To this day, even traditional dancing is prohibited for its allegedly suggestive nature (cf. Crawford 1981; Wilde 2003). The territorial homelands of the Bamu are a bit further east and inland, up the Aramia river. The several different tribes of the Kikori, a gloss for three separate linguistic groups, come from neighbouring Gulf Province to the east. Australian missionaries and business people roundly repudiate their morality to this day. All four peoples began to migrate to Daru in the mid-late 1960s, as did quite a few Marind-anim refugees from Indonesian incursions across the border, many of them not returning until 2003 (see also Kirsch 2006: 2). Lacking 'traditional' rights of access to water, garden space, or land on which to live, however, and possessing little in the way of educational attainments or occupational skills, these and other in-migrating peoples began to gain a foothold through relations of friendship, Christian worship, marriage and other forms of sexual networking and the sale of small goods and services (such as firewood provision). One Kiwai informant said to me 'So, when [Wabuda villagers] come down to town, they see all the things in the store and so they sell their body, the *pamuku* way' (author's fieldnotes, Doumori village, 1991). Ian Willis noted a similar process occurring in Lae regarding the in-migrating Ahi-Hengali, 'whose landless state was impressed upon them and has remained to the present day despite considerable intermarriage' (1974: 29). *Ol Tari meri* (Huli-speaking women from the Tari Basin of Southern Highlands Province) selling sexual services exist in seven provincial capitals I've visited and are reminded of their landless status by security guards, customers and accomplices.

A sex industry emerged on Daru just as it did for similar (and for different) reasons in Tabubil, near the Ok Tedi mine-site; in Kiunga, which is Ok Tedi's river-staging port downstream; and at logging camps such as Kamusi. In each case those selling sexual services were members of already despised social groups, and they sold them in locales where they didn't own land. Mining and mine-sites have long attracted in-migrating women who engage in sexual service provision. Mine-site authorities and restrictions tend to discourage the movement of entire, intact families, and so provide 'a good impetus for female fortune seekers to migrate to mining settlements for the purpose of earning a living through prostitution' (Aderinto 2006: 315–16). Women from the Oksapmin area and beyond, the so-called *pasindia meri* from Huli-speaking areas of the Tari Basin, have migrated to Tabubil (Clark 1997; Wardlow 2006a, 2007).

Daru's many 'labour forms' of prostitution began slowly to form and consolidate, but each one springs from different sources and tells a different story (for ethnographic and sociological details of each, see Hammar n.d., 1996a, 1999a). While *tu kina bus* is more about migration, inter-ethnic rivalry and husbandly prerogative, the 'family' form has to do with child sexual exploitation and grinding poverty. Sometimes it has also to do with ethnic and other divisions in local sex industries on which male relatives play, for example, the preference currently in Port Moresby of expatriate males for lighter-skinned, longer-haired Papuan females (and some males) over those females of New Guinea highland physiognomy. 'Freelance' and 'sex-broker' forms have more to do with the emergence of public drinking locales, changing marital norms, divorce and the mass exodus of expatriates at and shortly following Independence (Hammar 1998c). 'White-flight' had a particularly pernicious effect on the Kiwai wives, daughters and girlfriends who were especially favoured by expatriate males but nevertheless often left materially and socially high and dry, 'spoiled' of status and ever-dependent on money. Having lost their virginity and innocence to Australians, Germans, Americans and British, they began to suffer the consequences of having 'fatherless kids'. They possessed little cultural capital (in terms of language and gardening skills and knowledge of village affairs) and suffered strained natal ties. They truncated tribal obligations of kinship and exchange by shacking up with non-reciprocating expatriate patrol officers, school-teachers, businessmen and administrators, which flouted the customary norms of at least cousin- if not sister-exchange (Crawford 1981; Knauft 1993; Ohtsuka 1983). Being taken out of school by boyfriends and husbands precluded further educational attainments and crimped their occupational options. Expatriate boyfriends and husbands who left Daru on holiday sometimes failed to return or they did so but with a new girlfriend in tow or with their 'real' wife from Down South (author's fieldnotes, 1990–92). Nagata (2004) describes a situation perhaps the reverse of what I'm showing here. He analyses relationships between Torres Straits women and the Japanese men who, despite having wives and 'real families' back home in Japan, also married locally, fathered children *and stayed on*. Not since the turn of the twentieth century, when five Portuguese brothers and their sister married five Kiwai sisters and their brother, have Europeans brought siblings to exchange in marriage.

White-flight also drained newly created provincial- and district-level bodies of key skills, capital, persons and their accumulated knowledge, which was either 'lost' (Lawrence 1989a) or dumped in the ocean or thrown away (said my informants in 1990–92) at handover/takeover in 1975. This vacuum was filled partially with Chinese, Indonesian, Malaysian and Japanese men and the tradestores they owned and services they provided, such as coastal shipping and the buying of crocodile-skins and *pisirimai*, or sea-cucumber. These expatriates, however, had even fewer reasons to court Kiwai, Gogodala, Pahoturi and Bine females and marry them appropriately, but even more money to burn on sex, drinking and leisure. Many of the Kiwai, Suki and Gogodala women who became my good friends in 1990–92 said that 'Kongkong' (Tok Pisin for 'Asians' of any nationality) were favoured customers and drinking mates for being generous and less violent than their Papua New Guinean counterparts in the provincial and national government who were their predominant sex partners, but they made worse boyfriends and husbands for their transience, lack of social graces and neglect of obligations. This behavioural factor, too, I suspect, has something to do with the slow commercialisation of sexuality, the picking and choosing by females of parts but not the entirety of male personality and comportment.

Papua New Guineans from other provinces took on substantial roles in health, politics and provincial administration on Daru, just as they did in 'all the main administrative and commercial centres' (Griffin, Nelson and Firth 1979: 30). They also brought new languages and social expectations and additional sexual desires. Richard Jackson (1976: 93) notes that 'the only important group of migrants from other districts (now provinces) [is] high ranking Administration personnel and policemen'. Money, alcohol, empty promises and new generations of 'mix-race' children further opened the gulf between 'new' and 'old' sexual ethics. However well the Daruan children and girlfriends and wives of expatriates may have mixed with local populations, lacking 'a clear path to prestige or land ownership in the village', they earned the bulk of their social capital in the cash nexus (Griffin, Nelson and Firth 1979: 31). Exchange networks altered by the infusion of a cash economy turned expectations of payment from an extended to an immediate form (e.g. Beaver 1920: 76). Perhaps in a way analogous to the situation in Southern Highlands Province that Jeffrey Clark described for the Wiru (1991), the introduction in and nearby the Papuan Gulf of cash and the subsequent decline in value of shell wealth enabled the emergence of sexual intercourse as a commodity and denigrated the relationships it once signified, rewarded and found expression in. The coming of rural enclaves of resource extraction in the 1960s and 1970s 'introduced the idea of bride price', leading to 'non-exchange marriages' (Ohtsuka 1983: 15) in neighbouring Oriomo Plateau cultures. Long-time Patrol Officer Jack McCarthy wrote similarly about the Kikori Delta area that had been affected by oil exploration in the 1930s and 1940s, noting that the 'old-time traditional way of bartering food and tobacco' had given way 'to a money economy as wages circulated and people went out in search of canned foods and western clothing' (1970: 10). Oil bore-drilling activities long ago in the Kikori and Bamu river areas brought new thoughts, behaviours, forms of political organisation and heretofore unimaginable amounts of wealth and goods. As one early prospector noted, 'we had so much, so many new unheard-of things as well as many they valued very highly themselves' (O'Neill 1979: 64).

Sexual fluids and sexual intercourse once had little monetary value but great social, medical and symbolic value (Knauft 1990, 1993, 1994; Serpenti 1977, 1993; Van Baal 1966). In a few short decades, however, *tu kina bus* had resulted from these and other sweeping changes and emerged at the extreme physical and metaphorical margins of Daruan society. Moving every few years between mud, market and mangrove, saltwater, cemetery and swamp, *sagapari* was where marginalised men (mostly single, mostly non-salaried) found cheap sex available on their terms (little talking, no obligations, but often preceded and followed by alcohol consumption with mates) and being provided by even more marginalised (Bamu) women (Hammar 1996a, 1998c). The emergence of Daru as a regional market for marine, riverine and garden products; for store-bought goods and deer, wild pig and wallaby meat; for exchange in guns and drugs and the purchase and resale elsewhere of cheaply available alcohol; and for the disbursal of resource extraction-related royalties and salaries put heretofore unheard of amounts of cash into the hands of males. That they spent them largely on drinking and sex began to drub the public health and strain already precarious social relations between genders and ethnic or tribal groups. Alcohol abuse and multi-faceted, ubiquitous prostitution have further spoiled Daru's already dicey national, even international reputation (e.g. Hammar 1996a, b; Lawrence 1995).[1]

Just like its equivalents in Lae, Goroka, Port Moresby, Mt. Hagen, Jayapura and Vanimo, Daru's sex industry shows the gendered and tribal contradictions of political-economy. Donald Schug concluded that '[e]thnic differences, intensified by decades of exposure to different levels and types of external social forces, have come to the forefront as various groups attempt to extend their economic and political control over a limited resource base' (1995: 21). These have worsened owing to widespread migration from Fly river delta villages to Daru, to the fact that payments are made to nominal heads of male corporations (euphemised as 'landowner groups'), and to wild spending sprees taken on Daru and also in Kerema, Mt. Hagen and Port Moresby. As well, there is the increasingly imbalanced gender ratio common in 'developing' contexts. Jackson's data for 1966 indicate a male:female ratio of 1.18:1 and for 1971 of 1.13:1, and I estimated that ratio to have changed to 1.2:1 or greater by 1990 (Hammar 2004b). The NHASP-sponsored social mapping study found in 2003–2005 that all districts in Western Province had a surplus of males and that sexual services were available widely (2005c). The photo here depicts a small mangrove-leaf 'bed' on the muddy ground, and a torn condom wrapper, in the new location of *sagapari*.

The fact that an entire people reproduce themselves through sale of and barter in sexual services shows the shallow, insubstantial nature of the

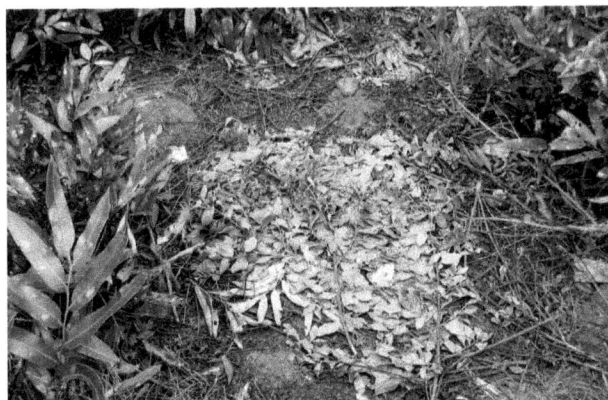

A mangrove leaf bed and condom wrappers

development process and what horrors it can mete out for women and girls. *Tu kina bus* has emerged owing to or coincidental with sometimes unexpected factors, including the presence of medical supplies, services and personnel. When I first visited Daru in 1988 *sagapari* was then dubbed 'Dokta Point' because of its close proximity to the base hospital. *Tu kina bus* emerged at Goroka's 'Maunten Kiss' across Greathead Road from the first base hospital. Port Moresby's Paga Hill became an outdoor site of sexual networking just opposite the first location of the Department of Health. Lae's current *tu kina bus* sprawls across an abandoned aerodrome just across the street from ANGAU Memorial hospital. Their equivalents in Moro, Tabubil, Kundiawa[2] and elsewhere are also located near medical facilities and personnel.

The dictates and behaviours of missionaries played their part, too. The women in Lae first dubbed 'prostitutes' were sometimes the second, third and fourth wives of men who, at the stroke of a missionary's pen, had become divorced (when polygyny was prohibited) and who had then turned to prostitution to support themselves. The anthropologist G.H.L. Pitt-Rivers made accusations in his 1927 essay in *Man* (and subsequent book), later confirmed by Hubert Murray, that priests, native converts and teachers had abducted second, third and fourth wives of polygynists and then married them off to monogamous Christians (Pitt-Rivers 1927). Others who had renounced polygyny and had accepted Christianity and monogamous prescriptions and then relapsed were shunned from the church, which often had disastrous consequences for especially the wives, a factor that came into play later during struggles over the Marriage Ordinance of 1912 that recognised polygyny (Langmore 1989: 124–5). Clark and Hughes (1995: 317) write also that '[c]ertain religious beliefs and cult practices, forbidden by the missions, are also believed to have benefited women's lives'. Ian Willis notes (1974: 57) that church-mandated 'release', as divorce was then euphemised, 'was hardest on divorced wives. They were left shamed and without support'. He notes further that mission converts posted away from their own homes frequently succumbed to sexual temptation in the villages to which they had been posted (1974: 57), those cuckolded husbands being away on labour service. Powdermaker (1971[1933]) also noted the frequent occurrence of extra-marital affairs in which Lesu women would engage while their husbands were away. By contrast, however, Lesu husbands didn't seem to mind so much because the *tsera* payments given by the lovers of their wives would sometimes come to them (1971[1933]: 245). Many of the 'released' women found support from mission converts and the alienated labour force that began to migrate to Lae and to other mission stations, plantations and financial and industrial centres and who, being unmarried, required domestic services, including sexual. One group of Awa (the Ilakia) of Okapa District in Eastern Highlands Province took part in substantial out-migration in the 1960s of up to half of the men in the villages who left to take up labour contracts on coffee plantations. Similar levels of out-migration of men have been seen in the 1970s and 1980s among Telefolmin peoples of Western Province and West Sepik Province, in this case to the Ok Tedi mine at Tabubil (Allen 1997: 121–2; Jorgenson 2005). In the Tari Basin the discouragement by mission officials of polygyny led Huli men (especially older ones) to abandon successive wives casually in a pretend form of serial monogamy (Clark and Hughes 1995: 321). This left women to suffer social stigma and a heavier burden in fending for themselves. The polygyny that once added to now compromises their (especially Christian) identity (Clark 1997; Wardlow 2006a, b, 2007).

Europeans, their carriers, constables and representatives stole women and sexual services (Kituai 1998; Singe 1989: 28).[3] In some places they introduced prostitution where it hadn't existed or yet hardened and become institutionalised forms of sexual networking, just as Americans and others did in other parts of the Pacific. Siosiua Lafitani (1998: 78–9), for example, writing of Post-WWII Tonga, notes that Tongan adoption of the Judeo-Christian ethic resulted in a sharp decline in production of illegitimate children, but a correspondingly sharp increase in STDs, which she says were 'unknown to Tongans until the Second World War when the sexual act acquired new dimensions of socioeconomic reward, and the institutionalisation of prostitution'. Australian kiaps patrolling the rural Papuan hinterlands made a practice of taking local girls for their amusement while on patrol (Willis 1974: 75). Wardlow has argued (2004: 1019) that 'the behavioural model for prostitution' was learned by Huli women from expatriates in the mining camps and towns of Southern Highlands Province. Among the Gende of the central highlands, the procurement of local women for Europeans and their native constabulary by the constabulary made their 'stomachs … heavy with grief', but the policemen had guns, said an elderly man: 'what could we do against such strong opposition except to suffer silently'? (Kituai 1998: 231). In other areas prostitution emerged because indigenous practices and expectations meshed sufficiently well with introduced ones. The commodity logic of prostitution may have only slowly dawned on the Huli (Wardlow 2004: 1028), but that dawn broke long ago for Bamu and others who already sexualised inter-tribal trade relations.

Bad reputations

When Kikori, Wabuda, Kenedibi (the name of one village of the Tabo ethnolinguistic group), Marind-anim, Keraki, Suki, Bamu and other so-called 'bush' peoples from the Papuan hinterlands began to migrate to Daru in the early–mid 1960s, they were criticised by Europeans for real and alleged promiscuity, either of a 'traditional' sort or that which they exhibited while in transit to new lands and the embrace of 'modern' lifestyles. Comparison was made with the putative sexual abstemiousness of Europeans or other Papuan Gulf and Trans-Fly peoples.[4] Wabuda men played a key role in the regional political-economy by brokering black-palm between Bamu and Kiwai, but they also offered their wives sexually to Bamu trading partners (Beaver 1920: 228), who returned the favour. As well, Wabuda also took part in *mouguru*-like events of ritualised heterosexuality until 'some of the women show signs of pregnancy' (Landtman 1954: 184). Jan van Baal (1966) publicized the fact that married Marind-anim engaged one another in impressively large rituals involving group heterosexual intercourse. Although he did not name them as such, Butcher was referring to the Gogodala when he imputed to them 'a dark streak in their social habits' (1964: 57), which was perceived to be sexual promiscuity broadly, and maybe worse. Gunnar Landtman noted (1927: 249) that for tribes east of the Kiwai, 'it is common for hosts to place their wives temporarily at the disposal of guests. In certain parts – for instance, in the delta of the Kikori and Aird rivers – this custom is practiced on a large scale'. G.W. Massey-Baker noted in his account of the 1911 patrols he led into Gogodala-land on behalf of Assistant Resident Magistrate Beaver that although there was no evidence of ritualised homosexual intercourse occurring in the context of male initiation, there was plenty of the heterosexual variety (Massey-Baker 1911: 12). Charles Wilde (2003), Carol Jenkins (2007a: 24) and others have established that ritualised homosexuality was once common among the Gogodala, too. Over Christmas holiday in 1991 I was treated in a Gogodala village to great hospitality and lessons in fishing with bottle, line and sinker. I was also treated to a memorable story-telling session; with one of his rather wide-eyed grandsons crouched nearby, a village elder who features heavily in A.L. Crawford's well-known *Aida: life and ceremony of the Gogodala*, revealed that insemination of other males was virtually required from age 16 or so on up (author's fieldnotes, December 1991, Balimo Station).

Europeans debated not just whether wife-exchange or wife-lending was good, but also in terms of its varied functions. Some argued on behalf of its reciprocal nature (e.g. Serpenti 1977: 183), others in terms of its efficacy as a method of collecting multipurpose sexual fluids (Landtman 1954: 185). Most others argued on moral grounds against it (e.g. Holmes 1924), but also whether it conveyed friendly or hostile intent. Beaver (1920: 128) saw possible treachery as Bamu men handed over wives to potential trading partners, imputing to those wives a sort of Mata Hari character. Patrol officers Hides and Woodward occasionally encountered similar events in the field, as men from opposing tribes offered good talk, better tobacco and use of their wives sexually at night to those whom they would later assault and murder. Williams (1969[1936]: 160), on the other hand, identified *wundewunde* (among many other forms of female sexual servicing) as 'an act of hospitality or friendship... [which] is a means of establishing or confirming the bonds of fellowship', which would be recognised and renewed at next feast or trading bazaar. That wives were sometimes handed over to police detachments suggests obeisance, friendliness or perhaps a bribe being lodged for the asking of favours later. One of the early Resident Magistrates for Western Division, Army Henry Jiear (1903: 12), interpreted friendly encounters between coloniser and colonised as being promoted by and through sexual favours being offered and accepted.

Kikori, Goaribari, Namau, Kiwai, Bamu and other lowland Papuan peoples were long ago denigrated for longhouse-style living, which was conflated with ritualised heterosexuality; for sexual reciprocity, which was dubbed prostitution; and for polygyny, which was dubbed concubinage (Butcher 1964; Haddon 1920; Holmes 1924). In critiquing the trade of sex for labour and goods, many colonial and missiological sources, however, missed the reciprocal, non-exploitive side of sexual practice, and of course the consensual, pleasurable aspects. Kiwai men were said to loan wives to visitors to obtain extra-powerful semen and other goods and services

(Landtman 1927: 249). Kiwai women were themselves said (Landtman 1927: 50) to loan themselves for the same purpose and to mark the cessation of warfare or to hurt enemies (1927: 165–6, 45). Similar attributions were made to Suki, Keraki and other tribes in the Trans-Fly (Williams 1969[1936]: 159). Goaribari women, says McCarthy (1970: 18), were among the first to protest to government authorities when the right of husbands to trade wives sexually had been brought to the attention of colonial officials who forbade it. An elderly Kikori informant told me during an audiotaped interview (conducted on Daru, 15 February 1992) that

> Our custom is, when the girls told you to work for them, if they cut a sago down, they will squeeze the sago. And when you work hard with them, they will tell you to come in the night ... So, first thing, the girl lying, put the mats on [down on the floor], and put her right hand, like this [holding her palms up in her lap]. How many boys. Four, ten, eleven, twelve, fifteen boys. Just come and put their head on her hand ... When they talk, finish, then he can sex ... [Lawrence: 'So then, every boy gets to do sex with her, every boy who put his head on her hand, they get to sex with her'?] ... Yeah, they do the hard work, maybe she must pay them ... Every house, is, that's a big village, the same, they do the same because, custom, if you don't work, you don't have sex.

Perhaps he has exaggerated a bit, but the sex/labour nexus is just as clear as the relative agency of the females involved, who with boys chose the timing and number of participants and constructed the meaning of sexual intercourse. Prostitution is now extremely common in Kikori itself, however, and along the Kikori river in villages such as Kopi and Kaiam and around timber camps and roadside markets. In 2004 I saw a teenaged girl from Paia Inlet No. 2 village, with her 8-year-old brother in tow as 'security guard', step aboard a Javanese cargo barge, having paddled three kilometres in the choppy waters of the Delta so as to trade sexual favours with the ship's captain for two large buckets of drinking water – that's how bad the water is and how poor are the conditions in her village after 15 years' worth of logging activity. Bystanders said that money was probably not involved. In three years I lost only six digital photographs, three of them during this event, but the scene remains vivid in my memory if not etched in my memory card.

The taint of prostitution was attributed broadly across the Papuan Gulf and South Fly peoples, but the Bamu come off as the worst of the bunch. Wilfred Beaver's 1912 contribution to the *Annual Report for the Territory of Papua* (Beaver 1912: 66) complains that 'at first sight' there would appear to be little to show for many years' patient labour. 'Some of these [Bamu] are certainly the most unsatisfactory in the Division', he says, 'perhaps in the Territory. The general conditions of living, their morals, and customs are about as low as can be found'. Dwelling in swamps and near rivers, Bamu came from a 'mysterious region', he said, filled with 'bad people' (1920: 210). The 'primitive' Bamu suffered 'ghastly living conditions' prior to the arrival of missionaries, said a more contemporary missionary voice (Staff Writer 1961). The photographer and diarist Frank Hurley pronounced the Bamu 'uninteresting and unpictorial' and so left them alone (quoted in Specht and Fields 1984: 140). McCarthy wrote that Bamu-land comprised

'10,000 square miles of rawness' and that the Goaribari were stuck 'among the swamps and the reeds, the jungle and the mud', where 'life remained almost undisturbed' (1970: 4). The Bamu Delta, said a cadet officer about his patrol in 1953, was the most neglected area of all, as tides of everything but development washed up and over 'these unfortunate people' (Geyle 1998).

The sources of such negative appraisals of Bamu are multiple and are split between the alleged sins then of Bamu forefathers (and mothers) regarding sorcery and head-hunting and the putative promiscuity of Bamu daughters and wives now in transactional sex. I remember vividly that during fieldwork in 1990–92 on Daru, both visiting Kiwai and 'town Kiwai' men would tell me while drinking at the public drinking spot adjacent to *sagapari* how much, when intoxicated, they enjoyed abusing Bamu women sexually. Inverting somewhat the famous shouted dictum of the Mae Enga as publicized by Mervyn Meggitt ('We marry the ones we fight'!), Kiwai men seem metaphorically to be saying 'We fuck the ones we hate!', 'killing them' with sex (in Tok Pisin, *'nekim'*, *'sutim'* and *'rekim'*), really 'spoiling them', as 'we really hate those Bamu ladies', those 'detty, detty Bamu ladies'. In another context, Knauft notes correctly that Marind-anim ceremonial life, at least in its sexual elements, evinced 'the intense sexual domination of young women by Marind men' (1993: 96). Knauft's argument regarding the 'yelled frustration' of the Western Province Gebusi is pertinent here. He insists that Melanesians generally are 'relentlessly material and bodily in their aspirations' (1994: 422).

The resort to pointed expressions of tribal or ethnic conflict, particularly in terms of the wanderings and works of well-known folk or culture heroes, offers further clues as to Bamu degradation today. Beaver reminds us (1920: 210) that '[i]t was here [in Bamu-land] that Sido, the great Kiwai hero, was killed', a fact that many Daruan Kiwai over the age of 60 can recite. The material culture expert David Lawrence notes that it was Dibiri village, at the mouth of the majestic Bamu river, from which Sido was expelled due to the 'power of his magic' (Lawrence 1989b: 99). That was where Sido originated, too, in Alfred Cort Haddon's telling of this famous but contentious myth. According to my Daru informants, it is important to note that Sido came from Dibiri, a Bamu village, in a canoe he neither carved nor built, that he had intercourse with two Kiwai sisters joined at the waist, and that, in doing so, he de-twinned, split them apart, killed them as twins, but in so doing, gave life to two individuals, through and literally by sexing them. Despite having tried many canoe diggings-out, the woods Sido used were too soft. Legends have it that during westward travels he was given women sexually in exchange for the various skills and magic he pulled out of his *bag* (scrotum?).

Mike Wood suggests (in a personal communication, April 2005) that this speaks of objectification of bodily fluids, parts and substances such as genitals, semen, milk and so on, but perhaps also of bodily labour in the form of intercourse, fertility and reproduction. Women's bodies are on Daru negatively metaphorised as *uba pe* ('no-good canoe'), a canoe that has many holes in it, a sexually promiscuous woman (Hammar 1996b). Perhaps Sido's wood (penis?) was too soft (flaccid?) for the hardwoods of Bamu canoe hulls (vaginas?). Tellingly, while Sido was shown *by Bamu* the skills and magical formulae needed to make fine drums, small, non-outrigger canoes and effective sorcery, his reputation was built upon the sexual prowess he had to learn (Murray 1902: 85; Beaver 1912: 65) but which he later exercised with *non*-Kiwai women.

Sido spread more than just pleasure and extended ties. Patrol officer Adrian Geyle reminisced in 1998 about a medical patrol he took in 1953 into Bamu-land to 'clean up venereal diseases which had spread right through [... the Bamu] as a consequence of a promise of affluence like the white man's if everyone practised unbridled sex'. McCarthy (1970: 15) also wrote painfully of an old woman in the Kikori Delta ravaged by venereal disease who had been hidden by her family in a long-house attic. She died shortly upon admission to hospital after she had been found by patrol officers. When the Second World War ceased and Bamu men returned from plantation work, there broke out a 'cargo cult of serious proportions [in] the Lower Bamu', Geyle says (1998), 'and sexual excesses with all taboos lifted had left the victims physically and mentally damaged'. Bamu on Daru are said now to be both cause and effect of what is 'bad' and 'dirty' about contemporary life and are treated accordingly; two large-scale, outdoor, public bush toilets on Daru are located directly adjacent to Bamu settlements, and another Bamu settlement is close to 'Perfume Point' from which hundreds of reeking pan toilet buckets are dumped daily.

These many references to 'dirt' suggest a physical, moral and metaphorical taint imputed to Bamu and other despised people. Butcher was roused to anger at seeing a young girl whose shattered femur he had patched up return to her mother's breast, 'to the dirt and ignorance of village life' (1964: 130). 'We ... reached the village of [BUNIKI] which is a good one, and on a new site. Notwithstanding their new village these people are dirty and do not know what sanitation means', said the then Resident Magistrate A.P. Lyons while on patrol in 1913. 'I sent for the V.C. and then I had a talk with the villagers, pointing out a few things for their benefit. I suggested that they plant coconuts which would, in time to come, give them the means of getting money and incidentally clothes, axes, etc. I am afraid that at present the Bamu people are not sufficiently civilized to grasp things, and only with time and patience will they be taught' (Lyons 1914). That most 'outside' of the 'outside men', Jack Hides, remarked casually that villagers up the Fly river whom he met in his infamous 1935 patrol 'were dirty', and that 'one could quite easily picture them eating human flesh' (1936: 13). 'The Bamu native, who loves dirt', said a mission doctor's memorial, 'would be completely at sea and deeply suspicious in anything so grand and white as a conventional hospital ward' (*Pacific Islands Monthly* 1950: 23). Such tropes of dirt and mud, moral laxity and so on were common, of course, in colonial discourses in other places at this time. The anthropologist Monica Hunter, writing about Pondoland in sub-Saharan Africa in the early 1930s, observed that 'If when the dogs bark as someone goes past and a child is asked by its parents, who passes, a Christian child will say, if it be a Christian who has passed: "*Ngumntu*" (It is a person); if a pagan: "*Liqaba*"', a smearer of ocher on one's skin (quoted in Steinberg 2008: 38).

Bamu were thought 'dirty' in the sexual sense, too, being 'raw' and 'shy', in Beaver's words, but still freely soliciting sex while in transit to regional markets. The Resident Magistrate on Daru in October of 1904, A.H. Jiear, remarked of Bamu that their 'willingness to pander is very noticeable even yet' (quoted in Beaver 1920: 228–9). Beaver found appalling but equally fascinating the existence of 'professional prostitutes' (1920: 149) and sanctioned prostitution among the Bamu, a form that he found during patrols 'to hold good from Buji [west from Daru] to the Dutch border and [north and east] along both banks of the Fly' (Beaver 1920: 140). While on medical patrol A.P. Lyons tried to test the truth of statements that Jiear had made previously about low birth-rate among the Bamu allegedly being due to induced abortion, but came to learn that coitarche closely followed menarche for many Bamu brides, and that polygyny was practiced. 'The BAMU polygamist', he blurted, 'is grossly sensual', and to such sensualists as Bamu men, 'nothing could make a greater appeal than a buxom wench' (Lyons 1914).

Coming to town

Given the backdrop of these ethnological musings, the fact of male labour migration, an increasing cash economy and rising consumerism, it is not difficult to see where Bamu were heading. Bamu began to arrive by canoe fleet to Daru in the early–mid 1960s. Wolfgang Laade did fieldwork between 1963 and 1965 among nearby Torres Straits islanders, and he mentions one informant, 'Aubera' (a Bamu name), living at 'Bamu Camp' on Daru (Laade 1971: 56). My Kiwai and Gogodala informants on Daru said that for the first decade or more following their arrival, Kikori, Bamu and other in-migrating peoples were consigned to camps and stayed on their canoes and were not allowed residence on land. In 1965 land grants given by the Area Council allowed Bamu to leave their canoes at the foreshore and build houses in 'Giwari corner' and 'Bamu corner' and then 'Tawo'o corner' (opposite Bamu corner) and 'Dibiri corner', which emerged on the eastern side of the wharf, opposite Giwari corner. Jackson (1976: 96) recalls that a 1968 Town Planning document noted the resettlement of Bamu from 'appalling shanty conditions on the Daru waterfront', but movement upon land didn't necessarily improve their living conditions, for the poorest settlement by the early 1970s was still Bamu corner (1976: 91).

The linguistic transition from 'camp' (temporary, literally and figuratively marginal) to 'corner' (named, belonging there) signifies this process. Only the temporary – or lonely – can park at Canoe camp. Only the homeless live in Mosquito camp. Only short-timers stay in Firewood camp. Were Daru a clock-face, Bamu would be located at 10, 2, 4 and 6 o'clock, but at its physical and aesthetic margins. An elderly expatriate businessman told me in 1991 that he vividly remembered several specific migratory waves of Bamu that occurred beginning in the late 1960s, a few years after he had established his hardware store and liquor shop. They pulled up their canoes to the foreshore on the west side of the wharf and quickly became his customers, he said, at the liquor shop whose fence abutted the eastern edge of *sagapari*. 'Shagging the blokes to pay for their grog', was how he put it to me, with considerable rhetorical slippage, since it was the husbands who drank the grog and wives who did the shagging. By 1970 *sagapari* was established in locale and public consciousness. It was located first adjacent to Giwari corner ('poison' in Bamu language) and then between Dibiri corner and the hospital compound. At this latter site it came to be known as 'Dokta Point' for its proximity to medical services and owing to the occupational niche of many clients. My fieldnotes from 1990–92 contain multiple references to Bamu women trading sex not just for money but for antibiotics, which they received from clinicians and medical orderlies.

Several migratory pushes and pulls led Bamu to predominate in *tu kina bus*. As for the former, Lawrence pointed out (1995: 16) that Bamu settlements on Daru were 'comparatively recent' and composed mostly of those who have 'moved away from the poverty and hopelessness of the Bamu [area] in search of economic opportunities in Daru'. My informants, Lawrence's, and other researchers and activists are of one voice: despite there having been logging activity for two decades, the Bamu receive few health services, attend few schools or churches, travel no roads, sell at no markets and seldom have their voices heard in national politics. The 1990 summary of the infamous Barnett Report issued in 1988 noted also that '[t]he Bamu people have a remote area mentality with limited access to education, health and other services, and little employment opportunities. They appear to be some of the least educated and enlightened people in PNG regarding knowledge of the outside world and business and industrial relations' (1990:48). By contrast, few Kikori remain on Daru, as Kikori station has gained new centrality as a staging ground for intensive industries in fishing, timber, oil and possibly natural gas, and has a well-maintained hospital run by the Gulf Christian Services. Garry McKellar-James was for nine years the Assistant District Officer, and with one other patrol officer patrolled the Biami, Bamu and Goaribari homelands. He complained recently that in 1968 they were unsuccessful in reining in the 'rambunctious' Bamu living in an 'unexploitable land' and who had 'failed' at insertion into the global economy (McKellar-James 2004). Prior to hearing from Phil Carr, who has for many years lived in the area, I had written that the 28 Bamu villages were serviced spiritually by two Catholic nuns, a priest and a Seventh Day Adventist church in nearby Mubami. Five schools, an equal number of trade stores, four badly crumbling health facilities and a poorly functioning government station at Emeti are expected to serve the 6,313 Bamu people enumerated at the 2000 National Census. Phil Carr, however, said (in a personal communication, 24 June 2007), that such numbers are out-of-date as soon as they are published, that the two Filipina nuns 'left the Bamu several years ago', that it has been years since a Catholic priest lived amongst the Bamu, and that the fellow still serving the Bamu splits his time 'between Daru and Kamusi'. He adds that a Bamu man was ordained 'as a minister of the United Church', the first, at Iowa/Emeti at Easter 2007'. The literacy rate, which the Summer Institute of Linguistics has estimated to be 32–43% nationwide, is estimated to be ~2% for Bamu women (Lennox 2000). There isn't and perhaps hasn't ever been a source of *clear*, clean, fresh water for the Bamu. Beaver (1920: 227–8) noted that 'there is practically no decent drinking water whatever to be obtained on the coast … You have to go nearly sixty miles up the Bamu before it is possible to get any that is quite above suspicion'. Sedimentation of these rivers and their tributaries is occurring, and rumours of chemical poisoning related to logging have circulated since the mid-1980s (Lennox 2000).

The ethnographic data regarding migratory pulls to Daru I collected in 1991 during census of Giwari corner are interesting but contentious. When I asked occupants of 60 Bamu houses why they had migrated to Daru, none, of course, replied 'Why, to engage in sexual toil at an outdoor toilet as part of the informal economy and so thereby to join in economic globalisation'. All but a very few responded, 'to collect *bili*-leaves'. Nevertheless, while *bili*-leaves, which are used in thatching, cooking and basketry, can be collected and bundled virtually anywhere along south coast New Guinea, really only on Daru can they be *sold* by Bamu to any great extent because Daru is the only large urban locale in the area lacking appreciable gardening. Others claimed to have come to Daru to sell garden, marine and riverine resources, but that is even less likely true, given the long distances and great expense involved in getting there. Moreover, the competition for such was high at an already desultory public market (Lawrence 1995), for example, in terms of mats and carvings that Wonie and other Oriomo Plateau peoples sold (Ohtsuka 1983: 25). In any event, the market has been further pushed aside by a huge Asian-owned hotel complex, and Bamu predominate there only in the selling of firewood. By permanently migrating to Daru, Bamu would have lost access to the collection of such resources back home. Even if this explanation is 'true', therefore, it can have been only temporarily so. Not being ethnic majority Kiwai, Bamu would have had traditional rights of access to neither *maza* (reef), *pari* (garden), *pisirimai* (sea cucumber), *boromo* (wild pig), *gamo* (turtle), nor *dubari* (bananas). Yet other Bamu said they came so as to '*sell* the firewoods', which they and others collect on neighboring, uninhabited Bobo island (although no one said 'to *sell* the empty bottles'). This seems truer, since firewood-selling, sexual servicing and bottle-collection and sale virtually exhaust income-sources for Bamu on Daru.

The coming of a cash economy led Bamu to buy clothing, engage in Christian tithing, eat tradestore-bought foods and pay school-fees, and allowed them to gamble, purchase petrol and dinghies and drink alcohol. As a result Bamu began slowly to migrate away from their ancestral homelands, first to other administrative and mission centres such as Balimo, Emeti and Daru, but eventually to timber camps, river ports, sawmills and oil exploration camps. My informants in 1990–92 said that Bamu families were already involved in Kiunga in the selling of sexual services to tug-boat and cargo-barge operators and to sailors and stevedores. They said that church, community and women's groups had begun to complain to the company and to national newspapers within two short years of the town's founding as a staging port (Nomelea 1986: 8; Matit 2005). Interestingly, Kiwai families were reported during the nationwide social mapping study to be engaging in the same thing. 'Young people (women)', it said, 'at Philip Corner and Parama Corner in Kiunga Town [two Kiwai settlements] were said to leave especially at weekends to visit seamen and employees "for sexual relationships"' (NHASP 2005c: 21). As of 1996 Rimbunan-Hijau was paying the equivalent of $2 (US) per cubic metre of harvested timber, and although they have paid slightly higher royalties since then, their 'company store' takes it right back. Lennox's summary (2000) of a report prepared by three Catholics suggests that Bamu families who had moved to Kamusi and other timber camps are easily trapped in cycles of drinking, gambling and prostitution. 'The husband is unable to bring home anything to his wife because he squanders it on drinking and gambling' she notes, but because the price of food is so high, 'the husband turns around and forces the wife into prostitution to raise money for the family's subsistence'. This is the position taken by contemporary observers especially in Port Moresby as regards gender and family relations in primarily Papuan settlements such as Tatana, Wanigela and Hanuabada, but it has a much longer pedigree (see Whiteman 1973: 138, n. 1, 141, 144). The Summary of the Barnett Report concluded that in the Bamu watershed cash in great volume is handed out and subsequently 'wasted on unnecessary and unprofitable expenditure. It means, at the moment, they are dressed better and they drink more beer, and probably have more access to trade store goods' (1990: 49). William Goinau's brief report (1995) is extremely grim regarding the likely future facing his own people in view of logging and the 'development' process. A brief trip Mike Wood made a year later into this area showed also that the Malaysian logging giant Rimbunan-Hijau had broken promises and left schools unfinished and airstrips unusable (Wood 1996).

Of mud and missions

Unexplored New Guinea was published in 1920, three years after the death on the battlefields of World War I of its author, Wilfred Beaver. Beaver was a long-time British hand who eventually became the Resident Magistrate for Western Division. He died, taking his men into the Polygon Wood of France. The caption to its frontispiece reads: 'The whole of the Goaribari delta is chiefly mud or sago swamp'. Mud, which the gentleman-explorer Theodore Bevan referred to as being 'bottomless' throughout the Papuan Gulf (1890: 237), was reviled in colonial discourse as slowing down or altogether precluding a civilising mission that needed unstinting, unbroken frequency of contact to be effective. The author of the Foreword to the second of Mabel Anne Bladon's two memoirs, *The Song of the Bamu*, commented that Bamu-land might appear to Australians as the last place on the planet they'd want to live: 'low lying river flats of humid heat, torrential rains and perpetual mud ... ' (Edwards 1964: iii). A lost opportunity to engage Bamu in the civilising process was thought lost forever, although it probably didn't appear that way to indigenes.[5] The Resident Magistrate in 1913, A.P. Lyons, gave instructions while on patrol to the Wapaura villagers he encountered to cut roads between villages. 'At present', he complained, 'one has to wallow in mud to reach them walking' (Lyons 1914). E. Baxter Riley remarked (1925: 21) that there is 'absolutely nothing to excite the emotion of admiration except the large quantities of mud'. 'The most depressing feature', he added, 'is the mud'. Beaver (1920: 212) described the Bamu river, a 'melancholy and lifeless river, as lifeless as one could imagine no tropical river to be', as the 'least attractive of them all. Whenever I go into the river I seem to catch the feeling of depression that hangs over the low, muddy mangrove swamps'. Bamu villages were 'impossibly muddy' to get to and navigate between, such as at Maipani village, where he found 'fourteen feet of steep slippery mud to climb up to reach comparatively dry land' (1920: 225, 213). He described the lower Bamu river villages of Damerakoromo and Oromokoromo as 'the muddiest in a muddy district ... both built two or three hundred yards in from the river, and when the tide is out there are two or three hundred yards of the thickest, stickiest mud it is possible to imagine' (1920: 214). The Bamu River Mission led by Harry and Eva Standen,[6] who were from England and Australia, respectively, was described as 'the Mission in the Mud' (Staff Writer 1961). When the Standens arrived in Bamu-land in 1936 they purposely selected Dibiri island, five miles long by two wide, as their headquarters, despite obvious evidence that high tides periodically flooded it. An early flood 'left behind ... revolting mud, peculiar to this Gulf country and into which it was possible to sink up to the knees, hips or further' (Staff Writer 1961: 45). One 'W.D.' penned an article in 1940 for *Pacific Islands Monthly* whose sub-title was 'it is not all mud', but also featured mention of 'the depressing, dirty rivers of the delta' (W.D. 1940: 44). Bladon's two memoirs, but especially *The Song of the Bamu*, are literally dripping with nods to heat, humidity and mud. 'Lord, I can't stand it!', she exclaims. 'My heart cried out in hasty rebellion. "It's mud everywhere, every day, and I can't even get my clothes clean. I loathe the mud"'. Her 'dear Lord' is said to have replied to her, however, 'Lo, I am with you always' (Bladon 1984: 68). A New Zealand doctor informant in nearby Balimo told me in January of 1991 that during his periodic medical patrols to Bamu villages, living conditions were still 'almost "barbaric"': 'every time the tide came in the village was awash in water; right up to the house level ... when the tide went out, they were up to their knees and beyond in mud. Their villages [were] not high up enough to be able to have decent gardens' (author's field-notes, Balimo, 1991).

Square kilometre after square mile of 'soft creamy mud' – this revolting ooze precluded the sedentary lifestyles built upon intensive agriculture a desire for which Europeans wished to instill in their charges. Beaver complained once (1920: 214) of having stationed six policemen at the Bamu village of Ibu so as to give them 'an object lesson in gardening', but that there remained 'about as much cultivation ... as there was twenty years ago and that is none'. Above Ibu, past Maipani and neighbouring villages (in the Middle Bamu river area), 'any pretense at civilisation is left behind ... Not a single tribe cultivates the soil' (1920: 214–5). Nevertheless, mud was for Papuans their bread-basket, containing shell-fish, prawns and crabs; forming a defensive barrier; and providing a good excuse for avoiding the approach of pesky Europeans. Mud might have been a useful defense against raiding of the Marind-anim from the west, too. Nomadism mandates that *temporary* homes be made anyway, that time spent cleaning up *temporary* villages is time wasted, that, in the midst of flooded, swampy land, sporadic efforts to work puny gardens will likely result in few surpluses. More positive assessments by Europeans are extremely rare:

> A marshland of mud and rain forest, river-glades and sago trees, home of the Asmat people. Regularly, once daily, twice monthly and more dramatically

twice a year, the ubiquitous mudscape slides beneath the surface as the seawater drifts inwards oozing inexorably up on the verge of audibility. Or rather the defenseless world seems to sink into the incoming slush as stumps and even scrubs and trees gradually sink into the mire. The muddy lunar tides are fertile, growth giving, alive with seafood and the providers of powerful, life-transforming spirits. Slimy, pock-holed, teeming with amphibious creatures, Asmat mud is a great absorbent taking in all comers, home to crabs and crocodiles, fish and prawns, snakes and frogs that shuffle, writhe, crawl, slither and then disappear into its welcoming womb. (Prior 2001)

For most Europeans, however, mud precluded the swift and proper flow of goods, services and people. Mud sat proxy for Papuan recalcitrance and European heroism in eventually surmounting it – if not actually drying it up.

Neither was fishing particularly central to Bamu economies. This, too, indexed for Europeans the Bamu unfitness for the civilising mission. Beaver notes (1920: 232) that he never saw a 'real' fishing net in the Bamu. They maintained fishing grounds, collected prawns and mud-crabs and netted and trapped mud fish with some ingenuity, but enjoyed no sedentary village life and had few resource surpluses with which they might have paid more taxes, tithed more generously and obtained other much-needed items. Bamu lived too leisurely and depended too much, thought Europeans, on sago, sago grubs and, as Beaver points out, *small* fish (1920: 214, 215, 232, my emphasis). Having 'nothing to do', which was for Beaver 'characteristic of most sago-eating tribes who do not cultivate the soil' (1920: 223), steered them toward desultory fighting, mindless head-taking and immoral prostituting. This appeared to be a problem for other Europeans. Lawrence has written that, like the Western Division, the delta areas scribed by the Aird, Omati, Kikori and Purari rivers 'remained isolated, inhospitable and threatening. The Delta Division was never "controlled" or "settled"' (2006: 18).

Another Bamu character trait Europeans found unappealing was their nomadism.[7] A patrol officer report from 1909 complained about the 'rawness' of the tribes of the upper Bamu, about the fact that their villages were not permanently settled, that their houses were miserable and that the 'general conditions of life [were] primitive'. This was contrasted with six lower Bamu villages whose residents were 'well acquainted with the ways of the Government' and whose 'villages are well built permanent places'.[8] Beaver remarked that 'almost every [Bamu] tribe is a wandering one', and claimed that the 'nomadic habits of these tribes' were partly due to 'death or a series of deaths occurring there either from disease or, I suppose I should say, sorcery' (Beaver 1920: 212, 216). William Goinau noted in his Masters Thesis that 'the people had no permanent locations for their village[s] until the early 1960s' (1995: 4). A reporter for the *Pacific Islands Monthly* (1953: 35) suggested that the missionaries Standen at Dibiri 'found that these semi-nomadic people who live on the muddy rivers and muddier banks of the Western rivers have some desire for learning but their manner of living, suspicion of other natives and wandering, preclude anything in the nature of a permanent school'. A.P. Lyons remarked in 1913 that the (Bamu) Sisiame 'are in the transition state from the nomadic to the settled life', and hoped that soon they would 'erect a settled village in accordance with my recommendation'.[9] Lyons patrolled the Bamu river in 1913, and at several villages or camps he remonstrated them for *not* staying in one place, as had their Kiwai neighbors agreed to do. At Bina he found them 'in a temporary camp [and] living in "leantos". Suggested that they build a permanent village at the place they were at, it being in every way suitable. Pointed out the benefits of having a settled village'. Upriver he met the nomadic Deravi people. 'Before I parted with them I tried to induce them to erect a permanent village, pointing out the benefits. I promised them if they did so, I would appoint a mamoose or V[illage] C[onstable] amongst them'. Further upstream at Wakau: 'Pointed out the advantages of having a settled village, of planting coconuts &c'. At Bimaramio, he 'had a long yarn with some of the old men and pointed out the benefits of having a settled village &c'. At Sisiame, he found nothing but 'poor nomads', but 'Got some of the old men to call the people together when I went ashore and had a talk with them pointing out that they were now sufficiently civilized to have a settled village'. At Asaramia he promised to appoint a particular man as V.C. 'if he would get his people to build a settled village on the river bank'.[10] Lewis Lett (1942: 173–4) blamed a too lenient natural environment for nomadism, since it provided them with surplus time (if not money) to think up and perform 'elaborate ritual' expressing 'the revolting customs that informed their lives'.

Several more decades would pass, but the dreams of Beaver and Lyon, Butcher and Lett never materialized. Phil Carr (in a personal communication, 24 June 2007) reminded me that no Bamu village is permanent. Iowa moved a few hundred yards in 1994, and then Amagoa, Etere and Asaramio 'have all moved a long way in from the river', with Bimaramio and Aniadae moving 'along their branches of the river', as did Kuria along the Aramia River and the Ibuo along the Bamu, who 'left their village empty and moved right across the mouths of the Bamu and a fair way up the Fly'. Carr shared with me that:

> Among the reasons I've been told for people moving their villages are that it was being washed away, that too many people had died at the former site and it was now a (spiritually) bad place, that it floods too often, that there isn't enough harvestable sago around the old location anymore.

Bamu were described, inscribed and denigrated as much for what they lacked (intensive agriculture) and didn't do (stay put) as for what they did (engaged in prostitution).

Deliverance

With regards to canoes, however – well, that's a different story. In the nineteen teens Beaver noted that one canoe was worth 'two large arm-shells and a small one, one melon shell, one dugong rib bone, and a string of dogs' teeth' (Beaver 1920: 77). He remarked (1920: 250) that Goaribari and Bamu natives were 'expert at building and handling canoes' cut from the solid logs that had been obtained from the upper Kiko[ri?] river (and from Dibiri island itself), and which were then further manufactured by villagers themselves. He marvelled at the sometimes 'twenty- or thirty-men canoe[s in which they] perform the most amazing feats of dexterity'. According to Beaver (1920: 228) and Landtman (1927: 208), the 'most famous' canoes (and drums – Beaver 1920: 210), were made by Bimarami (lower Bamu) and Miriwo (Middle Bamu) villagers, and were exported 'to such far distant places as Torres Straits' (1920: 228). While once patrolling the Bamu region, A.H. Jiear found at one such canoe bazaar well over 1,000 people[11] and remarked that 'Without doubt, the most important form of native trading is that of buying and selling canoes' (1905: 69).

Several scholars (Lawrence 1989a, b, 1990a, b, 1991; Barham *et al.* 2004; Shnukal 2004) have shown that the extent of this trade prior to 'European contact' has been underestimated due to European ethnocentrism. Anna Shnukal (2004: 326) has written perceptively about trading routes and relations 'on contact' and argued that Torres Straits islanders provided 'surplus fish, dugong and turtle taken from their reefs; human skulls seized in battle; stone-headed clubs; pearlshell, *Melo* shells for balers and saucepans; armlets and necklets finely crafted from mother-of-pearl, tortoiseshell and coneshell' to Papuans in exchange for 'yams, sago, canoes, thick bamboo for water pipes, mats, drums, bows and arrows, and cassowary and bird-of-paradise plumes for ornaments and bone for arrows'. Singe adds that the Papuans also traded shredded sago leaves and bundles of freshly made sago, being especially anxious to receive pearlshell in return (1989: 4–5). The Meriam (from Mer, or Murray island) took voyages called *wauri* to obtain canoes directly from Kiwai (ultimately from Bamu) in exchange for names, food, small ornaments and other gifts, which would be returned the following year by Kiwai partners (Sharp 1993: 28, citing a mis-referenced Haddon). In the social environment of mutual need they created, one partner vied with another to add more and more presents so as to be favoured in the next round. Some of the presents and small items received by Kiwai on the outward-bound trip were then turned over to Bamu and other partners on the return home. One can easily imagine sexual services being provided at overnight stops along the way in an environment of mutual need but non-identical availability of natural resources. Sharp calls it a 'form of exchange of the equivalences of dissimilarity' between people who sought and traded in marriage partners, canoes, fishing and gardening tools and the like (1993: 28). 'Exchange', she notes elsewhere, 'knotted people together in reciprocal ties necessary for life, for spice to life and for meaning' (1993: 31).

Many great surveying voyages to and through this area were taken in the mid–late eighteenth to the late nineteenth centuries. Sailors, hydrographers, navigators, missionaries and ethnologists noticed not only a great eagerness of all for trade with Europeans but also between various Papuan mainland peoples, between them and Torres Straits islanders, and between both of them and even some Australian Aboriginal groups. Torres Straits islanders from the eastern portion directly and indirectly obtained from Bamu people canoe hulls, bows, masks, arrows and stone suitable for being turned into clubs, axes and other tools and weapons (Allen and Corris 1977: 33–7; Landtman 1927: 34; Lawrence 1990a, b, 1991: 7; McNiven, von Gnielinski and Quinell 2004). Its importance is obvious on the face of it. Nonie Sharp asserts (1993: 28) that Torres Straits islanders were shown by Kiwai villagers at Mawat[t]a the magic, so to speak, of the double-outrigger canoe; once they grafted gunwales onto them (Landtman 1927: 211) they could go just about anywhere, unlike the swamp- and river-dwelling Gogodala. Nonie Sharp has shown that Erub peoples (Darnley island) made *wauri* voyages in two directions, one being to Op Deudai (the New Guinea mainland) 'for canoes, cassowary feathers, dogs' teeth necklaces and other dance ornaments ... ' (1993: 27–8). One of the clerks from the mid-nineteenth century expedition of the HMS *Fly*, John Sweatman, was sent onto the HMS *Bramble* for a second survey of the area (c. 1861) and commented on the extent, beauty and meaningfulness of the pearl and cowrie shells given by Torres Straits islanders ultimately in exchange for canoe hulls (Allen and Corris 1977). Haddon (1914: 613) travelled to this area in 1888 and 1898 and remarked several times with admiration that 'superior' canoe hulls came from Dibiri.

For Bamu, Wabuda, Kiwai, Gogodala and Torres Straits islanders, the canoe facilitated travel and socialising and the production and distribution of marine, riverine and agricultural resources. Before he learned of the importance of Bamu input in such, Haddon's first of many disquisitions on the 'canoe trade' (1890) isolated Wabuda village as the origin of large canoes used throughout the Torres Straits (cf. Lawrence 1989a: 85–6), although canoe *hulls* originated elsewhere. Wabuda relationships with Torres Straits islanders were also founded upon ties of naming and mythic creatures and heroes. A hill on the Eastern island of Mer is said to resemble a dugong (Gelam), who is said to have originated in Wabuda (Singe 1989: 3). Lawrence notes (1995: 12) that '[c]anoes are still obtained from the Dibiri Island or from the Balamula areas and traded down to Daru and the coastal villages', suggesting continuity in need and source of canoe. Kiwai men once feared the spirits dwelling in large trees (Landtman 1927: 65; cf. Wood 1998: 236), which may explain their reticence to cut them down. Hardwoods in sufficient size and density were unevenly available and not at all available on any of the Torres Straits islands (Singe 1989: 5), although sometimes tree-trunks float past there when the wind is right. *Shells* Kiwai had, in abundance, and could provide, too, by the canoe-full – if they only had one. For that, they needed Bamu carvers, Wabuda middlemen and perhaps a Bamu woman or two.

Trafficking women

Unlike Kiwai men, Bamu men were virtually powerless viz. European newcomers. Being located up Papuan waterways, not along the coast where they might have competed for employment, status and exposure to European ways, they also were relatively less powerful in terms of regional political-economy. Nevertheless, they provided black-palm used to make tools, weapons and finery; some stone; hardwood species (e.g. *gagoro*) required to make canoes and canoe hulls; and eventually, women and sexual services. From the Kiwai and Gogodala, the Bamu received bundles of probably cultivated, not wild sago; fresh barramundi and dugong and turtle meat; and *bidi-bidi* (cowry), *mabuo* (armshells), *sagera* (pearl shells worn around the neck) and dogs' teeth shells, each of which figured prominently in marital and other sexual transactions. The manufacture and exchange of such utilitarian items and meaning-rich finery enhanced their lives and those of others, providing the ways and means of ceremony, nutrition, material existence and a social life. 'From the Dibiri side', noted Gunnar Landtman, the Finnish ethnographer who lived on nearby Kiwai island from 1910 to 1912, 'come carved bark belts (*epora*) beautifully ornamented, the back ground generally filled in with white' (Landtman 1927: 27). Dibiri is a Bamu village, and those *epora* were treasured and worn by Kiwai during ceremonial dancing and feasting.

What kind of 'custom', therefore, underwrote the eventual emergence on Daru of *tu kina bus*? How 'customary' was sexual networking? Beaver used the term 'custom' frequently, but in reference to Bamu, quite neutrally: 'I should rather say [Bamu] are non-moral. Custom is custom, and that is about all one can say' (Beaver 1920: 229). A.P. Lyons (1926: 354) referred to Gogodala in the same fashion, as 'unmoral', in reference to their canoe races, which he described as being 'of a pornographical nature'. It was one of the first things that missionaries forbade – and one of the first traditional practices that emerged in the 'cultural revival' analysed by Crawford (1981). McCarthy wrote similarly of the Goaribari that 'he' [*sic*] lived as he did within his own tribal framework, [and] could not be classed immoral by our standards'. 'Rather', he argued, the Goaribari man 'was unmoral for he regarded certain forms of sexual license as perfectly justifiable and would probably have been shocked to learn that in other societies, of which he knew little or nothing, his own convictions on sexual freedom would have brought severe criticism, his actions, punishment' (McCarthy 1970: 17). Bamu men told me in 1991 that in Bimaramio and Torobina, men catching women stealing sago grubs from their downed sago palms could keep them as temporary wives. McCarthy noted (1970: 17) a court case in which 'An old man had wanted the young man's pig and had made an agreement that the young man could use the old man's wife – who happened to be quite young – in payment for a certain number of times [of sexual intercourse], a normal village transaction which raised no eyebrows'.

In the broader context of Papuan sociality, the Bamu penchant for sexual networking hardly seems unusual. Beaver argued that such customs were well-nigh 'universal[,] and [that] the women themselves seem to regard the position with equanimity' (1920: 229). Though Butcher lived in the Kikori river delta at Aird Hills, he many times witnessed performances of the *buguru* ceremony in Bamu-land and complained about a tribe [the Bamu] 'notorious for the shameless traffic of its [*sic*] women' (1964: 180). In the Kiwai language, this was rendered *muguru* or *mouguru*. Riley's account (1925: 189–240) is the most lengthy (but completely sanitised) version of much early colonial commentary thereupon. He complains elsewhere (1925: 260) of a dance that is 'very disgusting and indelicate'. Flint (1919), Beaver (1920), Butcher (1964) and my Bamu informants each noted that new Bamu brides made two-weeks-long canoe-paddling 'tours' with their husbands to and between other Bamu and non-Bamu villages, having sex with as many admirers as they fancied and keeping the shell valuables and other wealth given them by admirers. The Reverend Holmes wrote of similar practices among the Papuan Gulf Namau (1924: 172, 175) and Government Anthropologist F.E. Williams (1924: 211–4) said the same thing about his hosts in the Purari Delta, pointing out specifically that shell wealth that went to women was theirs to keep (1924: 56), though they shared such profits jointly with their husbands. To what extent this added prestige value to the women as persons (or added to their value to their husbands as wives) is just as difficult a question to answer as that of the extra material value now burning holes in the trouser-pockets of their husbands. Ethnological data don't clarify how much shell or other wealth Bamu husbands accrued thereby or to what (new) ends they put it. On other occasions, Beaver saw Wabuda men in canoe fleets in the Bamu river delta trading these shells to Bamu, husbands exchanging wives and wives, husbands.

When Knauft says that Purari and Kiwai women 'engaged in extramarital heterosexual intercourse with pleasure, equality, and esteem' (1994: 410), perhaps it was because their exchange relations had not been so severed and persons demeaned by having K2 thrown at them. Even the Reverend Holmes had begrudgingly to admire Purari women's skill and pride in taking lovers, engaging in extra-marital liaisons and receiving shell valuables in return. Lawrence remarked (1989a: 467) that both 'historical documentation and oral testimony' confirm that 'the exchange of rituals, legends and stories was accompanied by exchange of artifacts and women'. This suggests a more reciprocal than exploitive function of sexual networking, but yet a male-dominated, sexualised form of reciprocity that was ripe for commoditisation. McCarthy (1970: 16) writes that Goaribari women were 'chattels in the true sense of the word, movable objects that could be used as commodities, as part of a business arrangement, or as a social gesture'.

Women in traffic

Because the question of female agency is so thorny, it requires the application of facts, the sifting of perspectives, the weighing of competing interests and far more testimonies from women than we currently have. Although there are a couple of exhaustive and sensitive treatments (Knauft 1993, 1994), much of the ethnography and most of the ethnology is male-biased and male-focused. Williams, for example, notes at the outset of *Papuans of the Trans-Fly* that his original title for the book had been *Men of the Morehead River*, 'with the emphasis on the "Men"' (1969[1936]: viii). Women's narratives from this area are extremely few in number. I confess to having been stumped for two solid years in the field and again in 2003 and 2004, with Bamu females appearing just as shy, reticent, fearful and silenced. Certainly, their agency structures them, however much (or little) pride or money they can win for themselves at *sagapari*. In Daru's version of *tu kina bus*, all manner of gender, class and ethnic relations are played out and shored up. There is, for example, the fact that, at least until recently, no Bamu *men* were customers there, they being more afraid of themselves *sexually* breaking kinship taboos than they are disturbed by seeing their sisters and wives brutalised. Of the Tari Basin Huli, Holly Wardlow argues that '[i]n their attempts to evade or undermine the trafficking of women through bride-wealth and marriage [by becoming *pasindia meri*, women] may eventually find themselves caught in the trafficking of women through monetized sexual exchanges' (2004:

1037). These kinds of paradoxes underscore the fact that sexual networking of all kinds and time periods must be put in cultural and political-economic context and that ethnographic insight and analysis must be given their proper place.

The commentators I have cited to this point have examined ethnological and other materials from the Asmat, Yei-anim, Marind-anim and Kimam across the border to the west; from the Kiwai, Bamu, Gogodala, Goaribari, Wabuda and others on and north and east of Daru; and from the Suki, Keraki and others in the Trans-Fly. With ethnographic particularity but not peculiarity, men and women clearly exchanged themselves and one another. The German medico called upon to aid Dutch emergency efforts in treating now hyper-epidemic Donovanosis among the Marind-anim, M.U. Thierfelder, noted that in Marind anim-land, 'one [sic] gave a present to the husband for being allowed to *approach* his wife' (1928: 394, emphasis mine). Who knows what 'one' might give to such a wife later, upon having approached her more closely? Butcher noted (1964: 180) that once 'traditional' prohibitions on travelling inter-village had been lifted by administrative and missionary 'pacification', Bamu began to travel in 'companies' (!) of men and women so that men could exchange women for tobacco 'and other articles of barter'.

Ritualised homosexuality among the Asmat has been driven underground by religious authorities (just as it was among the Gogodala – see Wilde 2003), but ritualised heterosexuality has flourished longer and was once common to Kiwai and other South Fly and Trans-fly peoples, to which both men and women eagerly flocked (Landtman 1927: 351–52). The Reverend J.H. Holmes complained of the commonness of wife-exchange among the Namau of the Purari Delta (1924). Alphonse Sowada and Gerard Zegwaard (in Knauft 1993: 99) disagree as to the *degree* of husbandly prerogative involved, but both wrote perceptively about the *kind* of wife-lending and -exchange involved for Asmat. Geyle (1998) reminisced about an overtly sexualised celebration over Christmas in 1953 that he witnessed and had inadvertently condoned by his presence: 'The performance of that dance caused a great deal of pleasure in [the Wabuda village of] Tirere and a great deal of consternation in mission circles as far away as Melbourne'. Laurent Serpenti, who worked in the 1960s with elderly Kimam informants from Kolopom (Frederik Hendrik island), wrote of the widespread practice just prior to *thubudubor* (head-hunting expeditions) of wife-exchange, a special form of sexual networking designed to bond males through a sexual send-off of sorts, of killers who might be killed (1977: 183). Regarding the Asmat, and according to the amateur ethnologist-cum-photo journalist-cum-tour guide, Tobias Schneebaum:

> wife exchange ... is still common. Bond or *papisj* friends exchanged wives on ritual occasions and at times of stress, such as the rebellion ... *Papisj* meant that Allo's wife, having agreed to spend the night with her husband's exchange partner, would go to the partner's house in the late afternoon. There she would cook sago and other food for the man who would be her sexual companion for the night, as well as for the rest of his family ... Allo would decorate the woman he was with and his partner would decorate his wife. (1989: 84–5)

Kiwai, Kikori, Suki and Bamu women clearly displayed sexual initiative, just as did their counterparts across the (then) Dutch border and among Purari Delta peoples. Williams was impressed with the sexual and marital initiative that Purari women took, with the shell valuables they received at marriage, and even with the extra-marital sexuality in which they engaged, though with their husbands' consent, often receiving gifts such as arm-shells in payment (1924: 53, 56). Serpenti notes that for the Kimam, 'the initiative for a liaison must be taken by the girl' (1977: 174). He tells later (1977: 178) of the myth of Koné, a Kimam woman who, being yet unmarried, 'tries to molest men whenever possible'. This must have been doubly dangerous for men, for she possessed and wielded apparently lethal vagina dentata. Beaver says that among Kiwai, 'the overtures in making love should come from the women' (1920: 63; cf. 65–6). Jiear reported in 1903 that 'The evidence in many cases heard [in Native Matters Court] would go to show that in a majority of instances the principal offender is the female, as the male participator in the offence [adultery] often takes a passive part. On several occasions, the offence has only taken place at the earnest and continued solicitation of the female'.[12] Hubert Murray once claimed that 'native women' who preserved their chastity did exist but were exceptional, and that rape of one did not approximate the rape of a European woman. He claimed further that European men rarely had to force their affections on native women, and that he was unaware of 'a case of the rape of a native woman by a White man in Papua' (Murray 1927: 10). Perhaps he had forgotten by then that one of his charges, Resident Magistrate A.H. Jiear, was forced in 1908 to resign for having raped a Bamu female who had just been released from jail on a charge of adultery; one may wonder what kind of defense he used at his trial (see also Inglis 1974). Bamu informants told me that Bamu 'women who have sex every day' (*eragabo mamio*=fire/path/woman) were by definition married,[13] were well known to all, and were exchanged and continue to be exchanged and exchange themselves sexually for *bidi-bidi* shells, *sagera*, food, the use of canoe and gardening tools, to cancel debts and to pay for garden labour. One elderly Bamu informant told me that husbands and wives together will 'go in a secret way', and another said that 'man will give his wife to another man and only those three will know'. There might not be payment were both couples to exchange spouses, but 'if a man gives his wife to another for sex, there must be payment' (author's fieldnotes, Daru, 1991).

What most complicates the analysis of agency and exploitation is that many Papuan peoples were known for more positive, less exploitive views of sexuality. Landtman (1927: 78–80, 90) wrote that Kiwai women rubbed stone-axes and plant shoots along their vulva, dripped vaginal fluids onto about-to-be-cultivated plots and added such to foods to provide strength, medicine and protection. Serpenti's analysis of the Kimam life-cycle includes many mentions of male initiation requiring that incisions be made with a bamboo knife into which were rubbed semen for strength and growth. 'Everywhere on the island', he says, originally in 1965, 'sperm is believed to contain great powers', possessing 'healing and invigorating properties' (1977: 164, 174). A more recent essay of his reiterates that semen is 'man's life-giving potency, powerful and beneficial' (1993[1984]: 304). To this day, pubic hair and vaginal fluids are on Daru thought capable, if administered correctly to one's actual or would-be suitor's food or drink, of inciting desire and inducing lifelong fidelity. The Marind-anim ritual known as *otiv-bombari* ('many copulation') had supremely deleterious effects upon fertility and social life *after* the arrival of European-introduced STDs, probably first in the form of chlamydial infections, but certainly then in the form of Donovanosis (Vogel, with Richens 1989; see especially p. 217, n.22). As well, it may have induced the chronic vaginal, cervical and uterine irritations that early medicos investigated prior to their introduction. Nevertheless, the ostensible purpose of its performance was to increase human, plant and animal fertility by facilitating the mingled collection of male and female sexual fluids and their appropriate application. Serpenti has remarked that when villages were struck by disease epidemics, 'promiscuous heterosexual intercourse involving as many people as possible is organized' so as to collect semen with which to do battle (1993[1984]: 304).

The doubled, complementary application of male and female sexual efforts and fluids may imply female agency or at least complicate attributions of male bias (see Knauft 1993: 53). Nevertheless, the complexity of historical perspectives, economic forces and ethnographic context do not unequivocally answer questions. Lawrence quotes another source quoting an earlier source such that, alongside items offered by their husbands seeking trade, women themselves offered *bidi-bidi* they had won previously (1989a: 71), perhaps following sexual encounters they had initiated. Whether in Portland or Port Moresby, on Friday night or Thursday island, for shell wealth, cash, or Mardi Gras beads, females can of course act agentially when copulating serially, just as they can be harmed irreparably. Serial copulation can mean money and pleasure, friendship and achievement in the best of circumstances, but also traumatic coitarche, ascendant infections, secondary infertility and pain and suffering, in the worst. Landtman allows (1954: 92) that even women but especially girls participating avidly in the *mouguru* ceremonies were traumatised. Jan van Baal (1966: 25–31) grieved for the young brides who crawled home on their hands and knees, so worn out were they by their ordeal. Serpenti didn't expect to see much consent of Kimam females who were expected to have intercourse with prospective fathers-in-law and their age-mates, owing neither just to the number nor just to the character of the relationships, but to their age; 'the girls who had to be available for sexual intercourse with a large number of men were ... young and sometimes very young indeed' (1977: 184), 'girls who were not yet or scarcely sexually mature' (1977: 184–5). Elsewhere (1993[1984]: 307) he notes that on the appointed day, a young girl will be grabbed by the waist and laid down in a canoe: '[s]he is not supposed to resist. The parents-in-law know that she is going to have sexual intercourse with the older men; however, they pretend to be ignorant of what is going on'. Knauft (1994: 410), however, points out that insofar as 'ritual sexuality formed a venue of creative experimentation', some women may have been uplifted thereby.[14]

The creativity and gender complementarity implied for some anthropologists when female or mixed male and female sexual fluids were applied to gardens to make them fertile and to human skin to heal wounds, strengthen resolve and protect it from harm may not be so easy to think about or express. Patrol Officer Adrian Geyle (1998), for example, writing of his experiences 45 years previously, can barely keep his disgust in check:

> They coped, privy as they were to all the deprivations, and the cult-induced, aberrant sexual activities of adults around them. Child abuse was practised by some tribal elders as they consolidated their claims to small girls as 'wives' promised in exchange deals made even before they were born.

While on patrol and in a similar vein, another kiap (McCarthy 1970: 5) came within fifty feet of

> about two hundred men and women cavorting in the moonlight and between the glow and smoke of fires, dolefully chanting a dirge as they stamped, one behind the other, in large circles. Somewhere in a darkened hut a drum beat out the time ... and there began a frenzied display of perverted eroticism and sexual indulgence, with men and women scrambling around on the damp soil like animals, with the drum still beating as the circles broke and reformed into snaky lines of men and women, still one behind the other, stamping and screaming in orgiastic desire. This was the Buguru, and there are few white men who have seen it in its entirety as it may go on for days and nights in a continuous unbridled round of sexual orgy until exhaustion sets in and the dancers lie where they drop.

The Unevangelized Fields Mission representative, Bernard Lea, happened in 1937 upon frenzied preparations being made by Gogodala in Balimo for some kind of ceremony, a 'rather sexy affair', he wrote, designed 'to promote fertility'. Eventually invited inside one of the stupendous Gogodala long-houses, he found long lines of boys and girls, kneeling and squatting, one in front of the other, whom he found out later would eventually marry one another. 'It is obviously done', he concluded, 'to make these young people realize that they had approached another stage in life' (quoted in Crawford 1981: 250). His description of a Gogodala ceremony is more 'neutral' than Geyle's of a Bamu *buguru* and also tallies with that of Reverend Butcher. Butcher is remarkably restrained regarding who in this Bamu ritual does what to whom sexually and why, and comments *almost* respectfully upon the beauty, splendor, dancing, cosmetics and general aesthetics of the ceremony. In noting that bridegrooms normally remain celibate during such ceremonies, he added that sex took place between an uncle and his niece, a man and his neighbor's wife, a bride and her male affines and between a recently initiated girl and virtually all other men who had access 'to her person'. 'At the same time', he notes, there was 'uninhibited promiscuity among the men and women filling the place, mingled with a most disgusting rite [almost surely he is speaking of male–male anal intercourse], carried through with definite ceremonial form as an integral part of tribal life and considered essential to its continuance' (Butcher 1964: 177).

Patrol Officer Flint's claim, that *buguru* ceremonies among the Bamu were performed so that 'children should learn how they came into existence' (1919: 39), is deliciously ambiguous. Perhaps he meant that children 'came into existence' insofar as physiological conception can occur between sperm and egg on the night of and in the midst of such ceremonies. Perhaps, on the other hand, children come into being *socially* in the midst of ceremonies themselves and following their ritual instructions in those dark, smoky, jam-packed long-houses. Perhaps in the midst of ritualised sexual activities, instead, children learned what it means to be a Bamu man or a Bamu woman or Bamu as against Keraki and Kiwai. Perhaps Flint meant that such ceremonies communicated the 'total social fact' of serial copulation or of sexual networking as an institution: to be Bamu meant to live within a social system whereby *young girls* will be *given sexually* to elder men for ritual and actual sexual instruction; female *children* 'come into existence', that is, insofar as (male) *elders* tell them so and make them so. Nearby on Kiwai island, similar ritual instruction of girls in sexual matters was carried out by older men in the *máure moguru* ceremony, and many girls shrieked in attempt to resist sexual intercourse, but to no avail. 'The girls', noted Landtman dryly (1954: 185), 'are generally married shortly after the *moguru*'. In his contribution to *Ritualized Homosexuality in Melanesia*, written some decades after first fieldwork, Laurent Serpenti noted that the promiscuous intercourse to which young Kimam girls were subject was something of a test. 'If they fell ill after intercourse', he notes, 'it was proof that they were not yet suited for marriage' (1993[1984]: 301). Maybe that's a bit too late.

Conclusions: full circle

These ethnological data and ethnographic musings may seem light-years away from the current situation of Bamu women. In 2001, four Kiwai men on Daru decapitated and dismembered a Bamu woman at the new locale of *saga-pari*. None were arrested, and while stories conflict on the issue, the murder seemed to have occurred either after they had sex with but without having paid her, because she had asked for payment, or because she refused them sexually altogether (author's fieldnotes, Daru, November, 2003, January, 2004). Holly Wardlow's exciting new ethnography, *Wayward Women*, plays with the idea of 'negative agency' introduced in another context by Corinne Kratz, but she noted in an earlier discussion of Huli *pasindia meri*:

> [t]hey are stigmatized by their communities, often repudiated by their natal families, attacked by other women who suspect them of having sex with their husbands, and sometimes become prey to gang rape and murder by men who resent the fact that passenger women claim [reference omitted] the right to reject a potential sexual partner for any reason. (2004: 1037)

If 'Bamu' is substituted for 'passenger', my fieldnotes and case studies from 1990–1992 are replete with just such examples. Between 2003 and 2006 while I was working on the nationwide study I learned of many, many cases of precisely this, from Lae to Port Moresby, Goroka to Vanimo. On Daru and nearby, Bamu women are prostituted mostly by their husbands, not for shells, pleasure or ritual knowledge, but for cold, hard cash. Money supports their family, to be sure, but also enables their husbands to drink. Bamu women are treated roughly by customers, rudely by townspeople, violently by husbands and by health workers not with the compassion they deserve (Hammar 1999a, 2004c). Extremely few Bamu women receive contraceptive and antenatal services, seek HIVab testing, receive STD treatment, engage with condom promotion and HIV prevention activities or benefit from legal and political representation. Fear, shame and desire for compensation for provision of blood and other biological specimens prevented many Bamu from receiving the services provided by the IMR study there in 2003 and 2004.

Bamu women stigmatised on Daru and elsewhere as *tu kina meri* (cheap, easily available, sexually promiscuous women) little resemble the 'public harlots', 'professional beauties' and 'ceremonial prostitutes' to whom Flint (1919), Beaver (1920), Roheim (1940, 1946 – regarding another province), Butcher (1964) and others referred. Sexual delight and service were formerly integrated with food-preparation and feast-giving (cf. Wardlow 2004: 1028), if not also food-eating itself, and in local and regional trade, one fleet meeting another, husband standing alongside wife, wood and sex for meat and shells for masks and sago for gossip and tobacco. Patrol Officer Jack Hides took one interesting account from KAUPA, who stated that Gumak and Jauni people used a typical ruse to cover murderous intent. 'One GUMAK man, who had on a big cassowary head-dress and who spoke [M]otu, I now recognise as DANU. They told us to sit down and smoke; they said – "We will smoke and to-night you will have our women"'.[15] Nowadays, male ejaculations terminate the encounters, cash goes mostly to the husband-pimp and stigma attaches to the woman. The sex itself is stigmatized medically, too. For example, the heading 'History of Sex' in Ruta Fiti-Sinclair's brief communication regarding the study she conducted in Port Moresby in 1993 with 22 women in prostitution dealt not a whit with sex *per se*, but with infection with and treatment for STDs (1996: 120).

Remunerated sex proliferated amidst the arrival of new commodities, religious practices, social conditions and political powers. By the time Adrian Geyle visited Bamu river villages in 1953 to conduct an emergency venereal disease patrol, he noticed the absence of young-to-middle-aged men, who had been conscripted to work on copra plantations on the mainland and in the Torres Straits on pearling luggers. More young men began to leave Bamu villages in the late 1980s for work in sawmills and timber and oil-exploration camps. Some never returned, having died or been transplanted permanently to settlements in Port Moresby and elsewhere. Surely the loss of male labour *in* the villages (required for tree-felling, canoe-carving, hunting and garden-planting) and *between* them (in terms of trade and travel) added strain to already heavily burdened female shoulders. 'Pacification' opened new spaces in and between people and peoples when cannibalism and head-hunting were prohibited and sorcery denounced. The introduction of and trade in 'steel axes, knives, calico and beads' increased contact between Gogodala and Kiwai (Crawford 1981: 53), for example, which probably touched Bamu hands, too, perhaps further commoditising and expanding the trade in female sexual services and grounding it in the hands of men *qua* husbands. By 2003 and 2004 I found that Kiwai men had begun to prostitute their wives at *sagapari's* newest locale on the other side of the island – set between cemetery and swamp. Until quite recently none but Bamu women on Daru could be called '2KB' (i.e., *tu kina bus*). Even this, the lowest rung on the ladder of prostitution's labour forms, had been wrested from them.

Some said in 2004 that this had pushed Bamu families back into their homelands. An SBS television special in 2001 broadcast disturbing allegations about the treatment of Bamu female workers recruited into timber camps owned by the Malaysian logging giant, Rimbunan-Hijau. Women workers were allowed to leave, said the report, only after they have been 'forced to have sex with company officials and the police who work for them' (Dateline 2001). These claims echo those made about tuna, oil, gas and timber industries in Vanimo and Kikori, Moro and Lae, Goroka and Madang. If Bamu women weren't 'traditionally' prostituted in highly exploitive and brutalising ways, they surely are now. At varying points and with differing frequencies along south coast New Guinea, dinghies and outboard engines replaced paddles, canoes and outriggers, just as shotguns, cartridges, sauce-pans, bullets and handguns began to replace bows, baler-shell pots, arrows and spears. The 'value' of Bamu women has become perverted under the combined pressures of a cash economy, introduced alcohol consumption, migration and capitalist relations of production that have disenfranchised all Bamu.

Rather than locating the origin of sexual exploitation in ill-defined, highly reified concepts of 'tradition', as non-Bamu Daruans and evangelists suggest we do, it is better to interrogate the political-economy. *Tu kina bus* on Daru has for several decades immiserated Bamu women, Bamu families and, in quite other ways, probably the once-proud Bamu men, too. Left now with little but sexual services to trade, Bamu began to accrue a bad reputation as regards sexual and health stigmas that have increased over the years. Pierre Dufour (the pen name of Paul Lecroix) commented in his *History of Prostitution* that prostitution always lives on good terms with ecclesiastical and civil authorities, that it always comprises an important part of the 'body social' (Dufour 1926: 91). Those words are just as true about nineteenth century France as about 1960s-era Daru as about Papua New Guinea generally today.

STDs have been present in this area for at least a century, but have been made worse by human traffic, ethnic struggle, anti-condom sentiments, prodigious alcohol consumption, collapse of health service delivery and high levels of sexual violence (Gunther 1990; Hammar 1998a, 1999a, b, 2004b; Hughes 1997). Daru became in 1915 home to the Division's first venereal 'lock hospital', which was erected to treat the devastation primarily in rural villages wrought by a single STD – Donovanosis. Lock hospitals had by then been set up by both Papua and New Guinea administrations (Gunther 1990: 72) that required that sufferers complete hospital stays of up to two years, at least in the case of Donovanosis. Then known widely as 'granuloma venereum' (but by at least 30 other terms – see Hammar 1997: 29, n. 1), it devastated the Marind-anim and others across the border and many other peoples in the Papuan hinterlands. Kikori got its own 'lock hospital' in 1917 and now faces an extremely dire future, if the research the IMR conducted there in 2004 and 2005 is any clue. The Bamu among others were the subject of mid-century venereal medical patrols (Geyle 1998), and were served beginning in the mid-1980s by a New Zealand-based mission presence in nearby Balimo, although that presence has been severed owing to security issues, to lack of interest of expatriate staff and to government-sponsored upgrading of medical facilities and standards (Phil Carr, personal communication, 24 June 2007). There was significant focus later in the Goilala District of what is now Central Province upon Donovanosis outbreaks linked by church authorities to what they perceived to be orgiastic celebrations following feasting and who 'sought to have these dances banned by statute' (Gunther 1990: 72).

HIV and AIDS are well established on Daru and throughout Western and Gulf provinces. When I returned to Daru in 2003 after an absence of 11 years I learned that many friends and key informants from 1990–92 had already died or were dying, mostly under the radar. One was a mail-order bride from Fiji who had become the second wife of a school inspector; their young son has also died. Another was the young bride of a former governor; she had turned to prostitution upon finding out that he already had two wives and then divorcing him. When three crayfish-diving brothers died of AIDS the community became fearful because of their reputation for sexual promiscuity and penchant for sleeping with wives of other crayfish-divers. As disapproving in-laws played cards nearby I watched a young widow dying of AIDS move with great difficulty from shack to toilet. Although both of her sexual partners had been husbands, her in-laws blamed her for their son's death. Only one family member visited her in the hospital as she died of AIDS in February of 2004. I made another friend in 1992 who had recently separated from her German husband. By Christmas of 2003 she was suffering AIDS-related dementia, convinced that she had been engaged as the 'spiritual advisor' to the Israeli government, and died in early 2004. Many other of my friends and informants had also died from AIDS on Daru or back in the village, I was told.

Not surprisingly, Western Province has become for the Australian government a 'high-priority' province in terms of HIV and associated infections and illnesses. Australia closely watches the fragile relationship Papua New Guinea has with Indonesia to the west, but Western Province also shares a border, health facilities, water and cultural, sexual and historical ties with Torres Straits islanders. Public health among the latter has been extremely worrisome for many years. John Singe, who worked as a school-teacher on Thursday island, wrote that 'V.D. is out of control' (1989: 227). After having been trapped in political limbo for several years an AusAID-funded Sexual Health Clinic has finally been constructed on Daru. It treats STDs, diagnoses AIDS, tests serologically for HIVab and offers counselling services for Torres Straits islanders, just as many Papua New Guineans are served in the Torres Straits facilities nearby. Little has been done to help women trapped in sexual labour, however, and even less to mitigate the massive exploitation of Bamu women by customers and husbands and other pimps. Sex is certainly public enough in context of norms of male socialisation and alcohol consumption, and women, music and sexual excitement are just as obvious. When it comes to policy, however, sex, like marriage, remains private. 'Tradition', Christian doctrines, husbandly prerogative and public health models each prevent critical scrutiny of sex and marriage.

We will see in the next two chapters just how true that is, as two decades' worth of public health models and messages have persistently refused to put plain-old marriage on the policy table.

NOTES

1. A recently published novel that has had something of an underground notoriety, *The Blue Logic*, is founded upon ethnic/tribal stereotypes and clashes in Port Moresby. Tellingly, the one mention of 'Daru' has to do with Kiwai living in Kilakila (Horse Camp) settlement who are involved in gun-smuggling with Torres Straits islanders (Yakaipoko 2002). Other fictitious depictions of Kiwai in novels (including one with the name 'Daru') are strongly negatively stereotyping in terms of drinking, promiscuity and quickness to fight.

2. This latter example was provided to me by my *tambu*, whose name I won't spell here.

3. Brett Hilder's extended commentary on *The Voyage of Torres* (1980: 75) notes that in the Warrior Reefs area, and after having wantonly killed a youth, '[t]o add a touch of gallantry to the display of chivalry, the soldiers then chose three of the youngest women and took them aboard "for the service of the crew of the ship"'.

4. Goaribari have been dubbed sexually promiscuous, but they didn't migrate to Daru, essentially for safety reasons, owing to some number of them in 1901 having killed and eaten most of the LMS missionary, James Chalmers, his right-hand man, Tomkins, and eleven Kiwai carriers.

5. Charles Wilde notes for the Gogodala experience nearby that the inability of government authorities to sustain their presence in the area gave Gogodala 'time and space to adapt and continue' (2003: 10).

6. Phil Carr says (in a personal communication, 26 June 2007) that they were definitely the Standens, although many sources and pronunciations have it as 'Staunton'. Mabel Anne Bladon's intimate familiarity with them (see Bladon 1983, 1984) makes evident that their Baptist River Mission had been active in this area since 1936 or thereabouts.

7. Interestingly, it was precisely the more heavily populated and sedentary Bamu tribes upstream that both European and neighboring Papuan feared the most. In 1900, for example, then Resident Magistrate of the Western Division, C.G. Murray, easily found guides westward from Gaima on the north bank of the Fly river all the way up to but not into 'the swamp that lay ahead' (Crawford 1981: 21). At Maipani village in 1906, at the mouth of the Bamu river, the Sisiame, a huge settled tribe upstream, were convinced by the government-appointed Village Constable to raid and massacre them.

8. Papua New Guinea National Archives, CRS G91, Item 191a, Daru, Western Division, Patrol Reports, 1908–1909.

9. Papua New Guinea National Archives, CRS G91, Item 194, Daru, Western Division, Patrol Reports, 1913–1914.

10. Papua New Guinea National Archives, CRS G91, Item 194, Daru, Western Division, Patrol Reports, 1913–1914.

11. Papua New Guinea National Archives, CRS G91, Item 183C (Part), Daru, Western Division, Monthly Reports, August–December, 1903.

12. Papua New Guinea National Archives, British New Guinea Annual Reports, 1902–1903, Daru, Western Division. Box 6522, Folder 181.

13. Holly Wardlow's sample (2004) of 18 so-called *pasindia meri* (passenger women) from the Tari Basin consisted of 15 married and three unmarried women. My sample in 1991 on Daru of Bamu women toiling at *sagapari* was composed of 30 married women and one widow.

14. Or, tellingly, the agency they exhibit in refusing to be bartered, for example, one Miriam Wilngal, an 18-year-old high-school student who refused to become part of a compensation

claim (alongside $15,000 and 25 pigs) for the killing by her people of an enemy tribe big-man (see Mydans 1997).

15. Papua New Guinea National Archives, CRS G91, Item 211 (part) Daru Patrol Reports 1931/32.

Chapter 3

HIV in history

Serosurveillance and other studies, 1987–2007

Acronyms and acrimony

... STD epidemic is also rising rapidly thereby threatening the lives with high incidences reported in 1996–68, 1997–448, 1998–473, 1999–362, 2000–301 and 2002–306. The infections were mainly genital discharge and genital ulcer. The spread of the disease is driven by mainly unsafe sex between men and women through pleasurable heterosexual intercourse ...

... [Ours] remains the only town to have turned a major epidemic amount. Its extraordinary effort of multi-sectoral mobilization [has] pushed the adult HIV prevalence rate down from around .18% in the early 2000 to .6% in 2002. Elsewhere in some corners ... prevalence rates are still in double digits. [T]he main residential areas [named] have managed to slow in transmission ...

... Provincial government is loosing its grip on the escalating criminal operations perpetrated by youths, sex trading, high consumption of alcohol by both men and women and are confronted with mounting expenses for health and impoverishment care, reduced revenues and lower return on social investment. (NHASP 2002a: 1)

These three snippets are from one of the many impassioned documents written by local representatives of the National HIV and AIDS Support Project. The NHASP was funded with K120,000,000 by AusAID to run for five years beginning in October of 2000 and then funded again in October of 2006 to continue on in preparation for the next phase of the fight against HIV and AIDS. Entitled 'An HIV Overview', it was used during 'HIV/AIDS Workshops' and at other venues to instruct attendees in the 'natural history of HIV' and its epidemiology in Papua New Guinea and to train new recruits, staff and volunteers. Its specific contents and institutional provenance are worth examining in closer detail to reveal the structure and functioning of one of the major components of the national response – the provincial AIDS committee, or PAC – and the understanding of and tenor of rhetoric about the transmission of HIV. By one name or another, in one form or another, singular and plural, possessive and not, provincial-level AIDS committees, PACs and PACS (sometimes the 'C' means Council, sometimes Committee, just as 'S' can mean Secretariat but also denote plurality) have existed in Papua New Guinea since the mid-1990s. They were launched in at least six provinces under the rubric of the AusAID Sexual Health and HIV/AIDS Prevention and Care Project, later named the Foundation Project.

In another PAC an employee had stolen money and computer equipment from the PAC and also the PAC vehicle, which he crashed in another province before fleeing. He then forged documents claiming to be a medical doctor and was hired by a faith-based organisation (FBO) to lead a project. Neither its expatriate head nor the Board of Directors adequately checked his references, and so he became their clinical epidemiologist and supervised a study involving HIVab screening and the presumptive treatment of STDs in women in prostitution. In addition to having stolen financial documents, computer software and stationeries from the FBO, he racked up 3,000 kilometres on the organisation's vehicle and another 300 on that of the expatriate. He was alleged to have had sex with seven of the (only nine) women he enrolled in the study. He popped up later, emboldened with newly forged documents, and began working for another AIDS-related agency. The new, incoming head of the FBO was completely unaware of any of this. He was later accosted in a petrol station in Goroka by people who knew of his shenanigans and were affronted that he would return home without making amends (author's fieldnotes, 2004–6).

One chairperson of a PAC had been the Town Mayor. He was well-known as a philanderer, drunkard and abusive husband. I first met him on the edge of a public, outdoor prostitution locale. He died in 2003 of immune system breakdown aided by diabetes and gangrene that required several amputations and by lifelong tobacco and alcohol addiction. (Years after his death, however, his name still graced the NACS web-site page listing 'current' PAC personnel and contact details.) Following a cursory background check during an otherwise lengthy and expensive recruiting process, a replacement was found for the deceased Chairperson, but he was sacked within days of receiving his first paycheck and, upon getting drunk, assaulting the driver of the newly replaced vehicle in anger at having been refused the keys thereto. The PAC had been without one for nearly three years. Their first vehicle, a brand-new Toyota Hi-lux, had been crashed as the PAC Chairperson was being ferried about with his cronies, sex partners and beer in tow. One of the PAC's HRCs (HIV Response Coordinators) had previously been its PCC

(Provincial Counselling Coordinator) and was later taken to court by his wife on a charge of adultery. The NHASP entrusted him with supporting its nationwide social mapping study by monitoring and helping to conduct local research. Against the recommendations of the leader of the project, he had pocketed the money and engaged volunteers and others I had trained on a separate project (NHASP 2005c: 1; author's fieldnotes, 2005; personal communication with a NACS official, Port Moresby, April 2006). As had also occurred with respect to the Southern Highlands PAC, he had taken computer and other equipment to his home for personal use. In the computer, and without password protection, he kept records of the HIVab status of hospital patients. He engaged in sexual harassment on the job, but that did not lead to his sacking but to the resignation of the PAC's administrative assistant (author's fieldnotes, November, 2003 and February, 2004). He was many times observed under the influence of alcohol, including while on duty, which has been noted of other PAC personnel but which is only occasionally reflected in official documents (NHASP 2003b: 49, 2004b: 15, 2006d: 30). None of that was sufficient to remove him from his post, however. Other HRCs have been allowed to move from one province to another without demonstrating skills in capacity-building or financial acquittals (NHASP 2004b: Annex 5). The rate of HRC and PCC turnover is at 18 and 24 months on average, respectively (NHASP 2004b: 22). A NHASP review (2003b: 55) of a counselling training course in 2002 noted that 'there was a problem with the PAC chairman. He insisted on using the PAC vehicle for his own use. He also went to the PAC office and threatened the YOC [Youth Outreach Coordinator], a young girl who was extremely scared of being hit by him'. Her male counterpart told me that he had been imprisoned for several years in Port Moresby for his part in a murder (author's fieldnotes, November 2003). In 2004 he was accused of taking part in a pack-rape attempt that was foiled at the last second. When I raised these issues to NACS and NHASP officials in Port Moresby they only shrugged their shoulders; one said 'what can you do? Local politics'! In the meantime he had attended peer education workshops and training sessions in Port Moresby.

This PAC's Treasurer had been suspended (but put on half-pay) owing to several cases of mismanagement and clear conflicts of interest. One case involved the approval at the local and funding at the national level of a rogue 'serosurveillance' study conducted by a local doctor married to the HRC. (In another province the provincial counselling coordinator [PCC] is married to the HRC [e.g. NHASP 2004b: Annex 5].) Although this project began as an investigation of sexual behaviours and of the alleged sites of 'high-risk' sex (NHASP 2002c), risk was proclaimed, not investigated, and it soon morphed into a strict prospective serological 'study'. He and the new PCC eventually collected 775 blood samples in the provincial capital in settlements and at work-places and in villages and out-stations. The PCC claimed that 'sex workers' and others had 'voluntarily' consented to be tested. This seems a dubious claim given the illegal nature of the former's work, the moralistic tone of townspeople and church leaders toward them and the punitive nature of their relationship to legal authorities. Nor could HIVab test counsellors have handled even a tenth of the 775 study subjects.

There are least 30 languages spoken in the areas covered by the study; one of the counsellors was a Masters-level student whose way around the linguistic barrier was, he wrote in his thesis, to 'speak very, very slowly in English'. Although the physician and counsellor drew blood samples for screening for HIVab, participants could not have given fully informed consent, for neither test results, post-test counselling nor treatment for other infections were later provided. As well, many blood samples deteriorated under the hot sun while waiting for transportation that never arrived and were compromised further in the barely working refrigerator at the base hospital, which rendered at least one-third of them non-viable (author's fieldnotes, September and November, 2003 and February, 2004, based upon interviews with PAC officials and health workers). The physician noted that one leg of the study had to be abandoned because he hadn't brought any test tubes. He noted also that two airline tickets had been wasted because they had been late to the airport. The NACS-approved HIVab test counsellor had done 'some awareness at the [outstation school], which was not appreciated by the students and the staff' (NHASP 2002b: 1–2). An official from Port Moresby eventually showed up and shut down the study. Nevertheless, the doctor returned to private practice without incident and later received a prestigious honour from the Papua New Guinea Medical Society. He disavowed any ethical violations, he was still puzzled as to why he had been stopped, and he spoke ill of the study participants' 'jealousy' and obstinacy (author's fieldnotes, February, 2004). The NACS-approved counsellor told me that he had been instructed not to speak further.

These activities compromised the success of many HIV- and AIDS-related activities in its wake, not least of which were the social mapping study of the NHASP and those of the IMR and also of several well-intended VCT (Voluntary Counselling and Testing) initiatives. It is not known to what extent attendance was initially affected at the AusAID-funded Sexual Health Clinic, which finally opened in early 2006 after having been stuck in political limbo for several years. Townspeople were angry at having been 'tricked' into participation in the study by employers but never being able to learn their HIVab status (author's fieldnotes, February, 2004). The importance of these matters was amplified by the well-publicised death from AIDS of two nursing sisters, of a Fijian mail-order bride and several of her known sex partners (one of whom was an influential PAC member), and of three highly sexually active brothers from the same 'corner'. One of the latter had once been the de facto husband of a VSO (Voluntary Service Organization) volunteer who had for two years taught English at the local high school. One of the two nursing sisters had on her death-bed made quite public pronouncements of the names of nine sexual partners, one being a health official and 'AIDS researcher', another being a medical doctor who had multiple times been disgraced but never punished, only being moved from health facilities in one province to those in another. Caught *en flagrante delicto* several times in an unused hospital office having sex with women procured for him by drivers and security guards (giving him the moniker 'Dokta Bisket'[1] in reference to what he dubbed his lunchtime sexual conquests), that doctor was also charged many times in gun- and drug-related scandals (e.g. Pac News 2005;

National Court of Justice 2007; *Sydney Morning Herald* 2005b), although evidence against him was repeatedly 'lost' by policemen and other cronies. He is alleged to have been a local broker for the 'Aliens' gang who dealt with the 'Titanic' gang in Torres Strait. He now holds a prominent position in the infectious diseases section of the hospital and has been sponsored in Port Moresby to attend workshops and conferences. He didn't even recognise himself when these events were publicised in a presentation to NACS and NHASP officials.

✳ ✳ ✳

These characters and stories do not reflect well upon the nation's health workers, many of whom are highly dedicated, greatly underpaid and who work under often extremely trying conditions. Nevertheless, having worked in half of Papua New Guinea's provinces long enough to know, similar stories can be told of other health centres and PACs throughout the country. The sexually provocative or predatory ways of some of these health workers, of politicians, of diplomats and of policemen and jail warders is well known. Two officers in the Gulf Provincial Administration were recently brought up on charges of filming themselves engaged in various sexual acts and then producing a pornographic CD, entitled 'Scabies Dog'. 'Kerema Queen' and others similarly titled but made by others 'remain at large' (Fairparik 2008). In late 2007 the new Health Minister Sasa Zibe instituted reforms in good governance and accountability in the NAC as part of his efforts to reform the Health Department more broadly. Five senior officers, including Acting Director Mr Romanus Pakure, were asked to step down pending investigations of financial mismanagement and corruption. Reporter for *Pacific Magazine*, Alexander Rheeney, quoted Mr Rod Mitchell, CEO of both BAHA (Business Against HIV and AIDS) and NASFUND (the former National Provident Fund), as saying that the sacking of the top leadership of NACS showed that the governmental response was in shambles: 'The last few months have seen the effective unravelling of the National AIDS Council through legislative, legal and bureaucratic wrangles, maladministration and malaise. The government response to HIV is now in deep trouble. Many current activities of NACS – like condom distribution – need to be outsourced to businesses and NGOs' (Mitchell, quoted in Rheeney 2008). The writer of a letter to the editor of *The National* applauded Zibe for 'shaking the comfort zone of selfish people, who have found a safe haven and easy money from AusAID funds channelled through the National AIDS Council' (Morobean Observer 2008).

Unfortunately, NACS officials took Mr Zibe to National Court for allegedly not following 'sector processes' in sacking them, and the five were reinstated. That a legal technicality had been used to cover over such serious allegations at the nation's preeminent AIDS body was greeted with much dismay in Port Moresby and throughout the country by health workers and expatriate consultants alike. Minister Zibe buried the hatchet with the NACS in a very public way in March of 2008: Pakure handed over to him a live pig, they signed a peace agreement and the NAC pledged to recall their court case against Mr Zibe, thus allowing all NAC and NACS staff to return to work (*BW* 2008b).

The composition of the NACS of specific PACs, their expected roles and functions, and the ideas and behaviours of their members are therefore particularly telling of the promise of the national response but also of many of its weak spots. Of the provincial AIDS committee system, quite early on, Malau and Crockett (2000: 59) said that while 'the health sector had recognised the urgency of developing effective prevention measures, coordination was problematic and political commitment inconsistent'. What little critical attention has been paid to these matters has been phrased in terms of resource shortfalls, not lack of supervision; on communications snafus, not lack of individual accountability; on the inability sometimes of foreign consultants to 'get' Papua New Guinea, not on the political football that an STD clinic or rural hospital or intervention programme can be. The expatriate consultant who guided the roll-out of the antiretroviral programme suggested that the STD clinic in Lae 'is administratively not under the control of the hospital' (NHASP 2005a: 11). He does not apparently know that that is the norm, not exception, owing to the legacy of the colonial administrative experience. Venereal disease was during the colonial era a different animal, part of a European attitudinal *cordon sanitaire* and so constituted more of a political than a health problem. For decades STDs didn't 'belong' in a hospital so much as under the Provincial Health Office (Hammar 1998a; Hughes 1997).

The three snippets from the document cited at the outset of this chapter show that policy discussions focused at the urban, highly visible, national level can sometimes have little relevance to the intimate, local, often rural levels, even just on grounds of keeping of statistics. One of the recommendations made during the first-ever HIV Prevention Summit, held in Port Moresby in March of 2006, was that somehow the prevalence of STDs would be brought down to 5% in the 'risk populations' and to 3% in the so-called 'general population' (GoPNG 2006: 30). The prevalence is currently estimated to range from around 30% to 40% or more countrywide. The PAC document was admirably composed in English, which competes with probably another 25 languages in the provincial capital where it was written and another 800 or so throughout the country. Using terms such as 'multi-sectoral mobilization', an idea that was introduced and underwent formalisation in 2001, it relates AIDS to social inequities and economic strife. Nevertheless, it doesn't hold responsible any individuals, such as 'Dokta Bisket' above, the former PAC chairperson, the philandering PCC, the head of the rogue serosurveillance study or the male youth activity coordinator. It does not hold accountable any major power-holders, such as the provincial government itself, which is the single largest institutional purveyor and consumer of alcohol, owning distribution rights and being able to grant liquor licenses. Nor does it finger the criminal operations carried out by those other than disaffected youth gang members, that is, expatriates or public servants who are frequently arrested in gun- and drug-smuggling operations (e.g. Alpers 2005). It doesn't seem to acknowledge the *apparent* steep rise from 68 cases in 1996 to 448 in 1997 (but which was surely a typo), and then declines, and mistakes the highly endemic nature of a huge STD caseload in this area for a recent epidemic outbreak (Hammar 1998a, 2004c). Nevertheless, it does accept links between STDs and HIV and affirms the sexual means of their transmission, that is, without in the process invoking God or malign social relations and declining tradition, as other journalists and researchers have found (e.g. Eves 2003a, b, 2008; Levy 2006: 11, 15; McPherson 2008; NHASP 2005g; Tobias 2007: 11; Wardlow 2008). Also, and remarkably unlike other NACS and NHASP documents, it doesn't overtly blame women in prostitution. On the other hand, it mentions 'unsafe sex' (and even allows that sex is pleasurable, which is an extremely rare admission) but not condoms or issues of gender equity. It claims that this local HIV epidemic has been turned around owing to extraordinary effort, though empirical evidence collected shortly thereafter by the IMR was sharply contrary. (When publicised, the IMR evidence was discounted.) None of the 'risk areas' identified by respondents in the social mapping study were in people's homes, where the bulk of unsafe sex takes place. Neither was mentioned otherwise unused hospital offices or any of the other locales of sexual intercourse, whether government buildings, private offices and abandoned buildings (author's fieldnotes, 2003–2006), police stations (Amnesty International 2006: 20), or other sites of punishment (Reed 2003).

More tellingly, it suggests that HIVab serosurveillance activities were being conducted, settlement by settlement, though they were not. A single round of HIVab testing in this antenatal clinic in 2003, for example, turned it into one of '10 active sentinel surveillance sites' (NAC 2007: 22) when no more test results were reported for four years (NACS 2006b: 10, Table 1.9). At this and other would-be 'sentinel sites', figures were not adjusted for age and gender (see also NHASP 2005b: iii). The figures were aired with great alarm by the Governor-General in a workshop setting but who mistook Repeat Reactive test results drawn from the antenatal clinic for ones later 'disconfirmed' in Port Moresby; even worse, he claimed a 30% prevalence, which alarmed workshop attendees, and he suggested that homosexuality should be even further criminalised. The 2004 National Consensus Workshop (NHASP 2005e: 5) also claimed that the IMR had conducted 'sentinel'-type, clinic-based studies on Daru, in Lae and in the Porgera valley, when it hadn't, since these were community-based, inductive and treatment-oriented exercises, to a one. The document also promotes the idea that numbers by themselves speak in terms of 'baseline data' against which emergent trends may be assessed. 'Trends' is a term that is similarly misused in context of singular events or reports of data (e.g. NACS 2006a: 6, 8, 50). So does the term 'prevalence rates', which incorrectly connotes movement (rates) and stasis (prevalence) simultaneously. In any event, *the numbers in this example* (.18 to .6) *are speaking in the wrong direction* – going up, not down – and by more than three-fold! Use was not made of easily available and extensive documentation about these issues (Hammar 1996a, b, 1998a; 2004b).

The document reiterates the extraordinary promise of the national response to HIV and AIDS, but that promise remains in many ways unfulfilled. Rhetoric is too often confused with action, accounts of blood tests over-running those of suffering and dying.[2] Claims of surveillance – whether serological in nature or behavioural – have for too long gone unchallenged. Risk has been asserted and proclaimed instead of investigated, produced rhetorically and then 'verified' in dubious announcements of 'successes'. The announcement of '28 sentinel sites in 15 provinces, including four sites in rural areas, with over 580 people trained in data collection' (GoPNG 2006: 31–2) raises a number of pertinent questions that few seem willing to address in view of how many data are missing from quarterly reports and workshop presentations. When Australia's Foreign Secretary Alexander Downer spoke in Sydney to announce the ramping up of Australian aid to Papua New Guinea and the remainder of the Asia-Pacific region, he specifically mentioned a 'need to do more including more awareness, transferring of information to people and building the capacity in order for the country to respond better in tackling HIV/AIDS. So far', he said, 'Australia through AusAID has helped train 10,000 people in HIV/AIDS awareness, care and counselling and had distributed 700 million condoms throughout the country' (*Post-Courier*, 24 July 2007). 700,000,000 condoms? Really?

Capacity-building has been problematic also in cases of underperforming local organisations such as PACs. To be fair, there is also and a corresponding sense of overload felt by those supervising all too much, by those suffering from 'wearing too many hats' syndrome (NHASP 2006d: 28) or in not knowing which hat to wear in the first place. Provincial government officials, sometimes out in the communicatory hinterlands, have tended to feel that everything related to AIDS is the business of the NACS who, so they say, don't pay sufficient attention to or support them sufficiently well. The NACS in Port Moresby, on the other hand, has tended to act (for understandable reasons) as if PACs (and to a lesser extent, DACs) should manage their own programmes on the local level. The latter are often missing the resources, skills, political support and mandate to do so. The NHASP review of capacity-building efforts, Milestone 38, noted that the NACS was 'unable to provide management and supervisory support to the PAC[s] due to limited resources and competing priorities. Support includes supervising the HRCs [HIV Response Coordinators] and PCCs [Provincial Counseling Coordinators], operational support and monitoring financial processes' (NHASP 2004b: 9).

The sources of such problems are many. NHASP officials have their hands tied by national-level politics: do-little PAC employees are almost impossible to sack. Based in Port Moresby, NHASP officials for good reason know little of personnel recruited to PAC positions or of difficulties between PACs, provincial government, local churches and hospitals. This has blunted accountability and resulted in too little attention being paid to capacity-building. The NHASP review of VCT initiatives, for example, revealed data-collection and record-keeping practices that varied greatly throughout the country, despite there being consistent protocols for such, clearly stated expectations and mechanisms for dealing with shortfalls. Five of the first cohort of people to go on antiretrovirals died, one of heart attack secondary to anaemia, but regarding her case and those of others, the cause of mortality 'was unclear. It is difficult to find notes, or determine the cause of death even when the notes are available. A more rigorous analysis of adverse outcomes would be desirable, but may not be achievable' (NHASP 2005a: 10). Anaemia was reported to be the leading immediate cause of death of AIDS patients as of 2006, with *pneumocystis carinii* pneumonia and tuberculosis being second and third (Treat Asia 2006). Having visited many STD and other clinics and health centres from 2003 to 2006, I can concur: data collection systems need to be strengthened and case-study and interviewing techniques can be improved. This is precisely where social scientific expertise can be put to good work. A NHASP review of the data collected at VCT sites concluded that:

> This data [sic] is mainly statistical with very little narrative component. Some centres visited had difficulty in sending their monthly reports on time, for others this had become routine. The written reports that were kept had very little information and the content was not immediately clear. There was little or no written institutional history in many of the centres. Most of the information about the work of the centres was 'known' by the staff, but not recorded. (NHASP 2006a: 21)

Another part of the problem is the extent to which the case reports themselves are unique. Many people seem to be getting tested twice, thrice and more but at different locations (Gerawa 2003), which clinicians may or may not know about. This is partly because people do not believe what pieces of paper tell them – in both directions. On the one hand, it hardly makes sense in the first place for people who are healthy to get tested for HIVab, and a 'positive' 'AIDS test' (which is actually quite negative, and which is not a clinical test for markers of disease, anyway) simply cannot, and therefore must not be true. Van Amstel and van der Geest (2004: 2092–3) have contributed valuable case studies showing for the Southern Highlands Province capital of Mendi how little compensation claims regarding injuries are based upon the facts of actual hospital records, compared to their rhetorical manipulation. 'A medical report proving that a person died a natural death', they argue, 'will not remove the accusation of sorcery (poisin)'. On the other hand, clinical, psychological and ethnographic literature is mounting that tells of 'the worried well', for whom persistently HIVab seronegative findings to the same extent simply cannot be true and who thus seek repeated tests (Biehl 2007). This problem has been aided and abetted each time HIV and AIDS are conflated (e.g. 'HIV/AIDS', 'HIV/AIDS test', 'HIV/AIDS virus', 'AIDS test' and the like). People cannot help but be confused by phrasings such as 'people living with the HIV/AIDS virus in their area' (Gumuno 2008), and yet that is the norm, even in so-called 'awareness campaigns'. This is also because of problems of logistics, communication and coordination. The NHASP review of the antiretroviral roll-out notes that 'the PMGH laboratory regularly did not have reagents for certain tests. There was a very high rate of test results that were not returned to the [Heduru] clinic. Some tests were simply not done. In other cases the laboratory claimed they had not received samples' (NHASP 2005a: 8). People go elsewhere to be tested again when they haven't yet received results from prior tests.

Telling stories

With these more intimate asides grounded in close personal experience I turn now in this section to painting in broad strokes a portrait of the history of HIVab surveillance in Papua New Guinea. I have been more or less intimately involved in these issues since at least 1990, having had the privilege of visiting and then living for five years plus in Papua New Guinea, both during

> *'In settings such as PNG, emergency action against HIV/*
> *AIDS is called for, but the nature of this emergency is long-*
> *term' (O'Keeffe, Godwin and Moodie 2005: 38).*

the early years of the HIV epidemic (1988, 1990–2) and when the national response was being greatly ratcheted up (2003–6).

The editorial published in 1996 by Carol Jenkins in the *Papua New Guinea Medical Journal*, a venue that more than any other has kept these issues at the forefront, still rings largely true in 2008. She notes (1996: 164) that '[i]t has been a long and difficult process to bring AIDS ... to the attention of the people of Papua New Guinea' and that, despite 'voices of alarm' having 'been raised in various quarters' (e.g. Hammar 1993a, b, 1996a, b, 1998a; Hughes 1991; NSRRT and Jenkins 1994), attempts made again and again 'to gain political support for a serious national AIDS prevention campaign [were] met with silence'. 'By mid-1994', she continued, 'most of the alarmed voices had declined to a whisper' and even much ballyhooed programmes and projects had been met, when met at all, with 'complacency' (1996: 164). Bill Bowtell's recent policy paper for the Lowy Institute similarly blames a 'failure of political will to translate scientific evidence into good policy in time to cap and control the spread of the virus' (2007: 3). Although O'Keeffe, Godwin and Moodie are right generally with the following claim, it doesn't apply to Papua New Guinea specifically. 'Especially in the early stages of an epidemic', they write,

> leaders will be more readily convinced to invest resources and attention to HIV/AIDS if they understand the epidemiological characteristics of HIV. This includes the long period of latency [which was well established by the early 1990s], the way it can spread explosively in vulnerable populations and then more broadly throughout the whole population [ditto], its incurability [which has long featured prominently in many campaigns], the complexity of treatment, and the way HIV/AIDS interacts with and compounds the impact of other prevalent diseases [known to medical officers since at least 1990]. (O'Keeffe, Godwin and Moodie 2005: 21–2)

The NACS has noted with admirable candour that, '[w]hereas global evidence indicates that strong leadership and honest political commitment and advocacy are vital to making a difference in HIV/AIDS epidemic, leadership is yet to become very vocal in advocacy in PNG' (NACS 2006a: 10). I would affirm in general terms the tone of this and like-minded documents but perhaps shift the wording slightly to read that since roughly 2003 the advocacy has been quite vocal – indeed, at points it has seemed alarmist bordering on shrill – but that it can yet be superficial. It seems yet to obsess over 'awareness' and individual acts of unkindness instead of showing concern for fundamental changes that need to be made in social-structure. Rhetoric has too often substituted for action, and Culture is invoked about as often as it is denied in the moralistic, preachy slogans and messages that oppose social norms and obligations around sexuality, fertility and gender relations. I accept that many of those latter realms of social life need to change in order on a mass scale to prevent HIV transmission. Claims about 'high-risk' this and 'high-risk setting' that, have too often preceded instead of followed empirical investigation. Such pronouncements seldom lead very far

> *'Not to develop a john-based strategy', said two social scientists some time ago, 'leads to misguided policy and ineffective intervention. The mistake is doubtless related to the cultural perceptions of the men who control such policy. After all, boys will be boys' (Hammel and Friou 1994).*

up the ladder to where powerful organisations set the tone and authorise the kind of language that can be used.

Although discussions in Papua New Guinea have since Jenkins' 1996 editorial been raised to a level above that of a whisper, many wonder whether too little has been done too late. Ballard and Malau (2002: 3) note that many politicians and health officials early on opposed the diversion of funds to AIDS prevention, although others in the late-1980s, including Minister Robert Suckling and clinicians such as Tompkins Tabua and Malau himself did their best to push public and private levers in planning for an eventual epidemic. Similar worries have been expressed more recently with regards to the advent of antiretroviral therapies and the fear that their considerable costs may cut terribly into prevention efforts (WHO-SPC 2004: 1). The Australian journalist Trevor Cullen notes that when he interviewed 10 current and former newspaper editors in Papua New Guinea in 1999, they 'revealed a lack of awareness and urgency about the potential consequences of an emerging HIV/AIDS epidemic within the country. Coverage was mainly limited to the latest figures, workshops and donations' (Cullen 2003b: 77). In 2000, the first Director of the NAC, Dr Clement Malau, and his colleague in the AusAID-funded Interim Sexual Health Project, Ms Sue Crockett, suggested that the national response had been 'slow to evolve' (Malau and Crockett 2000: 59) owing to political sensitivities, to an inability to 'visualise' AIDS by extrapolating from STDs (see Hammar 1998a; Hughes 1997; Richards 2004; Riley 2000) and because of a lack of coordination between church, government, business and community. Consequently, the National Executive Council failed, despite many presentations thereof, to pass the National AIDS Council Act, 'and programmes lost technical and funding support when the Global Programme on AIDS was withdrawn' (Malau and Crockett 2000: 59). Jenkins noted also that '[m]uch complacency still remains, despite far greater awareness in the general population' (2002: 7).

HIV and AIDS in Papua New Guinea at a glance

The first newspaper article about any of these topics, so far as I am aware, was published in 1985 in the *Post-Courier*. To this end, I do not agree with Cullen's claim as I understand it that the first AIDS-related article published in a Papua New Guinea newspaper was published on 12 June 1987 by *The Independent* (Cullen 2000: 130), a newspaper then wholly owned by Papua New Guinea's four mainline churches. 'Test Kits Here for AIDS' [sic] noted the first arrival in the region of HIVab test kits. Right from the outset, therefore, HIV (the Human Immunodeficiency *Virus*) and AIDS (the Acquired Immunodeficiency Disease *Syndrome*) were confused and conflated. Newspaper stories, government documents, academic researchers and policy papers in about equal measure can still be careless with words and imprecise in phrasings, confusing HIV with AIDS and suggesting that AIDS is a singular disease. The ceaseless use of the imprecise and confusing 'HIV/AIDS' wouldn't be quite so bad if the speakers weren't at the same time usually condemning the knowledge bases and attitudes of the people whom they are supposed to be serving. The Director for the Enga University of Papua New Guinea, Mr Raphael Tombe titled his 2008 presentation to the Papua New Guinea Association for Distance Education biennial conference 'Zero Effectiveness on HIV/AIDS Awareness and the Need for a Separate HIV/AIDS Curriculum in Papua New Guinea'. In it he expressed surprise that 'a vast majority of people were still confused and cannot differentiate between HIV and AIDS' (Kanu 2008). His presentation didn't either. The results of the 2004–2005 Second Generation Surveillance of six Pacific island countries were published in 2006 to great fanfare, but one of the proxies of 'correct' knowledge of Pacific islanders was 'Number of respondents … who know that a healthy looking person can transmit AIDS' (WHOSSP 2006: 13, Table 1.3), when of course AIDS can be transmitted by neither healthy nor unhealthy people, although HIV can.

So far as I am aware, the next two articles in which AIDS is mentioned were published on 7 January 1986 ('VD Shock: It's Out of Control') and 17 January ('Youths Main VD Target'). The set of articles published in the *Post-Courier* later that year and into 1987 represent well the kind and allowable parameters of discourse about HIV and AIDS. For example, AIDS was early on constructed as a 'Sex *Abuse* Disease' (18 August 1986), not so much implicating mere sexual transmission of HIV as implying immorality and sexual promiscuity. Florid metaphors were published early, too, such as 'The Plague Sweeping' (19 December 1986) and 'AIDS Creeps Across Asia' (4 February 1987). Article titles implicated migration and alcohol consumption, sexual immorality and abuse and especially the promiscuity attached to being expatriate or involved in prostitution. Women already dubbed *pamukus* and *tu kina meri* by two decades' worth of newspaper articles were further constructed linguistically and serologically as harbors and reservoirs and carriers of infection, and worse, as the signs and signifiers of rapid socioeconomic change and breakdown in family values. 'Prostitution Rife in the Urban Areas', said a *Post-Courier* headline from 1 November 1990, the story behind which told of a Family Planning Association press conference held the previous day. The origins of AIDS were assumed to lie elsewhere, even though the specific diseases usually mentioned – *pneumocystis carinii* pneumonia, tuberculosis, anaemia and the like – were sufficiently well known to most Papua New Guineans. Papua New Guinea was represented as something of a blank (but absorbent) slate upon which infections washed as akin to a tidal wave or a spreading stain. AIDS was in the early years rhetorically located primarily in the bodies of despised people such as women in prostitution, although others blamed for it were not so marginalised, such as expatriates and homosexuals. These were contrasted with those dubbed 'innocent' (babies and infants). Notably, and quite unlike the situation in other countries, there has yet to occur a report of a case in which HIV was acquired through transfusion of blood or blood product. Jenkins (2000: 23) attributes this partly to a switch to ever younger school student donors. Not all blood donations, however, were screened up until 2000 (GoPNG 1998: 7; WHO-NAC-NDoH 2000: 4). Nor are high school students necessarily the studious virgins others hope of them.

Table 3.1 AIDS-related articles in the Papua New Guinea Post-Courier, 1986–7

Date	Title
(1986)	
7 January	'VD Shock: It's Out of Control'
17 January	'Youths Main VD Target'
18 August	'Fight to Halt Sex Abuse Disease'
19 December	'The Plague Sweeping'
(1987)	
4 February	'AIDS Creeps Across Asia'
16 April	'AIDS Action'
6 May	'Students Warned About AIDS'
11 May	'AIDS Lessons Get the Chop'
27 May	'Bishops Urge Action Now'
6 June	'Politician Calls for AIDS Checks'
2 July	'AIDS Victim in P.M.'
3 July	'A "Killer" That Can't Be Bested'
6 July	'PNG Prostitute Has AIDS'
10 July	'New Aspects to the AIDS Furore'
22 July	'AIDS Test or No Entry'
24 July	'AIDS: When Its Murder'
30 July	'Catholics Condemn Condoms', 'Sydney Meeting on AIDS'
8 August	'Churches Urge AIDS Actions'
29 September	'Another AIDS Carrier'
1 October	'Rabaul AIDS Rumors Denied'
5 October	'Premier Fears AIDS in Isle of Love'
23 November	'AIDS Testing: MPs lead way'

Source: Lawrence Hammar, Author's fieldnotes, 1991–2, based upon manual searches of back issues of the Post-Courier.

The early emphasis in newspaper reporting upon women in prostitution is hardly surprising, for prostitution-related tropes had for a long time featured heavily in the pages of *The Independent*, the *Post-Courier*, the *Times of Papua New Guinea* and the *Wantok* (in Tok Pisin). 'Pamuks on the Rise' was the title of a feature story based on changes that had occurred on market day in West New Britain Province around pay-day. An authority local to the market-place, however, noted that it was not local women from his block who were coming in droves to do this, but 'women from other provinces on the block' (*Post-Courier*, 18 August 1973). 'Prostitution: the Great Debate (Again)' was the title of a commentary in the *Times* (11 January 1986), and it noted that most women in prostitution prosecuted for such had been charged under the Vagrancy Act instead of the Summary Offences Act. Tellingly, the author had difficulty distinguishing typists and clerks from 'professionals' and 'part-timers' from school students and housewives in attempting to define prostitution and describe the contours of Port Moresby's sex industry. The first several years' worth of AIDS-related coverage was no different. Four of the first six articles published in the *Post-Courier* once an HIVab+ case had been reported (2, 3, 6, 10, 22 and 24 July 1987) implicated prostitution without presenting any evidence of HIV transmission dynamics or apparent concern for the woman, her sexual partners and her family or the conditions under which she might have been infected. Trevor Cullen's quantitative assessment of newspaper coverage of HIV and AIDS shows clearly enough the same dynamic at work well into the late 1990s, with articles titled 'Forty sex workers test HIV positive', 'Prostitution and the AIDS dilemma', 'Sex Workers High Risk for AIDS', 'Brothel Fears in Rabaul' and 'Sex workers: high-risk group for HIV' (Cullen 2000: 168). Jenny Hughes noted in 2002 of work she conducted a decade earlier that women in prostitution in the Tari Basin of Southern Highlands Province have been a convenient scapegoat for local communities. 'Regular commercial sex, reported by 70% of men, was seen by the men as the source of their infections' (Hughes 2002: 131). The Summary Report for the nationwide social mapping study concluded that '[a]nother common misconception, found in all provinces, is that the virus only affects prostitutes or people living in towns and cities while people in rural villages are safe' (NHASP 2005g: 14). Hughes commented in 1991 upon the existence of a 'strongly held belief among the Huli population' that a 'small infected pool of prostitutes (*pasendia meri*)' was responsible for the bulk of sexually transmitted disease in the area. This attitude has led to a cavalier attitude to prevention, she says, men claiming that 'the women they sleep with do not fall into this category and therefore they are not at risk' (Hughes 1991: 134).

This kind of attitude, however, is just as evident in high as low places. More than a decade after the first diagnosis of AIDS in Papua New Guinea, the then Health Department Secretary argued that prostitution was 'on the rise, resulting in an increase in HIV/AIDS diseases' (quoted in Tobia 1998: 31). This was a most unfortunate phrasing since neither 'HIV' nor 'AIDS' are 'diseases' and because it implied that somehow tuberculosis and malnutrition and pneumonia and cytomegalovirus and diarrhoea also result from prostitution. As well, by this time it was becoming well known that 'housewife' had nearly three times more infections attached to it than 'sex worker' in emerging epidemiological data, although 84% of the cases had no 'occupational' status attached to them (CIE 2002: 83). No shortage of ethnographic and other data existed as to the special risks of marriage (Hammar 1996a, b; Hughes 1991, 1997; NSRRT and Jenkins 1994; Zimmer-Tamakoshi 1993a, b, 1997). Not surprisingly, the very next article published in the *Post-Courier* condemned condom usage and another published the same day indicated the likely future of AIDS prevention campaigns: overseas aid. Trevor Cullen's work in this regard (see especially 2000) is important for confirming quantitatively what I am suggesting also qualitatively. He finds also in the early years of the HIV epidemic in Papua New Guinea a decided slant in newspaper coverage with stories that place HIV and AIDS '"out there" rather than "within the country"' (2000: 125). Just as others have found with regards to press coverage in other countries, Cullen finds between 1987 and 1997 an almost inverse relationship between extent of newspaper coverage and the number of new infections being reported. Interestingly, 1993, which was a busy kind of year in other ways, was one characterised by greatly decreased frequency of *Post-Courier* published articles, letters, editorials and other items regarding HIV and AIDS. Cullen concludes that between 1993 and 1995, 'when HIV infections began to make a significant increase within the country, press coverage of HIV/AIDS in the *Post-Courier* reached its lowest point' (2000: 127).

The fact that 'HIV' is mentioned in none of these articles is notable. Condoms are stigmatised. Fears were expressed as to potential harm to traditional custom and the tourism industry (i.e., the Yam Harvest Festival in the Trobriand Islands). More tellingly, the fact that the first person in Papua New Guinea reported to have died of AIDS was a policeman, neither a sex worker, an expatriate, nor a homosexual, was not highlighted in the press. In similar fashion, the first person in New Caledonia found to be HIVab+ was a French soldier, in 1986, fully three years before an indigenous Kanak person was found to be so (Salomon and Hamelin 2008: 83). Interestingly, the policeman was from the Morehead District area in Western Province, and he died at home after having been hospitalised both in Port Moresby and on Daru. This was followed close upon by the deaths of his wife and child (Hammar 1998a: 264). Indeed, the well known mobility and sexually active nature also of Papua New Guinean policemen, politicians and businessmen was routinely suppressed in the public press in these early years. The suppression to some extent persists today, although scandal breaks out periodically when Papua New Guinean diplomats and politicians misbehave. It was reported in April of 2008 that 'a certain PNG diplomat' had been discovered 'luring professional women and underage children into a PNG High Commission office abroad and sexually abusing them' (Joku 2008).

The relatively lengthy incubation period for HIV was well known by 1987, which pushed back the longevity of HIV in the country and region. Nevertheless, newspaper stories represented the emergence of HIV as if it was a complete surprise. This enabled the externalisation of risk and fuelled the growing tendency to blame. By 1988, the seventh Papua New Guinean had died. Two of those first seven, it was pointed out, were females with histories of 'multiple, expatriate and Melanesian sexual partners' (Currie *et al.* 1988: 100). Again, however, *no evidence of transmission was presented*. Most Papua New Guinean *men* have multiple Melanesian sexual partners and that some of them also have multiple expatriate ones many of whom also have multiple Melanesian sexual partners. Unfortunately, this has figured in neither popular nor public health understandings of HIV transmission dynamics or its epidemiology. When a new condom designed for and marketed to the Papua New Guinea Defence Force was announced in 1992, one Colonel Ani encouraged all his soldiers 'to use condoms in all their "encounters"' (*Post-Courier*, 21 February 1992). Was this supposed to include wives and girlfriends?

The following year George Nurse and Diro Babona, the latter of whom came to head the Central Public Health Laboratory in the Port Moresby General Hospital, published an article (Babona and Nurse 1988) that brought to the attention of health officials the seroprevalence of antibodies to human T-cell lymphotropic virus type I or HTLV-I (where today's 'HIV-I' and 'HIV-II' were once 'HTLV-III' and 'HTLV-IV') and raised the important issues of serological cross-reactivity. In 1989, Michael O'Leary and colleagues (O'Leary *et al.* 1993) commenced a pilot study of serological evidence of HIVab and found three HIVab+ samples among the 1,233 tested, for a seroprevalence of .0024%. The study proper was carried out from June of 1989 to May of 1990 and tested 7,948 blood samples collected from what were assumed to be 'low-risk' (antenatal clinic attendees) and 'high-risk' (STD clinic attendees) populations, though none were found to be HIVab+. This *seeming* paradox – zero prevalence in a 'high-risk' population – didn't budge prevailing models of the constitution of risk. Neither did people appear to accept that antenatal females might also have STDs (but weren't attending the STD clinic or that some STD clinic attendees might be pregnant). By May, 1990 there had by other means been identified, however, a total of 45 HIVab+ blood samples, but again the authors were somewhat puzzled by the seronegative findings in ostensibly high-risk populations. They proposed three reasons why, but discounted the third, which was laboratory error. Further but also limited attempts at serosurveillance occurred in 1991 and 1992, this time finding five more HIVab+ cases of 6,035 samples screened by ELISA (Enzyme-linked Immunosorbent Assay), but all five having been found from among 2,000 attendees of the Port Moresby STD Clinic, resulting in an HIVab seroprevalence of .0025%.

Outside the STD clinic, through the blood donation service and in other clinical settings, 118 more people were diagnosed with HIV infection by the end of 1992. Researchers found 21% of the males and 19% of the females to be suffering from genital ulcers; the prevalence figures established were highest in Mt. Hagen and lowest in Wewak. Almost 8% of the STD clinic patients had a reactive test for syphilis, as did nearly 4% of antenatal clinic attendees. Perhaps this suggests that the latter were not necessarily the hoped-for 'low-risk' subjects against whom could be pitched expectations of 'high-risk' rates later. Quite sensibly, they warned that, already by 1993, Papua New Guinea had a 'recognized AIDS problem' that was going to worsen because of relatively low levels of accurate knowledge of STD signs and symptoms and transmission routes and because relatively few people attended clinics to treat the extremely high levels of especially ulcerative STD found in the country. The same point was made sharply by Mary Louise O'Callaghan in 1995, who noted that, of the women surveyed in the 1991–1992 nationwide study, '65% said they did not know how AIDS could be prevented and only 16% were aware that it was fatal' (1995: 3). The researchers employed the 'tip-of-a-much-larger-iceberg' metaphor to underline the fact that the greatest bulk of clinical diagnoses of AIDS and serological ones of HIVab had been made in a passive case-finding system; they had not been found, that is, through highly regulated and carefully conceptualised serosurveillance. From these early clinical and serological findings had sprung in 1990, just as importantly, an 'STD-AIDS Unit' located within the Department of Health, which in name sponsored my research on Daru from 1990–1992 and which made available a small stipend in recognition of work I completed on Daru. It was later abandoned, however, for lack of funding and political sponsorship, because positions went unfilled, because quarterly reports were no longer being written and because bills were going unpaid (Jenkins and Passey 1998: 247). Initial efforts at surveillance and monitoring 'focused on ensuring safe blood supplies and establishing HIV antibody testing throughout the country', and the health sector 'established a National AIDS Surveillance Committee in 1986' (Malau and Crockett 2000: 59) so as to develop policy guidelines and investigate the future of surveillance and monitoring. This body became critical for the later overseeing of the 'the activities prescribed in the Short-Term Plan for 1987–1988' (Ballard and Malau 2002: 2–3).

Table 3.2 AIDS-related articles in the Papua New Guinea Post-Courier, 1988

Date	Title
6 January	'AIDS Trio Vow to Leave Disco Scene'
7 January	'Precaution Talk is All Rubbish'
12 January	'Night Clubs Worry', 'AIDS Tops Agenda in London Conference'
4 February	'Church Tackles AIDS'
23 February	'AIDS Top Priority'
10 March	'AIDS is Not Our Worst Problem'
4 April	'An Alarming Increase in Diseases'
14 April	'PNG Health News: AIDS in PNG – the Facts'
9 May	'AIDS Alarm: Victims go into hiding'
10 May	'Expatriates Face AIDS Test'
11 May	'Close Nightclubs: MP'
13 May	'AIDS: Control Still Lacking'
16 May	'Doctors Gear Up for AIDS Campaign'
19 May	'Papua New Guinea and AIDS'
20 May	'Sex Habits the Key to Prevention'
23 May	'AIDS Fight Started'
24 May	'Visiting Senator', 'Ambassador Dismisses Epidemic Allegation'
27 May	'Disease Threat to Pregnancy'

Date	Title
1 June	'Health Chiefs Call for AIDS Action'
16 June	'Sexually Transmitted Diseases'
1 July	'Meeting on AIDS'
7 July	'Workshop on AIDS'
21 July	'Can Mosquitoes Cause AIDS?: a letter'
28 July	'AIDS: Tests Find Four More'
3 August	'Doctors Warn of More Cases'
5 August	'AIDS Test for Single Expats'
9 August	'Why the Tests Are Needed'
10 August	'Disco Boss'
12 August	'More Heat on Suckling's Discos'
15 August	'VD Cases Highest in Highlands regions'
18 August	'No Prostitution'
19 August	'AIDS Policy Soon'
23 August	'Anti AIDS Move'
29 August	'Rabaul Fears AIDS'
31 August	'Help Us to Halt AIDS'
1 September	'AIDS Reports Rile Leaders'
7 September	'Getting a Look at AIDS', 'Rabaul Moves on AIDS Awareness'
20 September	'Questions About AIDS: Letter'
21 September	'Two Here to Fight AIDS'
25 October	'2000 AIDS Carriers'
1 December	'Massive Campaign Starts Against AIDS'
2 December	'War on AIDS Begins at Home'
5 December	'Anis: Moral Decline'
15 December	'Group Tackles Condom Image', '20,000 AIDS Posters'

Source: Lawrence Hammar, Author's fieldnotes, 1991–2, based upon manual searches of back issues of the Post-Courier.

Table 3.2 presents article titles from 1988. 'HIV' has yet to appear, nightclubs are once again fingered as feared hot-spots of infection, women who frequent them are dubbed AIDS 'carriers', 'AIDS tests' are proclaimed (when none such exist) and risk has been projected outward toward single expatriates (presumably males). In New Caledonia at this time local notions of risk were projected outwards toward French soldiers, and thus AIDS became 'white people's sickness' (Salomon and Hamelin 2008). The Papua New Guinea public was again comforted by news reports that blood transfusion services were reporting remarkably few HIVab+ blood donations; among healthy blood donors, the rate was only 0.005% in 1990, although it had risen by 1998 to 0.024% (NHASP 2001: 12). By 1996, according to Tozer (1996), only 11 blood donors had tested HIVab+, although eight of those had been detected in the previous year and a half only.

Table 3.3 depicts article titles from 1989 and 1990 in the *Post-Courier*. Anti-condom sentiments were aired at this time and later, by both men and women in the street and high-ranking politicians, religious leaders and health officials. At the first national AIDS seminar, Papua New Guinea's Attorney-General at the time, Bernard Narokobi, for example, said 'I don't believe condoms should be made available to the young people as it only promotes promiscuity and adultery' (quoted in the *Post-Courier*, 20 February 1992, p. 12). Though not the first equation of condoms and promiscuity, it was especially powerful because it came from the national leader associated with 'the Melanesian Way', a respected leader and legal expert.

Table 3.3 AIDS-related articles in the Papua New Guinea Post-Courier, 1989–90

Date	Title
(1989)	
1 January	'Health Workers Meet to Plan'
12 January	'Sexual Diseases Gaining Ground'
23 January	'AIDS Update'
1 February	'Rampant VD Alarms Madang Author'
3 February	'Chinese Herbal Medicine for PNG'
2 March	'Plague of AIDS'
7 March	'Daru in Major Health Worry'
17 March	'AIDS Warning: Control Habits'
1 August	'28,000 in PNG, STDs'
6 October	'Authorities Fear Outbreak of AIDS in Highlands'
17 October	'Baby is Among PNG's AIDS Cases'
2 November	'Condoms Aren't the Answer to AIDS: Minister'
10 November	'Campaign Combats AIDS'
1 December	'Health Officials Appeal for Caution'
15 December	'AIDS Poster Winner'
(1990)	
28 February	'Youths Must be Protected'
15 March	'Two Babies in List of 16 AIDS Deaths'
26 March	'AIDS Awareness Exhibition Begins'
6 April	'Expat in Lae Found be AIDS Carrier'
23 April	'Contraception Now Available Without Spouse's Consent'
3 May	'AIDS Scare Serious'
4 May	'More than 3000 visit AIDS Exhibit'
9 May	'AIDS Fight'
10 May	'AIDS Epidemic Looms: Forum'
17 May	'Sexual Diseases on the Increase in Morobe'

Source: Lawrence Hammar, Author's fieldnotes, 1991–2, based upon manual searches of back issues of the Post-Courier.

By my manual count of scrap-books maintained by the *Post-Courier*, there were another eight stories published in 1991, for example, 'Break the Custom on Sex: Kwarara', and another 11 in 1992, such as 'The Young More Prone as Carriers'. During this initial period, 1985–1992, the pattern is compellingly clear. There shall be no mention of putative cause, only terrifying effects. There shall be (rightfully) enthusiastic coverage of workshops, campaigns and visits of foreign consultants and ambassadors. There shall be alarming note taken of worsening statistics, especially as regards untreated STDs. Condoms shall not be spoken of positively, when spoken of at all. Youth, expatriates and women in prostitution shall be targeted. Neither marriage, male sexual privilege, nor powerful businessmen and politicians shall be mentioned. In this latter aspect *Post-Courier* coverage in the late 1980s and early 1990s was simply following precedent: I counted over 150 articles published about prostitution from 1972 to 1986 (author's fieldnotes, September, 1990). Representative titles included 'Synod Against Brothel Idea' (1973), 'Independence Day Upstaged by Prostitution Worries' (1974), 'Women's Meeting Against Prostitution' (1976), 'Schools Used as Brothels at Night' (1978), 'K2 Bush Business is a Disgrace' (1980), 'Can the Rapes Stop by Opening Brothels?' (1982), 'Modern Problem' (1984) and 'Don't Legalise Prostitution, says Church' (1986).

During these first few years when blood samples were being screened for HIVab the Central Public Health Laboratory adopted the then routine strategy of doing so first by ELISA and then 'confirming' them, in case of a Repeat Reactive test result, by use of a Western Blot test performed in Australia. A WHO recommendation made during 1992, however, was adopted in Papua New Guinea in 1993 such that two different, additional ELISA tests were to be performed in case of a Repeat Reactive. Discrepant test results were then to be resolved by application of either antigen tests or Western Blot assays performed at the Australian National Reference Laboratory at Fairfield (Babona *et al.*1996: 201). Assurances were made then that *clearly* 'negative' and 'positive' test results would then be given back in seven days (Babona *et al.* 1996: 203), although slowness in provision of test results and the frequent loss thereof has been noted all along. Carol Jenkins noted in her 2002 review that test results were six years later still taking upwards of six months to be returned owing to funding and communication snafus and other factors (2002: 21–2). The NHASP review of the introduction of antiretrovirals throughout the country found that 'receipt of confirmed results in provincial areas can be six months or more' (NHASP 2005a: 15). This places physicians in the awkward position of having to commence patients on therapies prior even to receiving test results. It compromises the care given to antenatal women, the prevention of vertical transmission and the timing of post-exposure prophylaxis. The addition of several regional confirmatory laboratories since then has greatly helped in this regard, and by all accounts the lag in test result provision has shortened.

Accumulating clinical data and puzzles were approached in a retrospective study published in 1996 (Seaton *et al.* 1996) but that built upon early, brief medical reports and aired suspicions. In his editorial published in a 1990 issue of the *Papua New Guinea Medical Journal*, Paul Mondia noted that then current data suggested that 'tuberculosis will play a major role in the way AIDS will express itself' (Mondia 1990: 81). This prediction has in fact been borne out. Twenty of the first 25 persons who were confirmed HIVab+ by application of both ELISA and Western Blot testing were handled in tuberculosis clinics. This wasn't surprising, because by the time of his writing 50% of all diagnosed AIDS cases were of people who were suffering from tuberculosis, and many others had 'non-mycobacterial chest infection, with clinical manifestations very similar to tuberculous infection' (Mondia 1990: 81). The paper he and his colleague read at the 26th Annual Medical Symposium, held in 1990 in Goroka, Eastern Highlands Province, showed that about 4% of 215 tuberculosis patients serologically tested positive for HIVab (Mondia and Perera 1990). This alarmed attendees but also alerted them to the eventual future of clinical aspects of HIV infection throughout the country. HIVab seropositivity prevalence figures from Ward 4B in the Port Moresby General Hospital are now routinely stated to be 30%, 40% or higher (author's fieldnotes, August, 2006; Cronau 2006). Seaton and his colleagues reviewed clinical syndromes suffered by patients admitted to one or another ward of this hospital between January of 1990 and September of 1995 and who had tested HIVab+. Most of the resulting client sample of 70 was composed of young, urban dwelling adults, as many female as male, from various social groups. They found chronic diarrhoea in 47.8% of their sample, terrible wasting in 94.2%, and another 68.7% to be suffering from oropharyngeal candidiasis. On clinical grounds they suspected tuberculosis in over two-thirds of the sample (68.6%) and cryptococcal meningitis was detected in 8.6%, with one patient found to be suffering from a rare form thereof. Over half of the sample died in hospital, and they concluded that mortality of HIV infection was high and that patients tended to present to hospital 'late in their disease course' (Seaton *et al.* 1996: 783). Noting clinical symptoms 'similar to those observed in Africa', they assumed heterosexual transmission and promiscuity as the major mode and contributing factor, respectively, but presented no evidence of either. These accumulating data and hunches mounting on clinical grounds, regardless of their degree of veracity, led eventually to an organised response. A strange irony engulfed the response from the start, however, since the knowledge bases of Papua New Guineans were frequently challenged or denigrated, but yet, of the first 745 cases of HIV infection, 547 of them were registered without any evidence whatsoever of transmission mode or route(s) (*Australian Nursing Journal* 1997).

The first government-sponsored plan of any substance for HIV prevention was the *National Medium-Term Programme for the Prevention and Control of AIDS in Papua New Guinea, 1989–1995*. It was drawn up in 1989 by officials from the Disease Control and STD/AIDS units in the Department of Health. Ballard and Malau (2002: 4) note a certain (and probably unavoidable) biomedicine top-heavy aspect to it. It possessed standard features such as expansion of training opportunities, the refurbishment of STD clinics and some attention paid to HIVab surveillance, each of the goals being still relevant to the national response but also deeply problematic. It also was drafted by an anthropologist who possessed intimate knowledge of and connections to

Papua New Guinea, Dr Katherine Lepani, and was informed by a number of ethnographic insights and sociological principles. The *Programme* died on the vine, however, because of lack of governmental commitment to funding, and so only a few staffing needs were filled. Even USAID pulled out from further support of their condom social marketing initiatives and later from other Pacific-based health programmes (Ballard and Malau 2002: 4).

Between 1989 and 1994 the reported number of HIVab+ cases rose from 17 to 69, and then in the ensuing four years rose nearly ten-fold to 634 (Caldwell 2000: 5). Because of the seeming fast increases in reported cases in the early years of the epidemic, AusAID was contacted formally in 1993 to initiate a programme that came to be known as the AusAID Sexual Health and HIV/AIDS Prevention and Care Project, which was launched in 1995 and which aided the National Department of Health with funding and technical and other support (Malau and Crockett 2000: 60). This assistance was greatly needed insofar as the only existing national surveillance system relevant to STDs and HIV had by 1994 ceased operation. Jenkins (2002: 22) notes that this was partly owing to breaches in confidentiality, which had so compromised the willingness of people even to be tested that the surveillance system became something of a stand-alone project. This is a problem, too, not just in otherwise isolated rural hospitals or health sub-centres, but in the nation's second-largest, ANGAU Memorial hospital, where there was, as of 2004, 'no identifiable area … where patients can access anonymous and confidential HIV testing' (NHASP 2005a: 11). This terrible paradox – for stigma of and discrimination against those living with HIV and AIDS to be lessened, people have to self-disclose – remains deeply embedded today. Leach *et al.*'s critique of the national response in this regard is quite telling: 'Some agencies and individual PLHA [People Living with HIV or AIDS] have wrongly assumed that in order for PLHA to make any contribution to HIV services they must disclose their status. Sometimes, this is associated with a desire on the part of the agency to publicly demonstrate its acceptance of PLHA' (2006: 20). If too much information was shared on one side of the ledger (the identities of those being tested), too little was being captured on the other: 71% of the cases of HIVab+ blood samples had by 2002 been registered *without any information whatsoever* about age, gender, place of origin, or transmission dynamics (NACS 2002).

Research highlights and lowlights

During the first decade following the appearance in Papua New Guinea of HIV, important social scientific research was carried out regarding the knowledge of, attitudes toward, and behaviours relevant to its transmission and prevention. Jenny Hughes contributed intriguing ethnographic data and insights from the studies she carried out in the late 1980s and early 1990s while attached to the Institute of Medical Research. The IMR once had a research station where now sits an empty building on the compound of the district hospital in Tari. Tribal fighting at and over the clinic drove IMR staff away. Of the Tari Basin, Huli-speakers of Southern Highlands Province with whom she worked, she wrote with great prescience:

To a people who have abandoned much of their traditional morality and had forty years of Christian morality overlaid on its remains, the provision of a device [condoms] which seemingly permits licence without penalty, appears to be problematic in some quarters. The almost total opposition of community women questioned on the topic indicates that if condoms are to be successfully introduced this issue will need to be handled very sensitively. (Hughes 1991: 139)

In this and in other publications (Hughes 1997, 2002) Hughes also showed that embodied knowledge of physiology, anatomy and STD signs and symptoms was sub-optimal, and that this and other factors contributed to late or to nil presentation to health facilities for treatment (cf. Hammar 2004b, 2006b; NSRRT and Jenkins 1994; Passey 1996; Passey *et al.* 1998a, b). In April and May of 1991 Carol Jenkins and Kerry Pataki-Schweitzer randomly selected nearly 900 informants in or near Lae and Madang on the coast and Goroka and Mt. Hagen in the highlands with whom they conducted interviews. They found that 93% had at least heard of the term 'AIDS', although only 3%, they showed, had good knowledge of HIV transmission, whether involving blood transfusion or vertical means, or of means of prevention. Although condom use by males seemed to vary with educational attainment, those who had university education being twice as likely as those without education to use them, fewer than half were convinced that condom use could prevent HIV transmission. The marginal status of social scientific knowledge was implied in their quite correct statement that '[m]essages stating that one is protected if there is only 1 sexual partner and avoidance of sexual intercourse with prostitutes' clash with the reality of contemporary sexual practice (Jenkins and Pataki-Schweitzer 1993: 192).

The study conducted in 1991 and 1992 by Carol and the National Sexuality and Reproduction Research Team (NSRRT and Jenkins 1994) was the bellwether research of the early–mid 1990s. Many of its findings, if not methods, have been retained, although in my opinion they continue to be overlooked at a policy level and with regards to church leaders and policies. With USAID funding, she and her colleagues trained teachers, housewives and public servants to conduct sexuality and reproduction-related research in their home villages and in their own languages, drawing upon more than 400 informants representing about 40 different language groups. Many of the findings were denied on the face of them by some members of some church groups. A decade later, other church leaders found it difficult to swallow the fact that fellowship gatherings, church conferences and evangelical crusades were also settings of densely patterned sexual networking (NHASP 2005g: 12). Probably little of that sexual networking was protected by condoms or involved non-penetrative sex.

There are many important findings to register here, among them the striking absence of embodied knowledge of sexual and reproductive anatomy and health. She confirmed this finding significantly in a subsequent urban-based study of youth (Jenkins 1997; and see Hammar 1992, 1996a, b; 2004b; Hughes 2002; Wardlow 2002a, b). She and the NSRRT team found that 44% of the women surveyed knew no specific signs, symptoms or transmission risks of STDs. The fact that nearly one-third of the single men had had sex with married women dents faith somewhat in the inordinate fidelity. Professor of Obstetrics and Gynecology in Port Moresby at the School of Medicine of the University of Papua New Guinea, Dr Glen Mola, has shown from statistics drawn from the antenatal clinic there that 25% of the women who test HIVab+ and who naturally suspect their partner's infidelity actually have HIVab- partners (2005: 22). Another relevant finding would be the staggeringly high levels they found throughout the country of sexual violence perpetrated against girls and women, often at coitarche and around pregnancy, just as is the case in the US and elsewhere (Hammar 1999b, 2006a). That sexual violence *was* marriage was one of the components of the monograph that the Papua New Guinea Censorship Board found 'obscene' (marked by stapled note inside the front cover). This would not have been so bad but for the implied sexual titillation at violence (not, that is, at eroticism). Now that's obscene! This was the same Office of Censorship that in September of 1992 required pharmacies wishing to sell the new state-sponsored 'Protector' condom to remove the instruction leaflets contained inside of a line drawing of an erect penis, which was deemed pornographic. The same thing happened in the US in 1995 involving Elizabeth Dole, then President of the American Red Cross, and the same drawing of an erect penis. With perverse irony, it was her husband, Senator Bob Dole, frequent candidate for President of the US, who early on stumped for clinical recognition of ED: erectile dysfunction. More recently, with much perversity but no irony, Mrs Dole supported legislation in the US Senate that would honour the notorious bigot and homophobe, the recently deceased Jesse Helms, for his work in AIDS! Yet another signal finding was that multiple acts of intercourse were thought necessary for conception to occur. Lewis Langness wrote of the Bena Bena, for example, that 'nobody believes that one act of intercourse can result in pregnancy' (1969: 42–3). Such notions encourage men (at least those who wished not to be saddled with fatherhood) to engage in multi-partner unions so as to escape responsibility, whereas women were consigned to engage in it to fulfill theirs, that is, to find through sex a man who would support their offspring. Culturally 'safer' sexual intercourse is, therefore, multiple and frequently so (NSRRT and Jenkins 1994:40; cf. Hammar 1996a, b; Wardlow 2006a). Extensive training in sexual physiology and health being precluded by both 'traditional' and Church-introduced taboos, sexual intercourse was not found to be protected by barrier methods of contraception and STD prevention.

Unfortunately, this *seeming* paradox laid bare by Jenkins and her colleagues in this and other publications and by other social scientists still has yet really to be taken on board. Instead, campaign slogans and attempts at BCC (Behaviour Change Communications) continue to try to reshape sexuality to fit ideals of single-partner, lifetime, heterosexual monogamy, hopefully Christian and condom-less. Naomi McPherson argues that such Christian values are expressed in 'authorised', that is, married sex and that is engaged in for creation, not recreation, and in prayer as frequent and constant as possible (McPherson 2008). Allowable discourse about sexuality and sexual acts remains in Papua New Guinea discourse about squanderable resources and gifts from God that can be 'misused' and so need to be used 'correctly' (Bonivento 2001a, 2001b; but see Bouten 1996; Farmer 1996).

These and other studies conducted in the early–mid 1990s by ethnographers (e.g. Clark and Hughes 1995; Fiti-Sinclair 1996; Hammar 1992, 1993a, b, 1996a, b, 2004b; Hughes 1991, 2002) augmented the significant research presence exhibited by national and international researchers employed or otherwise sponsored by the IMR. If there was a consistent finding of these studies it was of extremely high prevalence of STDs amongst presumed 'low-risk' populations such as village-dwelling adults in 'remote' areas, antenatal clinic attendees and 'rural women'. Unfortunately, that signal finding has been just as consistently overlooked by national health bodies and officials in formulation of models of high risk. As if high rates of infection weren't bad enough, sub-optimal understanding of transmission routes and risks, little compliance with treatment regime, staggeringly high rates of secondary infertility and widespread disavowal of condoms were among the other significant findings. A partial sampling of this important research would include Lemeki *et al.* (1996), Mgone *et al.* (2002), Passey (1996) and Passey *et al.* (1998a, b). These and other important studies established in the mid-1990s that few community members used condoms and that STD infection rates ranged from 30% to 40% or more, sometimes even reaching or exceeding 60% or 70% in case of assays for multiple infections. A majority of women suffering from STDs were found not to recognise their associated symptoms, or if they were, not to know of their sexually transmitted nature and so infrequently or not at all attended clinics and received follow-up treatment. Megan Passey found that symptoms were considered so 'normal' (see also Garg *et al.* 2001) that it was thought unnecessary to attend a clinic (1996: 257). NSRRT and Jenkins (1994: 125) found that men did not associate urethral discharge and genital sores so much with STDs as with sorcery, poor sexual hygiene and menstrual blood poisoning (see also Hammar 1996a, b). Other IMR-sponsored researchers found that women perceived genital mayhem, if at all, as resulting from 'dirt' and semen and extramarital sexuality *per se.* They expressed shame at attendance at clinics when rarely they attended, so great was the judgmental attitude toward their patients exhibited by health workers (Hammar 1996a; Hughes 1991, 2002; Passey 1996; Wardlow 2002a, b). The study conducted in Port Moresby by Ruta Fiti-Sinclair in 1993 of 22 women in prostitution found that 20 of them had been treated for STDs but that '[n]one sought regular check-ups; all stated that they went only when symptoms manifested' (1996: 120). This finding helps to explain why it is that HIV infection is so frequently in Papua New Guinea diagnosed in terms of something else, that is, in an Emergency Department visit for oral thrush or in a newborn baby who fails to thrive.

A clinic-based study conducted in 1992–93 in the Porgera valley (Kramer 1995) found extremely high rates of especially gonorrhea and Donovanosis and gendered equivalents of pelvic inflammatory disease among 300 consecutive patients at the STD clinic. This researcher found that six of 10 male clients had had an extramarital sexual contact in the previous quarter and that nearly half and fully two-thirds of all males and females, respectively, had at most heard the term 'AIDS'. Only 1% of the female clients were aware of the efficacy of condoms in preventing STDs and HIV. Both males and females exhibited what the clinician felt were poor rates of compliance with treatment regime, although access to health services in this area is extremely difficult in terms of distance, cost and difficulty of terrain. Kramer also called for widespread condom promotion despite evident opposition from Christian groups. A 1996 Demographic and Health Survey in Papua New Guinea showed that, of the 65% of the women surveyed who claimed any knowledge at all about such issues, only 19% correctly noted the HIV and STD transmission preventive properties of condoms, and that 73% of women overall did not perceive themselves as being at risk of either (NHASP 2001: 19). Misconceptions of risk continue to be fuelled by church leaders, such as that 'HIV/AIDS [sic] is a punishment by God', which promotes understandings that 'the virus [sic] only affects prostitutes or people living in towns and cities while people in rural villages are safe' (NHASP 2005g: 14). Papua New Guinea and the Cook Islands are the only two countries in the insular Pacific in which HIVab testing in public clinics is not free (Rupali *et al.* 2007: 217), and though the fee is minimal, it and the associated costs of food, bus-fare and the like are beyond many would-be clients. Surely this presents a significant problem with regards to expanded roll-out of antiretrovirals, in that '[n]ear-perfect pill taking is required to achieve viral suppression and to avoid the emergence of viral resistance' (NHASP 2005a: Annex 1, n.p.). These and similar issues informed a later turn of health authorities toward using principles of syndromic management of suspected STDs and showed many likely challenges thereto. There are significant clinical and technical requirements to consider, and many, many women don't report or have or know they have symptoms.

Mounting a 'national' response

Most reviewers of the response made in Papua New Guinea to HIV and AIDS agree that the years 1993–1997 were extremely quiet ones, save for the publication of important research documents such as the monograph published by the IMR in 1994 by NSRRT and Jenkins. Some form of a National AIDS Council was proposed as early as 1993 that would employ its own personnel and other resources to launch what came to be known as a 'multi-sectoral' response. Senior health officials, researchers, policy-makers and politicians attended a conference in July of 1993 that was designed also to enlist NGOs in the fight against AIDS, but space was denied them on the Parliamentary agenda that year (Ballard and Malau 2002: 6–7). The recently resigned Minister of Health, Sir Peter Barter, who was made to look foolish regarding medicine distribution in the ABC Four Corners programme, 'Sick No Good', aired in August, 2006, was 12 years prior also Minister of Health under a different Prime Minister. Julius Chan rejected calls for government support of HIV prevention, although K100,000 were given to Carol Jenkins to support programmes in research and education (Ballard and Malau 2002: 7). Unfortunately, healthcare and policy-making branches of the government cut or attenuated HIV and AIDS related programmes. Educational messages and programmes that were designed to speak frankly about sexual matters and positively about condoms (harking back to the efforts in 1988 of the

Minister of Health, Robert Suckling) were shoved aside or discouraged by church and health officials and the Censorship Board. Consequently, say Ballard and Malau (2002: 7), the period from 1993 to the founding of an operational National AIDS Council and Secretariat by 1998, was one of 'reduced funding, reduced staff and no political commitment to AIDS'.

What came later to be named the Foundation Project was in 1996 launched as the Sexual Health and HIV/AIDS Prevention and Care Project from within the Department of Health. Then Health Minister Sir Albert Kipalan launched it in Port Moresby on 21 February by noting its three-year duration and funding of K7,000,000. 'I am determined that we need not waste any more of our precious time on talk nothing', he said, 'it is time for real action' (*STD Nius* 1996: 1). This was the first initiative supported by AusAID with major funding and which revived somewhat dormant interest shown by Australia in Papua New Guinea in view of expected epidemic outbreak of HIV (Jenkins 2002: 4). At this time were established several early templates for what came to be known as the Provincial AIDS Committees, each of which were to be linked in more than just name to the Provincial Health Advisers and to the various provincial administrations. This was much later noted as a serious organisational shortfall (NHASP 2006d: 7), but yet it commenced the process of thinking about HIV in terms other than the microscopically small and of AIDS as being something more than an inescapably fatal, contagious and morally stigmatising form of illness. These early initiatives were key to the process of bridge-building, awareness raising, grant proposal writing and political engagement. Out of these forward-thinking initiatives came the so-called Transex Project (Jenkins 2000), which incorporated sex workers and male employees in the transportation industry, including highway drivers and stevedores, sailors and security guards. It was founded upon a 1995 pilot study of issues of methodology and logistics. AusAID's funding of the project and institutional support provided by the Department of Health were augmented by support provided by the WHO, UNAIDS and USAID. This project more than perhaps any other deserves credit for conceiving the first targeted interventions in terms of knowledge, condom usage, STD treatment and awareness-raising and -changing.

From these new forms of cooperation, although not informed by emergent ethnographic data about sexual matters, the National AIDS Council and the National AIDS Council Secretariat were established formally in 1997. An important plank of the establishment of the *National AIDS Council Act* was that from that point forward school-based policies were to have mandated teaching about sexual health matters. Of the 11 Asia-Pacific countries that Smith *et al.* (2003) surveyed in their study of sexual health education policies and practices, however, Papua New Guinea had the lowest enrollment of school children, by far, in both primary and secondary school (2003: 11, Table III). Of those 11, Papua New Guinea is one of only four that even mentions condom use as a means of HIV transmission prevention (2003: 12). Over 350 new reports of HIV infection were made that year and another 642 were reported the following year, in 1998, indicating a fairly grim future for Papua New Guinea. Prime Minister Bill Skate was criticised at this time for financial mismanagement and budgetary shortfalls that negatively influenced healthcare and health policies and for a series of diplomatic and other blunders, including committing state monies to a crusading evangelist.[4] Nevertheless, Skate is credited for in a sense rescuing HIV and AIDS from the backburner to which they had been consigned by his predecessor, Julius Chan. Prime Minister Skate and his wife showed direct and sustained interest in them and associated health issues, as did his Health Minister, Ludger Mond (1999), and then Secretary for Health, Dr Puka Temu (Tobia 1998), who is a lay evangelical preacher. Dr Temu is a member of a prominent Central Province family (his brother was once head of the National Research Institute) and would again be made Secretary for Health and eventually be named in 2005 Minister responsible for 'Assisting the Prime Minister on HIV/ AIDS'. Both made several notable public pronouncements about the gravity of the situation soon facing Papua New Guinea. Malau and Crockett (2000), Ballard and Malau (2002) and Jenkins (2002) each note how quickly was the NAC brought into being and how forceful was the language used to enlist the support of government bodies, churches, business groups and NGOs in the renewed fight against HIV and AIDS. High-level political support was required to unleash potential funding streams and to develop and consolidate new forms of national and international cooperation.

The Medium Term Plan drafted in 1998 after extensive consultations contained significant input from multiple sectors, including academic research. In the Foreword to the Plan, Skate pledged his administration's full support to the NAC and to formulating a 'multi-sectoral strategy for HIV/ AIDS' to 'help contain the potentially devastating impact of the epidemic on the country's development' (GoPNG 1998: n.p.). The Plan was aimed at improving sexual health, reducing the suffering to individuals and families of HIV and AIDS in terms of care and treatment and social stigma, enabling a supportive legal and ethical environment and strengthening the national response to HIV and AIDS. Particularly progressive about the Plan was the fact that absent and incorrect knowledge of STD signs and symptoms and of transmission routes and risks of HIV were themselves noted as 'risk factors' (GoPNG 1998: ii). 'High Risk Behaviour' was defined as '[a]ny behaviour, sexual or otherwise, that is capable of transmitting HIV' (GoPNG 1998: 51). Would that it had stayed that way! The half-a-dozen high-priority topics defined then have for the most part remained today:

- *Education, Information and Media*, which shaped messages, posters and campaigns, but which have gradually morphed into Behaviour Change Communications (BCC).

- *Counselling, Community Care and Support*, which underwrote VCT initiatives, and since 2005, an upsurge in interest in prevention of mother-to-child transmission (PMTCT).

- *Legal and Ethical Issues*, which led eventually to the 2003 HAMP Act legislation.

- *Social and Economic Impact*, which put AIDS in its proper development context and warned of the consequences of a likely dying off of well educated teachers and health workers and of the huge dent that would likely be made in rural enclave projects.

- *Monitoring Surveillance, Evaluation and Research*, which established guidelines, case reporting systems and sentinel sites from which were to be reported new infections.

- *Medical and Laboratory*, which identified technical and training needs and shortfalls, from lymphocyte counters to clinic upgrades, from courses for prescribers of antiretroviral therapies to the development of regional confirmatory laboratories.

In 1999 the National Department of Health ceded its control over the national response to the NAC owing to lack of monitoring, surveillance, reporting and financial accounting capability.

The first Consensus Workshop was held in 2000. This underwrote the development the following year of an HIVab serosurveillance system. In March of 2000 Australia announced that it was between 2000 and 2005 going to fund (with dates later being adjusted) the National HIV/AIDS Support Project, to the tune of K100,000,000. The Consensus Workshop reported surveillance figures obtained from serological study of blood samples provided by sex workers in Lae and Port Moresby and also expressed alarm that seroprevalence had risen two-fold amongst antenatal and STD clinic attendees in Port Moresby between 1998 and 1999 and almost three-fold during the same time period in blood donors (WHO-NAC-NDoH 2000: 2, 6).

By April of 1999, the Director of the NACS had been appointed, Dr Clement Malau. His relatively frank talk about sexual matters earned him much ignominy among church leaders and led also to the humorous moniker, 'Dr K', for either *kondom* or *koap* (sexual penetration), depending on one's perspective. Quite sensibly, he launched NACS goals and objectives in public settings with straight talk, for example, in 2001 when he was quoted as saying: 'The issue of sex cannot be underestimated. There is no question that HIV is being transmitted through sex and therefore everyone is at risk. We cannot afford to joke about this anymore' (*Post-Courier* 2001). (This was also the time at which the NAC launched a new, state-sponsored condom, Karamap, which many found sensible and timely but which many others found offensive and squeamish, with many Tok Pisin speakers wanting instead a word in Motu or Tolai to be used.) Unfortunately, the opposition was as swift as it was widespread, and two newspaper editors mandated a blanket prohibition on coverage of the new media campaign (Vulum 2001).

Similar situations have been noted in the Marshall Islands, in which mixed-company discussions of sex are prohibited (Westaway 1989: 4). Tongan, Samoan and Fijian broadcasts and print media presentations of sexual and reproductive health issues are notable for avoiding explicit discussion of sexual acts and body parts (Winn and Lucas 1993). In Papua New Guinea parents instructed their children to turn away from television spots airing the ads or to close their ears when they came on the radio. It should not therefore surprise to note that only two editorials were published about HIV and AIDS in the *Post-Courier* from 1987 to 1997 (Cullen 2000: 128). This created a difficult climate for Dr Malau as for other committed health officials and politicians. During a 3 July 2002 interview conducted for 'The World Today' by Ian Townsend, Dr Malau responded to a question about AIDS control. 'The structures are there, and I believe they are good ones', he replied, in reference to the NACS and PACs and DACs (District AIDS Committees) and NHASP, and continued: '[b]ut really what happens out there is really a major problem I think. I don't think we are making much difference to the epidemic at this stage' (Townsend 2002).

The fact that these remarks came only two years following commencement of the NHASP programme is relevant, especially given the set of conditions the NHASP inherited and which to a certain extent remain today:

> At the time of NHASP inception the PNG health system was impacted by the overall decline in the institutional capacity of national government, decentralisation and the general economic downturn. Many provincial and district centres, and STI clinic buildings were either non-existent or inadequate. Basic client confidentiality and physical assessment-treatment needs could not be provided. The NDoH's capacity to conduct, collate and manage STI and HIV surveillance was not adequate for reporting, monitoring of the epidemic or planning and there was no capacity for STI and HIV/ AIDS program planning, management, and monitoring within the Disease Control Section. Additionally, there were major problems at all levels with the distribution and availability of pharmaceuticals, laboratory supplies and equipment including infection control supplies. Public health laboratory planning and management at the national level was very limited and in-country training programs for laboratory staff were unavailable. In some provinces, there were long delays in the transportation and reporting of HIV antibody screening tests which impacted on both clinical management and counselling and care. (NHASP 2004b: 7–8)

From this perspective the accomplishments from 2001 to 2004 are quite remarkable. When the second Consensus Workshop was held in 2004 it reviewed the objectives of and findings presented at its 2000 predecessor and examined in close detail what had transpired since then. Goals and objectives of the 2004 workshop were to 1) review available clinical, behavioural and serological data relevant to HIV and AIDS and STI; 2) estimate the current prevalence of HIV; and 3) recommend ways of improving the surveillance system (NHASP 2005e: iii). It was reported that the number of new HIV infections having been diagnosed had more than doubled, from the 1,062 reported in 2000 to the 2,373 reported in 2004, such that now a 'relatively clear picture of the trends in the epidemic' was available. More worrisome, it was noted that now fully half of all ward beds at the Port Moresby General Hospital were occupied by AIDS patients. By this time national policies had not yet been drafted that would mandate the routine screening in antenatal clinics of pregnant women (Rupali *et al.* 2007: 218). Beginning in January of 2005, however, nevirapine prophylaxis was administered post-natally to both mother and child, as in the controversial HIVNET 12 trial conducted in Uganda. It was estimated by a Papua New Guinean medical doctor that the HIVab seroprevalence at this time in antenatal women was 0.0025% (Rupali *et al.* 2007: 220), which even then was a dramatic undercounting.

Having attended and participated in the workshop, however, and for many reasons, I cannot endorse the conclusion above. I would for starters mention the fact of incomplete reporting, logistical difficulties related to 'confirmatory' testing and the change in testing techniques and algorithms that had taken place. For example, the Serodia test of blood samples that in case of an Initial Reactive test result is performed again in provincial laboratories is said to be 'confirmed' at the Central Public Health Laboratory by application of Abbott Determine, Immunocomb and ELISA. Elsewhere, however, it is said itself to be used for 'confirmation' (NHASP 2005a: 15, 17); this is a misnomer in that one cannot 'confirm' a test result by application of the same test. One could also mention the inconsistency of analytic units, the fact that some provinces provided no surveillance data whatsoever, and that even a marked decrease in new infections, quarter by quarter, had been reported (NHASP 2005e: 3, 4, 6). This last was assumed to be an artifact of decreased testing, not proof of lessened transmission, although increases are seldom if ever viewed this way. Province of origin of testing subject was still known for only 24% of the entire sample, too, but at other times this analytic category became fetishized , was made an object almost of worship, to the extent it was held necessarily to explain anything. At one point one of the consultant epidemiologists, faced with a situation in which three contiguous highlands provinces provided only two sets of surveillance data, decided to average the combined prevalence reported for the westernmost and easternmost province and impute it to the one in the middle (Simbu Province)! None of the people to whom I spoke afterward expressed any misgivings. The fourfold increase estimated to have taken place from 2000 to 2004, pushing the overall prevalence to 1.7%, was considered to be based on 'reasonable assumptions' (NHASP 2005e: 8). I suggest here and argue in the next chapter that they were anything but. Presentations indicated such problems as mentioned above, and there remained substantial confusion from private industry representatives (medical doctors) who still confused Initial with Repeat Reactive test results and both with a 'confirmed' HIVab test result, thus setting back discussions greatly. For example, a medical doctor working in Western Province noted a massive increase in the span of two years but became irate when asked to discuss and explain it. Understandable regret was expressed at missed opportunities to conduct serological, clinical and behavioural surveillance at sentinel sites (NHASP 2005e: 10). There was no public commentary upon the disturbing clinical data presented regarding the initial enrollees at the Heduru Clinic, specifically as regards their late diagnosis, their difficulty negotiating the toxicity of the antiretrovirals then being prescribed, and the hastening of their early death by heart-attack, anaemia and weight loss. Several medical doctors present reacted indignantly to requests for clarification.

The year 2003 was momentous in ways good and bad. That year marked the end of the three-year tenure of its Director, Dr Clement Malau, who left to pursue international public health research and advocacy work at the Burnet Institute in Melbourne (and who came back in 2007 to become the Secretary for Health). It marked the ascension of Dr Ninkama Moiya. After four years at the helm he took over the 'rebranded' *Tingim Laip* (Think

Life) Programme.[5] The year 2003 also witnessed the passage of the HIV/AIDS Management and Prevention Bill, which was enacted later that year (see Stewart 2004). It wasn't until 2009 that the HAMP Act was tested in court,[6] however (see Chapter 4). The NACS report from 2008 puts the problem at the feet of the victimised: 'no known cases of abuses being registered' (NACS 2008: 91), although later in the same document (i.e., 2008: 122) it would appear that many cases of abuse and discrimination have been collected, so it must be a problem of either reporting them (unlikely) or not taking them sufficiently seriously. Nicole Haley's revelation of what happened to several Duna women (2008) was by this time well known in manuscript form and had been presented several times publicly and had circulated on the Internet and in the Australian press (e.g. *Sydney Morning Herald* 2007a). Ditto, my attempt to tell Susan's Story (Hammar 2008) and Christine Stewart's telling of the events at Three Mile (2004), to mention only three of the more obvious stories well known to NACS and NHASP officials but about which nothing was done.

This again raises questions of the disjuncture between the rhetoric of often quite progressive stances taken toward issues of stigma and discrimination and access to condoms and confidential testing, on the one hand, and lived realities, on the other. The HRSS, or High-Risk Settings Strategy, was launched in early 2004 after lengthy deliberations. It was designed to move top-heavy, 'top-down' approaches that had characterised NAC initiatives to that point, ones that aimed for an overall, population-wide awareness-raising, toward specific interventions among specified sub-groups in a more horizontal, participatory way.

Thus we have a double irony of the national response: although formulated at the top level if not offshore, HRSS was designed to be a 'bottom-up'-style approach (NHASP 2006e: 7); and just as the HIV epidemic in Papua New Guinea had been recognised as a 'generalised' one ('we're all at risk'), so did rhetorics of risk become the more acutely focused on already vulnerable, often stigmatised people. Social vulnerabilities transmuted into biological ones: 'women and girls are especially vulnerable', 'homosexual intercourse is especially risky', and the like. 'High-risk'-type discourse and programme initiatives cannot help but enable stigma and bad feelings for those on the receiving end. They have been the focus of sustained critique by social scientists and members of so-called High Risk Settings alike since their inception. Finally in 2006, during the first-ever HIV Prevention Summit, a number of these complaints were aired publicly, although not by the major proponent of HRSS, who has since left the country. 'A key concern is that the use of the term "high risk" for a behaviour change strategy', said one consultant as the strategy was being ironed out and implemented, 'is likely to reinforce existing stigma, discrimination, and abuse of the people associated with targeted settings and groups, and result in the continued blame of HIV infection on certain sectors of the population, particularly female sex workers, settlement dwellers, and unemployed youth' (Lepani 2004: iii; see also 2007b, 2008b). One of the so-called high-risk settings was the Red Scar neighbourhood of Madang, which I know reasonably well. In Red Scar sexual (and other forms of social) networking is omnipresent, just as it is in hundreds of other neighbourhoods or settlements throughout the country, but condoms are also easily found, people are friendly, and the streets and pathways are packed with people until the wee hours of the morning. The HRSS review (NHASP 2006e: 30, 42) noted that the women selling sexual services 'at Red Scar were strong women and the KAPB Study showed that they had both the strength and skills to negotiate for safe sex, even when they were drunk, and clients just had to accept' (NHASP 2006e: Annex 6, p. 44). Similar examples could be cited from my experiences in Goroka, Tabubil and Vanimo. Once again assertions of 'high-risk' sexual activities there trumped demonstration of them.

> *'You don't think he's a man?! He's a man, alright! Of course he's had sex with us. He's had sex with all the girls, he and his cronies. Oh, when he was posted here, he was one of the biggest players of all' (35-year-old peer educator and former sex worker, Goroka, commenting on one of the touring members of the Special Parliamentary Committee on HIV/AIDS).*

The year 2004 also witnessed the formation of the Special Parliamentary Committee on HIV/AIDS with full parliamentary support and which was headed by Dr Banare Bun, then Member for Parliament from Henganofi. Dr Bun chaired the public airing and recording of testimony throughout the country throughout the following year. It elicited often quite compelling and vivid testimony about sexual violence and sexual networking and about lack of coordination between government, business, research, church and community efforts to prevent HIV transmission. During this time I gave a deposition in Port Moresby on behalf of the IMR and shared an apartment and many beers with the UK-based private consultant who arranged the itinerary and managed the documentation of testimony. The exercise was to my mind rather underwhelming in its presumption that anyone could find much of the public testimony at all surprising, although it was, of course, quite grim. The nation gave an audible gasp the day following presentation of the fact that there were '53' 'known sites where sex takes place' in Port Moresby. No way! This, however, is how participating parliamentarians, news reporters and their reading public took the reports of sexual violence, church shenanigans with regards to condoms, the mismanagement of funds and the good deeds of little known persons and organisations. 'Poverty is the key issue in the fight against HIV/AIDS', Dr Bun was quoted as saying (e.g. *Post-Courier* 2006), even though untreated STDs and sexual violence rank consistently above poverty in terms of health priorities. The day following one of the first public airings of testimony he was quoted as saying that guesthouses and motels were also 'growing like "mushrooms" and had become places where sexual activities were taking place on large scale' and that they are 'providing girls for their customers'. 'This is very alarming and this committee will address this issue very seriously', Dr Bun also said (*Post-Courier* 2005). I am not quibbling with the facts save to complain of their late airing; evidence of such already existed in droves at no expense but the time spent reading it. Nothing has been done since then about those motels and guest houses, hotels and semi-brothels, either, nor about the male politicians, programme managers, taxi-cab drivers and businessmen who congregate there and arrange and take part in associated sexual activities.

The NACS was relocated to the Prime Minister's Office in 2005 to increase political support, under NEC Directive 124/2004. Dr Temu was appointed in 2005 to be responsible for assisting the Prime Minister, Michael Somare, in areas related to HIV and AIDS. This was seen as giving greater priority to the issues, which was confirmed the following year when the government endorsed HIV and AIDS as key priorities in the *National Medium Term Development Strategy for 2006–2010*. In 2006 also occurred the first-ever HIV Prevention Summit, during which 'evidence-based policy' emerged as the new buzzword. Papua New Guinea was represented graphically and otherwise as being at the epicentre of insular Pacific HIV epidemics. The NAC, UNAIDS and the Special Parliamentary Committee on HIV/AIDS chaired by Dr Bun, in collaboration with and with sponsorship by AusAID, its New Zealand equivalent (NZAID), the European Union (EU) and the Asian Development Bank (ADB) held from 7–9 March a Summit on Intensifying HIV Prevention in PNG. Over two hundred participants were invited from business, donor agencies, health research and government bodies to summarise and probe more deeply into the wide range and degrees of efficacy of HIV prevention efforts throughout the country, to contextualise them in terms of well-known 'international best-practices' and to provide guiding recommendations. Scheduled by way of plenary sessions and significant small-group discussions and presentations thereof, the Summit was organised around five main themes:

- *Leadership and Advocacy in HIV Prevention*, strengthened in partnerships, spanning multiple sectors, and requiring improved education, planning and coordination.

- *Managing the National Response: Challenges in Implementing a Decentralised Response*, which is no easy feat amidst health systems collapse and a greatly Port Moresby-based staging ground.

- *Critical Issues in Education and Behaviour Change*, including those of community mobilisation and making the face of HIV more personal, for example, by inviting the greater participation of people already infected.

- *Treatment, Care and Support in HIV Prevention*, especially the gradual roll-out of antiretroviral therapies.

- *Need for an Evidence-Based National Response* (GoPNG 2006: iv).

As the report makes evident, the Three Ones were promoted during and following the Summit. Great political commitment was suggested in attendance by the Prime Minister, the Governor-General and the Chair of the Parliamentary Special Committee of HIV/AIDS. Dr Puka Temu received the draft summary report and recommendations on behalf of the Government. The recommendations fit nicely into the 'goals, objectives, and strategies of the National Strategic Plan on HIV/AIDS' (GoPNG 2006: iv). Particular highlights included that people living with HIV should be given the more prominent place in policy development and implementation that they all along deserved, and that parliamentarians, as a condition of service, be provided with information about HIV and AIDS and be strongly encouraged themselves to undergo voluntary counselling and testing (VCT). Renewed cooperation with police and other security forces was called for by Carol Jenkins, and churches especially were encouraged to become 'centres for HIV and AIDS information, education, care and healing' (GoPNG 2006: 4, 13). Elisabeth Reid delivered a quite moving speech that showed the great promise of attitudinal changes on the part of health workers who were faced with sick and dying patients. Great care was taken also to obtain promises from national, provincial and district level governments regarding funding of AIDS committees and secretariats and to apprise stakeholders of the existence of the HAMP Act and its provisions to challenge stigma and discrimination. People in education called for a move from 'general awareness' to more focused interventions and forms of community engagement. Behavioural surveillance data were presented by Dr John Millan that showed that so many people were becoming sexually active at such young ages as perhaps to rethink when sex education should commence.

Other high points included a public airing (for the first time, in my experience) of doubts about the efficacy of the ABC approach, recognising that it had 'limited effectiveness'. More sound evidence was presented of the special risks for women of and in marriage, which had long been held as the bulwark (along with 'family', which is tirelessly promoted by Bruce Copeland of AIDS Holistics) against HIV infection (GoPNG 2006: 4, 5). The Poro Sapot Project sponsored by Save the Children (in Papua New Guinea) was introduced by Christopher Hershey and Thomas Kauage in terms of lessons it had learned in its progressive work with the especially vulnerable in Goroka, Kainantu, Lae and Port Moresby. Their presentation pushed the envelope of moralistic approaches to HIV transmission prevention (GoPNG 2006: 22). Their condemnation of everyday usage of pejorative language to describe gay and bisexual males (such as *geli-geli*, akin to the American 'faggot' or the Australian 'pooftah') was well-received.

Behavioural (if not yet serological) surveillance was to provide the foundation for an evidence-based approach, which was perhaps the most radical of the many ideas discussed and presented throughout the Summit. That, and the call by Dr Temu closing the Summit that the government stood behind a '100% condom use' approach to preventing future transmission. Dr Temu's request that churches 'put aside their biases' in these matters (author's fieldnotes, 9 March 2006) was badly misquoted the next day in newspapers as that churches had been 'demanded to ignore their beliefs'. (I know this because I overhead a newspaper editor attending the seminar call his paper and read to it the headline he wanted the next day.) This soured the intent of Dr Temu's message and led three days later to him pulling back on his message on Em-TV and changing the wording to mean '100% condom usage *outside* marriage'. It has since then transmuted further to goals of 100% condom *accessibility* (NACS 2008: 92). Another success of the condom social marketing campaign conducted jointly with NACS and NHASP was the message, 'no condom, no sex', but which was aimed primarily at urban youth (NHASP 2006f: 5), not at unsafe sex *per se*.

There was another truly notable absence on the programme. Just recently there had been published by Chris Curry, Paul Bunungan, Carolyn Annerud and Diro Babona an article in *Emergency Medicine Australasia* (Curry *et al*. 2005). The authors expressed concern at the seemingly fast increasing number of anecdotal reports among attending physicians and nurses of patients in the Emergency Department of the Port Moresby General Hospital who were presenting with evidence of opportunistic infections, with intractable diarrhoea and with acute respiratory illnesses. They conducted an anonymous survey of HIVab seroprevalence in 300 consecutive Emergency Department patients who, between April and July of 2003, already required venipuncture for other reasons. 'There was no linking of results to patients and therefore there was no follow up of positive results', say the authors (Curry *et al*. 2005: 360), but their findings of 18% HIVab seroprevalence among victims of snake-bite, car-crash and domestic assault, broken bones and the like are truly alarming. They found also a 44% seroprevalence among their youngest cohort (aged 10–19), second-highest (at 29%) being amongst 40–49 year-olds (Curry *et al*. 2005: 361). At least the pattern to these alarming data supports IMR and scattered other findings, for example, of 10% and 8% HIVab seropositivity among 15–19-year-old antenatal clinic attendees in Port Moresby in 2003 and 2004, respectively (Carol Jenkins, quoted in NHASP 2005b: 3). Especially disconcerting was the fact that Dr Babona heads the national reference laboratory, but NACS officials have consistently undercut the message of the Curry *et al*. article by claiming that the seroprevalence figures weren't confirmed (author's fieldnotes, Port Moresby, 2005–06).

Secretary for Education, Dr Joseph Pagelio, introduced also in 2006 a first-ever critically minded *HIV & AIDS and Reproductive Health* course for lecturers and student teachers funded by AusAID, the NHASP, the NACS and the EU. It was especially supported by VSO TokautAIDS, an NGO managed by Carol Dover and was working in tandem with the Madang PAC that has emerged with significant capacity, expertise and goodwill. Yanga Treppa and Rich Jones, of Fresh Produce Community Development and VSO, respectively, acted in training and project management capacities to produce a thoughtful, conceptually clear and attractively laid out guide for use in designing educational curricula around sexual and reproductive health (Department of Education 2006a, b). The Lecturer's Guide contains many interesting lessons, topics, strategies and suggestions regarding the struggle to educate Papua New Guinea teachers about not just HIV and AIDS and even STDs, but also issues of discrimination and stigma. One lesson has it that the HAMP Act was 'based on human rights and Christian values' (Department of Education 2006a: 55), a claim that is only half-right, since the latter word does not appear in the Act (GoPNG 2003), and there are other debatable assertions of anatomy and physiology (such as that females living together necessarily menstruate simultaneously), but it is in many, many ways an extremely important and progressive document and course. Unfortunately, the resource guide eventually became the personal whipping boy of Bishop

Bonivento (see Chapter 5). He reported to Agenzia Fides in Rome that this educational resource was guilty of 'encouraging them to engage in sexual relations', that it contained scientific errors and that it is 'educationally and morally deceiving' to boot (Agenzia Fides 2008). Scientific errors? Shall we talk of physiology and conception theory in the books of the Old Testament? He asked that the government withdraw the book and suggested that all concerned parents should enroll their kids in Catholic schools. There, he argued passionately, they would learn, among other things, that 'a person is able to avoid HIV/AIDS infection [sic] not only if she/he receives adequate information regarding the origin, the nature, the deadly gravity of this infection, but also and above all if she/he lives the Christian values ... These Christian values are the best protection against HIV/AIDS [sic] ' (Bonivento 2008: 2). Worst of all, he belittled the instructors of such courses for using the term 'life skill' to denote the learned negotiation of safer sex practices such as masturbation.

The reproductive health course was no doubt strengthened by field experience and findings collected by volunteers and paid staff members of VSO, who had conducted an initial study in early 2005 and then a follow-up study in 2006 (see Levy 2005, 2006) in three districts: Jimi, Raikos and Ambunti/Dreikikir. Tour and training reports from the theatre troupes who accompanied or preceded or followed them were also called upon to attempt to measure changes in knowledge, attitudes, practices and behaviours relevant to HIV and AIDS; to condoms and their usage; to stigma and discrimination; and to community mobilisation around these issues. These reports speak favourably about progress made in these areas, that is, in terms of lowered stigma, greater sexual agency exhibited by women and the identification of positive change agents. Nevertheless, the study found still significant disjuncture between knowledge and awareness, perhaps increasing association of condoms with 'risky' behaviours (see Chapters 4 and 5) and little distinction between HIV and AIDS. This greatly ups the ante as to the communication of 'risk' and denouncing of stigma, since the two are often held to be identical.

> 'Most PACs list representatives of women's and youth organisations among their membership, however in only a few cases are these representatives able or encouraged to play an active role in the committee. Few women have executive roles on the PACs, and none of the 9 provinces visited had a female PAC chair' (NHASP 2006d: 13).

The Papua New Guinea National Strategic Plan for 2006–2010 was finalised in 2006 with support from UNAIDS, who also pitched in to support the national Monitoring and Evaluation Framework. UNAIDS also guided the construction of the Workplace Policy Tool Kit on HIV/AIDS, which is being used in settings of both public service and private industry, and another critically important document, the Gender Policy on HIV/AIDS, although its planned insertion into the 2008 national budget never occurred (NACS 2008: 34). UNAIDS also spearheaded the Papua New Guinea Alliance of Civil Society Organizations, which was formed and launched in September 2006.

Another welcome development was the construction of a new web-site for the NACS (http://staging.nacs.org.pg). It is flush with downloadable versions in PDF of key reviews, evaluations and monitoring and surveillance documents. Contact details are still missing, however, for several score individuals, PACs and DACs, and I have yet ever to receive a reply to my queries by facsimile or e-mail. It still defines AIDS as 'a disease' (instead of as a protean disease syndrome) that can be 'spread' (which is physically impossible), and states that one can get an 'HIV/AIDS' test, which is also physically impossible and further confusing. It claims to want '[t]o improve social behavior research in PNG so that it complements epidemiological and other information and informs the development of strategies for behavior change'. Once again, the dubious nature of much of what passes for epidemiological knowledge about HIV and AIDS in Papua New Guinea (see Chapter 4) is let off the hook, and it fails to acknowledge the routine overlooking of social research findings (e.g. NHASP 2003a: vii) that challenge the status quo. Critical social scientific data are kept generally at arm's length anyway, so it's difficult to see how they can 'complement' anything.

However much improved, the web-site provides no *evidence* that the staggering amounts of money that have been spent have led to discernable outcome in terms of reduced transmission. It rightly trumpets the tremendous scale-up in VCT services for which Papua New Guineans and their donor agency sponsors can be justifiably proud, but it doesn't address the more difficult question as to the extent to which such scale-up has led to declines in HIV transmission, and how that links to transmission dynamics has yet to be addressed. Experience elsewhere suggests more than a note of caution, that HIVab testing and counselling do not have the hoped-for impacts upon reduction of transmissive risk behaviour (e.g. Higgins *et al.*, 1991; Ickovics *et al.* 1994; Dawson *et al.*, 1991). Susan Kippax has argued that 'while it may be true that [antiretroviral] treatment roll-out will reduce HIV-related stigma and discrimination by turning HIV into a treatable and chronic, rather than a deadly, disease, it is also possible that increasing testing – especially testing of the "routine/opt out" or mandatory kind – will increase HIV-related stigma' (2006: 231). The South African journalist Jonny Steinberg tells in the 300+ pages of *Sizwe's Test* of the personal idiosyncrasies of the doctors, nurses, chiefs, health managers, politicians and villagers who do and don't, who want to but can't obtain HIVab testing and counselling. By book's end, Sizwe hasn't yet been tested. Despite taking a year to screw up his courage to do so, when he does go, there is neither electricity nor running water and healthcare workers are in short supply. 'People arrive at a health-care facility frightened and unsure', says the architect of one local treatment initiative, Dr Hermann Rueter, but if 'you turn them away, they will not come back' (quoted in Steinberg 2008: 325). Alongside the tremendous scale-up in Papua New Guinea in VCT services are recurrent logistic shortfalls. Curry *et al.*'s study based in the country's premier hospital, Port Moresby General Hospital, and involving the shortest legs of transportation in the country, had this to say:

> Even so, collection of samples was irregular and unsystematic. Logistic difficulties in the supply of specimen bottles, in getting samples to the laboratory and in testing samples impacted on the number that were processed. Limited patient information was sought but even then collection of data was incomplete. For many patients age was unknown and therefore estimated by a member of staff. (Curry *et al.* 2005: 361)

Even Edward Green, the conservative advocate of the A and the B in ABC (and member of the US President's Advisory Committee on AIDS), concluded recently that VCT is 'a measure that has been shown to have no effect in preventing new HIV infections, however important it is as a gateway to treatment' (Green and Ruark 2008: 24).

Many downloadable NHASP- and NACS-sponsored documents and reviews peel back at least the top layers of what are supposed to be transparent results and processes. Even then, however, legitimate questions can be raised as to the degree of transparency achieved. The Provincial AIDS Committee system, for example, is seen in one report as 'varying' in levels of performance, as having 'inherent weaknesses' and as 'underperforming' PACS are said to be so for being under-resourced and perpetually short of staff (NHASP 2006d: 1, 2). Those familiar with PACs, however, know that the problems are systemic more than fleeting. Local politics and idiosyncratic personalities (neither personnel nor lack of money *per se*) determine shortfalls in coordination of outreach activities and reporting schemes. Multiple vehicles have been crashed, but only the one time that a woman was driving one was the driver sacked. Computer equipment has in several provinces been absconded with or destroyed, but neither is that necessarily a sackable offence. HRCs have been moved sideways from one province to another but without having had to demonstrate capacity in the province left behind. In one province a theatre group rival to the one sponsored by the PAC was disallowed entry owing to the personal jealousies of the HRC anxious to protect his fiefdom. Condom promotion has been blunted by church opposition to it, but only rarely have NACS officials confronted such opposition squarely. A recent salvo of anti-condom rhetoric, not this time from Bishop Bonivento (see Chapter 5) but from United Church pastor Reverend John Ravusiro (Gerawa 2008), was answered once again by a lone medical doctor, Glen Mola (Mola 2008), that is, by neither NACS, NHASP nor AusAID officials. Dr Mola's clear-thinking response was couched in part-medical, part-Biblical terms, suggesting that Jesus but not contemporary anti-condom crusading pastors 'dined with prostitutes'. This reveals some of the tension between religious and what passes for secular approaches to HIV transmission prevention in Papua New Guinea. I am suggesting, therefore, that NACS and NHASP and NGO documents have focused far too much on the sociology of pathology (on epidemiological models, on allegedly deficient lay understandings of transmission dynamics, on ill-tempered local responses, and so on) at the expense of the sociology of the response itself. Relationships between PACs, religious leaders, provincial health officers, the local hospital and FBOs, and between all of them and the NAC and NHASP – these are sociological issues, too.

Conclusions: toward a sociology of knowledge

This chapter has attempted to tell in broad terms the story of the response to HIV and AIDS and associated issues that occurred in Papua New Guinea from roughly the mid-1980s to 2007. There are currently taking place many progressive actions engaged in by well-meaning people and organisations. If grasp doesn't always exceed reach, at least it can be said that government organisations, NGOs, churches and their leaders, and even the private sector have begun to get serious about a likely devastating epidemic of suffering, death, confusion and blame. Undoubted successes have occurred, just as remain many intractable problems. For example, when the NAC was transferred to the control of Prime Minister Michael Somare's department, no 'PLHA' (Person Living with HIV and/or AIDS) representative went with it (Leach *et al.* 2006: 14). Fortunately, since then several prominent PLHA groups have formed, for example, in Alotau, Mt. Hagen, Lae and Madang, in affiliation with the national Igat Hope office (NACS 2008: 36). Only one of the seven focus areas of the National Strategic Plan, however, in this case, the Research Advisory Committee, has a board/council member known to be HIVab+.

To introduce the topics and critical spirit of the following two chapters, I'll mention a few here. First, the sexual behaviours of Papua New Guineans are denounced and pitied by other nationals from the pulpit and conference room, village men for their roaming and violence,[7] females for their promiscuity and vulnerability, and the less heterosexual for their transgressions and deserved come-uppance. However, while they cry 'foul' when expatriate politicians or policy brief-writers say so, national politicians, women's group leaders and public health authorities call disaffected settlement-dwelling youth and highway truckers 'animalistic', 'high-risk', 'dog-like' and worse (see also Zimmer-Tamakoshi 1997). Just before he passed away the late Sir William Skate said that entire settlements and villages had become 'saturated with all "the three evils" [meaning home-brew, poverty and AIDS]' (quoted in Waiut 2005: 4). Seldom is the sexual prerogative of male health workers or aid workers critiqued, and pastors and members of the House of Parliament always get a free pass. There remains silence about the specifically sexual double standards in Christian doctrine and specifically gendered ones of Christian practice. 'Traditional' and introduced property concepts that keep land, employment, money and decisions about family planning in male hands are similarly absent from programme directives. Health bodies and officials refer only rarely to (and usually so as to dismiss) data and insights that would help contextualise contemporary sexual behaviours – if only to show why 'behaviour change' is so difficult to instill and monitor. Those are rejected as being introduced foreign things and behaviours, although Boxing Day, evangelical Christianity and the ABC message seem to do okay. The inconsistent grounds on which some concepts and practices are valorised and others pilloried aren't yet the focus of sustained critique.

Second, the fact that Papua New Guineans adhere to the Christian tenets that were instilled in them by evangelising missionaries but which don't prevent infections isn't surprising. Only distant journalists and marginalised social researchers can say so in public, however. Probably not intending the pun, a NHASP report noted that '[r]espondents in all regions also mentioned church gatherings, crusades and night fellowships as risk occasions where lots of people come together for several days' (NHASP 2005g: 12). Butt, Morin and Numbery (2002b: 27) found in Indonesian Papua, too, that church crusades were among the '[f]requently mentioned events or places at which youth congregate and arrange for opportunistic sexual encounters'. It seems that, unlike in Tanzania (Dilger 2007), New Guinean females are flocking to Pentecostal churches and gatherings not seeking salvation from compulsory heterosexuality so much as support and the possibility to maximize options in it. 'Christian fellowship' has not yet been dubbed a 'high-risk setting' in policy documents, however, and neither have the 'campaign houses' where votes are bought with beer and sex (Polly Wiessner, personal communication, June 2007). Perhaps they should.

Third, 'housewives' have not emerged as a 'high-risk group' in mainstream epidemiology although they are accepted as being especially 'vulnerable', just as are 'girls' and 'young, unmarried females' but on whom are blamed HIV prevalence in mobile males. 'Husbands' and 'male relatives' have yet to be targeted as such for behavioural or serological surveillance, though they're getting infected from someone, somewhere, and certainly infecting their wives, nieces and daughters. In the strange logic of risk assessments, 'high-risk' sex is that which takes place at 'high-risk' settings between 'high-risk' people no matter the number of used condoms littering the scene and despite the absence of any, much less good ethnographic data to sustain such assessments. Sound ethnographic data to the contrary in droves has been swept aside. By contrast, that which has *not* yet been dubbed 'high-risk' – unprotected, often coercive sex in companionate relationships – *is*. Watch how quickly it disappears from normative assessments: 'Generally low levels of condom use, a rise in extra-marital and premarital sex, and low levels of awareness and knowledge about HIV/AIDS contribute to the country's potential crisis' (ABM 2005: n.p.). Poof! The Governor-General, Paulias Matane, recently called for people to follow the Ten Commandments (but marriage is apparently infection-free): 'There is a big increase in HIV/Aids cases in the country', he said, 'because of adultery, despite knowing it's wrong' (*BBC News*, 16 August 2007). Poof! An otherwise progressive article published in the *Post-Courier* yet said that '[s]taying negative means never having any "risky sex" again. "Risky sex" is any sex that is not with your lifetime partner (that is wife or husband). If you don't have a life-time partner, then this means abstinence. But if you do have any risky sex, then you should make it less risky by using a condom' (Mola 2006). Poof! Marital sex again gets off scot-free, but condoms are for 'high-risk' sex. Logical gymnastics are required to dub something that is categorical (sex either with or without a condom) in rather more fluid, sliding terms ('less risky') and without disturbing the normative paradigm. By whatever measure, the normative paradigm excludes marriage from settings of high-risk sex. The WHO defined it thusly: 'Risky sexual practices such as *casual and commercial sex*' (WHOSSP 2006: 27, emphasis added). Poof!

In the following chapter I dig more deeply under the surface level of structures and linkages to reveal ideology and significant disjunctures between the rhetoric of the national response and the lived realities of individuals and communities being affected most directly by HIV and AIDS. I critique the assumptions that guide and underpin the response, whether those be of funding stream requirements or the tendency to prefer quantity of data no matter their quality or degree of completeness. I aim to help strengthen a national response that has not shown yet much desire critically and reflexively to examine itself and adjust accordingly.

NOTES

1. Christine Stewart cites in her recent fine essay, 'Men Behaving Badly', a source of Clive Moore for the contention that 'rock-hard durable navy biscuits' were given during wartime by soldiers in exchange for sex with, in this case, young boys (2008: 83).

2. There is no shortage of reports of the incidence of HIV in medical and more popular literature, in government documents, in NGO press releases, in unpublished conference presentations and in radio transcripts. Clinical literature about AIDS is in Papua New Guinea not perhaps as well developed as in other nations, but as elsewhere, the clinical manifestations of AIDS are multiple and complex but have tended to cluster around contagious diseases such as tuberculosis, around immune system dysfunction related to malnutrition and otherwise easily treatable bacterial infections and especially around respiratory ailments including pneumonia. Anaemia is heavily implicated in the 'side effects' of the toxicity of antiretrovirals, both pre-existing and those that are expressed in slight decline or reconstitution of the immune system (e.g. NHASP 2005a: 9) and will no doubt become the focus of more clinical reports akin to that of McBride and Bradford (2004). We can only hope that more reports are published as to the clinical successes and remaining challenges of such therapies, not just as access to them increases toward the hoped-for 'universal' coverage but also as their supply remains unstable.

3. In 1986 the National AIDS Surveillance Committee (known briefly as the NASC) was formed and four years later, in September, if I remember correctly, the National Department of Health published its first National Medium-Term Programme for the Prevention and Control of AIDS. This was sponsored and informed by the Disease Control Unit, whose members included two national doctors and also two expatriate social scientists and an epidemiologist who would later go to Suva, Fiji to work for the South Pacific Commission in related matters. One of the objectives of the first Medium-term Plan was to 'establish a baseline on knowledge, attitudes, beliefs and practices related to AIDS and HIV infection' (quoted in Fiti-Sinclair 1996: 117).

4. For example, he chose for interests of short-term gain to recognise the government of the Republic of Taiwan in Taipei. As well, he earmarked at least K180,000 of government money for the Filipino Christian televangelist, Benny Hinn, who during his crusades in 1999 promptly termed Jesus Christ the real Prime Minister of the country and himself, its Ambassador (Sullivan 2007: 72).

5. Tingim Laip, or 'Think Life', is a programme sponsored and supported by Save the Children (in Papua New Guinea) that has been implemented in 36 sites split between 11 provinces so as to accomplish the following: 'to facilitate and sustain behaviour change to minimize HIV/AIDS and STI transmission and increase awareness in high risk settings and communities in PNG'. Tingim Laip is grounded on four pillars: 1) ensuring accessibility and availability of condoms (male and female); 2) referrals to user friendly STI services; 3) referrals to user-friendly services of voluntary counselling and testing; and 4) care and support for PLHIV.

6. Only a few weeks after I wrote these words I was given a manuscript to review for the *South Pacific Journal of Law* written by an author claiming that at this point four such cases had been put to the Ombudsman Commission but that no records or reports were available

about their outcome, if indeed they had already concluded. The source listed was a personal contact.

7. Tobias' statement is typical of such constructions: '[m]en drifting to towns and travelling along highways sleep with infected prostitutes and pass the virus on to their wives when they return home' (2007: 2). Given the rural-to-urban-to-rural-to-periurban-to-rural nature of mobility and migration in Papua New Guinea, reverse scenarios are just as plausible. In any event, transmission dynamics are never observed, but only proclaimed.

Chapter 4

HIV in discourse

Problems and prospects of the national response, 1987–2007

Prospects and problems

> [P]articular features of the HIV/AIDS epidemic demand the reappraisal of much that is taken for granted by social scientists engaged in development policy and practice. The most striking of these is the way HIV/AIDS challenges borders of all kinds: the folly of analysing the phenomena according to political and administrative borders is most marked yet ... the intellectual borders posed by categories of analysis that are taken for granted are equally fraught. (David Plummer and Doug Porter, 1997, p. 41)

The narrative I told in Chapter 3 about efforts in Papua New Guinea to understand the introduction of, monitor the spread and prevent the transmission of HIV is but one of many that could be told. Perhaps the preferable narrative is one of Papua New Guinea achieving slow but steady progress toward a capping and reduction of transmission and of thus meeting Millennium Goals and winning renewed confidence from WHO. This narrative would tell of 'multi-sector collaborations' and 'innovative, participatory programmes' that build on 'community goodwill' in 'culturally appropriate' ways to achieve '100% condom usage' and 'universal access' to antiretrovirals for 'the most vulnerable among us'. These kinds of narratives tend to be told at press conferences and in opening workshops because the claim of success, the appearance of success is perhaps even more important than actual success. The Hon. Paul Tiensten proudly displayed the UNGASS 2008 report at its launching ceremony on 15 July 2008, holding it up for all to see, and noted that 'we [are] only two-years away from the goal of universal access to comprehensive prevention, treatment, care and support' (*BW* 2008b).

Others seem to prefer bloodier, gloom-and-doom scenarios, which emanate especially in the foreign press. As much as she claimed to want not to apportion blame, Miranda Tobias claimed an 'absence of commitment by the Papua New Guinea government' that was leading Papua New Guinea to 'a humanitarian disaster' (Tobias 2007: 1, 14). These claims are flatly contradicted by much of the previous chapter. For good measure she interpreted levels of suffering of tuberculosis to be so low as to need to impute reporting errors (Tobias 2007: 5), when in fact tuberculosis infection is extremely common in Papua New Guinea and also quite well reported. Matthew Carney's reportage in the ABC-Produced Four Corners programme, 'Sick No Good' (Carney 2006; Cronau 2006) opened with the alarming prediction that 'Papua New Guinea is sliding towards a disaster – an epidemic of African proportions' and that 'Australia may have to take the fallout'. Peter Sims' letter to the editor of *BMJ* (Sims 2003) reported upon AIDS figures and related deaths as rising 'remorselessly' and depicted urban settlements in Port Moresby as living Hells, especially for health workers and those suffering from AIDS, a situation that he argued required a 'law and order approach' to remedy. Bill Bowtell (2007) has charged that governments in the Asia-Pacific, despite for a long time knowing how to curb and reduce HIV transmission, have proven unable or unwilling to do so. The most recent Country Cooperation Strategy published by the WHO (WHO 2006) writes of numbers of HIV infection increasing 'hyperbolically', not just exponentially.

In this chapter I address the efficacy of leading messages and programmes and show how little attention has been paid to critical, reflexive thought about them. Whether or not its proponents and documents would say it this way, the national response in Papua New Guinea to HIV and AIDS, among many other things, constitutes a 'system of signification'. Sociologists and semioticians who pursue the scientific study of the meaning of signs and their communication and reception by listeners and viewers expect those listeners and viewers to 'complete the meanings' intended by advertisements. See an image of a car, buy it. Be instructed as to behavioural comportment, model it. For example, in the next chapter there are presented several AIDS-related posters that feature drawings or cartoon likenesses of humans that, given the signs and expectations we have from prior campaigns remind us of our obligations toward heterosexual monogamy and to warn against its breaching. In *Sign Wars: the cluttered landscape of advertising*, Robert Goldman and Stephen Papson suggest that American audiences have entered a realm of 'hypersignification', a profound shift in the ways in which consumers relate to products and services and advertisements about them. 'Advertising', they argue, 'instead tries to turn the "code" itself into a sign' (Goldman and Papson 1993: 57). I suggest in this and the following chapter that in Papua New Guinea ABC functions something like that, just as do similar alphabetic constructions elsewhere. The South African loveLife programme offers a similar message called PRD, which stands for 'Protect (with condoms), Reduce (your partners), Delay (your sexual debut)' (Epstein 2007: 148). Little discussion has occurred regarding its constituent parts, for example, what 'abstinence' might mean in a male-dominated and compulsorily heterosexual state, or what 'fidelity' means to men who can have more than one wife or to the wives who marry them. No serious debate has ensued regarding the particular and obvious illogic of the code itself, since neither abstinence nor fidelity squares with current political-economy or traditional social-structure.

That does not preclude its effective rhetorical deployment. Adherents wear it as a badge of sorts, a shield against implications of impropriety, and utter it as a slogan signifier of one's modernity. And that's of course only the ones who can cop to the C part of the code.

'It was impossible even to find someone in the National AIDS Council Secretariat or UNAIDS to discuss the data that had been given to me. I was not satisfied with the assumption that the adult [HIVab] prevalence rate would level off at under 6% but I was unable to find anyone who could explain how that assumption had been arrived at. People were always away at meetings, on leave or otherwise inaccessible' (consulting demographer, in a personal communication to me, April 2008)

Moreover, the relationship of code to code-master (i.e., the international consultants, the national health officials, the church leaders) is restricted from view. For 15 years now settlement-dwelling Papua New Guineans or their rural brothers and sisters have had their 'knowledge bases' regarding HIV transmission prevention tested in terms of apparent 'awareness' of ABC and other slogans such as 'stay faithful', 'high-risk settings' and 'avoid sex with prostitutes'. What such awareness may mean in terms of HIV prevention has not really been addressed squarely, and neither has it been set forth what it may mean to health officials and policy planners. (I have yet to hear a NACS or NHASP official say that ABC prevents transmission.) The technical, administrative system known as the 'national response' (and its many sub- and sub-sub-systems on the provincial and district and local levels) uses words, acronyms, references, definitions, statistics and exhortations to do what it does. Nevertheless, there is meaning communicated by silences and gaps, too, in omissions as much as in commissions. While national health authorities join foreign consultants in lamenting the cultural taboos that surround discussions of sexual matters, the average conference, workshop, seminar and press briefing is noticeably tidy and sanitised in that same regard. Attendees seem no less squeamish about sex, but yet no one has made them the targets of cognitive or behavioural surveillance. In other words, the national response has yet to turn this system of signification back upon itself, to reflect upon itself, to make itself its own object. The subject (the proponents, consumers, agencies and donors) and the object (HIV transmission and AIDS-related miseries) have not fused into one cohesive analytic unit so as to be made known to others. The national response has been weakened to the extent it is unwilling to generate knowledge of itself suitable for viewing by others.

My critique is therefore not designed to point the finger of blame at individuals so much as to encourage the appearance of the missing reflexive component and to ring the death knell of ABC. It must go. If there has been graft involved in cases pertaining to the HIV/AIDS Management and

Protection (or HAMP) Act of 2003, for example, by insiders selling what should be a free manual of its implementation, then that harms the national response. If policies regarding condom distribution are not being adhered to, then that also harms the national response. If the policemen who raided Port Moresby's Three-Mile Guest House and assaulted and detained innocent people have still, six years later, not been prosecuted (HRW 2005; Stewart 2004), then the efficacy of the law and people's faith in it have been blunted. If bribes were sought in this and related cases, for example, in bailing out detainees, then confidence in authorities is weakened. Their denial by NACS and NHASP and other officials, no less than the acts themselves, are harmful.

This larger point I'm making is implicated in a number of ways. A persistent weakness of the national response is its imbalanced approach to research, one that has tended to collect and promote numbers that are of often dubious quality and that don't aid so much as preclude the development of critical theory about transmission dynamics. The fact that Papua New Guinea's HIV epidemic is considered a 'heterosexual' one that is 'about' promiscuity and prostitution (e.g. AusAID 2004; Caldwell 2000; Caldwell and Isaac-Toua 2002; CIE 2002; ESCAP 2005; Middleton 2006b; NACS 2006b; WHO 2001a; WHO-SPC 2004;WHO-NACS-NDoH 2000) is partly owing to the politics of epidemiology, but partly owing to the squeamishness of national officials who are none too anxious to air what is perceived to be 'dirty' laundry, for example, about the state of data collection, the extent of male–male sexuality or the real location of most infections: between spouses. On some levels epidemiologists have followed the lead of national health officials in wanting *not* to have the real facts of transmission shared, for example, that X number of transmissions might be attributed to sexual assaults occurring in families and prisons, that Y number can be chalked up to marriages and politicians, and that Z numbers of people have been infected *multiply* and through *multiple* risks and modes.

Nevertheless, we should not underestimate national and especially religious sensitivities about sexuality, for they also play their part. In asking so little of the real state of sexual praxis (and in so ignoring substantial research findings about it), they have all too willingly hidden behind a dangerous assumption regarding the roughly equal male:female ratio that exists in reported cases of HIVab seropositivity. Despite that 'epidemics' have neither sexual identity nor orientation to begin with (since neither germs nor infections are 'heterosexual'), the assumption that Papua New Guinea's HIV epidemic is 'heterosexual' *merely for this reason* is as unforgivable as it is unnecessary. Epidemiologists have in this way hidden behind national health authorities. Routinely reported male:female ratios of 3:1 or 5:1 or 8:1 in STD prevalence, for example, are seldom if ever used to promote notions of a 'gay' epidemic. The rhetorical appearance of the slow 'feminisation' of its HIV epidemic (thus adding 'gender' to the prior 'sex') does not mean that increasing numbers of lesbians were becoming infected, either, to which such phrasings would logically lead. In any event the sexual component that should be democratising discourse about transmission hasn't done so. What I mean is that the 'heterosexual' signifier should capture also aunties and politicians and religious leaders in its net instead of 'targeting' already vulnerable people.

Those who promote the prevailing model of HIV epidemiology can't have it both ways: if equal male:female ratios are to mean that the transmission mode is heterosexual intercourse, then Members of Parliament, expatriate timber barons and aunties (who are heterosexual) need to be targeted, too, and about equally so. I make clear throughout the chapter that *certain kinds* of heterosexuals are still targeted, not heterosexuality *per se*, which is what the discourse ought on other grounds to be saying. What emerges especially in more 'public' forms of discourse in the national response (workshop presentations, addresses, letters to the editor) is that health, political and particularly religious leaders seem so uncomfortable about one facet of a 'Western'-style epidemic (in which male–male sex accounts for far higher numbers of infections) that they prefer the more obfuscating 'African'-style alternative in which the roughly equal number of cases in men and women means that at least *heterosexual* sex is occurring. In fact, of course, neither a 1:1 nor a 5:1 ratio yet tells us much about the kinds and extent of sexual transactions that are taking place and the social and economic contexts in which they occur. Therefore, a more forthright spelling out of the contours and details of a Papua New Guinea-style epidemic is lost track of.

This suggests a certain confusion resulting from the ways in which data are collected and analysed in clinic settings, which are relatively new things. Moreover, and in contrast to countries such as Brazil or Mexico, Thailand and Indonesia, sexual identity formation is thought by most social scientists to be weakly developed in Papua New Guinea. There is little acceptance of or support for third or more genders, and few communities are arranged or function according to sexual object choice or erotic practices. Some movement is occurring with regards to sexual transgression, for example, the *pasindia meri* of Wardlow's *Wayward Women* or the commercialising transvestism of Port Moresby nightclubs. Until recently, when they were brought by WHO and FHI consultants and others, there were few words to describe or great facility with concepts of sexuality, sexual identities and sexual scripts. 'Bisexual' and even 'heterosexual' have little parlance in indigenous language (*tok ples*). 'Gay', 'straight', 'lesbian' and 'homosexual' and other such terms apply more to FHI-sponsored workshops and AusAID-funded conference settings than to families, villages and indigenous research. This is why such terms and their associated acronyms trip so neatly off the tongues of NGO representatives but who haven't yet grounded them in social scientific research. That's not to say that there aren't laudable amounts of diversity and contingency in sexual practice, only that they haven't congealed into identities or been used effectively to guide more appropriate HIV transmission prevention activities. The term 'bisexual' dropped out of epidemiological parlance as a discrete category sometime post-1995. At that time, of the 308 known cases of HIV infection registered, only four were chalked up to 'bisexual' (*The Health Worker* 1995: 3). What that meant more precisely remains a mystery. A bisexual male infecting a bisexual female? A bisexual male being infected by a homosexual male? A heterosexual male infecting another heterosexual male via anal intercourse?

Father Paul Duffy's criticism of Australian funding schemes – that AusAID funds what it is interested in, not what Papua New Guineans themselves say they want or what is likely to work (Greer 2006) – is repeated often and loudly but with seemingly little effect. This leads to understandable frustration on both sides. Some say that the problem is accentuated by donor country initiatives that are pitched to work directly parallel with communities instead of partnering with government departments. Others complain instead of the difficulties of working with precisely those government departments but that are understaffed and that have little experience with proper accounting and monitoring functions. For example, the surveillance and monitoring function that ought properly to have been the responsibility of the Department of Health was taken from them for precisely this reason. It has since been returned, but yet the same kinds of criticisms are being made currently. Private companies and many NGOs and CBOs seem to 'get things done' in that regard, but political exigencies, such as that real financial power rests in Kuala Lumpur and Canberra, not Port Moresby, require that donor agencies make use of private management consultants and companies to oversee and supervise such projects. ACIL Pty., Ltd., for example, won the private bidding to manage the AU$60,000,000 NHASP project that commenced in 2001 and that was extended again in 2006. ACIL received AU$323,000,000 in 2003–2004 by managing 31 Australian government aid contracts alone (AIDWATCH 2005: 4). The Asian Development Bank-sponsored Rural Enclaves Project grant application had more money slated for consultancies (over $US5,000,000) than equipment, trainings and workshops and project management combined (ADB 2006:12). '"It is boomerang aid," says one PNG official contemptuously – "much of the cost of the [aid] programme will go straight back to Australia in salaries and contracts to Australian companies"' (quoted in *Sydney Morning Herald* 2005). When foreign aid becomes an ATM (the phrasing is Epstein's; 2007: 202–9), there is really no sense in blaming health officials for financial mismanagement or the proliferation of managed speech about 'high-risk settings' and 'multi-sectoral responses' and 'strategic plans' (see especially Katz 2002: 136).

Quantity over quality

As I showed in the previous chapter the national response to HIV and AIDS began in the clinic. I argue in this chapter that it has to a large extent remained there. A heavily quantifying research tradition has since 1987 virtually ignored qualitative data and approaches and shown little interest in questioning assumptions. Most health officials and many politicians and church leaders can recite the fact that HIVab was first detected in a blood sample collected in 1987. Nevertheless, few seem aware of the impressive array of *relevant* social scientific and historical research already conducted regarding, for example, ritualised homosexuality (Herdt 1993a, b; Knauft 1993, 2003), ethnomedicine (Glick 1977; Lewis 1975), clinic attendance (Hammar 2004b; Hughes 1991, 2002), anti-condom discourse and practices in health care facilities (Hughes 1991; Wardlow 2002c, 2006a), serial copulation (see Chapter 2), conception beliefs (Mallett 2003) and appropriateness of research method in handling sensitive topics and collecting high-quality data *in context* (Hammar 2004c; NSRRT and Jenkins 2004). Granted, those are not topics generally taught in medical school, but since 1987 they should have been. There is even less excuse now for not including them in policy discussion and workshop presentation. The NHASP review of antiretroviral roll-out recommended that '[b]arriers to HIV testing in hospital settings should be investigated' (NHASP 2005a: 19). My response is that *relevant* findings regarding precisely that should first have been investigated ... in the library.

Thus far in the evolution of the HIV epidemic in Papua New Guinea, NGO and especially government documents have tended to blame *the patient* and a background in *village ignorance,* not the health worker and the legacy of the colonial experience in medical matters, the practices of segregation of European from Native on church mission stations or in health facilities. Passey *et al.* (1998b: 401), for example, argued that WHO guidelines for the syndromic management of STDs needed to reflect the fact that '[c]ultural barriers, as well as poor understanding of the significance of the symptoms may also reduce care-seeking by women' and that the vast majority of women (and even many men) didn't even seek treatment. Although true in itself, the statement only presents one side of the ledger. They point out later in their essay (and correctly) that a woman may be confused at being dubbed 'high-risk' but without ever having had any laboratory tests done on her behalf. Nevertheless, this is also true of all 'sex workers' the first time they are seen in a clinic and of 'MSM' who for various reasons have also never seen the inside of a clinic or been told that their sexual predilections have been acronymised. The sexual behaviour of the patient and her or his alleged cognitive deficits are blamed along with his or her tendency to abscond. The other determinants of sexuality or clinic attendance have seldom been implicated, for example, the shame and fear induced by church policies or the confidences that are compromised there. A survey of 19 country-level STD services programmes in the Pacific was carried out by Sarda and Gallwey (1995: 37), who found that the constraints of such programmes most commonly reported by programme officers included 'inappropriate health care seeking behaviour'. It's sad that they didn't obtain patient reports about some of those same officers.

I say this no longer with rancor, but five times since 2002 I have helped consultants hired by NACS, NHASP, the National Research Institute and other NGOs to collect bibliographies and assemble knowledge about these relevant issues. Despite asking several times – and nicely – I have never received the courtesy of acknowledgement by their employers or even a copy of the work produced. Apart from the ill feelings that this breeds in social researchers, it results in old lessons needing to be learned repeatedly, in the reduplication of work that wastes precious resources, and in the blunting of much needed coordination of individuals and agencies. Nevertheless, study after study, one review upon another keep finding the same facts – and then little is made of them. The NHASP review of social science research priorities that was written by a well-respected expatriate ethnographer concluded that this last deficit is most notable in research proposals put to the Research Advisory Committee. 'Most show little awareness of the current literature on HIV/ AIDS', he concluded, 'including that on sexuality and gender, either for PNG or more widely' (NHASP 2003a: 55; see also IRG 2007: 13). Nevertheless, review after review complains of '[l]ack of behavioural and social research' (UNAID-AusAID-NAC 2004: 24; see also WHO-NAC-NDoH 2000: 14; NACS 2007: Recommendation 4). Who is lacking here? Social scientists?

The loss to the national response is incalculable. Policy makers and health planners have lost sight of, if they haven't themselves elided, the contextual nature of sexual acts and motivations for which they keep calling. The narrative component to sexual scripts (the anguish and silences) and outcomes (unwanted pregnancies, spoiled reputations) that help to explain precisely why individualising messages about HIV transmission risk don't 'work' is consistently ignored or under-appreciated. Put bluntly, they don't understand why men choose to risk transmission in terms of misconstrued models and emerging masculinities (Reed 2003; Wilde 2004, 2007; Wood 1998) and why women *have* to risk transmission as the price of survival.

A more fundamental problem is the fetishization of numbers and the seeming unwillingness to ascertain their veracity or conceptualise their relevance. The 2007 Consensus Workshop report, for example, which appears to have for the first time been penned by NDoH staff, specifically prescribed 'the use of "official" statistics by all stakeholders', which would 'ensure consistency of information' (NACS 2007: 5). That's good, so long as that consistent information is also truthful. When the interviewer for Radio Australia's 'Pacific Beat' programme, Geraldine Coutts (GC), interviewed the national health official (HO) responsible for such, she let slide his many conflations of HIV and AIDS and statistical errors on the order of magnitude:

HO: The objective of the [most recent Consensus] workshop basically first was to do an estimate of the national prevalence, and then the second one was also to do an estimate of how many people actually are living in PNG with the virus [which are the same thing]. So we're talking about both asymptomatic and symptomatic cases, but also to give us some idea of the extent of the problem we're currently dealing with on a national level. I'm talking about 2–3.5%. When you're talking about say for ten people we're talking about two people infected with HIV, out of every ten [thus moving from 2% to 20%]. So it could be between two to four people that's arranged [thus sliding from 2% to 40% in a single paragraph!].

GC: Now that's very high[;] is this higher than the last time it was estimated?

HO: Yes it's higher.

GC: And so at what rate is it growing?

HO: The rate we also calculated it anyway, because we've had two workshops [in 2000 and 2004], this is the third one, so we definitely can give some rate of how we are going at the moment. But that I can't give you at the moment.[1]

GC: So if it keeps going at this rate … [although there has not yet been stated a rate].

HO: If you're talking about the national level, yes, if you're talking about regions, there are two regions that are not as bad as the other two [expression of hope?]. So if you're talking about the southern region and the highlands region which actually have the gravest problem. If you're talking about the

Momase and the New Guinea islands the problem we know that was but what we're trying to do is, there's a lot of factors that drive it here and one of the things that they'd be actually discuss at length to identify most of our high-risk groups. (Radio Australia 2007)

This was a less than convincing recounting of the findings that emerged from the 2007 Consensus Workshop (see NACS 2007); my inquiries to Port Moresby officials have gone unanswered, even to the media specialists at NACS whose job it is to handle such queries.

Papua New Guinea is paying the high costs of such naïve empiricism by the erection of debatably constituted risk groups that compromises national HIVab seroprevalence data. In 2006 a NACS spokesperson quite highly placed was quoted at a press conference held in Australia to the effect that '[d]uring the course of finding the estimate figure, nearly all the people interviewed said they have *multiple* sexual partners' (Franklin 2006: 1, emphasis added) despite that the NACS' own figures show 'faithful housewives' to be at particularly high risk, accounting for more than twice the numbers of infected 'sex workers' (CIE 2002). Moreover, if they're all having multiple partners, then why has so little conceptualisation of multi-partnering occurred, why have members of one putative group (sex workers) been so consistently singled out, and why have ethnographic insights into sexual networking been so ignored? Data quantity and quantitative data, regardless of their completeness or veracity, have thus been promoted over qualitative data of a high(er) quality.

The accuracy of reports and releases from government and private research authorities seems immune from criticism but is used anyway to denigrate the knowledge bases of Papua New Guineans. The 'HIV/AIDS Quarterly Report' from December of 2006 says that 'All cases of HIV and AIDS have undergone confirmatory testing' (NACS 2006b: 2), though of course there is no such thing as an 'AIDS test', and despite that a large clinical sample of 'AIDS diagnoses' in the Port Moresby General Hospital were characterised by *11% of them coming with no evidence whatsoever of HIV* (Lavu et al. 2004). The NACS 2007 Consensus Workshop report expressed but did not attempt to explain why it was that, of the 18,484 people who 'tested HIV positive' by the end of 2006, 'data was [sic] not reported for the majority [9,709 (52.53%)] as to whether they were classified with HIV infection or with an AIDS defining illness at the time of their diagnosis'. This opens the door to rather different interpretations of what 'AIDS' is since once again an HIVab+ test result is not necessarily part of the equation. Cases of persistent tuberculosis or diarrhoea or unexplained weight loss stand proxy for 'HIV infection' even despite lack of serological testing. An editorial published in the *Pacific Economic Bulletin* by a well-known international consultant in these matters stated that in Papua New Guinea, a country characterised by 'low literacy', 'HIV is *directly caused by*' (that is, instead of 'potentially transmitted during') unprotected sex, birth, breastfeeding, blood product transfusion and drug injection (Butcher 2007: 158, 160, 159, emphasis added). The Director of the New Zealand AIDS Foundation, Rachael le Mesurier, was quoted as saying that half of the recent steep rise in numbers of HIV infections was '*caused by* gay sex' (Donald 2007, emphasis added). Miranda Tobias reported in her inflammatory policy paper published for the Centre for Independent Studies that '120,000 Papua New Guineans are likely to have HIV/AIDS'. Well, which is it?, since that 120,000 figure could be divided by eight or multiplied by it. 'Infection rates are now estimated to be 2% to 3% of the population', she wrote, just before writing that '[a]t least 1%, and probably 2%, of the population is infected' (2007: 1, 2). Nevertheless, she criticised the specific content of HIV and AIDS related theatre performances as 'problematic' in this 'barely literate society' (2007: 11, 12). A team of three Japanese researchers worked in the Republic of the Marshall Islands to study 'cultural barriers to talking about sexuality' that made the provision of sex education difficult. One of the means used to assess 'knowledge' of 'transmission routes' was the assertion, 'AIDS can be transmitted by oral sex' (Suzuki et al., 2006: 141), even though it cannot. That 81% of boys and nearly 86% of girls answered in the affirmative means that a great 'teachable moment' was probably lost. Bill Bowtell decries the fact of HIV and AIDS prevention strategies that are founded upon theology instead of scientific, empirical evidence, which is fair enough. Then he argues, however, that 'the HIV virus' [sic] is 'not nearly as contagious as, for example, the influenza virus' (2007: 3), when in fact HIV is not at all contagious, but is, of course, to varying degrees infectious. A media release issued from the Wycliffe Australia-sponsored conference in 2006 estimated an 87% rural population in Papua New Guinea, many of whom were only 'semi-literate', thus requiring special educational programmes and messages. Nevertheless, the media release many times conflated HIV and AIDS and thus allowed to stand an estimate that there were upwards of 400,000 cases of AIDS in the country. Moreover, it claimed that a more God-centred family life would lower transmissive risk and lessen the impact of AIDS (Franklin 2006: 1–2). The PAC Beat radio interview in March of 2007 (see above) included the following explanation by the national health official: ' ... because a lot of the people who could potentially be infected with HIV/AIDS are a-symptomatic, and they are the ones who are actually spreading the virus' (PAC Beat 2007). One cannot be infected simultaneously with cause and effect of disease. One cannot be suffering from AIDS and be asymptomatic. The deathly ill are not highly sexually active. Those about whom one knows nothing (those 'potentially infected') cannot fairly be assumed to be 'spreading the virus'.

Such missteps and conflations are common enough in government documents, too. Table 1.2 of the March, 2005 Quarterly Report suggests that 268 cases of AIDS had been reported from 1987 to 1996 but only seven cases of HIV and that the cumulative total of AIDS reports by 2005 outstripped those of HIV by over 500 (NACS 2005: 4), despite that elsewhere one 'symptom' of an AIDS diagnosis is required to be an HIVab+ blood test. 'AIDS is not well reported' by health authorities in Fiji and Papua New Guinea, according to Tim Sladden (2005: 28). Noting fairly enough that '[d]eath notification and case classification are major problems', the report also showed graphically that 70% of the case reports were 'unclassified' (that is, that they didn't specify either an HIVab+ test result or a death from 'AIDS-defining illness') (NACS 2005: 4). The same document claims that increasing rates of infection from 2004 to 2005 were due partly to improved testing, but that 77% of the case reports were still 'unknown' regarding transmission route and that an equal percentage were unknown regarding 'province of origin' (NACS 2005: 7, 5). A NHASP document published the same year but based upon the 2004 Consensus Workshop (NHASP 2005e: 11) complained of precisely these kinds of mistakes and others, but which were apparently not corrected prior to the holding of the workshop or even prior to the publication of the ensuing Quarterly Report. The NHASP review of the 2004 National Consensus Workshop findings noted that '[t]here is a need for a regular review and interpretation of quarterly surveillance data by a small group of specialists from NACS and NDoH, with additional technical support as required, *prior* to the publication of the quarterly reports' (NHASP 2005e: 11, emphasis in the original). Another NAC document defines 'epidemic' as 'a *disease* that spreads rapidly through a demographic segment of the human population in a geographic area' and claims further that epidemics 'can be spread from person to person or from a contaminated source such as food or water' (NAC 2007: vi, emphasis added). I am not trying to play 'gotcha', but rather, suggesting that these missteps can no longer remain immune from criticism, that they must be analysed and be treated *the same way* as are assertions made by the 'common folk' that receive such bad press, especially the ones attributed to lack of education.

Many other untrue claims have been made regarding 'surveillance'. Upon closer look, this often means a one-off bleeding in an institutional setting, the taking of X number of blood samples consecutively several years ago or two-off but with many intervening years. This makes the resultant samples as little repeatable as they are representative. Surveillance is supposed to mean the constant observation, the close monitoring of people, places and social processes, not simply the periodic extraction of data from 'well-matched' subjects. There appear to be no debates over meaning, no framing of hypotheses regarding transmission dynamics, and no recognition of the problems of interviewer transference in the clinical setting, for example, by imputing heterosexuality where it doesn't belong, assuming fidelity in married females, assuming only single infective sources, and the like. Damian De Walque studied serodiscordant couples in Burkina Faso, Cameroon, Ghana, Kenya and Tanzania. He found that it was the wife who brought the infection into the marriage somewhere between 30%–40% of the time (De Walque 2006). Vinod Mishra also found female HIVab seropositivity in HIVab serodiscordant couples in 11 African countries to range from 32% to 62% (Mishra 2007). By 2006, therefore, it was not true to claim that '26 sentinel sites [are] giving good quality sero data' (NHASP 2005b: 80), when one review after another says the opposite. As of 2007, for example, Daru's antenatal clinic contributed only once, in 2003. When data from it were aired in a workshop setting the resulting figures (5 of 150 blood samples being found Repeat Reactive to HIVab, but only one of which was 'confirmed' serologically, for a true prevalence of 0.7%) were misconstrued by an attending politician as meaning a *30%* seroprevalence, not even 3% (5/150). He then used the occasion to argue for conservative realignments of sexual matters and decried the presence of homosexuals in the country. His homophobic comments then and on other occasions went unopposed by the many NHASP and NACS officials and others present, including those who are gay, lesbian and bisexual (author's fieldnotes, Port Moresby, 2004, 2006). The same document notes hopefully that new protocols will be put in place to begin filling in the considerable data-collection and -reporting gaps, but only if data can begin to be disaggregated by age, sex and other sociodemographic variables (NHASP 2005b: 80). These would be welcome developments were they to occur, and social scientists could be put to good service in this endeavour.

❋ ❋ ❋

It is now time to examine more closely the empirical claims made about the shape, pace and tenor of Papua New Guinea's HIV and AIDS epidemics. Table 4.1 replicates information presented at the 2007 Consensus Workshop (NACS 2007).

Table 4.1 Key HIV and AIDS indicators

		Years in Question			
		2003	*2005*	*2006*	*2007*
People Living with HIV/AIDS	Adult and children	19,738	32,904	46,275	56,175
	Adults 15+	19,117	31,864		54,448
	Adults (15–49) rates (%)	0.64	1.02	1.28	1.61
	Women (15+)	10,806	18,407		31,883
	Children (0–14)	621	1,040		1,727
New HIV infections	Adult and Children	5,227	8,531		14,638
	Adults (15+)	4,874	7,954		13,684
	Women (15+)	2,819	4,666		8,174
	Children (0–14)	353	577		954
AIDS Deaths	Death in adults and children	2,185	3,871	4,935	5,995
Orphans due to AIDS	Orphans (0–17)	1,549	2,704	3,326	3,730
ART Treatment	Number of Adults (15+) in need of treatment	2,437	3,204	4,238	5,712
	Number of Adults (15+) on ART		80	1,098	3,000
	Number of Children (0–14) in need of ART	233	384		636

Source: Author's adaptation of figures provided in NACS (2007)

Many tough questions may rightly be asked of the information presented here. For starters, one could make allowances for those aged 15, 16, or 17 being dubbed an 'adult', although socially, economically, sexually and occupationally few such are, especially boys. However, Table 4.1 suggests that one can be both an 'adult' at 15, 16 and 17 but also simultaneously an 'orphan'. Elsewhere the same document notes that 24-year-old females are still 'youth' (NACS 2007: 8). Second, the row header entitled 'Orphans due to AIDS', which is to say, whose parents have died of AIDS, seems to switch subject to those orphans *who have AIDS*. Moreover, the grounds on which both parents can be said to have died from AIDS, given the loose definitions of 'mama' and 'papa' and the accepted problems with data collection and reporting, are neither firm nor given. Peter Barter says in the Foreword to this document that 3,700 are predicted to die in 2007 of AIDS, leaving 3,700 orphans (2007: iv). Is that logically possible? Third, there is no explanation of the missing data in terms of who, what, why and where. Was it insufficient training of data collectors, late reporting, logistical difficulties that prevented coordination, or what? Fourth, it is not clear to what extent, regarding data from 2007, these are reported numbers or are estimates thereof. The estimate regarding how many patients are on antiretrovirals, for example, 3,636, is three times more than the published number announced by the leader of the country's antiretroviral programme, Dr Goa Tau, as of 7 June 2007 (Rei 2007: 26). The estimate of 14,638 'New HIV infections' in 2007 would then push the cumulative total wildly past the total of 16,104 as of June, 2006, published by the NACS (2006b: 2). Given the often repeated estimate that reported infections are one-fifth to one-tenth of the real totals, this would completely reshape the suspected epidemiology of HIV in Papua New Guinea and would necessitate the restructuring of counselling, care and treatment

What seems to be the case is this: so long as tables and charts, graphs and PowerPoint presentations are loaded with statistics and numbers, they come to have an 'aura of validity and rigor' (the phrase is Holly Wardlow's) even though they are riddled with internal inconsistencies, and despite that many data are missing and others, suspect. Moreover, despite that social researchers have collected and verified data collected by qualitative, often long-term means and usually in context, they are dismissed insofar as they cannot be made to fit into a table or onto a PowerPoint presentation. Poor-quality, quantitative data are endlessly repeated.

Similar kinds of questions can be asked of the seeming disconnect between low estimates of national HIVab seroprevalence (1.28%) and the often markedly higher figures established at sites of Voluntary Counselling and Testing (VCT). Those are shown in Table 4.2 (adapted from NHASP 2006b: 11, Table 1.11).

Table 4.2 HIVab seroprevalence in sites of voluntary counselling and testing

Province	Site	Type	2004 (%)	2005 (%)	2006 (%)
ESP	Center of Hope (FBO)	VCT+		2.4	1.3
MP	Bethany (FBO)	VCT	9.0	4.5	6.3

Province	Site	Type	2004 (%)	2005 (%)	2006 (%)
SP	Nende (FBO)	VCT		6.8	
	Mingende (FBO)	VCT		12.1	4.0
SHP	Kumin (FBO)	VCT		7.9	14.0
NCD	Clinic 6 (PHF)	VCT	19.0	20.0	
	Anglicare (FBO)	VCT+	3.3	9.3	6.5
	Poro Sapot (NGO)	VCT+		14.8	6.3
	St Theresa (FBO)	VCT			3.5
	St Mary's (FBO)	VCT+		7.9	2.7
GP	Kikori (FBO)	STD		11.1	
EP	Yampu (FBO)	VCT		11.8	1.0
WHP	Tininga (PHF)	STD	7.0	12.0	
	Shalom Care (FBO)	VCT+	12.0	13.5	8.4
	Rabiamul (FBO)	VCT		19.2	11.0
EHP	Michael Alpers (PHF)	STD	4.0	5.0	12.0
	Kainantu (PHF)	STD	8.0	20.0	20.0
CP	Vei'fa (FBO)	VCT+			0.0
MP	Friends (PHF)	STD	8.0	7.0	8.0
	ADRA (FBO)	VCT			4.2
Totals 1*			8.8	10.9	6.8
Totals 2**			7.0	10.3	6.0
			48/728	311/3016	258/4292

Legend: PHF=Public Health Facility; STD=STD clinic; VCT=Voluntary Counselling and Testing; VCT+=Voluntary Counselling and Testing plus other services such as food, clothing, housing, etc.; *=average of HIVab seroprevalence reported at sites providing or not providing numerators and denominators; **=HIVab seroprevalence, where numerators and denominators are provided. Complete notes on funding sources and services offered can be found in UNAIDS-AusAID-NAC (2004).

Source: Author's adaptation of figures provided in NHASP (2006b: 11, Table 1.11)

The December, 2006 Quarterly Report (NACS 2006b) included data being reported from 20 of the 75 sites of VCT. Those included two sites run by NGOs, eight that are private clinics, 34 that are supported by churches and another 31 that belong to the public sector (NHASP 2006b: 11, Table 1.11). These data are difficult to assess critically for all the gaps and omissions, but they do reflect the obvious ramping up of the number of facilities providing VCT and of numbers of people being tested. In 2005, the numerators and denominators were unfortunately not provided for the tests performed at the so-called Friends Clinic (Lae), the Michael Alpers Clinic (Goroka), the STD clinic in Kainantu and the Tininga Clinic (Mt. Hagen). Each clinic exhibits high and increasing levels of testing, seroprevalence of HIVab that is many times higher than what is accepted as being the national average, and high prevalence of STDs. Each is an ostensibly 'secular' clinic run by the government, but which is funded greatly by AusAID. Neither the Friends Clinic nor the STD clinic in Kainantu provided numeric data for 2006, and data are missing altogether for the Tininga Clinic. This means that true seroprevalence, were those data added, would almost certainly be greatly higher than the 6.0% figure obtained otherwise. In any event, taken together, and thinking also of the high figures of seroprevalence reported for the Porgera valley, Wabag, and so forth, they surely call into question the estimate of 1.28% offered at the 2007 Consensus Workshop (NACS 2007). A report by the American Foundation for AIDS Research from the Port Moresby General Hospital has said the true seroprevalence would be 4.4% were surveillance strategies (the tools, the software, the assumptions, the data sources) better developed (Treat Asia 2007). I would suggest that similar improvements could be made were the gaps in surveillance to be honestly accounted for. For example, in the Foreword to the Consensus Workshop Peter Barter claims that 'This report was compiled with data collected and gathered from all the surveillance sites in the country', but the document itself notes later that data from only 47 of the country's surveillance sites were reported (63%). In 2005 the HIVab+ prevalence figure cited for Papua New Guinea's blood donors was 1.49% (NACS 2007: 11). Granted, figures from other years are lower, but still, it raises questions; I know of no other country in which blood donor seropositivity outranks that accepted for the 'general population'. Does this mean that blood donors should now be targeted?

It is a fair question to ask, then, why that 1.28% figure became official. Other notable features of this quarterly report include the statement that reports of new cases had 'slowed down' because numbers are 'not growing exponentially' (NACS 2006b: 2), when in fact they were *never* rising exponentially but are frequently *said* to be (e.g. McBride 2005: 304; Sladden 2005: 22: Vinit 2004; NACS 2007: 28; NACS 2008: 17, 18), when they are not said to be rising *hyperbolically* (e.g. WHO 2006: 12). Since roughly the mid-1990s, the number of reported cases has risen about 30% annually or less, and notable apparent declines in testing or the reports of results thereof have occurred, for example, in 2004. What explains the allegedly steep decline from 2006 estimates? It's difficult to say, for official pronouncements about it are extremely confusing. For example, then Minister for Health, Sir Peter Barter, in introducing the 2007 Consensus Workshop findings in its Foreword, wrote that 'The trend of the epidemic is showing a *high increase*, especially in rural areas where 85% of the PNG population lives. It is projected that *starting in 2007* the prevalence among the rural population *will become* higher than in urban areas. The new 2006 prevalence estimate, when compared to previous estimates, shows that while the *prevalence is lower* than what has been previously estimated; the trends in the epidemic are *increasing more sharply* than what has been previously documented' (Barter 2007: iii, emphasis added). The Executive Summary of the same report also concludes that data collected from VCT, ANC and tuberculosis clinics 'are showing a high increase in the level of the epidemic' (NACS 2007: viii). It says that 'the new 2006 estimates, when compared to previous estimates, show lower prevalence; however these new estimates have a steeper increasing trend than what has been documented before' (NACS 2007: ix). Elsewhere it concludes that the decline of seroprevalence from the 2005 figure of 2% to the 2006 figure of 1.28% 'does not in any way represent a decrease in the epidemic', that 'while the HIV prevalence is lower, there is a sharper increasing trend' (2007: 26). If there had occurred a 'high increase', then why were the new estimates so much lower than previously suspected? If they were lower, then how can they be said to have 'increased more sharply' and to exhibit a 'steeper increasing trend'? If the previous estimates were incorrect, on what grounds were they found to be so, why were they allowed for so long to stand, and could the same kinds of mistakes be being made yet? A related concern, evident at many points throughout NACS documents (e.g. NACS 2007: 13, 28) is that declines and increases in HIVab testing are often cited to explain seemingly declining or increasing *prevalence*, when such could only affect *incidence*, that is, based upon absolute numbers. The Acting Director of the NAC, Romanus Pakure, was quoted by a reporter for *The National* covering the Pacific Countries Ports Association conference as having said that HIVab seropositivity was currently in Papua New Guinea 1%, not even the 1.28% figure discussed above. The newspaper article says that he said the 'generalised HIV/AIDS epidemic prevalence rate is 1%' (Satoro 2008), which is confusing and incorrect on too many levels to count.

These kinds of discursive slippage and confusions regarding fundaments of epidemiology help to explain the frequently alarmist tone and sometimes quite wild predictions that are made. For example, in 2006 Wycliffe Australia issued a press release in which it was said that '[t]he HIV positive rate in PNG could jump from 2% to 25% within several years. If current infection trends continue, by 2010 Asia-Pacific will have taken over from sub-Saharan Africa in HIV/AIDS prevalence' (Franklin 2006: 1). McBride's editorial made the same point, suggesting that the results of a hospital-based study 'tell us that HIV prevalence in the country is well on the way to reaching the levels seen in Sub-Saharan Africa' (2005: 304). Trends, rates and patterns are in Papua New Guinea difficult to assess because seronegative findings don't tend to get published, because seropositive tests are often not adjusted for the total number of tests performed. Thus, the best for which we can hope is to know reported cases with certainty, but not about overall infection and disease burden (e.g. Sladden 2005: 34). Contrary to the optimism voiced above, the increase among males from 2004 to 2005 was of 158 (to 1,310 new cases) and then of another 401 new cases the following year (to a cumulative total of 1,711). Of the cases between 2003 and 2006 in which female sex is reported, there occurred increases from the previous year of 56, 394 and 378 (NACS 2006b: 2). Moreover, a cumulative total from 1987 to 2006 of only 58 cases was reported for Gulf and Central provinces combined. Only 0.16% of the total number of cases ever reported, therefore, have come from two provinces marked by remarkably rapid social changes, oil exploration, intense sexual networking, logging activities and widespread mobility. The social mapping team in Gulf Province, for example, found that:

> Disputes between communities or tribes can also lead to risk behaviour. A group from Kaintiba (Kerema) said that women might become victims in conflicts between two villages, where the men from one village, once the opportunity emerged might rape women from the other village as payback or as part of the "argument". The mapping team also added "line up sex". At times during parties or whenever there was an opportunity men might arrange line ups where they lure a woman or girl into taking drugs or alcohol and then all men take turns having sexual intercourse with her. In such cases the men would not think of using condoms or they simply do not want to use them. (NHASP 2005i: 21)

Additionally, 76.85% of all case reports during this quarter came without listing province of origin (NACS 2006b: 4), so it is difficult to know what to do with such figures. Not surprisingly, the age group 15–19 exhibited a markedly higher number of cases seropositive in females (63) than in males (14), and the next two age-groups (20–24, 25–29) were marked by the same imbalance (147–70 and 148–84), although these need to be adjusted slightly to reflect the fact that females out-tested males by the ratio of 1.1:1. Missing data regarding age are particularly hampering the ability of the national response to be guided by epidemiological models because the assumptions made regarding transmission dynamics are not likely to be true sociologically. Sladden (2005: 24), for example, distributed HIV infections but of unknown age across the known demographic profile of Papua New Guinea so as to allow for age-adjusted ratios; he would surely agree that this robs epidemiological models of explanatory power, since humongous statistical artefacts (men don't attend antenatal clinics, boys aren't raped by much older female relatives and family friends) could be responsible.

Further evidence of HIV transmission seeming not to be slowing down and thus contradicting the figure of 1.28% was provided by Table 1.10 of the same document (NACS 2006b: 10), adapted here in Table 4.3. Data are unfortunately missing for 2006 for three extremely busy STD clinics, in Kainantu, Mt. Hagen and the Port Moresby General Hospital, but prevalence figures are high and seemingly getting higher.

Table 4.3 Select STD clinics (% patients testing HIVab+)

Province	Site	2001	2002	2003	2004	2005	2006
EHP	Goroka	<1.0	1.6	3.0	4.0	5.0	12.0
EHP	Kainantu			2.0	7.4	19.0	
MP	Lae		5.1	7.1	8.3	6.9	7.3
WHP	Mt. Hagen	1.7		6.3	7.2	11.5	
NCD	PMGH	9.0	9.6	10.8	19.9	20.0	

Source: Author's adaptation of figures provided in NHASP (2006b: 10).

How dynamic is your transmission?

> In Melanesia and South-East Asia, the diversity of physical environments, histories, cultures, practices and beliefs; demographics; social, economic and political relationships; and farming systems, coupled with extremely rapid change, suggest that predicting the impact of HIV/AIDS will be at least as difficult as it has been in Africa, and probably more so. (Bryant Allen, 'HIV/ AIDS in Rural Melanesia and South-East Asia', 1997, p. 123)

The section and chapter above have in different ways shown that we do not know enough about transmission dynamics in Papua New Guinea even were data to be more consistently reported. Were we asking better questions in more appropriate contexts, however, and were we willing to give up cherished assumptions, we could easily strengthen the national response. The single most intractable problem with *usage* of data seems to be with their modelling. Returning to the 2000 Consensus Workshop, of special note is that all of the various groups enunciated and enumerated at this time – soldiers, antenatal and STD clinic attendees, sex workers and blood donors – were considered to belong categorically so and in non-overlapping fashion. There was no attempt then or since, so far as I know, to theorise or conceptualise how and of what were 'groups' conceptualised. It is worth asking how much of the seropositivity established in so-called 'high risk', STD clinic patients perhaps belonged to two or more categories. This would have the effect of decreasing some of their stigma perhaps and making the authorities think differently about 'low-risk' populations. What of, for example, STD clinic attendees who were also pregnant? Of antenatal clinic attendees were also sex workers? Of soldiers who were blood donors? Of pregnant women who complained not of the STDs with which they were yet infected? Of 'sex workers' who are, five days each week, petty marketers? Of disaffected youth who have been incarcerated briefly for sexual offences? Of 'villagers' recently emerged from long stretches in prison? These kinds of seeming conundrums and paradoxes are not complicated once one gives up cherished notions, as Helen Epstein found in sub-Saharan Africa. 'So, am I to understand', she asked a South African nurse, 'that the "low-risk" people are at higher risk than the so-called "high-risk" people'? '"Yes" was the reply' (Epstein 2007: 92). The epidemiologist was stunned, she says, by the sociological insight that miners preferred longer-term mistresses in town than 'wet tussles in the grass with prostitutes' (2007: 92).

Epidemiological models to date poorly fit the dynamism and contingency of Papua New Guinean sociality and sexuality. The conclusions that Plummer and Porter drew regarding the use and misuse of epidemiological categories were not drawn from, but they certainly apply to Papua New Guinea. They argue that the 'internationally accepted epidemiological categories do not adequately reflect the diversity of human behaviour: they make human sexuality, motivation and life choices appear simple and homogeneous. Because they are ill fitting', they continue, 'they can disguise important social dynamics' (Plummer and Porter 1997: 49). Key questions are thus not being asked regarding overlapping, contingent, negotiated membership in multiple social groups and regarding those 'important social dynamics' to which Plummer and Porter call. Assumptions are not being challenged and competing possibilities are going unasked, for example, that it is or might also be boyfriends and husbands and girlfriends, not just customers, who were infecting sex workers. The prevailing epidemiological narrative today is one uninterested in the highly contextual nature (if 'nature' is the right word) of sexual networking and of its great ubiquity. To take 'sex work' seriously as marking membership in a 'risk group' requires that certain kinds of data need more fully to be taken on board. Jenkins (2002: 11) reported a 1995 survey of young (under 21) unemployed females in towns and cities that 'reported that 49% stated that selling sex was their main mode of earning a living'. My own data from a study of sexual networking on Daru found that nearly 44% of 250 people surveyed in brief focus group discussions involving male and female alike, had been given or had given money, food or other material items or favours the last time they had sex (Hammar 1998a, c). Hughes concluded of her work in the Tari Basin that '[t]he reality is that many Huli women receive money and gifts for sex occasionally, if there is no alternative income source' (2002: 131). Wardlow has shown (e.g. 2004, 2006a, b, 2007) that many Huli women have taken to exchanging sexual services for material existence, owing to economic declines, absentee husbands and double-standards in employment, education and Christian doctrine. If 'sex work' is to be a viable epidemiological category, and if agency and choice are to be imputed to 'sex workers', then current databases in Papua New Guinea are completely inappropriate.

Questions about *with whom* sex workers used condoms 'last week' is another example of lost opportunities to make more of the epidemiological data we do have. The material, linguistic and social factors that denote the same sexual partner relating different ways to the same woman, as 'customer', 'boyfriend', 'pimp', husband', 'client-becoming-boyfriend' and so on, were not allowed in previous Consensus Workshops to infuse surveillance initiatives with any nuance or insight grounded in ethnographic particulars. The data presented in terms of 'mode of transmission' were extremely problematic in clinical terms, since AIDS was still constructed as a 'disease' and not a disease syndrome and as something that could be 'transmitted'; absence of information about HIV transmission was claimed in 38% of 'AIDS reports' (WHO-NAC-NDoH 2000: 19). Nor were any data published as to the setting in which questions were asked of the relatively few people providing blood samples about whom relevant information was being collected. Like doctors in other countries, many doctors in Papua New Guinea are for similar reasons uncomfortable with sexuality *per se* and with giving back test results for which their patients aren't ready. Nurses often presume information about their patients instead of gathering it. Heterosexuality is the only sexual orientation and identity allowed by law and so tends to be assumed unless demonstrated otherwise. In a clinical, counselling, employment or evangelical conversion setting of largely Christian sensibilities about sex, deviations from the ideals of monogamous heterosexuality must be extremely difficult to voice for gay men or for other kinds of men who have sex with other men. They must be even more difficult for the many tens of thousands of females who have been victimised in sexual violence committed by family members or church or legal authorities. Nor would it be easy for women sexually active extra-maritally, for whatever reason, to tell of their apparent 'indiscretions'. Many thousands of women periodically exchange sex for money and for food with which to feed their families or who must engage in such as a condition of their employment or promotion or ridership aboard a P.M.V. Otherwise straight men who from time to time have sex with other males, with and without their consent, as for example in institutional settings, must not feel much better about divulging their intimate secrets. Public scandals in Papua New Guinea involving national politicians and expatriate health advisors and television personalities have shown this vividly.

There were in 2000 estimated to be nearly 14,000 HIV infected Papua New Guineans (WHO-NAC-NDoH 2000: 11). Workshop attendees forthrightly noted the glaring omissions in surveillance systems, the reporting snafus, the inconsistent monitoring of infections and the still low number of sites providing surveillance data. Condoms were promoted but only sparingly so, and mostly to sex workers and their clients. The knowledge bases of members of the 'general population' regarding HIV and AIDS were assessed in 1996 and recounted in this 2000 report, for example, that 75% and 45% of males (and only 16% of females) had 'heard of' AIDS and knew that AIDS was fatal, respectively. Knowledge deficits were implied in that only 52% of males 'knew' it was transmitted sexually and only 7% that AIDS was transmissible via sex and also in blood transfusion (versus 36% and 5% of females, respectively). Insofar as AIDS cannot be transmitted by either sex or blood transfusion, however, perhaps the wrong population was being questioned. Certainly, the wrong questions were being asked. When media reports surfaced claiming that 12% of graduating University of Papua New Guinea students were HIVab+ (a completely unfounded charge, it was uncovered), an educational authority claimed that 'The disease is spreading like wildfire due to *ignorance* ...' (Anonymous 2006: 21, emphasis added). The fact that neither unprotected sex *per se* nor students specifically have *ever* been targeted (but in other contexts, school students are sought as blood donors – Jenkins 2000) does not yet seem part of the equation. A KAPB-style study published in 1995 but conducted in Morobe Province from July, 1993 to January of 1994 asserted that only 33% of residents of Kaiapit and 55% from the Coastal Lae area 'demonstrated knowledge of AIDS' and that 'the knowledge of HIV/AIDS of the majority of people was inadequate and inaccurate' (Karel 1995: 20, 23). Nevertheless, the researcher himself judged as a 'correct' answer 'one partner' regarding 'prevention of AIDS', which is factually incorrect. Moreover, he measured knowledge of participants against the phrase 'spread of AIDS', thus confusing cause and effect, and he dubbed 'prostitutes' a 'mode of transmission', which is wrong, illogical and misogynous. Siebers and Lynch (1998) contributed a valuable study of 'HIV and AIDS Knowledge Among Medical Laboratory Technologists in the Pacific'. One of the questions they asked study participants, however, was 'Which is more easily contracted – AIDS or Hepatitis B'? (1998: 25). They concluded that it was answered correctly only 65.4% of the time, but AIDS can't be contracted in the first place, nor is an acquired immunodeficiency disease *syndrome* (AIDS) parallel to a *virus* (HBV, in this case). The NHASP-supported Social Marketing campaigns involved interviewing respondents who were asked to respond to hypothetical positions, such as 'I feel I have no control over whether or not I contract HIV or AIDS' (2006h: 13), when the latter cannot at all be contracted, which was asserted in many other hypothetical scenarios or direct questions. Researchers and policy-makers cannot have it both ways – imputing knowledge gaps in their charges, but exhibiting them themselves all the time – though they frequently try.

✳ ✳ ✳

These examples show that there are many and interlocking strands of confusion that have hindered the good intentions and undoubted great efforts comprising the national response. Let us begin from the true premise that no one has ever seen transmission occur, that no one ever will and that probabilistic guesses are what we make, not observations. Let us assume further that those probabilistic guesses need to be more accurate. The normative AIDS paradigm in Papua New Guinea is evident in both academic research and in government and NGO documents. The article published in 2002 by John Caldwell and Geetha Isaac-Toua but which was founded on an essay the senior author presented two years prior (Caldwell 2000), concluded that in Papua New Guinea, 'the mode of transmission of HIV is ... almost entirely heterosexual' (2002: 104). Many government sources concur (e.g. NACS 2005: 7, 2006b: 5; NHASP 2006e: 23; WHO-NACS-NDoH 2000: 2) and like many score press releases and newspaper articles, they do so without critical comment.

However intuitively correct this may appear, in the interest of poking and prodding much-needed debate, several points can and need to be made in challenging these and other unfounded assumptions. First, Caldwell and Isaac-Toua claim that the then coming major epidemic in Papua New Guinea couldn't have been foreseen until 'very recently' (2002: 106) and that disease first 'takes hold in a major urban area of the country and then spreads from there' (2002: 106). Well, not so fast. I am certainly not alone in having predicted over a decade ago just such a major epidemic – it's just that no one wanted to listen to such predictions. I have met only few NHASP and NACS employees who showed any familiarity whatsoever with epidemiological and ethnographic data from prior to the terms of their employment. It is simply untrue to assert that the epidemic was unforeseeable.

Second, as for the Urban first, Rural second claim, I suggest that, in terms of the old saw, the drunk (the national response) has been looking for his keys (evidence of HIV infection) under the streetlights (in urban centres), where the light is better (where most HIVab testing is done), instead of where his keys (the real bulk of infection) are more likely to be, which is to say in the bushes next to the driveway (in marriages especially and also in rural areas). The same mistake was repeated in the UNAIDS, UNICEF, WHO summary of data for 2004, when they reported that 'infection appears to be concentrated in the capital city of Port Moresby' (2004: 2). *Appears*, in what sense? Sheri Fink's 2006 *Frontline World* essay, sub-titled 'No Escaping the Virus', shows the blind spots typical in Australian reportage about Papua New Guinea: 'While it's easy to see how HIV reached the capital, and spread through poverty and the sex trade, it's harder to understand why HIV is now beginning to devastate secluded rural areas'. Fink quoted Dame Lady Carol Kidu, who surmised that, 'Since people are mobile, if an individual becomes positive in an urban area and goes back to a community that has no knowledge of this, there's the potential it can almost wipe out the reproductive age group in communities' (Fink 2006; see also Hayes 2007: 11). Okay, I'll bite: how *did* HIV reach the capital? Could it have come from diplomats infected overseas and who return to infect village-bound and multiple wives? Could politicians be infecting women in rural-based campaign houses where beer and sex are traded freely for votes? What of missionaries, miners and aid workers posted to rural areas? If rural areas are so 'secluded', how does one explain the presence there of

'There was one thing that happened to us that I did not enjoy. That was anal sex, which took place during the initiation ceremony. We initiated boys were f***ed by a number of older men in a special hut (bidi gena) built for the purpose just before the ceremony took place. It did not have any windows and was quite dark inside. We did not know who f****ed our ass but we were told not to refuse because the purpose of this sex was to make us grow up to be strong men. The sperm is supposed to go into our bodies and make us strong and fearless. Well, when this was all over, my ass was very sore. It was bleeding from skin tears. You young people are lucky it disappeared before you were born ...We were told not to have sex before marriage, but sexual activities did take place in the men's house. This was anal sex and I did take part in these. All you had to do was arrange with one of the boys and take turns in f***ing each other's ass. As for sex with a female, only those boys who had sisters got married quickly, because to get married one's sister had to get married to your intended wife's brother. In other words, there was double marriage. As I have mentioned before, the couple had sex after marriage except for some cases where they married secretly because the time to wait was too long' (70-year-old male elder, Gogodala; Jenkins 2007: 24).

high-speed Internet, Malay fishermen, helicopters and Halliburton workers? Why can't people get infected in rural areas and transmit the infection when they travel to regional markets, provincial capitals and Port Moresby? Others have not found expected differences in the values and behaviours of urban versus rural youth (NSRRT and Jenkins 1994). As was shown also in detail in Chapter 2, there is much precedent for questioning the Urban first, Rural second scenario of infection (Hammar 1998a; Hughes 1997; Riley 2000; Thierfelder 1928; Vogel, with Richens 1989).

Third, not all of the sexual activities that occur in Papua New Guinea or that involve Papua New Guineans can rightfully be described as 'heterosexual'. An enormous literature has amassed over the years regarding 'traditional' and often highly ritualised forms of sexual intercourse between males, as often as not between younger boys and junior, but still unmarried males, and that doesn't necessarily stop when such males marry. In at least 35 different cultures throughout Melanesia, 'homosexuality' and/or 'bisexuality' (if you want to term it that) *were once normative* (see esp. Herdt 1993[1984]; Jenkins 2006; Knauft 1990, 1993, 2003; Wilde 2003). The fact that Christian missions and missionaries have prohibited such and that many Papua New Guineans continue to deny their existence or claim not to know of them in the first place does not mean that such norms and practices did not and do not exist. The health authorities guiding the national response never mention this vast literature.

As is vividly evident in the text box here, Carol Jenkins has shown that both coercive and consensual sex takes place between boys and between men, but it can happen in traditional, village settings as well as in institutional settings. Adam Reed's monograph about male prisoners in Port Moresby's Bomana Prison (Reed 2003) notes that '[s]exual thoughts drive them to masturbate endlessly, to have erotic dreams that cause involuntary emissions and sometimes to seize other men and forcibly penetrate them. The bodies of male prisoners are believed to be full of unreleased semen waiting to be ejaculated ... they will do anything to relieve themselves, including the rape of cellmates and men from their own language group' (2003: 116). Nevertheless, somewhat unlike other culture areas throughout the world, 'traditional transgendered roles are rare in Melanesian societies', says Jenkins, despite such sex being mundane, pleasurable, ritualised and sometimes coercive. 'In no case', however, 'did these practices have any implications for personal or community identity and apparently, prior to Christian missionaries, no major stigma. Almost all men married and had children, while some continued a behaviourally bisexually active life, as do some men today' (Jenkins 2006: 9).

Things have changed, however, in the shadow of homophobia. When the Christian Men's Network was founded in 2003 the launch was boosted by an inflammatory speech given by then Deputy Prime Minister, Dr Allan Marat. He claimed that gay men and lesbians, in their alleged promotion of 'sex hatred', caused straight men to spend their money on beer and assault their wives and girlfriends (John 2003). He took potshots at the NAC, too, in their promotion of condoms. The writer of a letter to the editor of the *Post-Courier* entitled 'It is moral to discriminate', signed by 'Anti MSM, Port

Moresby', rebuked a previous letter writer who had criticised Dr Marat's misogyny and homophobia. He concluded that, because 'our forefathers' practiced one of three heterosexual marital forms, 'monogamy', 'polygamy' and 'polyandry', 'thus, MSM never existed in PNG, until recently' (Anti-MSM 2003). The problem is that neither monogamy nor polygamy need be either heterosexual or even sexual. Males can be monogamous with other males and females with females, obviously, and millions of marriages around the world are virtually or completely sexless. Ironically enough, the only inherently heterosexual marriage form is polyandry, a term in anthropology that means one woman having multiple husbands, often brothers married in descending fashion. Not surprisingly, this marriage form is considered by many to be the only one that routinely provides women reasonable sexual choice. At a regional meeting held in 2001 and sponsored by UNGASS the health official delegation from Papua New Guinea 'raised objections to the inclusion of the phrase "men who have sex with men"', and so, in order to appear as a united front, the Health Minister from Tuvalu was required to use the phrase 'vulnerable groups' instead, but without even defining it (Pareti 2001: 5). Bruce Copeland, the Australian leader of the Port Moresby-based AIDS Holistics, has argued that it is not the responsibility of the community to take care of those living with HIV and/or AIDS and who have been rejected by their family: 'perhaps they have been trouble-makers in their family' (Copeland 2007). He claimed further that there is a 'gay hate campaign' against him, that the Fiji HIV and AIDS programme has a 'homosexual focus' to it, and that well-known expatriate NGO workers in the country were gay and lesbian, which is to say, paedophiles.

It is true that the acronym MSM is new. Nevertheless, the list is long of ethnic groups or culture groups throughout (Papua) New Guinea in which some form of sexuality between males (typically oral, anal, or masturbatory, compulsory here, erotic there) was considered the right, good and proper developmental precursor to heterosexuality, in addition to being pleasurable in and of itself for males in many groups. There is a culture alive-and-kicking in the nightclubs and discos, car parks and guest houses of Port Moresby, Lae and other towns that involve gay, bisexual and lesbian youth. Most of them are sexually active not just with and amongst one another but also with other erstwhile 'straight' Papua New Guineans and with expatriates, not all of whom themselves are gay or homosexual or identify as such, who may themselves be married and/or also have girlfriends with whom they are sexually intimate (Jenkins 2007; Yeka et al. 2006). How common male 'bisexuality' is (in the western sense of males who routinely have sex with women but also with other males) is not yet known because it has yet really to be defined and contextualised ethnographically or otherwise. The recent Second Generation Surveillance Study of Tokelau showed that 30% of the male youth surveyed had had sexual intercourse with other males (Peseta 2007: 5). Nevertheless, if one had in one's sights the institutional settings of sexuality (dormitories, barracks, timber camps, compounds and prisons, for example), as well as the often highly ritualised and homoerotic settings provided by *lainap* sex and pack rape, one would surely conclude that lots of Papua New Guinean males are 'bisexual'. In Port Moresby, 223 men who claimed to have sex with other men were interviewed, over 18% of whom either were currently or had been married. Only 23% of the total identified as gay or homosexual; 10% said they were heterosexual and two-thirds identified as bisexual (NACS 2007: 18). Carol Jenkins (2004) has suggested another reason beyond various nationalist or Christian grounds for why male–male sexual practices tend to be denied. Their denial, she argues, obscures otherwise stigmatised behaviours such as sexual aggression towards women, sex with transgendered people and homophobic attitudes and behaviours. In public forums such as newspaper articles and church settings, denials of male homosexuality 'sound good' and help to paper over the extent of (heterosexual) male domination of females, especially that which is Christian doctrine-inflected.

Spokespersons for national health bodies and NGOs have worried publicly about the 'nightmare' scenario of MSM-related transmission should it 'take off'. 'MSM' and 'gay' have already emerged as transmissive 'modes' to some doctors (e.g. Tau 2007), not just as a categorical marker of sexual behaviour. Relevant questions may be asked about the infective burden that MSM constitute in Papua New Guinea when compared to discourse about it. On ethnographic grounds, Papua New Guinea doesn't seem to match up to other Pacific Island Countries and Territories:

> Levels of reported MSM contact [as imputed source of HIV transmission] vary between different PICTs and in different sub-regions, with relatively high levels in Guam (64.9%), Tonga (58.3%), French Polynesia (38.5%) and New Caledonia (37.1%), and minimal or zero reported cases via this route in other countries (Fiji, Kiribati, Marshall Islands, PNG, Solomon Islands and Tuvalu. Numbers of cases are too small in many countries to infer any clear MSM exposure patterns. (Sladden 2005: 32)

Nevertheless, an extraordinary emphasis has in Papua New Guinea been put upon MSM knowledge bases, infection risks and intervention efforts. An extremely low number of cases of HIV has been registered to them, even though there is an extraordinary discourse about their infective burden. The exceedingly dense historical and ethnographic data relevant to male–male sexual networking dynamics yet goes without discussion. If they are rhetorically to constitute the 'bridging population', as is frequently asserted, then why haven't both sides of the ledger been scrutinised the same way, and why not also Asian fisherman, expatriate consultants, foreign aid workers and 'disciplined' forces? I note with no little irony the truth of Holly Aruwafu-Buchanan's statement recently (2007: 96) that 'no formal research has been done on MSM', despite that there has been mountains of evidence collected about men having sex with, well, at least other males (e.g. Herdt 1993[1984]; Knauft 2003; Wilde 2003).

The mental gymnastics required correctly to use even such seemingly straightforward terms as 'heterosexual', 'bisexual' and 'homosexual' in such an epidemiological setting as Papua New Guinea would make spin the head of an average person. Jenkins (1997, 2006, 2007) has written extensively about male–male sexuality in Papua New Guinea, and has added careful caveats about such not necessarily meaning anything about sexual identity. Nevertheless, MSM and 'at-risk population' discourse races ahead unimpeded.

It's too bad that such questions aren't asked, too, in that it remains illegal in Papua New Guinea to provide condoms to prisoners. A NACS document claims that condoms are now being distributed in prison settings (2008: 112), but my queries to NACS officials on this point went unanswered.

Fourteen years ago David Plummer and Doug Porter wrote compellingly about the specious assumptions of epidemiology when it comes to human sexuality. Although their comments were not aimed at Papua New Guinea, they are nevertheless just as apt today as in 1997 – perhaps even more so. They wrote:

> In addition, the epidemiological term homosexual does not readily accommodate people who engage in traditional practices where there is a transitory, male–male sexual element; or situational sex in male-only institutions such as the military, prisons, or sporting clubs; or culturally valued, religious transvestite traditions. All of these possibilities are conflated into one category, 'homosexual', and are thereby inappropriately related to the contemporary Western homosexual identity. (Plummer and Porter 1997: 43)

These facts should wake us up to expansive, not restrictive human sexual possibility and to healthy sexual diversity. They should be prodding us to ask behavioural and epidemiological questions differently. What, for example, does 'bisexual' transmission mean? If it means male infection of another male, then why doesn't that get slotted into the 'homosexual' category? If it means bisexual male infection of a woman, then should not it be enumerated in the 'heterosexual' category? If infection of one male has occurred by another but both of whom identify as heterosexual, or at least as neither 'gay' nor 'homosexual', then what role do sexual orientation and identity have for epidemiological categories? If both the males (one infecting, one being infected) identify as 'bisexual', then isn't that 'heterosexual' by the logic of the epidemiological assumptions (those of similar sexual orientations or identities being implicated in infection)? When a gay man has sex with a lesbian (in the US, such women are referred to with no necessary derision as 'fag hags'), does that belong in the 'heterosexual' category, even though neither participant is? Anecdotal evidence suggests that such exists on Daru and in Popondetta, Lae and Port Moresby (author's fieldnotes, 2003–2006). Over one-quarter of the MSM cited above had actually *sold* sex to female clients, not just had sex with women; and another quarter had had sex with 'female sex workers' (NACS 2007: 18). Are the young boys who present to the STD clinic with anal lesions because they have been sexually assaulted by elder males in fact 'homosexual'? Does that make the men who sometimes do such things gay? Can people not be infected multiple times by multiple routes and through sexual and other contacts with multiple others? In the language of epidemiology, anal intercourse trumps vaginal if no woman is involved. Thus, infections by males of other males is highlighted and exaggerated, but male infections of other females (by that route) are correspondingly buried. The Second Generation Surveillance Surveys sponsored by the WHO still counts 'homo/bisexual' as a transmissive mode, when the sexual acts in which they engage are to some (often great) degree 'heterosexual', by the logic of their terms, that is, those males also having sex with females (e.g. WHOSSP 2006). By means of the same algorithm, intravenous drug-using trumps sexual intercourse in terms of transmission risk, unless there is male–male intercourse involved. When men come into contact with infected semen by engaging in serial intercourse with a single, uninfected woman (most often non-consensually), known elsewhere as the 'milk-brother' phenomenon (e.g. Magaña 1991) but brought to our attention in the Papua New Guinea context of *lainap* sex, is that necessarily heterosexual transmission? Really? This would allow females to infect males, males to infect females, and males to infect other males via females, perhaps even both males and females becoming infected in the same encounter. 'Heterosexual' just doesn't cut it. Two Australian research teams conflated 'Male homosexual contact' with 'sexual contact between men' (Dore *et al.* 1996: 496; Kaldor *et al.* 1994: S170). In order for heterosexual male prisoners to remain that way but remain sexually active, institutional settings such as prisons require that other males be feminised and regendered through prison rape (see Reed 2003).

A fourth problem with epidemiological modelling is that the mode of transmission is largely unknown anyway by the terms of the epidemiological data themselves. For example, the September, 2002 Quarterly Report (NACS 2002: 3) noted that the mode of transmission was *entirely unknown* for 71% of the then 6,103 case reports of HIVab+ blood samples. Summary reports and government-sponsored estimates each show that information about province of origin and occupation were unavailable for 71% and 84% of HIVab+ case reports, respectively, well into the new millennium (CIE 2002; WHO-NAC-NDoH 2000). 'Where they were infected', said the Center for International Economics (CIE 2002: 14–15), 'and where they are now living and possibly infecting other people are the important, but unknown, matters'. Age was unknown of 41% of the HIVab+ case reports in August of 2003, according to the NACS statistical officer (Gege 2003). At the same Women in Mining Conference at which were presented such figures, it was also noted by Gege and two colleagues that mode of HIV transmission was unknown for 73% of the reported cases. By 2004, authors of the second Consensus Workshop summary report could not say whether there had been an improvement in recent quarters in terms of completeness of reporting upon province of origin, age, gender or occupation (NHASP 2005e: 5). By 2005 the percentage was 77% (NACS 2005: 7). Even as late as 2008 it was accepted that, still, '[t]wo-thirds of all of the recorded infections lack information about mode of transmission' (NACS 2008: 21). What to make of the remaining percentages is of course anyone's guess, but it had better be a good one – the number of reported cases has already topped 30,000. Former Minister for Health, Sir Peter Barter, closed the most recent data collectors workshop by calling attention to the problems noted in 2000, 2004 and 2007 that appear to be ongoing: 'We don't seem to have advanced very far in 12 months ... ' (*BW* 2008c).

A fifth problem compounding assumptions about sexual transmission is the uncritical acceptance of what and who constitutes 'high-risk' and why. They have been associated, for example, not just with high-risk sexual transmission *per se* but with institutional arrangements, for example, being 'geographically restricted to areas covered by each PAC' (NHASP 2005f: 29). One NHASP review noted that although 'social mapping and IMR studies have identified unsafe sexual practices right down to the village level' (eegads!), the HRSS would nevertheless focus on urban centres, ports and mines and 'well-known' risk groups (2005f: v). Carol Jenkins has rightly pointed out that such geographically limited approaches may be inappropriate for Papua New Guinea. Nevertheless, she adds the very proviso – '[e]xcept for *specific* high-risk groups, such as sex workers' (2007: 5, emphasis added) – that is undercut by her own data and the remainder of this document. She refers to a particular study of 'self-described FSW' (Gare *et al.* 2005) who *weren't* and who showed a zero HIVab seroprevalence! Two former and one current IMR employee shared with me (personal communications, 2003–2006) the conditions under which study eligibility was explained to local community settings. No one, I repeat, no one in rural village settings stands up and throws one's hands up and says, in effect, 'I am an FSW'! Such a phrasing, which is common in quantitative but not qualitative approaches to HIV research, too neatly covers over the often extremely complicated procedures involved in soliciting study participation and attempting to disentangle questions of language and meaning. Several women specifically rejected such a designation when they were informed of it, and said, in effect, that they thought the researchers were merely asking about 'women's sicknesses'. Government documents, press releases and NGO web-site postings frequently conflate intent to have sex, negotiations in that direction, the sex itself, the people who have it, the settings in which it occurs and the moral status of the sex they have. One document reporting upon 'HIV/AIDS Stakeholder Mapping' identified lack of social services and HIVab test-related counselling for 'high risk populations (eg. sex workers, MSM)' (UNAIDS-AusAID-NAC 2004: 24), reflecting longstanding biases that appear in one government document after another (e.g. NHASP 2005k: 9, 65). The 2006 WHO Country Assessment asserts that STD prevalence is rising in sex workers but that blood donors and antenatal clinic attendees remain 'low risk' in terms of HIV (2006: 12). The UNAIDS-UNICEF-WHO 'Fact Sheet' about Papua New Guinea defines 'higher-risk' sex as that which occurs with a 'non-regular partner', and *regardless of condom use* (2004: 10). Another NHASP review defined 'high-risk settings' as 'those where there is the greatest likelihood that transmission of the HIV/AIDS virus [*sic*] will occur' (NHASP 2005k: 85), but no attention is paid to the degree to which condoms will or won't be used there or how greatly or little consensual will be the sex. Instead, *who* or *what kinds* of people are going to be engaging in it is what counts, for example, 'commercial sex workers' and STD clinic patients and others who have 'high risk backgrounds' (NHASP 2005k: 9, Annex 4). In another NHASP review (2006g: 18) the high-risk settings were admittedly 'pre-defined', and yet that has not come out openly for discussion and reflection. NHASP and NACS officials have reacted defensively when invited to reflect critically upon such phrases and processes.

Of late, transportation workers and members of the disciplined forces have been added to the 'high risk' list but without addressing the more fundamental conceptual issues involved. 'Sex workers' could potentially be dubbed 'high risk' on a population-level, but only if 1) they were in fact as tightly knit a group as they are assumed to be; and 2) the sum total of their various kinds of partners were caught in the same net. Many of their security guard, policeman, truck driver and businessman partners have equivalent numbers of sex partners, lifetime, and exhibit the same frequency of sex partner change and rates of alcohol and other drug use. 'High risk' must logically therefore include the men who infect them, whether those are parliamentarians, male relatives, their customers, criminal gang members, expatriate consultants, or their husbands and boyfriends. 'High-risk' persons are in Papua New Guinea assumed to be so because they are highly mobile and residentially transient, such as *pasindia meri*, miners, soldiers and transportation workers. 'Low-risk' persons are typically understood and categorised on institutional grounds, for example, antenatal females, school students and 'village-dwellers'. The assumption seems to be that home is a haven in a heartless world and safe from sexually transmitted disease and that all 'commercial' sexual transactions are about equally unsafe. For one round of BSS (Behavioural Surveillance Survey) special focus was trained upon mobile, cash-earning men, and the results showed how dangerous it can be to flatten the patterns of sexual praxis. For example, when asked about past-month payments for sex, only 33% of the 70% of truck drivers who said that they had done so had used condoms, whereas 69% of the only 7% of Ramu Sugar workers surveyed had done so (NACS 2008: 25).

Risk, agency and struggles over meaning[2]

These kinds of assumptions have been detrimental to serosurveillance activities in the national response. Risk has been portrayed along lines of social desirability and ease of management, not along sociological lines of sexual acts and behaviours. Sentinel surveillance has tended to involve easier-to-manage antenatal mothers and military conscripts, or already stigmatised people such as incarcerated men. In like manner, many Kanak women in New Caledonia have been tested for HIVab while pregnant, but do not report so, for they do not know what the test is and how it is used (Salomon and Hamelin 2008: 84). The consulting physician who worked in the Heduru Clinic remarked that nearly 100% of all antenatal patients there wished to have an HIVab test, but more than 95% did not want to know the test result (Pathanapornpandh 2005: 29). Surveillance activities pit 'high risk' against 'low risk' so as to maintain the euphemism of 'the general population' (e.g. GoPNG 2006: 30; NHASP 2005e: 7, 2006e: 4, 5, 53; WHO-NAC-NDoH 2000: 14). The epidemiological concept of a 'general population' contradicts sharply with the facts of geographic isolation, the existence of over 850 languages and the presence and effects of at least 300 Christian ministries, sects and denominations. Here are a just a few of the many, many examples that could be cited:

- 'To determine HIV prevalence in low and high-risk population in Papua New Guinea, an anonymous serosurveillance was conducted in Government-administered antenatal and STD clinics ... '. (WHO-NACS-NDOH 2000: 4)

- 'Antenatal mothers are a low risk group who access the health facilities frequently so are easier to monitor' (Mr Marcel Burro, in *BW* 2008b)

- 'Although the HIV prevalence rate remains low in groups at low risk such as blood donors and ante-natal women, the rate is significant among people with high-risk behaviours, especially in Port Moresby'. (United Nations 2001: 50)

- '"Low-risk" means general population and "high-risk" refers to persons attending STI clinics or employed in commercial sex'. (Caldwell and Isaac-Toua 2002: 105)

- 'Sero-surveillance is done to monitor the epidemic in the low risk population (antenatal mothers) and also in the high risk group (people who attend the sexually transmitted infection clinic)'. (NACS 2005: 12)

- 'Guideline[s] for HIV serosurveillance [will be followed] at STI clinics (high risk population), and at ANC (low risk)'. (Limpakarnjanarat 2000: 114)

- 'In population groups that may be considered to be at lower risk (blood donors and pregnant women) the prevalence of HIV infection remains low, but it is already high in groups at higher risk (sex workers and STD clinic attendees)'. (WHO-NACS-NDOH 2000: 4)

Four objections must be raised so as to set aright the function of epidemiological categories and surveillance in Papua New Guinea. First, I have no great knowledge of the 'screening' questionnaires used in the blood banking services in Papua New Guinea, although I have spoken informally with many who work in a capacity of pre- and post-test counselling. In addition, having worked for a time as an Infectious Diseases Investigator for the American Red Cross, I do know how poorly designed are their equivalents in the US, where Blood Donation Records clearly reward would-be donors for providing The Right Answer instead of The Truth about sexual acts and identities and risk behaviours (Hammar 2003). In any event, by the time blood donations in Papua New Guinea have been obtained donors have already been pre-screened for current or past infections, for real and spurious high-risk behaviours, and often over a long period of time. Thus, the degree to which they stand proxy for anything, much less inherently 'low-risk' is something of a statistical artifact. It is for this reason that data obtained from blood donation are of little use in nationwide-modelling (e.g. Sladden 2005: 36). Rising rates of infection among them, however, must surely raise an eyebrow or two.

Second, insofar as many tens of thousands of pregnant females never receive antenatal services anyway (estimated at between 40% and 50% or more), it is difficult to accept how the ones who do can be allowed to stand proxy for the ones who don't, much less for most of the remainder of the nation. The latter are made the more difficult to get at in this regard because such figures are seldom if ever adjusted for age or gender, so we know even less about how representative they are and about the important factors that led them there. Many times this obvious bias has been pointed out, but it has not yet factored in risk algorithms. Its proponents seem to want to have it both ways. When 'antenatal mother' HIVab seroprevalence is considered 'low', it has seemed desirous to allow it to stand for the remainder of the 'general population'. Now that prevalence in several antenatal clinics throughout the country has risen quite ominously, however, its generalisability seems less desirable in terms of agreed-upon categories and assumptions. For example, the 2007 Consensus Workshop figure accepted for HIVab seroprevalence of the 'adult' population (that is, those 15 years of age and older) was an extremely conservative 1.28%, but figures from the antenatal clinics in Central (1.5%), Manus (1.9%), Eastern Highlands (2.0%), Morobe (2.5%) and Western Highlands (3.7%) are rather higher (see NACS 2007). Recall also how low were the numbers reported in Central Province.

Third, assumptions about 'high-risk' and 'low-risk' can be and quite frequently are empirically false. This has been shown time and again in studies conducted in sub-Saharan Africa. Epstein quotes a South African woman who worked in a project in Mothusimpolo saying that 'This is what we know. This has been shown by the World Health Organization and by USAID, by everyone. You have to target high-transmission groups in your approach to prevent HIV in the community in general'. Epstein added herself that '[a]nd yet I had recently learned that evidence from the very same mining region where Mr. Moema worked suggested that high-risk groups did not entirely explain how HIV was spreading in southern Africa' (Epstein 2007: 92). She pointed to epidemiological data, for example, showing that 60% of women aged 20–30 in the town near the mine were HIVab+ (Epstein 2007: 92). Curry *et al.* (2005: 360) found an HIVab seroprevalence of 18% in 300 consecutive patients, ranging in age from 18 to 60 (53% male, 47% female), admitted to the Emergency Department of the Port Moresby General Hospital. Presumably drawing broadly from the entire if not 'general' population, this figure was *more than double* the figure (7%) of HIVab seroprevalence then being reported in the STD clinic. Many more examples than the four below of prevalence findings that should have dislodged mainstream epidemiological categories but didn't may be cited (e.g. ABM 2005: n.p.; Lemeki, Passey and Setel 1996: 240; Olivier-Miller 2004: 821; Rupali *et al.* 2007: 218, Table 1; Toliman *et al.* 2006: 19; WHO-NACS-NDOH 2000: 6; WHO-NACS-NDOH 2000: 6, 17, Table 1.4):

- 'Among selected, presumably low-risk groups, estimated rates in the range of 18% to 80% for gonorrhea, 4% to 30% for syphilis, and 17% to 44% for chlamydia have been reported … '. (Gare *et al.* 2005: 466)

- 'In this community based study of an apparently "low risk" population of rural women [in EHP] we found an extremely high prevalence of STDs'. (Passey *et al.* 1998a: 124)

- 'STI prevalence surveys in Papua New Guinea show a high STI prevalence among both high-risk and low-risk groups'. (UNAIDS-UNICEF-WHO 2004: 2)

- 'High rates of STDs have been documented among apparently low-risk women, with reported prevalences in antenatal clinics, family planning clinics and rural community-based surveys in the range of 1–29% for *Chlamydia trachomatis*, 3–49% for *Trichomonas vaginalis*, 0.3–22% for *Neisseria gonorrhoea*, and 0.3–18% for syphilis'. (Passey *et al.* 1998b: 401)

> If the most important criterion for assessing HIV transmission risk is 'being sexually active', as one NHASP representative correctly has it (Paradi 2002: 2), then one is certainly obliged to ask the question as to the collective risk that Members of Parliament pose to others, or, let's say, all members of provincial governments. At least three MPs are well known to be HIVab+. While we're at it, insofar as their seroprevalence is higher than that of the putative 'general population', why haven't MPs been dubbed a 'high-risk group' and the House of Parliament, a 'high-risk setting?'

Fourth, while for two decades the low HIVab seroprevalence in antenatal females was used to justify assumptions of low seroprevalence in 'the general population' (and to pit both against 'high-risk', socially despised people), it is now all of the sudden accepted as 'well-known' that antenatal figures lead to an 'overestimation' of true prevalence (NACS 2007: 25)! So much so, in fact, that an 80% calibration rate must now be used. The fact of the suddenness of the appearance of this new equation, alongside absent commentary upon previous estimates, certainly raises many new questions.

Examples such as the above suggest something of the huge disconnect between empirical evidence of infection, on the one hand, and on the other, the notions of risk and epidemiological modelling of groups embodying it. None of these documents cited have said, in effect, 'Hmm. Consistently high prevalence of STDs in what we've been calling "low-risk" people; guess we're gonna hafta stop sayin' that'. Another NHASP document, Milestone 44, recommended that efforts needed to be made to include 'basic risk-defining behavioural questions' regarding such things as 'use of condom with last *non*-regular partner' (NHASP 2003a: x, emphasis added), suggesting that 'regular' partners don't pose a risk to others. The 2004 Consensus Workshop summary report urged similarly that '100% condom use must be vigorously promoted among men and women for all sexual encounters with *non*-regular partners' (NHASP 2005e: 9, emphasis added). Reports of double-digit HIVab seroprevalence among miners at the Porgera Joint Ventures mine-site in Enga Province were blamed by health officials on sex workers (People and Planet 2006). Neither wives nor girlfriends featured here, however, and the transmissive risk that miners pose to those 'sex workers' (or their more 'intimate' partners) was not acknowledged. That these men were miners trumped the fact that they were also mostly husbands.

These remarks suggest that HIV- and AIDS-related policies are ill-suited for a country that is so diverse, for a population that is so mobile, and for peoples whose acts, identities and social groupings confound 'risk-group'-style epidemiological modelling. The theme that emerged from the first HIV Prevention Summit was the usefulness of 'evidence-based approaches'. Dr Clement Malau applauded the decision made in 2008 by the National Research Institute to begin a three-year behavioural monitoring study by saying that health department decisions should be made 'based on evidence only' (*The National* 2008). Whether or not this constitutes tacit admission that prevention programmes had theretofore not been based on them (it clearly is) is less important than the fact that critical, reflexive approaches to emergent data are still not taken by epidemiologists, much less by Christian churches, policies and representatives. One NHASP review (2006c: 17) concluded that church leaders tend not to appreciate the complexity of the issues raised, that their response 'tends to simplistic platitudes or vitriolic sermons against the demons of lust', that 'they look to simplistic responses based on a theological world view that is radically out of step with the reality of HIV and AIDS'. Pastor Daniel Hawali frankly opposes condoms in the ABC platform that is mandated by his PAC's sponsors. Several other HRCs and even provincial governors have followed suit (see Chapter 5).

Milestones and millstones: toward a sociology of knowledge

The examples I have cited in the long section above call for a sociology of the knowledge produced and disseminated in the national response. By focusing upon the articles published in the *Post-Courier* about HIV and AIDS from the early years of the epidemic to about 1992 I shown in Chapter 3 that newspaper coverage tended to follow the same prejudices as typical in Western press a few years earlier. In this chapter I have showed that health officials have followed suit. Elias *et al.* (1990: 182), for example, claimed that 'having sex with prostitutes or "two-kina Meris" increases risk'. Ruta Fiti-Sinclair claimed on the basis of her 1993 study that '[p]rostitutes are considered a high-risk group, because of the multiple sex partners they have, so they are an important group to target with educational efforts' (1996: 118). Many housewives, of course, also have multiple sex partners, and the majority of their husbands are also engaged in multi-partnering, but yet neither 'wives' nor 'husbands' is targeted for intervention, despite that their number wildly outstrips those of 'sex workers'. Papua New Guinea itself, however, was assumed to be virgin territory, a blank slate upon or across which HIV began increasingly to be transmitted.[3] As infections seemed to rise, alarm increasingly spread, though that didn't seem to translate to sincere or dedicated attention being paid by politicians and health officials but for a small handful. Interestingly, Cullen finds that 'by late 1999 there was a noticeable decline in coverage, and this at a time when the epidemic was becoming more visible and widespread [reference omitted]. Recent interview with newspapers editors in PNG revealed that there are no plans to increase coverage of the disease [reference omitted]' (Cullen 2003b: 67). Thankfully, those plans were changed, and newspaper coverage from 2003 to 2008 of workshop summaries, intervention efforts, surveillance data and visits by consulting experts began to occur weekly, if not daily.

There are limits, however, to such newspaper coverage that are telling of the discursive limits of the national response itself. Media releases and e-mail based, list-serv discussions on AIDSTOK, for example, warn frequently of the negative consequences. I mentioned near the outset of Chapter 3 that the results of an FBO-sponsored study were presented at the 2004 Consensus Workshop. The high rates of HIVab seropositivity reported (17%) made their way into newspaper and Internet-based stories and now stand proxy for the entire country's 'prostitutes' and 'sex workers'. Similar figures from a 1998 survey conducted in Port Moresby and in Lae (e.g. Mgone *et al.* 2002; Tobias 2007: 6) were put to the same ends, implying a certain inevitability of infection. 'About one in every six sex workers in Port Moresby has already contracted HIV', says Sharon Fink (2006). In an article titled 'For *Goodness* Sake' (emphasis added), The Anglican Board of Missions warned visitors to Papua New Guinea that '[t]rends in HIV/AIDS [*sic*] prevalence rates [*sic*] indicate a considerably high level of HIV infection [17%] among sex workers' (ABM 2005: n.p.). This again confused notions of movement (trend, rate) and of stasis (prevalence, level). Another assessment asserted without any discussion whatsoever that '[s]eventeen per cent of sex workers in Port Moresby are HIV-positive' (WHO-SPC 2004: 3), a figure repeated also in statements by Zenner and Russell (2005) and McBride (2005). Matthew Carney's report aired on 'Sick No Good' included the claim that 'The most recent study on prostitution in PNG found 17 per cent of sex workers are HIV positive' (Carney 2006). When Health Ministers for the Pacific Island Countries met in Apia, Samoa, in March of 2005 the claim was repeated again and even more baldly in an uncommented-upon bullet: 'Seventeen per cent of female sex workers in Port Moresby are HIV-positive' (WHORO 2005: 3). UNAIDS reported the same figures but also took credit for them: '[i]n 1998, *UNAIDS reported* HIV prevalence rates [*sic*] among FSW at 17 percent in Port Moresby' (FHI 2007: 9, emphasis added), when the figures were collected by IMR staff.

There has occurred no critical commentary on the scandal I mentioned, however, nor of the sour taste it left behind in Port Moresby among study participants, nor of the veracity of the findings. One might as well be attempting to count cloudiness. The project head later (and rightly) decried the fact that, in the wake of the infamous police raid on the Three-Mile Guesthouse (see Stewart 2004), people weren't sufficiently aware of the negative public health consequences of police action. Nevertheless, she neglected to mention those of the sexual shenanigans of 'health officials', including her own, a 'clinical epidemiologist' who forged documents and credentials and who allegedly had sex with seven eventual or would-be clients of the nine he is alleged to have enrolled (author's fieldnotes, Port Moresby, 2004, 2005; personal communications with project staff). When several of us IMR staff in Goroka challenged him about the allegations and prior car crashes and equipment and money theft, he refused comment, but was already doing consultancy work in another province. Certain areas of coverage are simply off-limits. One multi-lateral document said that '[this NGO] considers that this model has been successful, and its findings will be useful in determining future interventions with CSWs' (UNAIDS-AusAID-NAC 2004: 18). Repeated attempts I made to contact staff of this NGO overseas and in Port Moresby were unsuccessful in locating a paper that was supposed to have been produced in collaboration with faculty from the Medical School of the University of Papua New Guinea. There has been to my knowledge no intervention, or even mention, since 2004, and no one I contacted claimed any knowledge of the study whatsoever, although it was apparently written up for formal presentation (Irumai, Bruce and Nonwo 2004). The study head did not discuss these issues at the 2004 workshop.

The same uncritical and non-reflexive attitude can be seen in periodic monitoring and evaluation of the PAC system. I mentioned at the outset of Chapter 3 the composition and foibles of a particular PAC, its uneasy relationship to provincial government and especially health authorities, and its questionable ethics and activities. My experience in 10 of Papua New Guinea's 20 provinces is that this PAC was neither novel nor extreme. The AusAID audit of NHASP (2005a, b) showed that other PACs had during their first few years of operation been rocked by setbacks and scandals, too, involving the same kinds of sexual shenanigans of youth group and response coordinators, other crashed vehicles, compromised communications, high rates of personnel change and financial mismanagement (see also NHASP 2004b). Notable exceptions included the PACs in West Sepik, Madang and Western Highlands provinces.

Internal audits and summaries, case studies and press releases by NACS and NHASP, however, have been rather more forgiving. The NHASP review of the PAC system, Milestone 104, is lengthy (at 82 pages) and is contextualised by reference to their equivalents in other countries. Nevertheless, it is stripped bare of sociological analysis. It tells in bloodless terms of the politics and rates of personnel turnover and misused resources and so makes for frustrating reading. It notes the 'inherent weaknesses' of PACs (NHASP 2006d: 2), that membership is broad but attendance at meetings low and that coordination of provincial-level activities, which is supposed to be their major responsibility, is limited and non-proactive (2006d: 3). AusAID noted that many PACs seemed to carry out activities only within close vicinity of their own offices. Townspeople in Wewak, Mendi, Kerema, Popondetta, Daru and Goroka told me that PAC officers and even some volunteers had assumed somewhat the reputation of health professionals who wish patients to come to them, on their terms. Their counterparts in Madang, Lae, Mt. Hagen and Vanimo, by contrast, praised their local PAC volunteers for their non-insular attitude. AusAID's review concluded that 'NHASP appears to have "cut their losses" on difficult PACs. Rather than trying to overcome their limitations, NHASP has often withdrawn resources, indicating a lack of awareness about the ramifications of nonfunctional infrastructure in PACs' offices' and of the likely costs of lack of supervision, busted equipment and social relations that need mending (2005a: xii). Each PAC was to have been outfitted with Internet-ready computers and e-mail addresses, but that was mooted owing to lack of training of personnel, to the theft of equipment and to unpaid telephone and other bills. At least five other PACs were judged by AusAID to have performed even worse than the one discussed in Chapter 3 (AusAID 2005b: 67–71). The NHASP review of the roll-out of antiretrovirals (2005a: 19) strongly recommended that e-mail and Internet access be guaranteed at each of the expanded number and refurbished character of VCT sites. This does not, however, recognise likelihood of further logistic complications and breaches of confidentiality as people's identities and test results are sent to and fro by e-mail and facsimile message. In like fashion a demographer consulting with the NACS assumed that estimates of HIVab incidence and prevalence would necessarily be better as the number of surveillance sites reporting data increased (Hayes 2007: 20). Without corresponding improvements and refinements in the means by which people are interviewed and transmission dynamics assayed, more data do not necessarily mean better data.

Biomedical approaches to HIV in Papua New Guinea seem contingent on similarly complicated technical issues that are neither supervised sufficiently well nor appreciated critically for the potential for misunderstandings. In February of 2007, for example, the government announced that medical circumcision would be pushed in Papua New Guinea to help the fight against AIDS. The CEO of Wewak's Boram Hospital, Sr. Joseph, was given the go-ahead by the provincial health office to launch a new programme whereby aid post workers would be trained to carry out proper circumcisions on males at all ages. The black market demand for circumcision that this would lead to, however, and the local mimesis occurring regarding circumcision in the form of supercision and superincision and other forms of genital cutting have not been discussed publicly. I discuss these issues in some detail in the Introduction to Part Two (see also Aggleton 2007; Berer 2007a, b; Dowsett and Couch 2007; Hankins 2007). Verena Keck's long-term ethnography of the Yupno, who straddle the border between Madang and Morobe provinces, is relevant here.

> In the traditional initiation of young men, which was given up decades ago on pressure from the Lutheran mission together with the men's houses, *mbema yut*, circumcision was unknown. Today, in a kind of revival, parts of this initiation are held 'undercover' in small, hidden *mbema yut* in the bush and strictly out of sight of church functionaries, and a new element is circumcision. This circumcision is linked to knowledge and power but also with the idea that it protects men from HIV/AIDS. (Keck 2007: 46)

One would certainly not know this from official documents, however, which have a decided Mission: Accomplished! character to them. The Annual Plan for 2006 published by the NHASP as Milestone 96, for example, mentions 'success' or 'successful' in terms of meetings held and interventions launched at least 10 times. Many documents are just like it in that regard, though neither 'fail' nor 'failure' appear even once. Most activities, regardless of degree of aforethought, prior consultation, cultural appropriateness, economic cost or *measurable* success in terms of changed behaviour and lessened transmission have become Milestones. Yawning deficits in use of existing social-scientific knowledge base featured in the release of Milestone 44, 'Social Science Research Priorities' (NHASP 2003a). This is a marvelously well-crafted document, but it has been reduplicated bibliographically several times by expatriate consultants and remains largely ignored in its recommendations. What does it mean, therefore? That that Milestone has been reached and passed? That social science priorities have now been addressed and valorised? Unduly lengthy waits for research funding have been aired but not dealt with frankly by other reviews. The updated review of the Grants Scheme process (NHASP 2006g: 8), for example, noted that only the members of the Research Advisory Committee who were external to the NACS and the NHASP regularly attended, owing probably to the low quality of proposals put to the committee. Lack of a Grants Manager has proved to be a real drawback. It has contributed to slow progress in improving the frequency and quality of reports that acquit grant monies properly. Only 71 of 207 funded projects had been at all monitored, and only 60 of those had been seen to have met their objectives (NHASP 2006g: 29) or to have adequately summarised research and other findings (2006g: 34). In some cases the funded groups did not appear even to have existed, or their leaders had made off with the money or side-stepped the purpose of the grants, for example, when religious messages dominated workshops ostensibly devoted to providing 'basic facts on HIV and AIDS' (2006g: 44, 42–3).

Other Milestones were notable for their frank admissions of partial completeness of task, for the too-short duration of their visits, for the collection of equivocal findings and for logistically nightmarish conditions (e.g. NHASP 2006a: 18). The review of the support by NHASP of community theatre responses to HIV and AIDS (NHASP 2006b: 2) mentioned that the review team was prohibited from travel to at least four field-sites owing to cancelled flights, security concerns and rough seas. Another review team, sent to investigate the availability and content of services provided at VCT sites, only visited four of 20 provinces, spoke with a total of five clients (all in the same focus group), and compared none of those sites with antenatal, tuberculosis, or STD clinics (NHASP 2006a: 25–6). It found extreme variation in the degree to which provincial-level theatre groups adhered to 'master scripts' approved by the NHASP or the NAC, including *how* to mention sex and *whether or not* to mention condoms (NHASP 2006b: 2, 13). This problem has been documented in some detail ethnographically and otherwise. Naomi McPherson (2008) has deconstructed the meanings communicated in AIDS 'action dramas' and that have little if anything to do with HIV transmission. The messages communicated in skits implicate behaviours and states of being thought immoral – adultery and promiscuity – and therefore provide no useful information about preventing transmission of a virus. The villagers with whom she worked in West New Britain Province read AIDS related posters as narratives of class and privilege, of urban-rural differences and of the special dangers of modernity and urban morality. Another drama performed in Trobriand islands communities in Milne Bay Province, according to Kathy Lepani (2007b), was titled 'Rasta Boy', and quite predictably located the source of HIV (and thus the cause of AIDS) in the body of a *maket pamuk* ('town prostitute') who infects a young village man who goes for a spin one day to the market, gets infected and brings it home to the village. Interestingly, whereas this drama would go over well in many communities, Trobriand islanders rejected it on the grounds of the absence of prostitution in the area, the generally free and available character of sex (Lepani 2007b: 250). The campaign launched by the NACS several years ago featuring new posters appealing to non-discriminatory attitudes and a reduction of fear (you'll never know who has it, she may look perfect, etc.) nevertheless unleashed yet more opportunities for interpretation and understanding different than those perhaps intended. I hasten to point out that the messages were not wrong, but rather, that care must be taken also in their reception and follow-up as such changing interpretations emerge. For example, the poster showing a clean-cut, well-dressed jazz musician warning viewers that one can't tell by looking who is and isn't HIVab+ (and therefore, please use a condom) induced in some the idea that 'those guitarists, that guy right there – that's the guy you wanna look out for' (translated from the Tok Pisin, a village counsellor to his neighbors, Wabag, April 2006).

Milestone 82 was the holding in 2004 of the so-called Consensus Workshop, but its 'findings', as indicated in the previous chapter and above, represented little if any consensus grounded in painstaking review of good evidence properly collected by those pursuing mixed methods research. Instead, there occurred the ramrodding by consultant epidemiologists of inconsistently collected and poorly conceptualised serosurveillance data into three epidemiological 'scenarios'. Those had absolutely no link to ethnographic or other contextual data with which to construct such a narrative. Good opportunities to assess frankly disturbing clinical data from the initial roll-out of HAART (Highly Active Antiretroviral Therapy) were not taken, either. It is well known that those who are already suffering from high levels of anaemia don't tolerate HAART well. Less than perfect adherence thereto can further complicate the treatment regimen. The nationwide study of such led by a consultant to the Asian Development Bank found that anaemia was extremely common but that it was being frequently misdiagnosed and allowed not to be treated, leading also to significant dehydration (Pathanapornpandh 2005: 4, 13, 27). The NHASP review of the initial roll-out concluded that patients 'for whom there is concern about adherence should not be commenced on ART' (2005a: Annex 1, n.p.). I should think that, based upon other evidence and issues raised here and at the 2004 Workshop, there is 'concern about adherence' for all but a small handful of potential clients. Pathanapornpandh (2005: 13, 27) noted that it was commonly found that people had not been adhering to their treatment regimen, especially the ones who presented to clinic all alone. Moreover, no consent form system was in place when he worked at the Heduru Clinic. The 2008 NACS report of to what extent Papua New Guinea had met UNGASS goals concluded that '[a]dherence rates are also low' (NACS 2008: 64). In 2004 it was noted by the WHO that critical criteria for participation in the so-called '3 by 5' programme had not yet been met in Papua New Guinea, including the 'patient monitoring system' and the 'drug monitoring system' (WHO-SPC 2004: 26). As such, and in the presence of much social and residential dislocation and challenged nutrition, physicians spoke privately at the Workshop of some patients being hastened to their death by loss of appetite, by heart attack, by their inability to be transfused and by persistent nausea. Others were consigned to suffer excruciatingly painful outbreaks of genital herpes and herpes zoster infections as their immune systems reconstituted slightly (e.g. McBride and Bradford 2004; Murdoch et al. 2007; NHASP 2005a; see also Steinberg 2008). Many studies have shown that those who commence HAART but from greatly disadvantaged social and nutritional positions die faster and suffer greater morbidity in the process (e.g. Lima et al. 2006). 'IRIS' is the cute new acronym for not-so-cute illness that has been given to the 'immune reconstitution inflammatory syndrome' from which new HAART patients can suffer as their newly restored immunity to infectious or non-infectious antigens is expressed. Murdoch et al. (2007: 1) have defined it as '[a] paradoxical clinical worsening of a known condition or the appearance of a new condition after initiating therapy'. Despite there being significant hallway talk about this among doctors in Papua New Guinea, a chance to air it was not taken. Neither were comments from the floor encouraged that would have challenged church-sponsored anti-condom and homophobic discourse. *Discursively*, most at this time were continuing to view the 12,000+ 'official' cases as clustering among 'sex workers', 'at-risk youth' and 'MSM'. *Empirically*, however, according to the evidence presented there and elsewhere, most infections were occurring in statistically average marriages, where the tenets of ABC least applied. The recording form in Heduru Clinic's PMTCT programme, sadly, noted a single 'risk factor' about which to inquire of antenatal mothers: 'have you ever been involve in commercial sex worker practice?' (form appended to Pathanapornpandh 2005: 44).

Social-scientific data have thus seldom been used to guide a more rational response, and I have shown this in multiple ways. The 'local history and epidemiology of HIV and AIDS' component in the initial HAART prescribers course which was by all accounts remarkably successful, was rated particularly poorly. Several of the comments provided by attendees ('less relevant than other points', 'no data/no analysis', 'data is [sic] poor', 'not enough statistics is [sic] available'; NHASP 2005a: Annex 3) indicate that even medical doctors know how badly needed are those kinds of data. Well-intended initiatives around HBC (Home-Based Care of those sick and dying) would be made more robust by ethnographic studies of death and dying in a village setting, for example, findings that 83% of the time the sick and dying are cared for by just one person, who was in one field setting with only one exception a woman (NHASP 2006f: 14). Just as access to clinics, doctors and therapies is a highly gendered process and one that is refracted further by issues of class and ethnicity, so do those therapies course through differently gendered and raced bodies. The morbidity and mortality due to HIV have gendered components to them, but the morbidity and mortality induced by HAART do, too (Huang *et al.* 2006).

The so-called Faith Communities Covenant on HIV, Milestone 107, was signed by representatives of Papua New Guinea's major church missions but has yet to be tested in any meaningful way. There are many reasons for this, including that the National Council of Churches was de facto defunct at the time it was to be tabled for discussion. Neither was it discussed meaningfully at the Heads of Churches Leadership Workshop that was held in Goroka in March of 2005. Just as with the importation of the ABC message and the unrealistically high expectations made of the functioning of the PAC system, the Covenant was not developed indigenously but by an expatriate 'faith based advisor', Bruce Gallacher, who was contracted by NHASP for 25 days (NHASP 2006c: 21), in addition to the three-year contract offered the Reverend Kerry William (Kim) Benton for leading the clergy-training workshops (Benton 2008). It accordingly fostered little sense of ownership, since churches were then in the awkward position of having to 'respond' to it and needing to deal with its 'uptake' (NHASP 2006c: 11, 12). More fundamentally, the Covenant would have required serious negotiation between faiths and denominations that are sometimes diametrically opposed in theological questions involving condoms, sexuality, gender relations and disease causation. The faith-based advisor engaged by NHASP admitted that by June of 2006 the Covenant was dead in the water (NHASP 2006c: 12). This is not the image promoted in the media, however, which reports on 'the' church response glowingly as if 'it' is so singular, progressive and uniform.

> '*Some church pastors and leaders will not talk about condoms unless it is in the context of marriage. This was revealed at the National Capital District Faith-based Organisations leaders network on HIV in Port Moresby yesterday ...United Church pastor Reverend John Ravusiro stated that putting a lot of emphasis on condoms in the HIV awareness was promoting promiscuity, especially among young. "As pastors we must at all costs not encourage the use of condoms in preventing HIV/AIDS. Otherwise, we will see a lot of young people just going out to do it. As a pastor, I do not want to talk about it", he said, adding the use of condoms was not safe anyway' (Gerawa 2008: 5).*

There would have remained serious limitations, too, even had it passed with flying colours. The Covenant (reproduced in AusAID 2005b: 72) fails to use the word 'condom' or to challenge sex-negative, homophobic and anti-condom discourse and policies that many Christian leaders and led promote, including in the health facilities they sponsor and operate. It mentions but does not define or contextualise 'sexual integrity'. It ends on a note of the very apocalyptic phrasing ('until the kingdom comes') that other social scientists (e.g. Dundon 2007; Eves 2003a, b; Wardlow 2008) have linked to the promotion of stigma, blame and isolation. Most fundamentally, however, the NACS-sponsored poster showing heads of several churches holding hands in the centre collectively to oppose stigma and discrimination belies theological rifts and jealous protectionism between them. The head Pastor of the 70,000 member-strong Revival Fellowship Church has claimed personally to have healed 40 people from HIV infection, but his method for HIV prevention is even simpler: 'Flee from sin, flee from committing adultery and fornication. If you are a church and you're issuing condoms, you are promoting sin and you're anti-Christ' (quoted in Bennett 2008). The relevant NHASP review (2006c: 14) noted that '[t]he faith based adviser spoke to all the heads of churches, [but] only the Anglicans were interested in Red Ribbon [an innovative approach to counselling and particularly care]. It was made abundantly clear that [the Heads of Churches] are all trying to address the issues by implementing their own programmes'. The same problems were noted in the Reverend Benton's curiously titled essay, 'Saints and Sinners: training Papua New Guinean (PNG) Christian clergy to respond to HIV and AIDS using a model of care' (Benton 2008). Who are the saints? Who are the implied sinners? Benton had difficulties getting these Christian clergy to take a more reflexive approach: '[t]he participants also expressed difficulty in accepting that a starting point for the model required them to take responsibility for their own behavior and their role as educators about HIV' (2008: n.p.). Benton thoughtfully presents some of the barriers that he encountered while leading these clergy training workshops, for example, the '[c]ultural and theological understandings of causes of disease based on concepts of punishment for sin and judgement', but fails to explain why the antidote for this, their 'need to be deconstructed and revitalized with a positivist [sic] approach' was begun in the workshops with more Bible study (Benton 2008: n.p.).

At a church-supported hospital in the highlands region I reported to the hospital CEO that a medical technician attached to the AusAID-funded Sexual Health Clinic there seemed to be engaging in ethically wrong and medically dangerous sexual activity. Investigation revealed that he had been using his skills in 'rapid' HIVab testing and his access to laboratory supplies and a spare room of the clinic on the weekends to, in a sense, 'screen' for his sexual contacts. Before I knew what was going on I had interviewed one of his recent conquests and found that, although she was later treated for other STDs, because he found her to be HIVab-, he didn't think it necessary to use condoms with her. Credit goes to the hospital CEO for sacking him, but the technician didn't believe his actions were wrong in the first place (author's fieldnotes, August, 2005).

With regards to faith-based initiatives, this has been nowhere more evident than with respect to the condom issue. Policy and personal statements about the moral status of condoms and their real and alleged efficacy vary by rank in church hierarchy (see Chapter 5). Some health services personnel refuse altogether to stock them, others do so but claim their dangerousness. Yet others rhetorically 'support' them in principle but not in the field, for example, the Evangelical Church of Papua New Guinea in Southern Highlands Province and in Western Province. They have been made political footballs of rural health facilities and of Australian monies designed to instill pro-condom attitudes and practices. The Salvation Army is not strictly speaking a church or denomination, but yet, just as with the US-based Focus on the Family ministry headed by James Dobson, some of its representatives believe in 'conversion' of homosexual desire following a spiritual experience and also in the STD curative powers of Christian prayer (MSIC 2006: 7). In August of 2006 I enjoyed an informal conversation with the supervisor of one of the peer educators allegedly 'converted' from homosexuality. He believed that STDs were physical manifestations of God's scorn upon immoral behaviour but that can be made to disappear upon rededication to God and worship and that using antibiotics to do so would be pointless, redundant, since 'Giving yourself to the church means that you have given your body to Jesus'. His supervisor told me that 'according to I Corinthians [6:9–11], transformation is possible: "And such were some of you: but ye are washed, but ye are sanctified, but ye are justified in the name of the Lord Jesus, and by the Spirit of our God'" (author's fieldnotes, Port Moresby). The NHASP review concluded that, at times, 'it seems the debate is not about condoms per se but a struggle for power and influence' (2006c: 15).

One is entitled to wonder, too, at the decision of the faith-based advisor to consult with no women (2006c: 23) despite that one of the provisions of the Covenant is to encourage their full participation. The NHASP review of the functioning of PACs revealed nary a single female PAC chairperson among the nine PACs the review team visited (NHASP 2006d: 13). The 'Programme for HIV/AIDS Awareness and Counselling Workshop for Pastors and Clergy' slotted an hour and a half for 'gender' issues, but was facilitated by a male pastor and included stories of women from the Bible (NHASP 2006c: 32). We all know how much safe, pleasurable and consensual sex *they* had. We can only imagine how they managed the obligations of virginity, fecundity and fidelity on their part. Lilith had a point.

Another high-profile Milestone but of yet unknown worth was the legislation drafted in 2002 as a Bill and enacted in 2003 called the HIV/AIDS Management Prevention (or HAMP) Act. This Act laid down the legal facts that, for example, neither HIV- and AIDS-related posters, pamphlets and brochures nor condoms and lubricants were obscene, objectionable or indecent under the Criminal Code. Of particular relevance here is that Section 11, dealing with 'Access to Means of Protection', makes it unlawful to 'deny a person access, without reasonable excuse, to a means of protection from infection of himself or another by HIV', including informational materials, condoms and lubricant. Nevertheless, none of the thousands of good opportunities to have by now mounted a test case thereof have been taken.[4] Somewhat ironically, the Catholic Health Services has for some time been offering *Post*-Exposure Prophylaxis (NHASP 2006a: 18) but not pre-exposure prophylactics. HIVab test counsellors from FBO sometimes refuse altogether even to have condoms or information about them on hand (Dundon 2007; Hammar 2006b, 2007b; McPherson 2008; NHASP 2006a; Wardlow 2008). 'Some health workers in government-run STI clinics', concluded another NHASP document (2005b: 83), 'not only refuse to give out condoms, but refuse information about them too, because they are "against the word of God". As one female health worker said: "When they ask about condoms, I tell them to think of their immortal souls"'. Even AusAID (2005a: 35) allowed within an otherwise fair but extremely tentatively worded document that health workers (of whatever stripe) and facilities who don't make condoms available (much less who discourage others from using them) 'probably' are engaging in an illegal act.

No matter: it's just discourse until the legislation is actually used. The case I reported to the NACS and the NHASP in the text box falls under the jurisdiction of Section 14(1b) of the Act, which prohibits anyone from performing 'an HIV test except on the request of a medical practitioner or authorized person'. Margaret Marabe is an HIVab+ widow and a prominent spokesperson for HIV advocacy. It was reported in the *Post-Courier* some time ago that during a telephone dispute a co-resident alleged that her HIV infection had made her confused and dishonest in their conversation. Ms Marabe attempted to bring a case against her, but the local judge who heard it encouraged the two disputants – the defendant being charged with using discriminatory language over the telephone, contrary to the provisions of Section 6(1) – to settle out of court. The serosurveillance study of 300 consecutive Emergency Department patients conducted by Curry *et al.* (2005: 361) was done altogether without pre-test counselling, obtaining of consent and post-test follow-up, which is precluded under Section 12(1) of the Act. One of the co-authors, Dr Diro Babona, is the Director of the Central Public Health Laboratory in Port Moresby, and the research was of course vetted by the Research Advisory Committee (although the findings were disavowed). In 2006 a woman from Tabubil in Western Province successfully convinced a District Court Magistrate to restrain her philandering husband from having sex with her unless and until he took another 'confirmatory' HIVab test, despite him having already tested HIVab 'non-reactive'. The District Court Magistrate, however, declined to use the relevant provisions of the HAMP Act (Section 23) that could have forced the husband to take another test, deferring instead to the National and Supreme courts (*Post-Courier*, 14 February 2006, p. 1), who let the case die. In 2001 Downer Construction Company mandated that new employees on their Highlands Highway reconstruction project demonstrate HIVab- serostatus and then sacked those who in Lae tested Repeat Reactive. The case was sent to the Solicitor-General, and the legal adviser in charge of the case was given a large fee, but the case 'died a natural death'. The same has occurred with regards to other charges in the Three-Mile Guest House raid and other cases of graft involving the HAMP Act manual itself (personal communication, a private consultant who chooses to remain anonymous, 7 July 2007). Such cases, however illegal or just plain wrong, are never going to be prosecuted unless the NACS grows legal teeth. Marge Berer concludes her recent essay about the search for biomedical quick fixes in the fields of HIV and AIDS intervention by saying that '[o]ur job ... will be to convince politicians, ministers of health, development and finance, and parliamentarians and judges that they must not continue to take account of, be intimidated by or legislate on the basis of these views precisely because of the damage to the public health and human rights that they engender' (Berer 2007a: 7). Many hundreds of opportunities have been lost to use the provisions of the Act to address and root out stigma and fear. Were NACS and NHASP officials to take its provisions seriously, then cases could be mounted every day involving church-run health facilities that deny condom promotion.

Vexing questions of privacy and confidentiality, too, have been asked of different kinds of medical settings, especially those sponsored and run by churches (AusAID 2005a: x, 13, 15, 59). In all fairness, many church workers and leaders want to do the 'wrong' thing, that is, breach confidence, but for the 'right' reasons, that is, to elicit support from church members in case of those diagnosed with HIV infection (for a compelling case study from Lesotho, see Makoae and Jubber 2008). Sometimes they do it in the 'wrong' settings, however, for example, in public 'confessions' asked of those who have recently tested HIVab+, or following street preachings or theatre performances (e.g. NHASP 2006b: 18). Similar cases have been reported for Tabubil and Tari (author's fieldnotes). Both myself and Wardlow (2006a; 2008) have interviewed the same hospital official who engages in such. On 27 August 2007, for example, the *Post-Courier* reported that '[o]n the day that the care centre was opened [in Tari] a total of 126 people with HIV declared their HIV status for the first time in public'. Why would someone lead 126 people to declare their HIVab test results in public? However one wishes to put it, by those who mean well, by those who mean poorly and by those who don't know they mean anything, confidentiality is breached: 'All staff professed to maintain confidentiality but in several centres people were introduced to the review team as "our first person living with HIV" or "this is our advocate for HIV, he is living with HIV himself"' (NHASP 2006a: 20).

> *'Greater sexual freedom among married and unmarried people is the reality in contemporary Papua New Guinea and, as such, prevention strategies must acknowledge this fact and place more emphasis on safe sex than on anti-promiscuity messages' (Koczberski 2000: 61).*

In such optimistic settings of donor-funded and -managed projects each box ticked becomes a Milestone reached no matter the sensibility of or the means by which or the difficulty of measuring the success of the activities to which it refers. The often-stated expectation is that through 'ramping up', 'scaling up' and aiming for 'universal coverage' the number of Papua New Guineans being treated for HIV infection by means of HAART will reach if not exceed international standards. Those standards were, if met, going to support Papua New Guinea's contribution to the international '3x5' drive by which 3,000,000 people worldwide were to have commenced on HAART by 2005. The target set in Papua New Guinea for the year 2010 was at one time to have been 10,000 people on treatment. A more reasonable goal was set in 2004 of 1,860 by the end of 2006 (NHASP 2005a: 12), but just barely 1,200 were on them even one year later (Rei 2007: 26). The 2007 Consensus Workshop indicated that the goal set for 2007 was 3,000 'adults' (those 15 and over, many of whom are decidedly not 'adults') and another 636 'children' (aged infant to 14), and despite there being no information presented for 2006 figures involving those children (NACS 2007). The 2008 UNGASS report for the progress made by Papua New Guinea in reaching treatment and reporting goals indicated that 2,250 had commenced antiretroviral treatment by December, 2007. However one slices it, this is a truly staggering rate of increase, not just in terms of the number of people who can now benefit from such treatment, but also in terms of what this must mean in terms of numbers of health workers trained, supplies moved and recording systems strengthened. Papua New Guineans and expatriates deserve credit for making these things happen.

In terms of the sociology of knowledge I am pursuing here, however, it is worth thinking past the rhetorical purpose of setting a figure of 10,000 as a realistic short-term goal and a long-term goal of 'universal' coverage. Given the 'generalised' status of Papua New Guinea's HIV epidemic, health authorities assume that 20% of all those HIVab+ need to be on treatment concurrently. In other words, 50,000 would need to be tested and found Repeat Reactive and then 'confirmed positive' and then 'confirmed' at an accredited regional confirmatory laboratory. Those 10,000 patients would need to be registered, put on treatment and then extremely closely monitored, by a very small number of doctors. The NHASP review (2005a: 12) quite liberally concluded that a 'reasonable estimate' of the personnel needed just for monitoring of patients was 'one doctor and one to two dedicated nurses per 200', which sounds impossible on the face of it, and which in any event means at least another 50 doctors and 100 more nurses are needed. This is by itself well beyond the current capacity of the health service, but even assuming the 'low scenario' of 2% HIVab+ prevalence growing annually by about 18%–20%, this would mean the screening of almost half the current populace (roughly 2,500,000 people) to identify those 50,000 candidates for HAART. Can the current health system handle such a testing burden? That would require at least two-and-a-half million sets of tests (requiring pre- and post-test counselling and two blood tests) and then another 10,000 cases in which third and fourth test result interpretations would be performed. Interestingly, O'Keeffe, Godwin and Moodie excepted Papua New Guinea from their expression of faith that access to antiretrovirals would be 'universal' in the Pacific by 2010, hoping instead that such would occur in Papua New Guinea 'as soon as practicable' (2005: 43). No matter: in the managed language of technical assistance, there are no failures, only Challenges. I should know: I have been called one! (by two NACS officials, March, 2006) for calling out several disjunctures between rhetoric in NACS documents and realities in the field.

With regards to the evaluation of programme efficacy, another factor in the sociology of knowledge production has to do with choice of interview subject. In addition to most reviews being prefaced with apologies as to the too-short nature of the time involved, the unavailability of this or that, the language barriers and the like, all of which is completely understandable, review team members have tended to meet with exceedingly few clients, patients, audience members and villagers. They have preferred instead to speak with supervisors, physicians, site-managers and their religious leaders (e.g. NHASP 2006a: 25). One NHASP mini-evaluation noted with admirable candour that a principal researcher and sponsoring university (the Divine Word University) had at the outset departed from the agreed-upon research protocol. Instead of investigating actual clinical competence and practice with regards to diagnosing STDs and treating them by means of principles of syndromic management, therefore, the review team focused on clinical facilities and supplies only (2005d: 4). It is with no little irony that I note also that NHASP officials rightly stood firm on principles of privacy and confidentiality in regards to clinical examinations in especially the settings of a sexual health clinic, which they could not therefore observe directly. On the other hand, there is good precedent for use of more 'extreme' research approaches under exceptional conditions of imminent harm (Hammar 1992; Rosenhan 1973; Van der Geest and Sarkodie 1998). Could not a female team member have surreptitiously sought consultation for a suspicious symptom? Could a male team member not have identified himself as a married man who nevertheless had a pocketful of money, a desire not to get infected and therefore a great need of condoms? Would he not likely be well poised to investigate what might be the disjuncture between policy and practice? Would she not have been well placed to observe normal clinic practice, for example, as regards speculum usage and sterilisation? I'm sure that they would be the first to agree that privacy is precluded and confidentiality is broken in many a health facility. Thus, the NHASP review team investigating the competence of district-level health workers to diagnose and treat STDs was faced with a terrible dilemma. They dealt with it in a practical, sympathetic way, as follows:

> They were asked to 'talk through' how they *would* take the history, conduct the physical/genital examination, discuss follow-up issues such as partner management, condom use to stay uninfected and provide appropriate treatment, using the recommended treatment protocols. If vaginal speculum examinations were conducted, questions on how health workers *would* disinfect the speculum and other instruments used in this procedure were asked of the health worker. (NHASP 2005d: 8, emphasis added)

This reveals some of the gaps in and especially politics of health systems research. The IRG review revealed that '[p]aediatric care and treatment, PMTCT and rural-based services are lagging in scale and coverage. Lack of sufficient health systems continues to be the key bottleneck and as yet there appear to be no national plans, activities and budgets to address this issue systematically' (IRG 2007: 7). It is not to criticise the NHASP review team or spirit with which they conducted their work, but rather, to indicate that such still does not get at *actual clinical practice* and the often vast gulf that exists between knowledge of policies and their enactment, between goals set for health systems and actual, existing states of repair. For the same reason, AusAID claims of the provision of 17,000,000 condoms to Papua New Guinea (see Chapter 5) fall short of investigation of their dispensation and use.

Critics of NACS and NHASP have charged also that little assessment is made of how effectively information has been communicated during outreach activities or retained later. There seems little follow-up to the good works accomplished during workshops and seminars. One NHASP review of church input to the national response (NHASP 2006c: 16) noted with admiration that during 'gender workshops' male church representatives 'reacted positively, by listening and seeking advi[c]e on how to support gender issues' but complained that 'without follow up, there is no continuity in training, educating or field work'. Special criticism has been aimed at the issue of how many of those trained to become HIVab test counsellors actually do some counselling when they return from training workshops, which is an issue that dogged our nationwide study. Taken together, the NHASP and the NACS trained between 2003 and 2005 over 1,000 people to become counsellors, but '[o]nly [a] few of these trained counsellors are currently working' (NACS 2006a: 19). Milestone 38 for the NHASP consisted of a 'Capacity-Building Status Report' that found, indeed, that many of those who had been trained at great NHASP expense had yet to deliver any services in return. The authors of the review wrote that '[i]n questioning the PCCs [Provincial Counselling Coordinators] regarding selection criteria it was not apparent that key criteria, such as having the time to undertake counselling services, were taken into account. Overall, PCCs did not maintain regular contact with trainees to provide ongoing support' (NHASP 2004b: 19, emphasis added).

Others have worried at the poor image promoted to potential donors of the fact that the NACS was audited only once (during 2001) in the lifetime of the NHASP up to 2005; the review team was unable to get information that would have verified whether or not the hoped-for goal of 15 of 20 PACs meeting minimum standards at project's end (AusAID 2005a: 40). More troubling is the current inability to show beyond discourse that the current programme 'works' to an appreciable degree, or at least in a way consonant with discourse about it. AusAID's evaluation of its support of NACS and NHASP notes that '[b]ehaviour change is a premiere outcome of any response to HIV', but that few data exist with which to assess how much

> significant behaviour change has occurred as the result of the NHASP activities. Informants acknowledged high awareness of HIV in PNG but were not confident of a corresponding level of behaviour change. The NHASP social marketing surveys do not show sustained or dramatic changes in key behavioural parameters such as condom use or numbers of partners. (AusAID 2005a: 62)

Yet others have pointed to the tendency to think that it is more important to acquit monies than to justify them conceptually or to have monitored and evaluated the efficacy with which they were spent. Still others have wondered at the usefulness in prevention of HIV transmission of piling one extremely expensive Leadership Forum atop another. No critical studies of which I am aware have established what those leaders do upon return to their villages and constituencies. This must be weighed against other inarguably more important issues, such as the reliability of the drug supply and the hygiene and general appearance of clinics and other settings in which matters of an intimate nature are to be discussed and biological specimens collected and stored. The IRG review, for example, noted that '[s]everal sites visited provide HIV activities within the STI clinic and there is crowding, long waiting periods and an unwelcoming environment. Many clinicians are also not well trained on providing STI services' (IRG 2007: 5). 'Environmental hygiene' was noted as 'a significant problem in all of the public health facilities, with some having no cleaner allocated to the facilities', according to one review (NHASP 2006a: 24). Another NHASP review (2005d: iv) noted that, owing to supervisory neglect and disrupted supply chains (see also NHASP 2006a: 20), '[i]n many cases, health workers provide just half of the medications for syndromic treatment and send patients away'. Another review (NHASP 2006a: 21) noted that at some VCT sites clinic staff routinely performed three HIVab tests before changing rubber gloves, and that the 'public health facilities were untidy, dirty and rundown. Staff at one facility said there were no cleaners and they were supposed to do their own cleaning of the entire clinic'. Yet another NHASP review (2005a: 19) found that the STD Clinic at the Port Moresby General Hospital for several reasons needed great improvement in appearance.

Conclusions

Words cannot describe how frustrating I have found the process of seeing that already difficult-to-follow surveillance data become increasingly fetishized the less reliable they become (see also IRG 2007: 6). Watching the wrong models be exported to Papua New Guinea with seemingly so little critical aforethought hasn't been any easier. Hearing the same pejorative mentions of 'bad' as against valorisation of putatively 'good' models of sexual comportment has felt no better. Neither has learning of yet another bibliographic collation of ethnographic and other forms of qualitative knowledge production that haven't been grasped or used in the first place. Reading yet another INGO or NDoH official deliver Keynote Addresses that purport to be news but that relate information already well known by social scientists makes me wonder where they've been all this time.

This chapter has aimed to produce a broad but critical start to a sociology of knowledge production about HIV and AIDS in Papua New Guinea. In this chapter and elsewhere throughout the book I have argued that the national response so far has not been marked by much critical or reflexive thought about itself. There has been precious little attention paid to the effects upon programme efficacy that institutional linkages to external donor agencies and funding sources can have – good and bad. There has been even less reflexivity shown toward the slogans, campaigns and messages that have driven the national response. Models of risk and transmission dynamics are assumed but seldom demonstrated or challenged. These and the anti-condom discourse I discuss next have blunted the good intentions and even better efforts of the organisations and individuals who have worked so hard to strengthen the system and make its programmes and messages effective in preventing transmission of HIV and STDs.

To summarise my argument to this point would be to say that models of risk in terms familiar to epidemiologists don't work well in Papua New Guinea because of false assumptions they make about group constitution, the extent of mobility, the contingencies of identity construction and maintenance and especially the ubiquity of sexual networking. Centralised means of data collection and reportage are compromised by shortfalls at the provincial levels; by inconsistencies of analytic unit; by lack of accountability in relations between health, private and government policy sectors; by lack of supervision that would strengthen capacity; and by both communication and communications problems. For reasons made more clear in the following chapter, imported messages such as ABC are destined to be problematic where social- structure and cultural norms and ideals preclude, in this case, abstinence and fidelity, where condom usage is precluded by people and policies, and where condom usage is constructed as something belonging only to bad, 'high-risk' people and non-regular, commercial or 'casual' partners. The joint publications of UNAIDS, UNICEF and the WHO in the form of their 'Epidemiological Fact Sheets', frequently elide the risks of transmission in marriages, for example, when they say ' ... behaviours (e.g. casual sex or condoms) that can spur or stem the transmission of HIV' (2004: 2), 'low levels of condom use in casual relationships' (2004: 3), and that 'higher-risk sex' was that engaged in with a 'non-regular partner' (2004: 10). A BBC report (Spiller 2006) alarmed viewers and readers with its claims of the extent of 'unprotected sex, both paid-for and casual', in Papua New Guinea, which was fast approaching levels seen in sub-Saharan Africa, the author said.

For these and many other reasons, I think it is fair to continue to ask hard questions about the current and likely future 'challenges' of and to today's surveillance systems. I believe it is important also to recognise its successes on many fronts, for example, in terms of funding streams and ties of collaboration and forms of capacity-strengthening. One of the central themes of the 2004 Consensus Workshop and then 2006's HIV Prevention Summit was the promotion of the approach introduced in 2001 and formalised later as The Three Ones. This model of national subservience to international authority mandates One coordinating body that provides the basis of cooperation, One monitoring and surveillance system throughout each country, and One strategic plan. Sounds good so far, but faith in their operation and efficacy, especially in resource-poor settings, has distinctly cooled over the years. Country-specific assessments have found years on just what was predicted to happen, namely, in some cases, the creation of a 'monster', a 'mechanism that is too large and bureaucratic to actually function, and within which, civil society is both voiceless and powerless' (IHAA 2006: 5). International surveys of the successes and failures of such approaches have revealed that while four-fifths of all independent countries had 'national AIDS authorities' that were recognised as the main coordinating bodies and persons given clear mandate to coordinate, only about half of them actually had the authority to allocate resources. This moots in practice the good ideas implied by adoption of a Three Ones approach. As well, the Three Ones was not supposed to install in power any single body (say, government) or enable the undue influence of external donors (which has clearly happened), and was designed to facilitate far greater influence of both civil society organisations and especially people directly affected by and with HIV and AIDS. Richard Eves and Leslie Butt commented recently that

> the effort there is set up according to the criteria of the Global Program
> on AIDS within the framework of global mobilization involving science,
> governments and agencies, which generally replicates the mistakes
> made elsewhere. This usually involves little more than an unquestioned
> importation of materials largely developed in and for other contexts. Despite
> an increasingly large literature that questions what Elizabeth Reid has
> felicitously called 'briefcase concepts', the importation continues of these
> ready-made and portable languages and tools that are carried anywhere an
> expert travels. (Eves and Butt 2008: 6)

Following the good lead provided by Eves and Butt, I would question the likelihood that a single national plan can be expected to respond effectively in the face of the diversities and complexities of social life in Papua New Guinea. Language, geography, health service decentralisation, communications, funding sources and ethnic jealousies are just a few of the challenges posed to the national response. Rural enclave development sites, for example, are presided over largely by expatriates (who often live elsewhere) and who jealously guard HIV registers. For many, many years large mining and other resource extraction companies such as Ok Tedi Mining Limited and Oil Search Limited didn't report any HIV infections among their employees to national authorities, but did do so to corporate headquarters in other countries. As well, the realities of often quite localised contexts can fall well outside the reach of The Three Ones in terms of Monitoring and Evaluation initiatives. HIV prevention initiatives can be launched and expected to work but amidst outbreaks of Pentecostal fever or tribal fighting. Rural health systems and facilities, their personnel and supplies, in about equal measure, have become footballs over which multiple teams fight. Whether it's a hospital in Kikori, Gulf Province, taken away from District Health Services by an expatriate FBO or its equivalent in Pimaga, Southern Highlands Province, where Provincial Health wants it back for use in political campaigning or a church organisation that wants no PAC counsellors to distribute condoms, each player currently has more to gain by competing than by cooperating. The Three Ones is more like the Sixty Ones – three for each of 20 provinces. The Three Ones is an approach that presumes too much about relationships between FBOs and NGOs, between them and the private sector, and between all of them and national and provincial-level government.

The model of the Three Ones was not designed to deliver the goods in such settings. Papua New Guinea stands currently at the threshold of conceiving, funding and implementing precisely the kinds of responses needed in towns and rural countryside to 'scale-up', but it has yet convincingly to demonstrate just what this means. Most would answer 'universal access to antiretroviral treatment' (the drugs, the doctors, the nurses), but that leaves the state of health services deliveries unaddressed, which is to say logistics, supply chains, reporting systems and the state of hygiene in clinics. These each have an individual impact upon the treatment of STDs, but which isn't yet organically connected to their prevention, since condom supply, access and attitudes are sub-optimal, and since improved education about sexual health is still roundly thought of as likely to promote promiscuity. Last on the list is the greater degree of consent and pleasure in sexual practice. At this juncture Papua New Guinea has yet completely to answer several challenges often posed by international development processes. First, donor strategies, national-level and local-level responses have yet to be aligned well. Second, as the number and kind of donor agencies who have stepped up to the plate have multiplied (NGOs, churches, INGOs, CBOs, businesses, GPA, and so on), the procedures employed among them to harmonise aid management have been the more poorly aligned. The research and activism initiative proposed and then carried out by World Vision in 2004–2005 is just one example, with appeals for support (to a university, to a research institute, to an INGO, in this case), going unheard. Many claims about universal access ('3 by 5', 'universal coverage has been reached', '2 by 7 by 10', and the like) have failed duly to acknowledge ways in which these ultimate goals are going to be aligned and harmonised among and between the various players in the 'national response'. 'Meaningful progress on alignment and harmonisation', write three authors of a *Lancet* editorial, 'depends on meaningful accountability' (Sidibe *et al.* 2006: 1853).

For The Three Ones to work, the national government would have to have a smooth and time-tested relationship with civil society, which is clearly not the case (e.g. Luker 2004; Hauck *et al.* 2005). One is also allowed to wonder whether yet another 'top-down', vertically arranged model (in the form of three singular strands each labelled the One) can work in context of competing discourse about horizontal, participatory approaches, for example, the HRSS. The gender-neutral language that tends to proliferate in such approaches ('mainstreaming' gender analyses, 'stay faithful to one partner', 'don't have sex' and the like) is inappropriate because it is precisely social-structure that needs to be challenged and gender- and sex-*saturated* language that needs to be used. That kind of language, however, doesn't tend to emanate from Washington, D.C. or Manila or Geneva. When Bishop Bonivento concludes that, '[t]herefore, if the uninfected spouse wants to remain so in the future, he/she has only one choice: abstinence' (2001b: 25), he shows how monstrously out-of-touch he is with the realities of sexual practice. Even the most fervent supporters of ABC admit that '[a]bstinence is near impossible without the helping hand of the Lord' (Emily Chambers, quoted in Epstein 2007: 195). Just as out of-touch are calls for 100% condom usage and 'universal access' to antiretrovirals. Neither speaks Truth to the Power of gender relations, since condoms have all but been prohibited in marriages, or to the real state of health services, which do not have that technical capacity, or to the true nature of struggles about sexual matters in an average community. An independent review concluded about this issue that '[t]here is as yet no evaluation of adherence rates and retention among the current cohort on ART. All ART is currently facility-based and beneficiaries require transport to collect drugs. Some units report occasional shortage of stock. There is as yet no rural delivery system and little linkage to community support groups (IRG 2007: 5).

'Mainstreaming' gender, making 'gender' shoulder the burden of being a 'cross-cutting issue' between multiple sectors often softens its sharp corners and robs it of its urgency. This is the more so insofar as gender is consistently imagined as an essence, usually pertaining to women mostly (or to certain kinds of them) instead of being seen as overlapping and hotly contested sets of relationships in which everyone is enmeshed. For the Three Ones to work in Papua New Guinea, it would require that NAC and PAC and DAC and NDoH officials possessed technical expertise and professional and especially political support for difficult decisions they have to make about medical policies. Those would involve the clinical treatment of HIV infection, the widespread use of 'bush' medicines and the absence of condoms in church-run health facilities. They would need to make tough decisions about resource allocation, too, for example, in assessing the merit of grant proposals and the costing of various programmes. They would need also to get on top of their priorities, that is, prevention over collaboration, treatment and care over political stability and blood supplies, sexual matters (e.g. pack-rape, the Julian Moti affair) over tourism, and questions of social-structure over those of xenophobia. It remains an open question whether the NAC in Papua New Guinea possesses the expertise (yet) in the specifics of development impacts of HIV and of their various drags on health, education, human rights and social justice initiatives. The Three Ones is a model that requires dedicated and highly skilled expertise in rural development schemes, foreign investment, statistical modelling, public health and gendered analysis. It has been difficult to get various mainline denominations to cooperate in a coherent HIV and AIDS policy. Having any of them, much less all of them collectively, be so coordinated as not to clash with government in terms of condom promotion, VCT initiatives and frank discussion of sexual matters is simply unrealistic. It is not to speak ill of Papua New Guinea to note how quickly the Three Ones can become hostage to squabbles over money, scope, voice and territory.

NOTES

1. According to two consultants who wish to remain anonymous, this was owing to the fact of upcoming elections, the wish not to release 'negative' findings too close thereto and the choice of epidemiology software that has a penchant for producing more conservative estimates of seroprevalence.

2. I want to acknowledge here in this section the especial inspiration provided by the writings of Brooke Schoepf.

3. Even as recently as 2005 Papua New Guineans and other insular Pacific islanders were represented as being collectively at particular risk of infection by those coming from neighbouring countries where seroprevalence was higher, or by their own people who had travelled abroad. By contrast, Vanuatuans and Solomon islanders were not so warned in their possible contacts with Papua New Guineans (Sladden 2005).

4. I reviewed a manuscript for the *South Pacific Journal of Law* in which it was claimed (by personal communication) that four cases had been brought to the Ombudsman's Commission but that they were not covered in the annual reports thereof.

Chapter 5

Foreign objects and cognitive dissonance

The strange waters of anti-condom discourse

Rubber wars

The evaluation team was concerned about the content of prevention messages, particularly those being disseminated by certain faith-based organisations. Some actively promote ambiguous and misinformed messages about protective behaviours, including re-configuring the 'ABC' prevention message, to promote the A (Abstinence) and B (Be faithful) components of the message, while equating C with Church doctrine. It is the team's opinion that this misinformation (at worst) and ambivalence (at best) is undermining HIV prevention in PNG and denying people a full range of proven protective choices. (AusAID 2005a: 13)

Rigid adherence to religious creed, in particular doctrine that prohibits sexual activity, seems to offer few coping resources to girls in the face of sexual situations. If sexual activity is strictly forbidden, perhaps girls fail to develop strategies for insisting on birth control, lack knowledge and access to birth control, or do not fully acknowledge the responsibility of intercourse. (Miller and Gur 2002: 404)

Resistance to the use of condoms in Melanesia, and perhaps elsewhere, is not merely a local manifestation of the distance between rational, scientific explanation and religious conviction but a statement about the cultural principles underlying knowledge and conduct. (Lindenbaum 2008: xii)

'Doctor, what you are saying about those things may be true, but you see, our ancestors didn't use them', said the well-dressed woman in Tok Pisin, one of Papua New Guinea's three linguas franca (alongside 852 other languages spoken). She stood alongside two other women and 35 other male colleagues at a mine-site workplace. They had assembled to hear me talk about Papua New Guinea's growing AIDS epidemic and what my IMR colleagues and I had found regarding sexual networking and STD prevalence in seven communities at or near her work-place. 'Those things are foreign objects', she continued, 'and against our culture'. I replied to this well educated, highly professional and articulate woman that 'those things' (condoms) weren't any newer to Papua New Guinea than beer, Modess and tin-fish. I said that Papua New Guineans seem to have taken readily enough to each of those, just as she had apparently taken to gold mining, hair gel and evangelical Christianity. She responded with the 'well-known facts' that condoms increase promiscuity, carry sickness and break up marriages. *Gumi nogat pawa* ('Condoms aren't effective'), she said, echoing the anti-condom sentiments of many health officials and religious leaders. 'We Papua New Guineans, we like it flesh-to-flesh, "natural way"', and as others added, to knowing chuckles, 'meat-to-meat', 'skin-to-skin' (e.g. Lepani 2007b: 258), just as those in the Solomon Islands seem to prefer their sex 'wire-to-wire' (Burslem *et al.* 1998). Unfortunately, there are consequences to unprotected sex The valuable study conducted in 2005–2006 by Pamela Toliman and associates of anti-gonorrhea drug sensitivities found an overall prevalence of gonorrhea infection among clients in four STD clinics throughout Papua New Guinea of nearly 53%. They found that '[many] of participants (41.5%) reported that they did not use a condom with their steady partner (Figure 8). Meanwhile, the majority of females (56.5%) reported that they had never used condoms [despite many suffering repeated infections from their husbands] and the majority of males (50.8%) reported that they only used condoms occasionally (Figure 9)' (Toliman *et al.* 2006: 16).

Condoms have been extremely contentious new technologies virtually wherever they have been introduced in the insular Pacific. There is a strange silence about them in government documents and research papers, however, usually with reference to 'cultural sensitivities' or 'taboos' likely to break were they to be mentioned. Myra White's presentation of Australia's contributions to family planning and reproductive health in the Pacific mentions condoms only thrice (twice in one foot-note), noting that most government condoms (in Papua New Guinea) end up in the hands of policemen, who leave them lying in the barracks (White 2000: 28, n. 105). During a recent Pacific Youth Festival held in Papeete, an HIV peer-educator from Kiribati, Tierata Taukabwan, was quoted as saying, 'One of the hardest things for us is to actually promote condoms. The Catholic Church is against the way we discuss sexual activity and condom use' (*Islands Business International* 2007). In Vanuatu, according to Zenner and Russell (2005), a woman who suggests condom use invites accusations of promoting promiscuity, and those accusations ratchet upwards insofar as the Ministry of Health promotes HIV awareness.

Condom usage has played an important but remarkably small part of family planning initiatives. For example, in Nuku'alofa, Tonga, only 35 of the 239 total new acceptors of contraceptive methods in 1973 chose condoms. Condoms were provided as a family planning device fewer than 6,300 times between 1971 and 1990 anywhere in Tonga (Ivarature 2000: 44–5). The Catholic Health Service there provides the greatest bulk of non-government based family planning services, so condoms do not currently feature heavily in Tonga in terms of HIV transmission prevention. Draftees of the first national surveillance plan in Tonga noted quite negative attitudes toward them and especially low rates of usage among sexually active youth. They also found inconsistent supply of condoms, attitudinal barriers of health workers to condom promotion, and a strong association between condoms and contraception, not disease prevention (SSPW 2000). Research conducted in Fiji to assess patterns of infection and reinfection found that even those suffering the latter still either 'never' or only 'sometimes' used condoms, owing to their short supply (Hotchin *et al.* 1996). The reported prevalence in Solomon Islands of child-bearing age women using condoms was only 0.5% in the late 1990s, whereas in Western Samoa and Tonga, the figures were around 12% (Chung 2000: 20). Of the New Caledonian Kanak women whose reproductive health histories were surveyed, fewer than half of those sexually active had ever used a condom, and substantial proportions of women who had used condoms in a prior relationship did not use them with a new partner (Salomon and Hamelin 2008: 92).

Examples drawn from the insular Pacific show that reticence to use condoms is seldom about only pleasure or even the attitudinal barriers of potential condom users; instead, it is more the attitudinal barrier of the potential distributors, whether those are government or church-sponsored clinic employees or other opinion leaders such as religious figures. Naomi McPherson writes on the basis of her extensive field research experience among the Bariai of West New Britain Province that 'Bariai feel that parents and children are "shamed" should their sexual matters be discussed in each other's presence' (McPherson 2008: 233). This led one Baria woman to 'read' an AIDS-related health poster as saying 'If you something, something, then put a something something if you something something' (2008: 235). In addition to local health workers seldom having any condoms to give out or showing willingness to instruct as to their use, condom-related posters are not infrequently found to be marked up, edited, if not also turned inward, facing the wall, which Holly Wardlow (2008: 197) found in the Tari Basin of Southern Highlands Province and which I have seen in that and other provinces in health centres, aid posts and clinics. Father Jude's pronouncement in March of 2006 following the HIV Prevention Summit (Ronayne-Ford 2006) was that '100% condom use' calls were 'a recipe for disaster by people who don't know what to do'. They exemplified, he continued, only the last-ditch efforts of 'desperate leadership [that] has neither the wisdom nor the moral authority to give the direction which is needed'. 'Experience in the South Pacific', wrote Margaret Winn and David Lucas some time ago, 'suggests that women want to talk about family planning and sexuality, and want to share contraceptive and sexual decision-making with their sexual partners. At the same time', they write,

> they are inhibited by a culture which places numerous socio-religious strictures on sexuality, which views much sexual behaviour as unnatural and shameful, which discourages an interest in acquiring or publicly discussing sexual knowledge and which has a limited sexuality lexicon. As a consequence, South Pacific women often feel they do not have the confidence, the permission, or the words to initiate a discussion of sexuality. (Winn and Lucas 1993: n.p.)

'Similarly, the sexual culture of Vanuatu encourages the concealment of sexual availability, condemning open talk about sex and any behavior that is perceived as blatantly sexual', says Maggie Cummings about Vanuatu. Not surprisingly, however, given such a publicly repressive sexual regime, Vanuatuans are apparently given to 'incessant – but furtive – talk about sex' (Cummings 2008: 134). Also unsurprising is that young women, who are demonstrably at risk of unwanted pregnancies, of STDs and of HIV transmission, are told merely to 'stay quiet' and not insist on condom use, 'for fear of being labeled promiscuous' (Cummings 2008: 138).

In like manner, Papua New Guineans who would like to use condoms often cannot find them or are in other ways discouraged from using them. That is because they live in areas too far from health centres or because those health centres refuse to stock and distribute them or do so but only to certain people or in certain contexts.[1] Sister Tarcicia Hunhoff, for example, a German Holy Spirit Missionary sister who leads the National Catholic AIDS Council from Port Moresby, was interviewed in 2006 by Stephen Crittenden for *The Religion Report*. Sister Hunhoff cares deeply about Papua New Guineans and her church mission, but was difficult to pin down in terms of her stance toward condoms. When asked whether or not her counselling centre 'had' condoms, she replied, '[w]e do have, as I said in counselling sessions – if there is a need. But you must understand we are not promoting condoms, we are promoting values, Christian values, we are not promoting condoms. There is a big difference in using a condom where there is a need, or promoting condoms'. She went on to assert that condoms and safe sex are not only anti-religion, but anti-cultural, 'not in tune with culture' (Crittenden 2006). The full context of her comments makes clear that condoms are to be a last resort, used only in context of *known* serodiscordant *married* couples. Given that most HIVab+ married persons do not know of their serostatus, it is difficult to think of such a strategy having any appreciable effect on dampening HIV transmission. Given the low levels of communication between couples about sexual health matters, it's difficult to understand her questioning the general existence of a need for condoms.

This problem has been noted far and wide throughout Papua New Guinea. One of the many NHASP review teams found, for example, in general praise of local-based efforts at awareness and prevention, that '[a]t the same time there were mixed messages being delivered by some faith-based groups regarding protective measures (NHASP 2005k: 9). Jenkins and Alpers found in their study of youth in Lufa, Morata and Goroka that '[e]ven if young people manage to seek treatment for STDs, few health workers will give them condoms' (1996: 249). Alison Dundon found in Balimo, Western Province, that nursing sisters had quite literally taken condoms 'off the streets' (Dundon 2007: 40–1). Church leaders oppose the idea and practice of providing frank HIV and sexual health education. Brother Joe Kewande, for example, scolded other activist pastors in Papua New Guinea not even to preach about, much less for condoms: 'Don't you know that the more you educate people about the use of condoms, you are encouraging them for more sex?' (Kewande 2008). Health workers in many areas of Enga Province 'said the government should ban condoms' (NHASP

2005l: 33). The independent review group that visited Papua New Guinea in 2007 concluded on the basis of many interviews and site visits that

> The contribution of the various Church-based groups to HIV prevention work is impressive. A distinction must however be made between those Churches that are contributing creatively and positively to the national response and those that may be misleading or doing harm. For example, some Church leaders have devised unique ways of condom promotion by 'turning a blind eye' to condom distribution, believing in it to be the 'lesser evil'. Others are involved in influencing more 'orthodox' clergy and training them for prevention work, including condom promotion. But many Church-based efforts do not move beyond awareness-raising, and are mainly about promoting A (Abstinence) and B (Being faithful), leaving reference to C (condoms) out of the equation. Moreover, there are mixed messages from some Church groups on what works (prayers and not medicines) ... Condom promotion and ART scale up have little scope for success if some local Church leaders and workers fail to support them. (IRG 2007: 8).

Moreover, many health workers and religious leaders yet believe and tell their congregation that condoms cause or promote promiscuity and facilitate transmission of or actually cause HIV (see below). Because of the extent to which churches subsidise education, however, confusion results over who is responsible for what, which services should government and which should churches deliver. Healthy debate is thus precluded. This can result in 'poor or no delivery of key sexual health messages even for young people who are accessing secondary education' (NZPPD 2006: 15). The role of churches in 'perpetuating women's ignorance as well as traditional religious gender stereotypes, subjecting women to subordinate and disadvantaged positions relative to men', say the authors of another critical review, 'contribute to making women particularly vulnerable to HIV infection' (ESCAP 2005: 4).

Many misconceptions of prevention methods and transmission routes and risks are fuelled by churches. The nationwide social mapping team found that such misconceptions were promoted especially by Catholic, Baptist, Seventh Day Adventist and evangelical and Pentecostal denominations (NHASP 2005g: 4, 5, 14, 15). In the Tari Basin of Southern Highlands Province AIDS is seen by many Huli as a sort of 'divine retribution', and so condoms are thought ill of. This is because their proper and consistent use (that is, in preventing HIV transmission) precludes the revelation of sin in the bodies and on the skin of AIDS sufferers (Wardlow 2007, 2008; see also Eves 2003a; Richards 2004). Across the border in Indonesian Papua, argues Sarah Hewat, women want to believe that men are serious about them, and so don't use condoms, just as men would like to believe in women's sexual loyalty and naiveté. For a woman to demand condoms of a male lover, she writes, 'would be to invite accusations of being a "slut" (*perempuan nakal*)' (Hewat 2008: 230). In the Talasea District of West New Britain Province the NHASP-sponsored social mapping team found strongly ambivalent community attitudes toward condoms and their distribution, especially to youth. Common beliefs included that doing so would lead youth into promiscuity with devices that 'are not 100% safe because there can be holes in them. A catechist at the Catholic Parish in Kimbe', they said, 'also worried about safety ... [insofar as] there is always the risk that there is a hole in the condom or that it breaks during intercourse' (NHASP 2005j: 27). Catholic Church members and health workers in Enga Province have said the same thing (NHASP 2005l: 42). The Catholic AIDS awareness group in Talasea misperceived condom usage, implying an ability of condoms to harm the family and to cause skin eruptions (because they were factory-made) and even brain injury. A university-educated student in the Kandrian area was convinced that one could see holes in the condom if stretched open (2005j: 27). This and every other report from the social mapping study shows how deeply entrenched is misinformation about the manufacturing of condoms, about their alleged role in inciting sexual desire and about their inappropriateness for married couples. Although scanning electron microscopy has been used to assess latex condoms and has found (infinitesimally small) pits and imperfections, laboratory studies have found neither that pores penetrate the condom's membrane nor that viruses pass through them, even when they are stretched and stressed (Conant 1984; Kish 1983). Nevertheless, this is the myth spread by many health officials and religious leaders in Papua New Guinea. And elsewhere: Epstein found that in southern Africa an oft-repeated rumour is consistent with the notion that condoms 'cause' AIDS. 'AIDS came from JeitO', said one young man in reference to a popular condom; 'if one hangs a JeitO condom up to dry in the sunlight for a day, one can eventually see the HIV virus squirming inside' (quoted in Epstein 2007: 148). The myth derives at least proximally, if not ultimately, from draft revisions of PEPFAR-related materials that 'contained the myth that condoms have microscopic pores that can be permeated by HIV' (Cohen 2005: 23–4). A NHASP review of training efficacy (NHASP 2005k) found that FBOs, in presenting the ABC message 'would not distribute condoms which are not … accessible at the village level. The effect of these actions was that a message was given but the means to react to that message were not available. Some instances were described where religious people delivering information about HIV/AIDS were actively promoting against condoms' (NHASP 2005k: 15). That disinformation is shared and promoted by health workers especially in those provinces (such as West Sepik, East Sepik and West New Britain) where health services are provided mostly by the Catholic Health Services.

The HRSS (High-Risk Settings Strategy) mandated the construction, placement and provisioning of condom vending machines, but few if any were promoted to the people between whom most infections occur: husband and wife, boyfriend and girlfriend. Despite that people throughout much of the Pacific have expressed fairly consistently the desire to learn more about their own and others' sexual and reproductive health, the appropriate health service providers are often 'acting as gate-keepers to information and services and deciding who should have access' (Chung 2000: 18). It would be ironic were it not so tragic that the people most needing sexual health information are the ones most missed in prevention programmes. Surveillance initiatives have focused most of their attentions on MSM and sex workers, despite that most STD and HIV infections in females occur in those who, in terms of epidemiology, relate as wives and girlfriends but in whom are expected abstinence and fidelity.

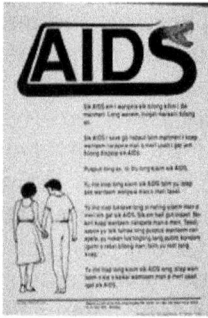

Early AIDS poster

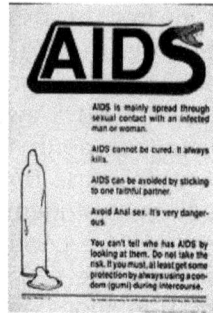

Early AIDS poster

Condom nation

The sources of these kinds of misconstrual of infective risk are many. This section examines some of the health promotional media in Papua New Guinea over the years that have formulated cognitive models that position the usage of condoms. Posters, pamphlets and messages have constructed condoms in ways that are sometimes consonant with certain, often conservative ideals. In the mid-late 1990s, however, they began to press on those ideals by reflecting sexual practice more accurately. The first poster depicted here, for example, in which 'AIDS' is spelled such that the 'S' is snake-like, says that AIDS is a lethal illness and indicates that 'transmission' (HIV is not specified) is not possible through close contact or kissing. First launched in 1988, the poster says straightforwardly that transmission is sexual and is therefore thwarted by using condoms. Interestingly, it uses two Tok Pisin verbs for sexual intercourse, *puspusim* and *koap*, the former of which never appeared again in a public health poster. Faithful monogamy is implied by the depiction of a couple walking hand in hand (though few such couples do so) and such that the male seems protective. Another 1988 poster of similar style and also featuring the snake motif suggested protection in the form of condoms, depicted in application and in use, and also instructed viewers to avoid anal sex, which it said was very dangerous, although without specifying why. Risk reduction was clearly linked, at least in words, with condom usage, but the poster seems on visual grounds to link AIDS and condoms and morally objectionable sex quite unhealthily. I am not aware of the extent to which these posters were also translated into Hiri Motu and Tok Pisin. A Department of Health-sponsored family planning poster in 1993, not depicted here, listed 'Ways to Help you Space Your Children', that is, not actually to prevent births altogether or STDs. Condoms were fourth on the list of methods or technologies for birth spacing. An expression of female agency, but set in a Port Moresby high-school, was evident in this poster from 1994, 'AIDS Prevention for Schools in PNG', in which 'John' and 'Mary' plan a Saturday night party rendezvous. She tells him to get lost, however, because he doesn't have a condom. Another poster depicts a sad looking school-girl, obviously pregnant, saying so, and asking the viewer: 'Should This Happen to You'? It would have been an extremely rare female in Papua New Guinea in 1990, however, to have been visibly pregnant and allowed to remain in school. According to

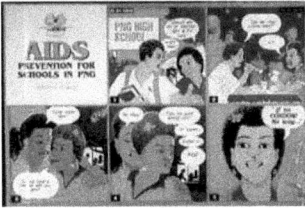

AIDS prevention for schools

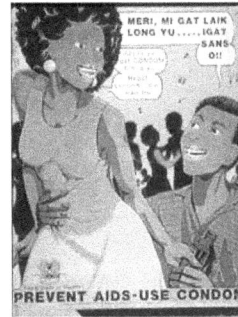

Meri Mi Gat Laik Yu

one of my adoptive mothers, on Daru, the Unevangelized Fields Mission in Western Province mandated topless female student attendance in school well into the 1960s. This was done, she said, so as better to monitor the possible signs of pregnancy that would have been sufficient grounds for expulsion.

One of several of its 1990 counterparts, not depicted here, features a dirty dress-wearing village woman in similar straits, but asking (presumably male) viewers the pregnant question: 'would you be more careful if it was you who could become pregnant?' Neither poster mentions STDs, neither mentions condom usage, and the reference in both cases is clearly pregnancy, but neither suggests an alternative. Two that might have been mentioned would be sexual practices other than penile-vaginal intercourse and the use of a condom. The I.E.C. unit of the Family Planning division of the Department of Health distributed a markedly different kind of poster, also in 1990, that was seemingly aimed at males. In Tok Pisin, it instructs viewers that male condoms are available here for only five toea, which then would have been about $.06US. The physiognomy depicted suggests a highlands man wearing, in stark contrast to the females in other posters, traditional clothing (of Melpa) and emboldened by traditional objects (that look to be from Simbu Province). Holding his spear in one hand and fingering an ankle-length waist-covering with the other, he appears confident and properly defensive. Whether contraception or STD prevention (or both) is indicated is unclear, but yet he appears strong compared the female vulnerability depicted in other posters.

A trial in 1992 by the Department of Health led in 1994 to the mass release of a cartoon-style depiction of a typical Port Moresby disco setting. Significantly, the poster was titled 'Prevent AIDS – Use Condoms'. This suggests that, at that point in Papua New Guinea's HIV epidemic, condoms were considered a viable, culturally acceptable option in preventing transmission. Nevertheless it located the potential of AIDS in a nightclub instead of in a village and between two anonymous persons, not intimate partners. The handsome-looking young male offers a skimpily clad woman a beer and expresses his desire for her: '*Meri, mi gat laik long yu. I gat sans, o?*' ('Hey, you're hot; do I have a shot?), to which she replies, translated from the Tok Pisin, 'well, if you've got a condom, sure, but no condom, no sex'. Whereas he is seated and she is coming astride him, suggesting something

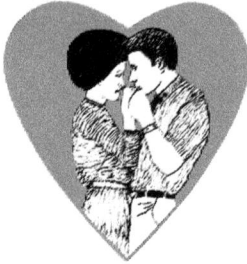

TINGTING PASTAIM BIFO YU LAIK SLIP
...WANTAIM NARAPELA MAN OR MERI !

AIDS

EM DISPELA SIK I SAVI KILIM MAN NA I
NOGAT MARASIN BILONG RAUSIM. SIK
KAMAP LONG TAIM WANPELA I SLIP WAN-
TAIM NARAPELA I GAT DISPELA SIK AIDS.

MAS ISTAP PAS WANTAIM WANPELA MAN
NA MERI TASOL.

Think first...

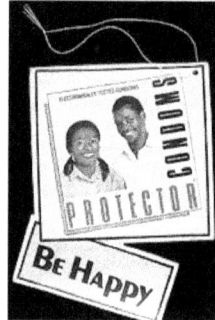

Protector condoms

of the fact of male prerogative, this poster yet affirms female sexual desire and agency. Instead of forcing himself on her, he *asks* her whether he's got a chance. On the other hand, he seems to be clasping her tightly and also plying her with alcohol, suggesting something of the context and constraints of female sexual agency.

In 1993 the Red Bank, New Jersey-based Ansell condom manufacturing company made a new one for Papua New Guinea dubbed the Protector, depicted here, but that didn't last very long. Each packet of three condoms came with an insert written in Tok Pisin advising on its handling and application but which was deemed by the Censorship Board to be obscene owing to the line drawing of an erect penis. The two people depicted on each packet could not look less Papua New Guinean, the female wearing a gingham-check shirt along with pink lipstick and styling her hair in pig-tails. Alternative depictions of those who had islander and highlander physiognomy, by contrast, were trialed but were apparently less appealing than this West African-looking couple. Indeed, the condom packet and associated paraphernalia were launched in Ghana. It is not immediately self evident from the condom packet with whom one should and with whom one does not need to use condoms, since there are no obvious signs of their relationship to each other, although they appear healthy and happy.

Another poster from the same time period relies heavily upon the signs and Western discourses of companionate relationships, framing an emotionally close, hand-holding couple who are poised inside a vividly red Valentine heart to embrace and perhaps kiss. It first instructs viewers to 'Think

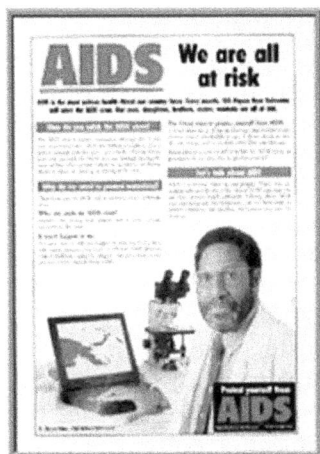

We are all at risk

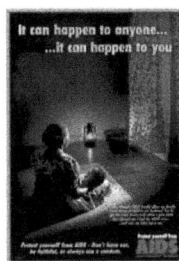

It can happen to you

before sleeping with another person', though not what to think about, and warns that AIDS is invariably fatal and without cure. Nor does it tell viewers to think before having sex with a spouse. Like most newspaper articles at this time and previously, it doesn't mention HIV. Further, it implies that AIDS can be transmitted sexually and that it occurs more or less on contact (*Sik kamap long taim* ...). It doesn't mention condoms at all, however, and implies that faithfulness is HIV transmission preventive: 'Stick to One Partner'. As well, the long incubation period of HIV ratchets up the effects of misstating one's and misinforming another's transmissive risk.

A poster promoted in 2001 was one of the first to democratise the risk of HIV transmission but at the same time call attention to the gendered nature of the expanding epidemic. Its predecessor in that first respect is the famous poster featuring Dr Clement Malau saying 'We Are All at Risk'. Text-heavy and designed in simple clinical colours, it certifies for the first time biomedical ways of knowing about HIV. Dr Malau is dressed in a lab coat, he is depicted as manipulating medical equipment in a laboratory setting, and his authority and knowledge are buttressed in appeals to scientific modernity by placement nearby of a laptop computer and gleaming countertop. Another poster from 2001, in stark contrast and in muted, emotional colour, comes with the tag line, 'It can happen to anyone ... it can happen to you'. A Papuan woman sits on a woven grass mat on the floor in a dark room lit only by hurricane lamp, seemingly in an urban setting, and holds a small infant. 'I never thought AIDS would affect my family', she says. 'I was always faithful to my husband, but he got the virus. It was only when I gave birth that I found out I had the AIDS virus ... and now my baby has it too'. The poster reflects a key feature of both the expanding epidemic – people learning of their HIV infection in reference to something else, child-birth, in this case – and of the national response to it: the ascendance to the level of policy of the ABC message. The injunction, 'Don't have sex', however, is too late, for she's married, and the 'Be faithful' component, according to her testimony, didn't work, either. We don't know whether she would have been able to negotiate condom use with her husband (there is no mention of physical abuse, religious affiliation that might have prohibited them, alcohol use or anything else) but yet she felt protected by her own fidelity. It was trust and faith, in other words, that crippled her self-assessment of risk, whereas these are two planks of the platform of the national response. At least rhetorically, then, two of the three victims here are rendered 'innocent', infected through no behaviour of their own, while the 'guilty', as in so many of these discourses, is (and apparently was) absent. No poster depicts a man (or a woman) saying, in effect, 'Yep, it was me. I did it'. Presumably, her husband was infected during condomless sex, which raises other issues of cognition and representation that aren't addressed. This is in stark contrast to other posters released in the following year, 2002, with the title 'Show You Care'. Again, risk was encoded in the message conveyed regarding sexual transmission of HIV. Because the word 'uninfected' doesn't appear, it falsely reassures that mutual faithfulness is HIV transmission preventive. 'Making love' appears for the first time, and the implied health and happiness of couples mutual in their desire for each other and for good sexual health was a real improvement.

The power to negotiate condom usage with an intimate partner was given a jolt of realism in a newer poster campaign launched in 2005 that put it bluntly and in three languages: No condom, No sex! The one depicted here, 'Nogat Kondom: maski long wip!' ('Don't have sex if you don't have a condom') is playful and colourful, featuring a young, hip and alive, urban, Papuan-looking woman wearing sporty sneakers, much jewelry and a sleeveless singlet. She tells the intended audience not to listen to one excuse after another from a lover who refuses to use condoms, whether boyfriend or husband. The importance of sexual negotiation is put front and centre. For the first time so bluntly, this poster situates risk in context of unprotected sex, pure and simple, instead of membership in a putative category. She calls out the ideals of companionate relationship, which can be dangerous, and with a smile on her face. That's just about precisely what we need.

In posture, content and perspective, this poster is light years from an earlier generation of other Department of Health-sponsored posters that blame persons, not specified acts, and that enable fear and stigma instead of attempt to dissolve it. Various NHASP reviews (e.g. 2005k: 76) have criticised this tendency of FBO-inspired anti-condom rhetoric. One poster says that to 'Abrusim AIDS' (Avoid AIDS) one must stay faithful to one partner, and it says specifically not to sleep with prostitutes. Another, titled 'Listen, Learn and Live', features a red Stop-sign inside of which sits the triple exhortation of the ABC message. Marriage is falsely assumed to be safe. The poster does not attempt to explain any of the contradictions implied, for example, both *not* to have sex (Abstain) but to have it only *in a certain way* (with one's spouse); to have sex only within marriage, but at the same to use a condom, when they are told elsewhere that 'one' (a male gender) doesn't use condoms with one's wives. Yet another poster is titled 'AIDS: what is it?' and mentions that 'multiple sex partners multiply the risk of STD/HIV infection', which isn't true. It conflates STD and HIV just at a time when consciousness is raising regarding the multiplicity of microscopically small pathogens. It puts extra pressure upon pregnant females, too, who are exhorted to 'responsible sexual

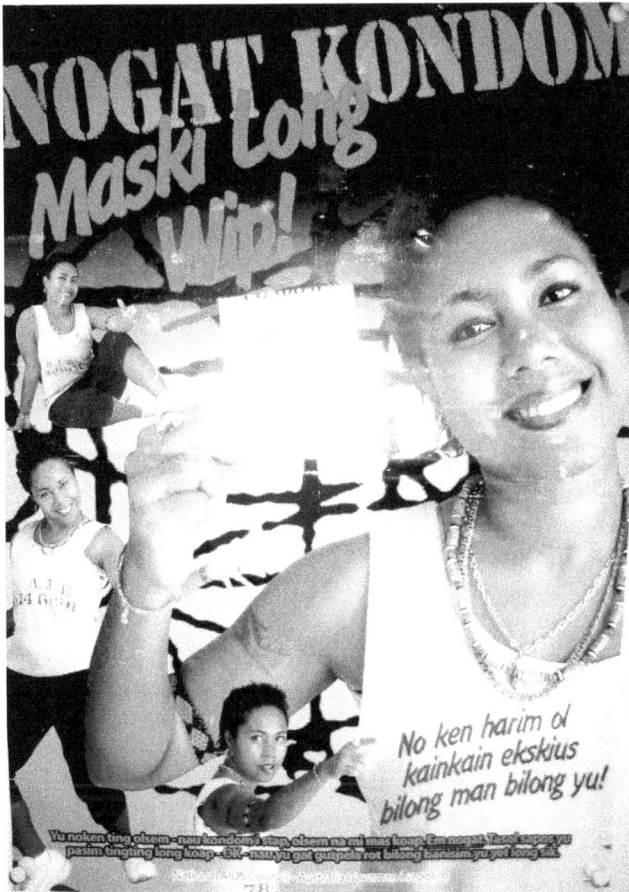

NOGAT KONDOM Maski Long Wip!

No ken harim ol kainkain ekskius bilong man bilong yu!

Don't listen to your partner's endless excuses

behaviour' to protect the life of the baby. In fact, it is not by and large the sexual behaviours of pregnant females in Papua New Guinea that endanger foetuses, but poor access to health services, abusive male partners, missing condoms and lacking sexual health information.

Thus have condoms been positioned cognitively in quite awkward fashion. Although the net effects of not using them are quite uniformly negative (unwanted pregnancy, school-leaving, HIV infection, maternal transmission, and the like), condoms are not yet positioned as our friend, as a tool, as a useful method. The contours of rhetoric about them suggest that condoms are in Papua New Guinea things not normally used by people who, insofar as their partners are infected, *should* use them. By the same token, and speaking as one who has spent a lot of time in the bushes and swamps of public sex locales (see also Lepani 2007b: 257), the fact that people use them in so-called 'high-risk settings' hasn't challenged much their designation as such by NGOs, the NACS and the NHASP. Each and every properly used condom lowers transmissive risk, that is, but condoms have been pitched at 'high-risk' people and 'high-risk settings' so as to become synonymous with

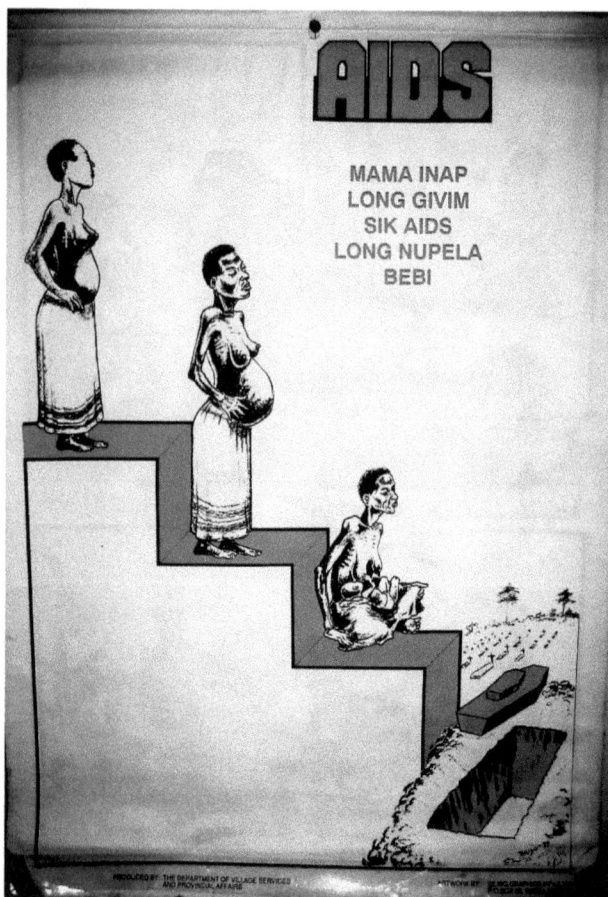

Mama can give AIDS to her new baby...

them. Condoms have been constructed over the years as being designed for morally 'bad' people or objectionable sex, despite that the vast majority of non-consensual sex, which can be painful and physically harmful for the female and be thus *truly* objectionable, takes place without them. Condoms have been constructed as pertaining to extra-marital sex, when the vast majority of marriages are not monogamous anyway and marriage-making often requires demonstration of fertility, that is, condomless sex. The consequences of such, both good and bad, featured in the earliest generation of AIDS-related posters. The one depicted here still graces the District Health Office in a highlands capital (April, 2006). *'Mama inap long givim sik AIDS long nupela bebi'*, it says. Once again there is no mention of HIV, and so AIDS is something said to be passed internally from mother to foetus. The finality and inevitability of death could not be portrayed more clearly or vividly, in bright red colour. The source of the infection, however, is contained internal to the woman herself and does not extend to her sex partner, which would presumably be a husband, given her traditional dress and the implied pastoral setting. Key to the rhetorical play of this and likeminded messages is the proper setting of condom usage – outside of marriage, not with a marital partner – and a certain confusion about the effectiveness of condoms.

These contradictions and ambivalences have been played out in the context of public health debates and policies, too, not just of individual choices. Condoms have been dubbed 'unsafe' by the very public health officials, community leaders and religious authorities who discourage frank discussions of signs and symptoms of STDs and of the positive aspects of sexuality. Some have claimed that condoms are like cigarettes (e.g. Bradshaw 2003). Bishop Bonivento claims that condoms won't protect people anyway who go against God (i.e., '*Yupela i no ken banisim yupela yet sapos yu agensim Lo bilong God*'; Bonivento 2005b: 1). In doing so, they have confused with regards to condoms the *real* issues of safety (let's say, of exposed electrical wires, worn brakes or dirty needles) with those of efficacy (in preventing, that is, unwanted pregnancies and STDs). Most gallingly, the straw man arguments they erect regarding condom usage fail at even elemental logic: even granting that condoms are not '100% effective', the fact that unprotected sex is just that – 0% safe – is never mentioned in public. Dr Thomas Vinit, now Head of the Lifestyle Diseases section of the Department of Health, said that 'the Government knows that condoms are not 100% safe and yet are going ahead and promoting its use' (Peter 2006: 3). He added for good measure that it was wrong to use condoms to prevent HIV transmission because condoms were originally designed for contraception. In this Dr Vinit was repeating a position long held by devout Catholics. In an American context, 'Catholics arguing against birth control', as Joshua Gamson has shown,

> continued to treat the condom exclusively as a contraceptive method, arguing that in using such devices to 'positively frustrate the procreative purpose of sexual intercourse' couples 'pervert the order of nature and thus directly oppose the designs of nature's Creator'. (Gamson 1990: 262)

Nevertheless, Dr Vinit supports the use of antiretroviral therapies but whose major component, AZT (azidothymidine), was synthesised in 1964 and was used originally to treat cancer (Arno and Feiden 1992: 40). Dr Vinit should not be allowed to have it both ways. Condoms are said by people such as Bishop Bonivento (see below) to be physically harmful, despite that sexual violence and other forms of physical abuse in marriage – *real* harm, that is – are in Papua New Guinea as frequent as anywhere else in the world, that coitarche (first vaginal intercourse) is for females often quite traumatic and that rates of infection inside marriage are astronomically high. Even granting that condoms were somehow harmful to the physical body, altering tissue or drubbing immune function, how does that harm compare to official estimates that one in five or one in four or four out of every 10 Papua New Guineans, or more, are already infected with an STD? Nearly 60% of two large groups of randomly selected women from rural communities in the Eastern Highlands Province were found to be infected with one or another STD (Passey *et al.* 1998b), and that was a decade ago. None of them belonged to socially despised groups such as sex workers or homosexual males or intravenous drug injectors and who are often held rhetorically to be at high risk of infection. These ambiguities are vividly portrayed in the text box quote from a letter to the editor of the *Post-Courier*.

'...*The AIDS prevention "awareness" campaigns have so far campaigned with double-edged slogans. On one hand, "AIDS is a virus [sic] that kills the human race by way of sexual contact". On the other, "It is okay to have sexual contact as long as you use a condom". The double-edged scenario here is that "it is okay by laws of this land or by any standards to have sex outside marriage and have fun. As long as one uses a condom he or she doesn't contact the AIDS virus and pass onto the married partner". It basically means that the laws allow sexual contact and adultery but it's unlawful to pass the AIDS virus onto your partner, as this would eventually be passed onto the other's married partner. What a joke! By any standard, having sex outside marriage is supposed to [be] unlawful and traditionally unethical and the law of this land prohibits that. Now the AIDS awareness campaigners and their agencies are promoting that sex outside marriage is alright as long as a condom is used, but is illegal to pass and multiply the AIDS virus to others. We should talk real and serious on this deadly virus by upholding any law on sex outside marriage and immediately put a stop to and make condoms an illegal commodity in the country*' (Eric 2005).

These contradictions haven't been subjected to much theorising and they are seldom opposed consistently and forcefully from top levels. The fact that anti-condom rhetoric wasn't nipped in the bud is an aspect of the sociology of knowledge of the HIV and AIDS epidemics that needs critical attention. To scrutinise public discussion in Papua New Guinea of pleasure, tradition, AIDS and condoms is to confront the many ironies of representation. Adherents to one foreign object (Christianity) are opposing another (condoms) despite the imminent threat of another (AIDS). Meanwhile, silenced Others (the less rhetorically Christian) are asking privately or secretly, sometimes desperately, for things – condoms and even the '*filins marasin*' (lubricant) that will *lukautim gumi* (protect the condom) and *hamamasim skin* (give pleasure) – that are pitched at the Other (sex workers and 'high-risk' people). Masturbation, meanwhile, is denounced as 'Western' and 'bloody useless'. For religious leaders such as Pope Pius XII, masturbation is seen as being a grave sin (e.g. Bonivento 2001b: 22), which Bishop Bonivento also castigates in his writings (e.g. 2008: 3). He goes further in claiming that '[a]dvising the students to negotiate safe sex like deep kissing, oral sex and intercourse with condom instead of penetrative sex [sic] ... is dishonest and dangerous, because they are not safe at all' (2008: 4). Sex toys, erotica, being gay or lesbian and the right of women safely and legally to choose to terminate an unwanted pregnancy, even in case of rape or sexual molestation, remain illegal in Papua New Guinea.

The woman at the work-place I mentioned at the outset of this chapter continued, 'we just can't use those things' (condoms) and said that STD and pregnancy avoidance are 'against our culture'. Nevertheless, similar claims that *sikAIDS, em i pe bilong sin bilong ol* ('AIDS is God's punishment for their sin') and that *tu kina meri* (promiscuous women) have been cursed with sickness by God for fornication and adultery (but not the men who are their sexual partners) clearly emanate from foreign sources and discourses. Politicians and petty marketers alike explain STDs in ontological terms as resulting from the aberrant acts (too much sex) of condemned individuals (*rot meri* and the like). Street preachers target migrating women, foreigners, homosexuals and even condoms themselves, usage of which, say some, will condemn one to Hell (Sue Crockett, cited in Eves 2003a: 261). Few have located the expanding HIV epidemics in the contradictions of social structure or of evangelical Christianity, in poverty, in sex-negativity, in the gutting of health services, or in corruption in high places. Fornication and adultery, neither polygyny nor male sexual prerogative *per se*, were the very definition of 'promiscuity', argues Dr Vinit, and he takes this promiscuity to be 'the route of transmission of HIV'. He encourages local cultural practices such as valorisation of female virginity so that 'they can get more bride-price'. 'Condoms', he notes, 'should only be used for the victim couples' (Vinit 2004), something that not even Bishop Bonivento allows (2001b). Dr Vinit decries the condom promotion efforts of the NACS as constituting a 'medical scandal' in that 'HIV/AIDS cells [*sic*]' are 500 times smaller than the holes in condoms, which are therefore 'not safe' (*The National* 2006). This was an increase in the estimate of 450 that was provided by Vatican Cardinal Alphonse Lopez Trujillo in 2003 and whose many other claims were repeated by Bishop Bonivento (see below). The funny thing is, how popular were the posters a few years ago that showed Dr Malau poking and prodding condoms filled (but not to bursting) with water. I have many score times in front of small or large groups of Papua New Guineans blown up condoms, filled them with water or stretched them over a wooden dildo or my hand to show how strong they are. Nevertheless, anti-condom sentiments seem often to have been strengthened instead of being weakened by such demonstrations, partly by deft movement to other positions: 'those are for *pamuk meri*, not for me', 'I'm faithful to my wife', 'I don't have a sickness' and 'I don't want a sickness'. Among the Bariai of West New Britain Province, according to Naomi McPherson, and in addition to the existence of already significant amounts of anti-condom rhetoric spawned by religious officials, there is the idea that to use condoms is to invoke further wrath from God: 'using condoms would presumably make God even more punitive, since the church condemns their use as sinful, and especially so in marital sex, where condoms are seen not as disease prevention but as birth control' (McPherson 2008: 244). 'Not only did condoms promote pre and extramarital sex', writes Holly Wardlow about the religious politics of sexual health matters in the Tari Basin,

> but they also prevented 'bad' people from getting the punishment they deserved and, further, prevented other people from witnessing and learning from their punishment. In other words, AIDS was a means used by God to force people to be good Christians, and condoms, because they enabled people to thwart his will and escape due punishment, were instruments devised by Satan so that sinners could cheat the divine scales of justice. (Wardlow 2008: 193)

* * *

It takes no great background in clinical psychology to suggest that cognitive dissonance underwrites such ambivalence, stigmatisation and disinformation as I've mentioned above. Theories of cognitive dissonance were developed by Leon Festinger and associates in their 1956 publication, *When Prophecy Fails*, to account for the psycho-social turmoil that ensues when values, beliefs and emotions conflict with one another and are contradicted by empirical facts. They showed why adherents to an Ohio cult built around the 'automatic writings' of Mrs Marion Keech *increasingly* believed in repeatedly falsified predictions that spaceships would land in her backyard and spirit adherents away from the imminent Armageddon. Parallels can be drawn to repeated refutations of the tenets of anti-condom discourse but that seem only to strengthen it. In the penultimate chapter to this marvelous text, 'Reactions to Disconfirmation', the authors write that the two leaders of this cult, Mrs Keech and Dr Armstrong, 'remained unwaveringly firm in their conviction. Though they searched desperately for messages that might guide them, never during this entire time did either of them utter a serious word of doubt or indicate in any way that they might have been wrong' (1956: 193).

During the work-place briefing I mentioned at the outset, the Papua New Guineans who out of nervousness laughed at mention of sexual pleasure and who out of Christian devotion denounced the efficacy of condoms were expressing their cognitive dissonance. When public health officials misinform about the tensile strength and degrees of porosity of condoms, they are exhibiting their cognitive dissonance. Medical doctors who believe that prayer or wooden crosses dipped in special water or consumption of healing waters from remote villages will cure HIV are expressing cognitive dissonance, too. Religious leaders who blame sexual promiscuity on condoms are also under cognitive dissonance. It's funny, too, how something so fragile and porous, so poorly made and misconceived, so ill conceived and poorly thought of, can yet display all this power, to cause AIDS, to break up families, to induce promiscuity.

Cognitive dissonance in several forms is hampering the best efforts of the NAC, the NHASP, the NDoH and many concerned NGOs, FBOs and CBOs. Though few themselves have been tested, mostly for fear of the test results and/or their dissemination, many nonetheless want those who have tested HIVab+ to be at least identified; some want them to be loved and supported, but others want them segregated and denounced. Health workers know that broken confidentiality damages individual and hospital reputations, but yet they break confidentiality and allow others to do so. Many throughout the country are calling for *mandatory* VCT, that's right, mandatory *voluntary* counselling and testing, just as have other communities in the Pacific, for example, in Suva, Fiji, since at least the early 1990s (O'Leary 1993). Others are calling for mandatory premarital testing for their children and relatives (NHASP 2005g: 7). Unfortunately, marriage is in Papua New Guinea and elsewhere more of a complicated social process than event. As such, it often follows, not precedes sex. One peer educator from the Trobriand islands, speaking extra forthrightly and truthfully because she was being interviewed

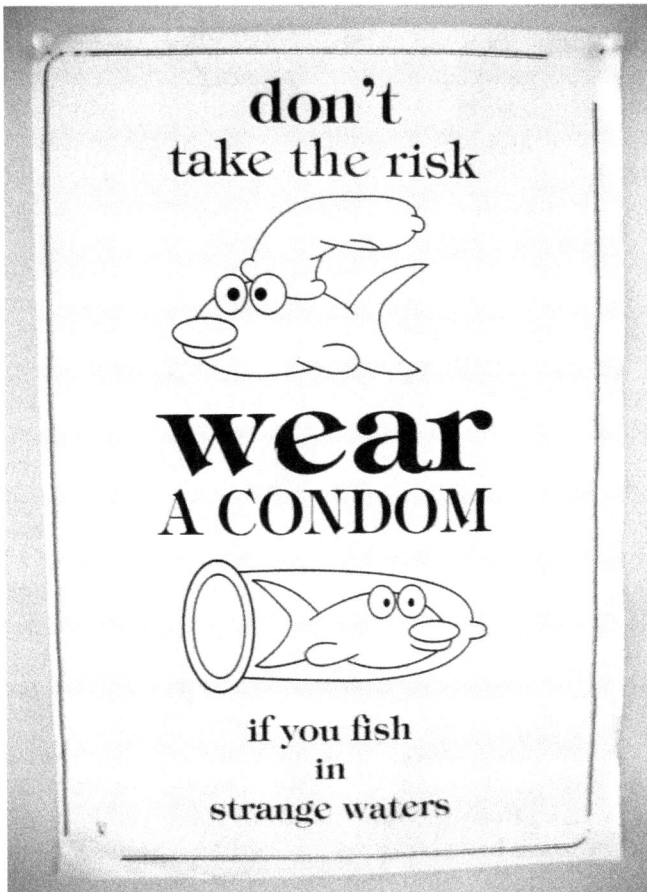

Don't take the risk

in church, said 'not one person has one partner only. Everyone has more than one boyfriend or one girlfriend, until they find the right partner to get married to' (quoted in Lepani 2007b: 252). Men and women about equally know that men 'bring sicknesses home' to 'innocent' wives and children, whether or not this is true, but if they have to blame someone, they will blame the young girls against whose charms the 45-year-old, cash-crazy, gold-panning landowners or mine-workers are apparently helpless. Letters to the editors of the national newspapers are written frequently by citizens who correlate rising levels of HIV infection with increased condom promotion. Community leaders and religious authorities also say that condom promotion is 'carrying sickness' into previously clean and 'good' communities. 'We don't want to use the condom', says Pastor Larry Koavea, who hails from one of Port Moresby's squatter settlements in Port Moresby. He is convinced that '[i]t brings disease into our community' (Fink 2006).

The situation in Papua New Guinea as regards condoms would appear to have sprung from the same sources of misinformation that confused others in the insular Pacific. In Tonga in 1990, for example, Roman Catholic Bishop

Patelisio Finau argued against condoms in a speech he gave to the South
Pacific Commission, suggesting that they were 'the main factor in the spread
of permissiveness in society', that AIDS was yet another example of what he
called 'the lethal rubbish of Western society,' and that condoms enabled its
spread. Wholly inverting logic, he dubbed 'safe sex' the 'road to death' and
suggested that in the bodies of those suffering from AIDS could be found
'proof of the correctness of the church's view on proper sexual conduct' (CDC
1990: 11; see also McPherson 2008; Wardlow 2008).

Cognitive dissonance has underwritten public discourse about condoms
for a long time. Public health posters such as 'Wear a Condom if You Fish
in Strange Waters', just as was suggested in the section above, suggest to
men that village girls and their own wives are 'safe'. More troublingly, such
constructions imply that condoms are both capable of risk-reduction (i.e.,
'don't take the risk' of not using one) and actually constitute risk itself (since
the sex one has with them is 'risky'). This kind of discursive double-helix runs
throughout the many writings of Bishop Bonivento (see below) and shapes
usage patterns. Most women involved in transactional sex nowadays use
condoms with customers fairly often (thus reducing risk), but still generally
not with the boyfriends and husbands whom they infect and/or who infect
them. In village settings condoms are 'bad' for women because using them
demonstrates social agency to the extent they prevent pregnancy and cuts
short the exchange networks in which their families and husbands involve
them. In urban settings they can imply promiscuity. Men distrust condoms
because they prevent 'full travel' of their semen, but yet get caught with
them in their pockets. Women in Guam involved in commercial sexual
networking seem caught in the same kinds of rhetorical contradictions that
result in condom usage being optional more than assumed, negotiated more
than fundamental. The selection process in which they engage 'is most often
based on stereotype labelling within the community: what's their ethnicity,
are they well-to-do, are they residents or tourists, can they pay cash?'
(Workman *et al.* 2001).

Church influence upon policies and public debate is felt throughout the
Pacific. In Samoa the editor of a national English daily newspaper remarked
during interview with the journalist Trevor Cullen that 'Churches have
considerable influence in this country and they do not like their people to
talk of condoms or [use] other explicit language' (Cullen 2000: 222). Cullen
found broadly that newspaper editors in Fiji, Samoa and Papua New Guinea
(all former British colonies) found it extremely difficult to speak frankly
about condoms even during private interview, much less encourage such
discussion in the pages of their newspapers. Prominent women's groups in
Fiji were able to strike references regarding homosexuality and prostitution
from official government documents announcing the implementation of
new, more progressive policies (Gibson 2006).

In Papua New Guinea, an installment of the popular weekly column,
Lifeline, featured a cry for help from 'Less Satisfied' regarding an apparent
decline in the level of sexual satisfaction he and his girlfriend had been
experiencing. Despite the obvious intelligence of the writer, despite that
their sexual relations had been founded upon love, consent and friendship,

and despite his having effected consistently an earnest, self-effacing tone, the column editors responded negatively and quite harshly with assertions that the writer and his girlfriend were only 'experimenting' with sex, that life-threatening diseases could result and that the spectre of unplanned, unwanted pregnancies was just around the corner. None of these are possible in marriage, it appears. 'Like most Christians', *Lifeline* responded, they 'understand sex quite differently'. Sex, they said, 'is a gift from God, designed and intended for married couples ... to use in bringing children into the world' (*Lifeline* 2004: 10). As in many of the AIDS dramas and faith-based presentations of 'HIV/AIDS Awareness' I've seen performed, condoms go unmentioned and sexual desire is erased, leaving 'Less Satisfied', well, even less so – and probably even less protected. Even when condoms are distributed and actually reach a health centre, they are often allowed to languish and expire there by the hundreds and thousands.

Negative Christian influence upon sexual matters can be seen also in terms of references in Tok Pisin to sex, to female body parts and to diseases said to result therefrom: *sin pasin* (sinful behaviour=sex), *ples nogut* (unclean body part), *sem bilong yu* (your shame=vagina), *deti bilong ol mama* (women's uncleanliness=vaginal secretions) and *sik nogut* (STD=a really 'bad' sickness). STDs are in Papua New Guinea, just as they are in New Caledonia (Salomon and Hamelin 2008: 86) gendered as *kan sik* (vaginal afflictions) and *sik bilong ol meri* (women's sicknesses), not as *kok sik* or *sik bilong ol man*. The room reserved for private prayer at a site of VCT is graced with a Tok Pisin Bible that when I visited last was open to the Book of Isaiah, in which is written (Chapter 1, Verse 4, translated): 'You people are really bad and your behaviors are sinful, too. You perpetually commit sin. Your own sin provided your downfall'. This particular site of respite and hospice undoubtedly does much good and is staffed by wonderful people, but this is not what I would want to be told upon my diagnosis.

Condoms and their usage are in Papua New Guinea so heavily gendered that to speak frankly about or use them is openly to challenge the gendered inequities of contemporary discourses. Women, not men, are supposed to bear the burdens of fertility regulation, moral dictates and disease avoidance. Men complain of condoms in terms of decreased sexual pleasure and of their potential harm through semen retention (Hammar 1998a) but may 'legitimately' beat wives who insist on their use, which is to say, get away with doing so. Condoms thus embody the difficult choice many women face between possible biological death caused by the results of having sex without condoms and the near certainty of social death caused by becoming spinsters and remaining sub-optimally fertile. This opens them further to stigma and community-level violence. Anti-condom rhetoric enables an environment in which those most at risk of STDs and HIV – God-loving, sexually faithful girlfriends and housewives – are the least likely to embrace condoms for what they are: their only means of protection. In Ruta Fiti-Sinclair's study conducted with women in prostitution Port Moresby, '[n]o one reported using condoms with their husbands, steady boyfriend, or friends they knew. All said they want to use condoms with men they do not know ... ' (1996: 121).

Given how much cognitive dissonance there is regarding condoms, it is unsurprising that such imbues the ABC campaign. Although it is comprised of markedly foreign ideas (Abstain from sex? What? Use condoms? Huh?) that clash with Papua New Guinean norms and forms of sociality – polygyny, pleasure, male privilege, young brides and demonstrated fertility, among them – it yet remains official policy. Like the failed prophecies of Mrs Keech, however, ABC shows remarkable resiliency to critique on logical and evidentiary grounds. The degree of sexual citizenship that females exhibit makes the A of 'Abstinence' problematic. Abstinence is quite literally anti-cultural. Norms of concurrent, multi-partner sexual networking preclude it. So do male-dominated political and social structures. So do religious double-standards.[2] Helen Epstein discussed these same issues with young men in South Africa: '[w]hen I suggested the idea of abstinence, or sticking to one sexual partner, hysterical laughter broke out all around me' (Epstein 2007: 71).

In any event, men don't abstain and females can't. Doctors who have long experience in Uganda have concluded that '[c]ontrary to what the evangelical Christians and African traditionalists maintain, abstinence-until-marriage seems to have made little contribution to the decline of HIV infection rates in Uganda' (Okuonzi and Epstein 2005: ii). As in Uganda, in Papua New Guinea, a political-economy driven by the needs of foreign capital at sites of resource extraction produces low wages, male employment mobility, sex-imbalanced villages and dependent females. Among the four factors Holly Wardlow cites in her explanation of Huli men's philandering is 'the role of male mobility and migration in creating social contexts in which extramarital sexual relations are the norm' (2007: 1008; see also 2006b). This renders the 'B' of 'Being faithful' similarly a pipe dream, and anyway, being full of faith means not to use condoms. Many researchers have shown that Papua New Guinean men are more likely to seek out and sustain extra-marital relationships when routinely separated from their spouses and families. Wardlow has over the years demonstrated in rich detail and with keen insight that disgruntled sisters and wives often enter transactional forms of sexual networking to protest gender inequities and experience of sexual violence that have gone unpunished and uncompensated. Marriage is valorised and prostitution excoriated, but few will admit how frequently married females engage in it or how many husbands women find in it. To do so would mean the admission of faulty premises, would be to confront and to overcome the cognitive dissonance that denies the degree to which contemporary social process disempowers and endangers many Christian women.

Not surprisingly, the 'C' of ABC has been replaced in alphabetic shenanigans. I attended one conference at which was presented by a Papua New Guinean health official a PowerPoint slide featuring a photograph of a t-shirt that read 'ABCDEFG' (A Boy Can Do Everything For a Girl), but 'GFEDCBA' (Girl Forgot Everything Done & Catches new Boy Again). A 'very critical elderly woman' (a highly placed nun in the national capital, in this case) suggested sarcastically in the face of ABC that when D is added, it ought to say 'DIE' (Tonny 2008). A writer of a letter to the editor of *The National* praised an HIV/AIDS activist who was himself infected via unprotected sex but who promoted the C in ABC to mean Change in Attitude, after having been 'inspired by the Lord' such that he now speaks with 'pride' and 'dignity' (Guss 2008). A pastor who appeared on an AIDS-related poster that promote condoms was removed from his ministry. Health policies about contraception and STD prevention that are mandated at the national or provincial levels are yet subverted at church-run health centres by health workers who are afraid to lose their jobs. Provincial governors campaign for monogamy and province-wide bans on condoms, though they use them in private and extra-maritally. Areas of low condom availability due to intense missionising against them are marked by staggeringly high STD rates, but yet 'high-risk settings' are the ones flooded with condoms. Governor of West Sepik Province, Carlos Yuni, called on 17 October 2004 for a countrywide ban on condom usage. The hallmark finding of Festinger and his associates was that people generally avoid information that causes discomfort.

Does condom misinformation harm or kill people?

Low rates of condom use can be explained apart from cultural taboo-related issues in terms of the ways in which anti-condom rhetoric has positioned their usage. This section looks in some detail at a particular example thereof, the writings of Bishop Cesare Bonivento of the Vanimo Diocese in West Sepik Province. Bishop Bonivento is most popular (and controversial) for two tracts, 'Do Condoms Stop or Spread AIDS'? (2001a) and 'AIDS and Condoms: the teachings of the Church' (2001b). The former was published in Goroka by the Liturgical Catechetical Institute but for the Vanimo Family Life Apostolate, whereas the publisher of the latter is not listed but was printed as a Pastoral Letter. Both are commonly seen throughout the country in people's homes, in used book sections of thrift shops and in Catholic Church-run bookstores. Additionally, they are cited and otherwise used in letters written to the editors of daily and weekly newspapers. Unlike, say, the writings that appear

'The minorities (like the Indians, the Negroes, the Puerto Ricans) record the worst condom failure rate: 36.3%' (Bonivento 2001a: 9).

'NACS/NHASP knows ...that the nightclubs are primary high risk sites in the nation for HIV/AIDS ...How many young people will catch HIV/AIDS after their visit to the nightclubs in the next few days? ...We ask PNG Foreign Affairs to withdraw the visas of [the Nigerian Christian family gospel group] Makoma. Now that they are making appearances in nightclubs, they have joined the enemy' (Bruce Copeland, AIDS Holistics, reported in The National 2004).

'100% of those having risky sex behavior and using condoms for more than four or more years can be predicted to get AIDS' (Bonivento 2001a: 25).

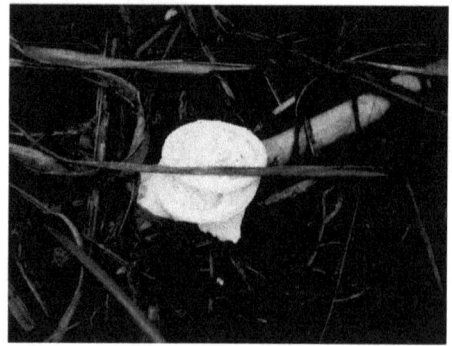

Doubled condom

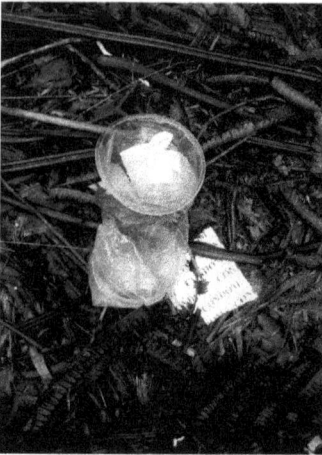

Male and female condom used together

on Bruce Copeland's web-site devoted to AIDS Holistics, which seem to be politely ignored in Port Moresby for their rants against expatriate consultants and raves for the tenets of Positive Living, the writings and speeches of Bishop Bonivento are quite influential in setting policy in and nearby Vanimo. His words do in fact matter. The Foreword to 'Do Condoms Stop or Spread AIDS?' (2001a) implies that it was other members of the Diocesan Health Services who wrote the booklet, and in another publication (2001b: 31) he writes 'the authors of the booklet'. (Does one write one's own Foreword?) This is difficult to accept, however, given the similarity of its tenor and phrasings to his other writings and to the statements of his colleagues to the contrary. Interestingly, the publisher inserted at the end of 'Do Condoms Stop or Spread AIDS?' a quite ambiguous disclaimer: 'The truthfulness of this information is left to those who state it'. Indeed, much was left to the Good Bishop.

It is not easy here in 2010 to assess precisely the ways in which Bishop Bonivento used his sources to argue against condom usage. Each of the 51 listed refers to an Internet web-site but the link to which is now broken. Nevertheless, it is quite relevant to the aims of this book to pay close attention to his argument, for he is a deeply thoughtful man who cares profoundly about Papua New Guineans. He claims to have wanted to avoid bias, moreover, by choosing to rely 'on information mainly released by Agencies promoting condoms' (2001a: 7), which is to say condom manufacturers and providers. In several ways it is simply not true to assert as he did, however, that 'negative' findings about contraceptive and STD preventive efficacy came mainly from condom manufacturers and organisations who promote them. When I was in Vanimo in November and December of 2005, repeated promises were made by a Diocesan Health Services official to provide me with photocopies of the articles in question (of which I saw two large stacks) but which went unfulfilled.

Closer examination of the provenance of the document's argument, however, revealed that four of the 51 sources listed are linked to the Westside Pregnancy Resource Center in Santa Monica, California. Speaking with

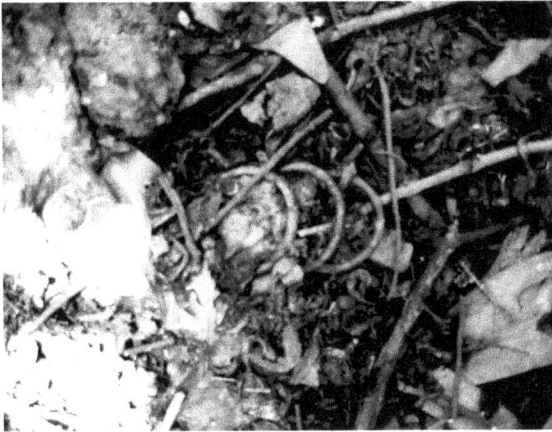

Tripled condom

the Director and pregnancy counsellor there (on 17 July 2007), I learned that they do no condom promotion or distribution whatsoever, although their web-site says that 'It has been shown that they reduce the risk of HIV transmission by 85%'.[3] The web-site also promotes the falsehood that there is no evidence that condoms 'reduce the risk of HPV' (Human Papilloma Virus). Using the same web-site (abcnews.com) that the Bishop used in supporting his stance against condoms *and on those grounds*, I found much evidence to the contrary, including a Columbia University Medical Center-sponsored study showing that females whose boyfriends used condoms while having sex with them even just 50% of the time yet reduced the risk of HPV transmission by 50% (Adlersberg 2006). Bishop Bonivento's claims are several other times buttressed by reference to an article, 'Condom "Safe Sex" Theory Full of Holes', adapted from a story published in *The Covington News* (15 March 1995). This newspaper is published in Covington, Georgia, that is, not by a condom manufacturer or its representative, as he several times implied. The story was written by a now deceased crusading evangelical, Diane Dew, an ex-Roman Catholic who left the church because she desired to speak directly to God instead of through church officials. Her web-site is still active, if not current, and it still rails against milk, secular humanism, coffee and Al Gore. It disinforms by repeating claims that HIV can 'readily pass through the condom' (see below), and which never emanate from condom manufacturers themselves.[4] These photos show some of the behavioral outcomes of the kinds of cognitive dissonance induced by condom disinformation: the first photo shows that a male and female condom were used simultaneously, the second shows the doubled use of male condoms, and the third, the tripled.

Other references in Bishop Bonivento's bibliography point to representatives of US-based conservative organisations such as Focus on the Family, Campaign for Our Children and Concerned Women of America. In no way, shape or form do those organisations stump for sex–or condom-positivity. Another three references are to Human Life International, a US-based Roman Catholic organisation founded in 1981 and which is also stridently against condom usage. Another three times the Bishop directed readers to Epigee.org, which is also opposed to condoms. Epigee.org explicitly warns clients not to rely upon either family planning clinics or pharmaceutical companies to educate staff members about contraception[5] but yet by rights had to conclude that '[i]f you are sexually active, though, it is necessary to use a condom every time you have sex to help prevent STDs'. Another page claims falsely that HIV 'does eventually develop into AIDS leading to death'.[6]

It would have been more appropriate for Bishop Bonivento to have said that he obtained 'negative' information about condoms from those already opposed to them. Indeed, close scrutiny shows that the original sources do not say what he says they say or that secondary conclusions drawn about them were not those drawn by the researchers themselves. One example is regarding the efficacy of chastity pledges extolled by Concerned Women of America (see below). The information he takes to be negative regarding condom efficacy is often upon closer scrutiny quite positive. A government health department concluded that '[u]sing condoms reduces the risk of becoming infected with most STDs, especially if they are used correctly and consistently',[7] but Bonivento cited (2001a: 21) an earlier version of the same reference in concluding that 'straightaway' one 'realizes the difficulty' of following instructions, for example, not to use damaged condoms or to store them in direct sunlight (Bonivento 2001a: 13). How many of you store condoms in direct sunlight? How many of you use damaged condoms? Several times Bishop Bonivento invokes the Sexuality Information and Education Council of the United States (SIECUS). Although the link to the web-page to which he referred readers was broken, a more recent one had this to say:

> In recent years, as a result of misinformation and insufficient research, the efficacy of condoms, especially in terms of STD prevention, has been debated in many forums. Research continues to show that condoms are one of the best methods of preventing unwanted pregnancy and are one of the only methods for sexually active individuals to protect themselves against STDs, including HIV.[8]

It is simply not possible to align the two positions, Bonivento's and that of SIECUS. Bonivento also cites information once posted on the web-sites of student health services centres and news organisations but that didn't and don't support what he says or implies they support. For example, he cites an article from an on-line encyclopaedia the link to which is now broken but whose more recent collection of related articles included one about condoms and specifically the ABC message in Uganda. It reprinted conclusions drawn from a 2005 article in *Science News* (Harder 2005) that concluded that neither abstinence nor monogamy deserve much credit for the decline in HIV prevalence: 'Of the three directives of the prevention mantra [ABC] only greater condom use appears to have coincided with a decline in the number of people living with HIV in western Uganda's Rakai district'.[9] Underhill *et al.* (2007) identified 13 US trials of sexual abstinence-only programmes to prevent HIV infection, involving nearly 16,000 youth. Their conclusion was that none of the programmes they studied in 'high-income countries' affected the frequency or incidence of coitarche, the number of sexual partners, the use of condoms, or even the incidence of unprotected vaginal sex. The Conclusions section of another article says that

> The methodological strength of the studies on condoms to reduce the risk of HIV/AIDS transmission far exceeds that for other STDs ... [and] consistent condom use decreased the risk of HIV/AIDS transmission by approximately 85%. These data provide strong evidence for the effectiveness of condoms for reducing sexually transmitted HIV.[10]

The reference that he makes to a web-site maintained at the Northern Arizona University Health Center is similarly now to a broken link, but the newer web-site of the Fronske Center for Student Health instructs students to 'Learn to use condoms correctly and they are a very reliable form of birth control and STI prevention ... [as] using condoms every time you have sex significantly reduces your risk of contracting an STI... . Latex condoms are recommended for best STI protection'.[11] I contacted the Director of the Duke University Student Health Services Center, Ms Lindsey Bickers-Bock, on 17 July 2007. When I read to her what the Bishop had construed her Center as having said about condoms she said that his was not an accurate assessment and neither would it have accurately reflected staff positions in 2000. Her staff and clients then and now are fully pro-condom and for obvious reasons.[12] The same is true of articles and information published on other web-sites that are news- or health-related (e.g. www.healthcentral.com, www.abc.news.com) or that refer back even to the adult porn industry (e.g. www.aim-med.org)! An article by Maria Cheng now appearing on the www. abc.com web-site warned public health practitioners and policy advocates not to 'put all your eggs in the abstinence basket', according to a professor of epidemiology at the London School of Hygiene and Tropical Medicine whose work she cited. Bonivento's reference to the University of Massachusetts-Lowell's student health services centre (2001a: 37) stated something that the centre, if it ever said, now doesn't say (that abstinence is 'the only perfect means for avoiding AIDS'). As well, despite his imputation to the centre of a negative stance toward condoms, its web-site currently offers blow-by-blow replies and retorts that students might make if their sexual partners opposed condom usage.[13] The State of Maryland public health department's web-site similarly urges condom usage by those who do not know the disease status of their partners.[14] References that Bonivento makes to healthcentral.com are now broken by non-working links, but yet it now concludes that '[i]t should be noted that only latex and polyurethane condoms, but not those made of natural animal membranes, effectively prevent the spread of viral infections such as HIV'.[15] Another story linked to the web-site reported upon a research study published in the *Journal of Adolescent Health* that followed 1,300 sexually active youth (aged 15–21) in Providence, Rhode Island, Miami, Florida, and Atlanta, Georgia, 65% of whom claimed not to have had sex with a 'non-regular' partner in the previous 90 days, whereas 35% said that they'd had sex with at least one 'casual' partner in the same period. Members in both arms of the study reported high prevalence of unprotected vaginal intercourse (21% and 19%) and many STDs. Interestingly, females were more likely to report 'main' partners and males, 'casual' ones, confirming something of the sexual behavioural paradox as has been covered in previous chapters.[16]

Similar findings have been reported in large-scale studies of serodiscordant couples in African countries and heavily gendered factors and issues that explained seroconversion. Women who seroconverted during one study were found to have been 'more likely to continue unprotected vaginal intercourse with primary partners if they were married, involved in newer relationships ... perceived greater difficulty in negotiating condom use, or reported more conflicts in their relationship'. Many men who seroconverted, by contrast, were found also to have consumed excessive alcohol prior to sex and expressed fewer concerns about the consequences of HIV infection (Coates *et al.* 2000: 4). Similar findings were gathered in rural Uganda over a 7-year period, with researchers finding that men were almost twice as likely as women to bring HIV into a new marriage and transmit the virus to their spouse – and twice as quickly (Carpenter *et al.* 1999). This is yet another of the many reasons why the gender-neutrality of Bonivento's stress upon 'chastity and faithfulness' needs to be challenged; it is unreasonable of expectation and flies in the face of what we know about human sexuality in Papua New Guinea (and elsewhere).

Bonivento has thus stretched credulity in asserting faithfulness to both the intent and the specific findings of these and other sources. It would take far more space than granted here fully to dissect his claims regarding condoms and their usage, and so I have for brevity's sake assembled representative examples of his facts that aren't and of rhetorical straw men. Three tables below list his claims and respond to them briefly, and a fourth table presents data regarding condom efficacy in serodiscordant couples that contradict many of his claims.

A less brief response may be registered here, however, to a categorical claim he makes 11 times in one way or another, such as that, '[a]nother surprise is that Chastity and faithfulness are acknowledged by everybody, including the USA, as the best means of avoiding AIDS and are used by a lot of youth' (2001a: 32). Bishop Bonivento frequently takes a longer-term view when it suits him, for example, in terms of condom or other contraceptive efficacy when examined over many years. It is thus important to examine chastity and fidelity as being often lengthy processes (not discrete things) that, from the perspective of deploying them rhetorically to promote this or that agenda, are fraught with methodological and other complexities. Nor are they the categorical events he seems to imply. It is true, for example, that chastity pledges have been undertaken *en masse* in the US, Pakistan, South Africa, Uganda and other sexually repressive countries and cultures. In addition to being founded upon misogynous ideals that are as often as not accompanied by quite sickening displays of fatherly (not motherly) prerogative and sponsorship,[17] they have also fuelled much misogynous backlash. That includes shunning of those who have been raped, the surgical closing of already broken hymens, the expression of a double-standard in demanding female but not male virginity at marriage, the cover-up of child molestation by male relatives and family friends, and even reinfibulation where such is practised. Some studies show *increased* sexual risk-taking when the abstinent break their vow (or have it broken for them). Those who take such pledges use condoms and other contraceptives less frequently, too, and they rely instead upon faith (in both God and their partner's lack of infection) to protect them. These have been documented in any number of forums and media, including the documentary *Abstaining from Reality: U.S. Restrictions on HIV Prevention*, a short film that puts a human face on the consequences of an abstinence-only approach to HIV prevention (Population Action International 2006).[18] The United States spent many tens of millions of dollars in 2004 alone to train 46,000 Ugandans to preach abstinence-only messages and recruit those who would sign virginity pledges. Randall Tobias, the man responsible in the US for directing the USAID's opposition to prostitution, which has had a chilling effect on support of progressive programmes world-wide, was forced to step down when it was learned that he hadn't honoured his own pledge. This is what he said on 18 March 2005 (Frontline 2005)

> It's abstinence really focused heavily on young people and getting them to understand that the best way to keep from getting infected is to be abstinent and not engage in sexual activity until they are old enough and mature enough and get into a committed relationship, such as a marriage. B is being faithful within that committed relationship.

In April of 2007, however, after his name and telephone number were found in the private files of a Washington, DC, madam, and after having once been the US Ambassador representing the President's Emergency Plan for AIDS Relief, or PEPFAR initiative, he admitted to having had received multiple massages. He said at that time that there had been 'no sex' ... As is already well known, the greatest bulk of PEPFAR monies have gone to Christian and Pentecostal churches and groups, most of whom hail from the US, and who preach an abstinence-only message. Many of those groups and churches are, of course, active in Papua New Guinea and elsewhere throughout Melanesia, and critics (e.g. Epstein 2005, 2007; Lindenbaum 2008) have charged them with gross wastage of monies on bankrupt ideas that do not engage so much as oppose indigenous ideas of sexual intercourse, commerce and fertility. Katherine Lepani, for example, makes much of the Trobriand islander propensity to reward consensual, pleasurable sex in terms of a wide array of social and genealogical linkages. Deploying a well known Trobriand island idiom for sex, she notes that 'questions of sexuality should not be concerned simply with the individual "itch" of individual sexual acts but with the meanings produced on the collective scale by intimate desires and pleasures' (Lepani 2008a: 252–3).

Regarding the US examples that Bishop Bonivento so glowingly cites, pledge-taking females have been shown, yes, to have delayed coitarche by some number of months, but also to have gotten married younger when they did get married and thus to commence unsafe sex earlier. In addition, looked at in the longer term, they also tend to have engaged in more receptive penile-oral and penile-anal intercourse to preserve vaginal virginity; only 2%

of those who didn't take the abstinence pledges had done so, but 13% of those who did, had (Bearman and Brückner 2001; Brückner and Bearman 2005). In this, they mimic their sisters in other religious communities and countries, for example, Recife, Brazil, where Catholic girls and women are subjected to extremely unfair double-standards of sexual comportment. The doctor-ethnographer Jessica Gregg found while studying cervical cancer suffering and rates there (which are the highest in the world) that Catholic girls end up engaging in oral and anal intercourse so as to preserve vaginal virginity, thus moving '[t]he boundary dividing "honest" and "shameless" behaviour' (Gregg 2003: 86). Tantalizing evidence on this point comes from Christian Nigeria, too, according to Daniel Smith. He notes that anal intercourse is for the Christian Igbo with whom he worked such an abomination 'that it was difficult to get people to discuss it candidly'. Nevertheless, he found that it might be increasing in incidence, especially among teenagers, 'and that HIV/ AIDS prevention messages in Nigeria may be partly responsible' insofar as they have obsessed over vaginal intercourse and preservation of virginity (Smith 2004: 435, n. 3). Elsewhere in Brazil, Paiva reports findings from her study of sexual health and knowledge among poor, less well educated, settlement-dwelling youth and their counterparts in local universities. She and her colleagues 'learned that anal sex as a means to avoid pregnancy was confused among [the poor] night-school students with a supposed efficacy of anal sex in avoiding HIV infection' (2007[2004]: 435). The four-state wide study commissioned by the US Congress of the efficacy of abstinence-only sex education was hoped by the Bush administrations in Texas and in the White House to support its having spent over $1,000,000,000 since 1998 to promote abstinence (in the form of educational programmes, posters, pamphlets and television and radio spots) in hundreds of thousands of girls and boys. Significant study findings include, however, that those exposed also to abstinence-only sex education showed no different predilection for sex as those exposed to information about contraception. Mathematica Policy Research sampled 2,057 teenagers from Florida, Wisconsin, Mississippi and Virginia and found that nearly one-quarter in both arms of the study 'had had sex in the previous year and always used a condom, 17% had sex only sometimes using a condom; and 4% had sex never using one. About a quarter of each group had had sex with three or more partners' (Pilkington 2007). 'Abstinence hasn't been given a very good chance', President Bush was quoted (by Pilkington) as saying, 'but it's worked when it's tried. That's

'A study was made not long ago of the male college students without experience in sexual intercourse. When asked if anyone had ever discussed their sexual behavior with them or indicated approval of their virginity, these young men said they had received no compliments, no approval, nor support from the adults around them ...' (Ashley-Montagu 1968: 126).

for certain.' Unfortunately, his own state of Texas, where he had as governor spent $10,000,000 per year in the 1990s, 'had the country's fifth-highest teen pregnancy rate' and since 2001 has been pumping ten times that amount annually into such programmes, even suggesting recently that the programme be extended to those aged 20–29, 'an age range in which 90% of people are sexually active' (Pilkington 2007). In any event, 14.9 was the average age of coitarche for members of both arms of the study. Members of the abstinence-only group reached it, however, armed with little information or supplies requisite to protecting themselves against unwanted pregnancies and STDs and HIV (see full report in Trenholm *et al.* 2007) and so suffered those more. The study of Miller and Gur (2002) of 3,336 adolescent girls in the US concluded that 'no dimension of religiousness in adolescents was associated with a decreased likelihood of sexual activity or sexual abstinence' (2008: 404). Worse, they found that '[u]niquely personal conservatism (a close or rigid adherence to religious creed) was shown to pose risk against sexual responsibility. Adolescent girls who scored high in personal conservatism were more likely to be exposed to unprotected sex, including forced sex, and more likely to allow males to control birth control use' (2008: 404).

These kinds of findings have been replicated in one evaluation after another of risk *avoidance* (abstinence-only) versus *harm reduction* (teaching abstinence but also methods of condom use) teen sexuality programmes. One early programme (1990) claiming to have delayed first intercourse for a cohort of 8th-grade minority US students by about 40% couldn't be replicated later (1997). An abstinence-only prevention programme reported in 1998 that although pre-test virgins delayed sexual initiation three months post-test, the delays did not stand up at six and 12 months. Another programme conducted in 1992, while reducing the rate in 'high-risk' high-school students of sexual initiation, had no effect on the 'low-risk' students. The 5 years-long mass media programme called *Not Me, Not Now*, seemed to have had an effect in reducing sexual intercourse in those under age 16, but not for older teens. Evaluation of the abstinence-only programme, *For Keeps*, found that reductions in frequency of sexual intercourse of already sexually active teens had 'no impact on sexual initiation' *per se* (Weed *et al.* 2008: 61; this resource and Trenholme *et al.* 2007 review the studies mentioned above).

In view of these findings about the limitations of abstinence-only programmes in the US, it is now time to examine use made of them by those promoting anti-condom rhetoric in Papua New Guinea, whether implicitly or explicitly. Table 5.1 depicts and comments upon just a few of the false claims made by Bishop Bonivento.

Table 5.1 Claims about condoms

Source	Claim
2001a: 34–5	'Advising people to use condoms means to put them at risk of getting AIDS and just spreads AIDS'

That is, of course, physically impossible. Telling people not to use condoms, however, increases the chance that people will forego their use when they most need them, that is, with an infected 'casual' or marital partner.

2001a: 31	'100% of those following abstinence before marriage will never get infected, except by accident ...'

Tell that to the many, many tens of thousands of girls and women in Papua New Guinea and worldwide who have had one and one partner only, lifetime – their husbands – but who infected them. Premarital abstinence *per se* confers no protective benefits when looked at over the longer-term. Heterosexual male domination of sexual cultures, whether in Italy, the US or Papua New Guinea, do not enable children to reach sexual maturity intact and healthy, anyway (Hammar 1999b, 2006a). Throughout Papua New Guinea, 'the husband is seen as the head of the family and the wife is expected to obey him in all things, including having sex with him even if she knows he may have an STI or HIV' (NAC 2006: 15). The Bishop's privileged position as a secluded, relatively wealthy white male protects him from the more earnest and honest exploration of real sexual risk in real people's lives.

2001a: back-flap	'Condoms may be one of the reasons why the incidence of HIV virus [*sic*] is rising not falling.'

The incidence of HIV is rising because the number of people newly becoming infected is rising. Unprotected sex by whatever route increases risk of transmission of HIV, especially in the presence of STDs. The vast majority of those were transmitted also during unprotected sex. Hundreds of studies have shown that condoms reduce risk. Nevertheless, many Catholic priests and bishops draw this false correlation. Those in Kenya, for example, where adult HIVab seroprevalence has reached 29% have argued that 'AIDS has grown so fast because of the availability of condoms' (quoted in Bradshaw 2003) and further, alleged that condoms are 'laced' with HIV.

2001a: 33	'If we consider all the factors in the use of condoms as prevention from AIDS, we can state that the risk of getting infected in the first year is as high as 100% among those involved in risky sex behavior.'

This is a specious use of statistics – risk cannot be said to be 'as high as' X% – but risk of HIV transmission drops each time someone correctly uses a condom. More needs to be done to enable more consistent condom usage, yes. Moreover, the Bishop's definition of 'risky sex' excludes marriage, which is terribly misleading.

Source	Claim
2001b: 32	'The HIV virus [sic] in an infected individual is present 100% of the time.'

Minimally, it depends on how one defines 'present', but viral load is differently constituted and exists in fluctuating degrees in various body parts and fluids, from the point of infection to death from AIDS. Long periods of relatively little viral replication are typical, including in context of use of antiretrovirals and other medicines. Viral replication is typically higher just following point of infection and near death. Bishop Bonivento's advice is particularly dangerous in view of these facts, especially for serodiscordant couples.

Source	Claim
2003: n.p.	'Papua [New Guinea] has no orphans.'

This is howlingly counter-factual. Children are orphaned every day in Papua New Guinea, and can be subjected to increased rates of violence, abuse and mistreatment (UNICEF-UNESCAP-ECPAT 2006). The 2007 Consensus Workshop estimated over 3,700 had been orphaned due to AIDS alone (NHASP 2007). Yes, many infants and children are adopted into loving families, but what happens to orphans, whether in the US, Uganda or Papua New Guinea, offers a particularly clear window in to the culture and the parameters of vulnerability.

Source	Claim
2005a: n.p.	Ineffective condoms 'are causing AIDS.'

Neither effective nor ineffective condoms are physically capable of causing AIDS. Unprotected sexual intercourse with an infected person or persons is what transmits HIV, which is similarly not caused by condoms.

Source	Claim
2005a: n.p.	'Condoms are a big risk of getting infected by HIV/AIDS.'

I'll be charitable and assume that this was a typo.

Bishop Bonivento has clearly made many confusing, contradictory and false claims about condoms, and I have merely brushed the surface. 'Condoms are not only ineffective', he has argued; 'they are also the cause of promiscuity', adding that condoms 'increase the mentality of promiscuity; consequently, it accelerates the spread of AIDS' (2005a: n.p.). This is perhaps the most jarring of the many claims of the *reductio ad absurdum* variety that dot his writings. It is, of course, physically impossible for condoms to do this, for they lack arms, legs, mouths, sentience or conscience, and neither does promiscuity possess a mentality. Sexual promiscuity is in the eye of beholder and isn't inherently wrong or unhealthy, but in any event social scientists highlight other issues and factors beyond condoms to explain it. Those include poverty, parental pressure to engage in prostitution, husbandly prerogative, media exposure and early traumatic experience of sexual intercourse (Bradley 2000; Hammar 1996a, b, 2006a; UNICEF-UNESCAP-ECPAT 2006; Wardlow 2006a; Zimmer-Tamakoshi 2004). Younger males abused by Catholic priests also have been shown over the years to exhibit elevated levels of suicidal behaviour and involvement in prostitution. Social scientists, public health officials, concerned physicians and activists see the 'spread' of AIDS, were they to use such a term, as related to structural adjustment programmes that gut health services, to the behavioural outcome of condom disinformation campaigns, to government inaction and to staggeringly high caseloads of untreated STDs (ADB 2006; Bowtell 2007; CIE 2002; Dundon 2007; Fordham 2005; Hammar 2007a; Keck 2007; Lepani 2007a, b, 2008b; Setel 1999; Tobias 2006; Wardlow 2002a, b, 2007; Wilde 2007).

Despite the publication over the years of massive amounts of evidence to the contrary of his claims, Bishop Bonivento also refuses to update his contentions. For example, he has claimed that 'experts agree that condoms are useless in the prevention of some diseases. One such disease is human papillomavirus' (2001a: 32). Actually, it's not a disease, but a kind of virus that comes in 87 different species, several of which are linked, yes, to cervical and uterine cancers. The American Social Health Association allows that condoms are 'less protective against STDs that spread through skin-to-skin contact, such as HPV and herpes ... [but] that is not to say condoms are useless. In fact, studies have shown condom use can lower the risk of acquiring HPV infection and reduce the risk of HPV-related diseases, as well as help prevent other STDs and unintended pregnancy.'[19] Another study of HPV transmission dynamics concluded that 'condom use blocks sexual HPV transmission by preventing reinfection and development of new penile lesions in men who are susceptible to the same type as present in the female partner' (Bleeker *et al.* 2005: 1388). Many more examples can be cited that challenge the Bishop's claims that condoms offer no protection whatsoever.

Bishop Bonivento's anti-condom positions can be addressed also in terms of opinions he has that masquerade as fact. Table 5.2 contains a few of many other examples.

Table 5.2 Confusion of opinion for fact

Source	Claim
2001a: back-flap	'a false sense of security can lead to an increase in sexual activity or risky sexual behavior.'

Prayer and denial of sexual risks in one's marriage, which are the hallmarks of many church positions in Papua New Guinea, also lead to a false sense of security, and there is no evidence that either prevents HIV or STD transmission. 'A woman who has remained abstinent until marriage and is faithful to her husband, for example, but whose husband is either HIV-infected or is sexually active outside the marriage, is in fact at high personal risk of HIV infection herself, notwithstanding her own monogamy' (Cohen 2007: 12).

Source	Claim
2001a: back-flap	'From the condom promoting agencies it appears that the only 100% effective means to avoid HIV virus [*sic*] is chastity before marriage, and faithfulness to the spouse once married.'

'Chastity' is not a word they ever use, although condom manufacturers do emphasise the benefits of abstinence and fidelity. Unlike Bishop Bonivento, who has not yet grasped the extent of untreated STDs in Papua New Guinea, they realise that lifelong chastity is freakishly rare and that condomless sex risks infection.

Source	Claim
2001b: 5	'We can summarize [different stands on HIV prevention] as follows: everybody is convinced that the best way to fight the spread of the HIV virus [sic] is chastity before marriage, and fidelity within marriage ...'

I disagree. I'm not convinced, and I'm not alone. Moreover, Bonivento's equation is gender-neutral when it needs to be gender-saturated, since chastity and fidelity are the burdens that females are specially expected to carry. The ABC message has been challenged and refuted in many African countries by too many researchers to cite (e.g. Brown 2006; Parikh 2007; Schoepf 2003) and in Papua New Guinea (e.g. Hammar 1998a, 2004a, 2006b, 2007b; Dundon and Wilde 2007; Keck 2007; Wardlow 2008). 'The ABC(D) prevention messages used in PNG and internationally therefore do not work for most women, especially married women' (NAC 2007: 5).

Source	Claim
2001b: 22	Masturbation remains 'objectively a grave sin'.

Virtually all atheists and agnostics and non-Catholics would disagree, and so too would many Catholics disagree. In any event, solo and mutual masturbation are linked to improved sexual health and heightened sexual communication with partners, and they carry no risk of infection or unwanted pregnancy. According to the World Association for Sexual Health (WAS 2007: n.p.), 'Sexual pleasure, including autoeroticism, is a source of physical, psychological, intellectual and spiritual well being.'

Source	Claim
2001b: 5, 6	Contraception generally degrades the 'dignity of marriage' and as such, 'is intrinsically wrong'; condoms specifically are 'harmful' to the body.

He is, of course, entitled to his opinion, but it is interesting to contemplate the rhetorical use of 'intrinsically' (11 times in this document) in context of discussions of quite culturally grounded ideas of human sexuality, for example, 'the Church teaches', 'evil by the moral law', and so on. As well, the billions of people who have preferred to use condoms and other forms of contraception and STD preventive measures instead of those that offer less or no protection whatsoever (e.g. withdrawal, rhythm method) will disagree. Use of either male or female condoms, moreover, minimises the harm done to women's bodies either by other invasive devices or by the tens of millions of unintended and unwanted pregnancies that have occurred.

Source	Claim
2003: n.p.	The teachings of John Paul II protect us by instructing us 'on the authentic way to fight AIDS, which necessarily includes keeping God's commandments'.

For believers (and non-believers, too), keeping sacred the Ten Commandments are good things in and of themselves, but they do not prevent HIV transmission. Bishop Bonivento again misleads the faithful.

Source	Claim
2005a: n.p.	'Condoms are immoral because they are against the sanctity of marriage.'

My marriage is sacred to me, but until my wife could no longer become pregnant, we used condoms during sex because they're far more effective than withdrawal or rhythm methods and because they don't harm her body. We choose to use condoms; condoms didn't choose to use us or anyone else.

Another category of disinformation relates to Bishop Bonivento's frequent confusion of his own opinion with empirical ways of establishing fact and proving falsehood. Homosexual intercourse he dubs 'frequently very violent' (2001b: 25), but heterosexual intercourse gets off scot-free. He has said that 'married couples using condoms have a great probability to infect each other in a short while' (2005a: n.p.), when he probably meant to say 'married couples *not* using condoms', right? Although here he does not indicate what he means by 'great probability', he has indicated elsewhere (2001a: 15, 2001b: 32, 2005a) that serodiscordant couples should *not* use condoms, that they are better off playing Russian Roulette, as he quotes the Westside Pregnancy Resource Center as saying in 2000 (2001b: 32). In this Bishop Bonivento is repeating claims made by anti-condom organisations such as Human Life International to whose web-site are linked articles implying dispassionate searching for the truth of condom efficacy but yet who show themselves not to be able to see the forest for the trees. Jacque Suaudeau (2007: 875), for example, argues that '[t]here is no true *"safe sex"* except in conjugal fidelity which renders the condom useless'. Jacque seems to have forgotten that, owing to the facts in Papua New Guinea of polygyny and something like 1,000,000 untreated STDs annually, neither premarital abstinence nor even marital fidelity can be said to be preventive, much less *safe*. Has the Bishop looked at rates of domestic violence lately? No matter: 'if the uninfected spouse wants to remain so in the future, he/she has only one choice: abstinence' (Bonivento 2001b: 25).

These opinions have been disconfirmed in many studies that have been conducted over the years of 'stable' (heterosexually coupled, whether married or not) but serodiscordant couples in which one partner is HIVab- but during the course of the study becomes infected. In European, Caribbean and African countries serodiscordant couples consistently using condoms have been shown to reduce HIV transmission by up to 90%, and in one meta-review of 12 studies, 'consistent condom use was 87% protective against HIV transmission compared with lack of condom use' (Shapiro and Kapiga 2002: 498). Another study conducted between 1987 and 1991 tracked 123 serodiscordant couples but who used condoms each and every time they had sex and who reported zero seroconversion, whereas 12 of another 122 couples who didn't consistently use condoms reported seroconversion. Several more are presented here in Table 5.3.

Table 5.3 Studies of HIV Transmission in HIV Serodiscordant Couples

	Study Details		% of participants infected by partner, by frequency of condom usage		
Author	Year	# Study Particip.	Never	Occasional	Consistent
Saracco et al.	1993	305	10.1	14.5	1.7
De Vicenzi et al.	1994	256		9.9	0.0
Deschamps et al.	1996	177	14.4	13.3	2.4
Hira et al.	1997	220		10.7	2.3

In that Bishop Bonivento has looked at the results of these studies and has concluded that using condoms is like playing Russian Roulette, he seems to think that only 100% risk reduction is acceptable. This is unreasonable in and of itself, but it is absurd in context of the failure rate of abstinence. Condoms should not be used, he argues, even in case of serodiscordant couples because condom usage is 'not fully safe' (2001b: 24). Having travelled to and worked amongst the good people of his parish, I can say with authority that he has successfully promoted the misconception that condoms are filled with holes to the extent they are ineffective, since that's what our informants told us he told them. He says, for example, that '**The HIV virus [*sic*] can go much more easily through the hole of a condom, since it is 500 times smaller than the sperm.** Condoms are not able to eliminate holes. Also the most perfect condoms have holes, big enough to let the HIV virus [*sic*] pass through' (2001a: 15, boldface in the original). The Bishop should have known, however, that US federal Food and Drug Administration teams have

'Another case of CSEC in Vanimo, involved a young girl sexually abused by two Indian Catholic priests while she was employed as their domestic helper. The case was revealed when she became pregnant. The priests allegedly offered the girl several hundred kina, gave her pills to try to abort and begged her to not reveal the facts of long-term sexual exploitation perpetrated by both upon her. The victim's family demanded K350,000 and a truck as compensation from the leaders of the Catholic church in Vanimo, for what the girl's father described as "damaging the girl's body and teaching her shameful sexual practices that she never knew before." The Vanimo District Court Magistrate showed the study team a photocopy of a cheque for K20,000 that was recently passed from the Catholic church to the family, thereby ensuring that the case remained out of the court. The two priest perpetrators have reportedly left PNG' (Help Resources 2005: 32).

several times conducted laboratory experiments designed to test condom porosity and permeability. Although correctly noting that condom usage does not reduce HIV transmission risk by 100%, they found that even if the condoms did exhibit some leakage, the amount of fluid crossing the latex membrane corresponded to 0.01% of a typical male ejaculation, an amount so small, they noted, that would in an HIV-infected person be expected still to be free of virus. The authors (Carey 1994; Carey *et al.* 1992) concluded that, even despite occasional leakage of an infinitesimally small amount, condoms would yet decrease HIV exposure by 10,000-fold. The National Institutes of Allergies and Infectious Diseases published a meta-analysis in 2000, when Bonivento was reviewing some of this same literature, and concluded from their exhaustive review of laboratory studies that latex male condoms were 'essentially impermeable to particles the size of STD pathogens, including HIV. Thus, they provide a highly effective barrier method when used correctly' (quoted in AMFAR 2005: 1). At many points Bonivento cites approvingly others who have cited the conclusions of Dr Susan Weller, a University of Texas researcher whose 1993 study has since been discredited by federal health officials. Her conclusion, that condoms reduced HIV transmission by only 69%, was rejected in 1997 by the Department of Health and Human Services because her analysis was flawed, because she had mixed data on 'consistent' use with those on 'inconsistent' use and had committed other methodological and procedural errors. Risk reduction has consistently been shown to be markedly higher.

Bishop Bonivento's writings about condoms also are rife with bogeymen and straw men arguments. For example, he claims the existence of 'political and economic support for false human rights like sex at any age, same sex marriage, pornography, sexslave rackets, paedophilia etc.' (2001a: 5). I am not aware of anyone who has promoted sex-slavery or sex-at-any-age as a human right, although I do of course support same-sex marriage. Lumping same-sex marriage in with paedophilia, however, as he does here and elsewhere, is also counter-productive insofar as the vast majority of the latter is committed by heterosexual, not homosexual males, including in the Bishop's own diocese. Indeed, one of the recommendations made by the authors of the large-scale study conducted by Help Resources and published in 2005 was that there needed to be Code of Conduct, a means by which training would occur and standards upheld specifically having to do with church workers and the issue of child sexual abuse and the commercial sexual exploitation of children. The same has been recommended in Uganda, where police reports indicated that the three groups of men most often reported to be having sex with minors were Christian pastors, teachers and policemen. Christian pastors were urged by a local NGO to use condoms 'because they were endangering their congregations' (Epstein 2007: 190). Recommendation 13 addressed both study findings and frequently occurring newspaper reports and legal cases 'indicating frequent cases of clergy and church leaders committing sexual abuse and sexual exploitation of children, in which the perpetrators' role in the church is referred to in appeals for and the handing down of lesser penalties or as a justification to pay to keep the case out of court to avoid a scandal for the church concerned' (Help Resources 2005: 119). Special care should be taken, they urged, to train Christian church leaders to deal with sexual assault and exploitation of children in all its forms according to 'existing laws, with no compromises or excuses and reduction of charges or penalties being made on basis of a perpetrator being referred to as a "good Christian" or a "good family man"' (Help Resources 2005: 119).

In view of that portion of paedophilic acts committed by homosexual males, one would think the Bishop might exercise a bit more caution, too, given the past several decades' worth of cover-ups perpetrated by high-ranking officials in the Catholic Church regarding the *many tens of thousands of cases thereof* reported to them and that are now the subject of hundreds of individual and even successful class-action suits *just in the US*, representing in many cases several score litigants at a time. The Diocese of San Diego, for example, settled 144 claims in 42 lawsuits for a total of $198,000,000 on 7 September 2007. Dioceses in Oakland (2005), Spokane (2007), Orange County (2004), Sacramento (2005) and Covington (2006) paid out $56,000,000, $48,000,000, $100,000,000, $35,000,000 and $84,000,000 to a total of 679 people. Meanwhile, the Archdioceses of Boston (2003), Portland (2007), Louisville (2003) and Los Angeles (2007) paid $84,000,000, $52,000,000, $25,700,000 and $660,000,000 to about 1,270 different victims (see Berry and Renner 2004; Associated Press articles, 2002–2007). This is a just a sample of the total devastation wrought by Catholic priests and those who covered up their abuse. The Catholic Church itself commissioned the John Jay Report (USCCB 2004) that estimated that at least 4% of all US priests had admitted to molesting their young parishioners. Much higher prevalence of such has been reported for Brazil, Ireland and Italy, among other countries that have confirmed the existence of mass perpetration and just as massive cover-up of paedophilic acts committed by clergy. In the Philippines, Catholic Church officials admitted in 2002 that hundreds and hundreds of cases of priestly paedophilia had occurred. In Ireland the so-called Ferns Report uncovered more than one hundred such cases involving 21 priests, including the rape of a young girl at the altar in a church. Condoms don't cause promiscuity. The ones who enabled the promiscuity of Catholic priests and deacons were other Catholic priests and deacons and other church officials.

Table 5.4 presents other of the many straw man arguments Bishop Bonivento engages.

Table 5.4 Bogeymen and straw men

Source	Claim
2001a: 9	'The longer the time for using condoms the higher the failure rate of condoms.'

What is the chance of infection over time *without* condom use? Which is more effective: using or not using condoms?

Source	Claim
2001a: 6, 2005a: n.p.	Bonivento frequently claims that health officials and agencies are promoting the idea of use by or more actively and directly giving condoms to 'children', such as Dr Glen Mola, whom he accused of saying that 'condoms are useful to the children'.

I have never seen or heard a health official do this, and Dr Mola did not say that condoms are 'useful to the children'. It is true, of course, that many young people are sexually active, many of them without their parents' consent, and that parents who do things they tell their children not to do might compromise sexual health education.

Source	Claim
2001a: 29	[quoting a healthcentral.com article quoting three British researchers] 'Condom-promotion policy could increase rather than decrease sexual exposure, if it has the unintended effect of encouraging greater sexual exposure activity.'

Hmm. Both religious and secular organisations and researchers have found that condom promotion does not encourage or sanction sexual promiscuity. In any event, the Bishop's charge would hold for every advertisement, depiction, ritual, custom and doctrine that promoted marriage, heterosexuality and, in it, condomless sex.

Source	Claim
2003: n.p.	Bishop Bonivento opposes 'sexual education' (he probably meant 'sex education' or 'sexual health education') that 'seriously threatens schools' and that allegedly pushes children 'to behaviour which seriously damages their dignity and health'. Privately, he has warned of the dangers of masturbation.

Pagan (me) and Christian researchers (my colleagues) showed the Bishop's own congregation what were the fruits of anti-sex education attitudes. They showed, for example, that fewer than one-third of the attributions that 195 respondents made to their STDs were to sex. The remainder was made to food, to drink, to clothes, to *kastom*, to water, to hospital and to nothing in particular. So, which damages people more: correct information or none at all?

Source	Claim
2003: n.p.	'…we find ourselves faced with pressing medical directives in favour of sterilization, the use of the condom as the only means to fight AIDS …'

I have never met anyone in Papua New Guinea, certainly no one from the NACS or the NHASP, who has adopted this stance. Additional means include information, antiretrovirals, behaviour change, drama groups, HIVab testing and post-exposure prophylaxis. Bishop Bonivento also opposes non-penetrative sex, a proven risk-reducer.

Source	Claim
2006: n.p.	[Bishop Peter Fox, in his letter opposing total condemnation of condom usage, gave] 'the impression that somebody is oppressing his freedom'.

He did no such thing, only disagreeing with the stance of the Catholic Church on condom usage, in this case, specifically with regards to serodiscordant couples, whom the Bishop tells to be abstinent. Nearby villages opposed to his policies humorously but also angrily asked whether he was going to be there when the man wants sex from his wife?

2006: n.p.	'Since condoms have been so greatly emphasised in the fight against HIV/AIDS, the menace has skyrocketed in our country.'

Firefighters are seen often at fires, but yet they do not cause them. As well, increasing rates of infection began to be reported long before the Bishop thinks they did. Nor has anti-condom rhetoric always been so pronounced.

2006: n.p.	'I humbly suggest Bishop Fox not to call upon the name of God in advising a man with risky sex behaviour to use condoms … We know that the teaching of Jesus on adultery is total[ly] different.'

Bishop Bonivento is confusing condom usage with adultery with high risk behaviour, which flies in the face of the known facts of transmission risk. As well, Jesus is not reported ever to have mentioned condoms. Bishop Bonivento should know that the fact that the silence has finally been broken about the extent of sanctioned paedophilia in the Catholic Church and has led to mass legal retribution does not mean necessarily that rates of such have gone up.

In flurries of publication of letters to the editor that engage him in dialogue with Dr Glen Mola, Bruce Copeland and the Bishop of the Anglican Church, Peter Fox, among others, Bishop Bonivento has made a number of other kinds of claims that are also contradicted by the facts, for example, that he had been falsely accused of preventing people from speaking (2006). One of his employees told me that he doesn't allow them even to touch condoms, much less speak about them to others, and he prevented other employees of and volunteers with the Diocesan Health Services from working with the IMR field research team for the same reason and because of our frank talk about sex, STDs and condoms. Moreover, he mandated the writing of a letter to us (copies of which I own) that attempted to prevent us from entering a village to conduct fieldwork with his congregation and to help inform them about HIV and AIDS and to treat the high prevalence of STDs we eventually found there. My colleagues took offense in the letter having stated that such work was 'anti-Christian' and was 'only contributing to the spread of AIDS'. That's right: research, too, and STD treatment, not just condoms, spread AIDS. He has also claimed that aid-post kits were never returned for this reason, when

Provincial Health Division officers told me to the contrary and showed me the kits (author's fieldnotes, Vanimo, 2005; see also AusAID 2005a: 15).

The Bishop's writings are rife with rhetorical flourishes that bend the truth further. For example, he quotes a condom manufacturer's web-site (www.durex.com) regarding condom slippage and breakage as indicating that, for example, '44% *are* experiencing slippage' (2001a: 13, emphasis added), suggesting an on-going, perpetual problem, when the reference is in fact to those who have *ever* experienced such, even once. (Moreover, 'slippage' doesn't mean breakage, an unintended pregnancy or an STD.) He cites the same web-site (2001a: 12) in view of 12 reasons why people found it hard to use condoms ('they smell terrible', 'they don't feel good' and the like). In fact the web-site refers to these as 'lame excuses' some people give, and counters them with common-sense replies. Bishop Bonivento uses specious statistics to support his position. For example: 'If we multiply the condom failure rate of 15.7% as contraceptive by 5 (which correspond more or less to the menstrual cycle), we obtain the conservative yearly rate of the risk of getting infected [with HIV] if the partner is already infected: it means 78.5. It seems incredible: however the calculation is logical' (2001a: 15). I leave it to the reader to formulate many possible replies, such as: 'incredible, yes, but logical?' Finally, when in Vanimo and confronted on the street by three Diocesan Health Services officials on the matter, they indicated to me during conversation that the Bishop had confused them by mixing talk of the allergic reactions that a small number (fewer than 1%) of condom users report (either to the latex or to certain kinds of lubricant) with an actual STD, most probably genital herpes (referring to it as *skin teikawei teikawei*). This, too, has enabled the 'condoms cause STDs/AIDS' talk that was so prominent in the area. These are the words the Bishop had to say in answer to the question as to whether or not serodiscordant couples should be using condoms: '[i]t is well known that the use of condoms cannot protect a person with high risk sexual behavior and much less the uninfected spouse; as for the uninfected spouse, it has been statistically proved that by using condoms he/she will get it in a short while' (2001b: 6).

Church and lay texts

Despite the tenor and the many inaccuracies of the claims made by Bishop Bonivento, both of which can be found broadly across the country, there is remarkable unevenness in the shape and extent of condom-related rhetoric. All manner of variations have been noted by researchers and in government documents. Variation exists between different Christian denominations, sects and ministries on the level of policy, for example, between Anglican and Catholic churches, between some United Church ministries and the New Apostolic Church denominations and evangelical Baptist denominations, sects and ministries. Fieldworkers have found great differences between stated policies, on the one hand, and realities on the ground at the local level, on the other. Even from within the ostensibly secular settings of NGOs and provincial AIDS committees there can be huge differences in attitudes to condoms. An NGO based in both Southern Highlands and Gulf provinces was by policy mandate engaged in condom promotion and distribution and supplied by the NAC, but in actual fact it opposed them and so hoarded them that male employees begged them from visiting IMR researchers. One of the posters they created changed the C in ABC to 'Christian Way'. Anglicare-STOPAIDS has taken a more progressive approach, with Bishop Peter Fox allowing condom use in some situations; despite still stumping for abstinence prior to marriage and opposing extra-marital sex, the Anglican Church began in 2001 to allow condom usage as a way of preventing STD and HIV transmission and founded Anglicare-StopAIDS. Not all Anglican churches are on-board, however (ABM 2005: n.p.) and Catholic bishops disagree with one another, too, as for example those in West Sepik and East Sepik provinces. The Bishop from Aitape allows for condom use in case of infected spouses, although not for infected sexual partners *per se*. Each of these variations is refracted further by considerations of the intended targets of policies and practices around condoms. In some places condoms are aimed at youth, but in others they are denied to them. Some clinics restrict their use to married couples only, but in other clinics they are for only single people. Hoarded here, excoriated there; demonised publicly, but privately sought after – condoms are an extremely multivalent symbol of sexual pleasure and anxiety now gripping Papua New Guineans as never before. One of the reports written by the NHASP social mapping team stressed the degree to which condom promotion was in Papua New Guinea at a log-jam, held hostage to conservative ideals of gender and sexuality:

> It was commonly known that condoms are a protection against HIV/AIDS [*sic*] and STIs. Yet when asked about risk behaviours, no mention was made that unprotected sex was a risk factor, and people seemed to think of sexual activities not 'approved' by the community as being risky, whether condoms are used or not. People generally associated condoms with promiscuity and increase in risk behaviour. (NHASP 2005l: 25)

The condom posters alluded to above, the ABC campaign, the current targeting of MSM instead of MSW (Men who have Sex with Women), the exclusion of high-ranking businessmen or politicians from critical scrutiny and the sexually repressive attitudes and legal statutes each attest to this. Throughout the past 12–15 years there have been increasingly frequent exhortations of the public to have less sex with fewer partners and to have sex for reproductive, not recreational purposes. Public health campaigns have therefore not helped over the years to underwrite more progressive approaches to safer and more pleasurable sex, especially those that are non-penetrative, as much as they have aimed to channel and restrict it. Regardless of the infectiousness or violence of intimate partner settings, Papua New Guineans (and especially females) have been enjoined to have sex in them. Directly and more subtly, they have been told not to use condoms when doing so.

Contemporary sexual practice is thus beginning to resemble that of decades ago. Sometimes even with good intentions, colonial powers wielded the spectre of STD and population control to stigmatise indigenous sexual ethics, to rearrange domestic life, to alter residential patterns and to instill

Christian attitudes to work, sexuality, trade, worship and fertility. Early colonial-era re-education campaigns, such as the one carried out among the Marind-anim in the wake of the Donovanosis pandemic (Thierfelder 1928), mandated nuclear living arrangements, instilled radical new notions of wifely subservience and crimped women's extra-household activities. This put females (many of whom were not yet women) in especially south coast New Guinea cultures in closer contact with the ones most likely to infect them – husbands and male relatives. With their heads filled with notions of 'trust' in the new Christian God, in the ideals of monogamous heterosexuality and in the proclamations of public health officials, such exhortations protected them then as much as they do today. When she visited Papua New Guinea in the mid-'90s the Reverend Elaine Farmer was told by members of one 'admirably active women's group' that they opposed the use of condoms 'because they believe a "no condom" policy will keep their men faithful and at home' (Farmer 1996: 215). Jenny Hughes writes that once condom usage was explained fully to Huli women from the Tari Basin, they 'declared their total opposition to [them]. Their reasoning was that if men could have sex with any woman at any time they would 'go wild' and all women would 'be used up"' (Hughes 2002: 131). A prominent spokesperson for UNICEF and other NGOs in Papua New Guinea told a reporter for *The Australian Magazine*, Mary O'Callahan, that he tells men to use condoms extramaritally but not with spouses, so that they will enjoy the sex more with the latter (O'Callahan 1999). I wonder whether he practises what he preaches. Few accounts exist of consensual, pleasurable, healthy marital sexuality, however, such that these injunctions and objections could take hold.

Today's exhortations toward faithfulness (e.g. 'Love Faithfully', *'Stap Wantaim Wanpela Tasol'* – 'Stick to One Partner' – and so on) are just as little grounded in social obligations and the realities of sexual practice now in 2010 as were their equivalents in 1910. The German medico M.U. Thierfelder, for example, was called upon by the Dutch to investigate the causes and treat the clinical sequelae of the Donovanosis epidemic that swept across the south coastal region. He helped to design moral-educational policies that would induce Marind-anim and their neighbours 'to monogamy, by building houses according to a given model and by combating superstition and sexual excesses' (1928: 406). The Dutch installed model nuclear family-type dwellings and exhorted them to a kind of faithfulness that was just as infectious as it was socially problematic. Although they meant well for the most part and were motivated by staggering levels of bodily suffering, especially by younger girls, their policies were yet counterproductive.

Things haven't changed that much in the past century. Indeed, the assessment made in 2000 by Ian Riley, a long-time contributor to the betterment of public health in Papua New Guinea, was that 'there had been no tangible progress in the prevention of transmission of sexually transmitted diseases between 1884 and 1984' (2000: 6). If this is also true, as I think it is, from 1987 (when the first HIVab case report was made public) to the present (during which time the latest long-term planning documents have been released by the government), it is because the messages hide precisely what should be revealed. The epidemiological models have yet to question their own assumptions about the clustering of risk behaviourally and geographically. Male sexual privilege is not yet fully on the table. A leading Christian parliamentarian, while denouncing sexual victimisation generally nevertheless concluded that women and girls were only 'sometimes' subjected to 'unacceptable' levels of abuse (Darius 2004). Another evangelical Christian and former (1999) Minister of Health, Ludger Mond, claimed correctly enough that 'The main cause of the spread of HIV/AIDS [sic] in Papua New Guinea is unprotected sexual intercourse', but still concluded that 'at this point of time the best and proven methods of protecting oneself is by being faithful to one sexual partner, on the part of married couples' (Mond 1999). Politician after health official, church leader after women's group representative, donor country spokesperson after foreign consultant keep repeating the same sad mantra about the *ideal* of faithful monogamy in the face of mountains of evidence to the contrary. The fact is that it is in the 'intimate' settings between boyfriend and girlfriend, husband and wife or wives, between (older) man and (young) girl that the bulk of HIV transmission is occurring and the majority of illness is being suffered. This is not yet reflected in the hard core of intervention programmes and surveillance initiatives, though it is nibbling in from the edges. The fact that power over wives, children, congregations, children and women has been ceded in Christian teachings to husbands, fathers, male clergy and men has yet really to be grasped in terms of the enormity of its relevance to prevention programmes.

There are many other reasons for this. Churches subsidise according to most estimates 40% of all educational services and have done an admirable job with regards to law and government reform initiatives, disaster relief and peace and justice work in relation to tribal fighting and interpersonal violence. They provide over 50% of the services in areas of primary health care, nurse training and health infrastructure. They provide in several hundred villages, settlements and towns sometimes the best, sometimes the only signs of law and order, employment, schooling and civil society and in general do so with extremely good hearts and intentions (Hauck *et al.* 2005; Luker 2004).

But that comes at a price. Verena Keck writes on the basis of long-term fieldwork she has conducted among Yupno people of the Finisterre Range that the Lutheran Church in this area 'has succeeded in maintaining its Christian monopoly among the Yupno; its sphere of influence includes a series of jobs and positions in the village that have to be supported and partially financed by villagers, from pastors, "tokples skul" teachers, church leaders as well as youth group leaders, and circuit president ... ' (Keck 2007: 45). Indeed, there is growing discomfort in HIV and AIDS work around the role of religion and church leaders in promoting notions of sex as sinful and unhealthy and of condoms as being flawed and immoral. The signs of this are ubiquitous in language, sign-board, poster and policy. Hauck *et al.* (2005), for example, estimate that over half of all church-run health facilities are Catholic Church-sponsored. These eschew frank talk about sex and body parts and functions, prohibit the distribution of condoms, misconstrue transmission risks and oppose safer expressions of sexual desire such as masturbation, use of sex toys, enjoyment of erotica and sex between women.

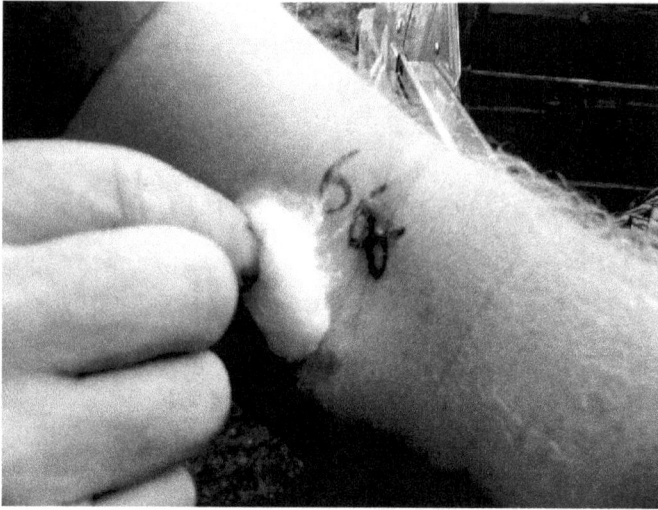

Mark of the Beast at the site of venipuncture

It remains difficult publicly, however, to suggest that the substitution in STD clinic settings of religious icons for clearly presented, factual information may increase isolation, may further stigmatise already stigmatised people. I have never heard a church leader say that church-sponsored public health messages regarding HIV and AIDS have drubbed the accuracy of people's self-assessment of risk. Trobriand island male youth will use condoms readily enough – but mostly only with girls they don't know, from other villages (Lepani 2007b: 259). A 20-year-old single mother from a Trobriand island village said to Lepani that '[m]aybe if you make a steady boyfriend, I don't think there is any danger of getting AIDS' (2007b: 259). Because of the extent to which churches subsidise education generally, however, confusion results over who is responsible for what, resulting in 'poor or no delivery of key sexual health messages even for young people who are accessing secondary education' (NZPGPD 2006: 15). Another review team concluded that '[t]heir role in perpetuating women's ignorance as well as traditional religious gender stereotypes, subjecting women to subordinate and disadvantaged position relative to men contribute to making women particularly vulnerable to HIV infection' (ESCAP 2005: 3). Many misconceptions of HIV and STD transmission route and risk are fuelled by Catholic, Baptist, Seventh Day Adventist and various evangelical and Pentecostal denominations and who then oppose sex education on various grounds (NHASP 2004a; NHASP 2005g). It is difficult to voice such concerns publicly, however, for fear of appearing anti-church, pagan and immoral, and I have seen this happen in the field many times. Youth in one Gulf Province village who had helped to organise IMR activities were rebuked by other youth from the Charismatic sect pastor's following and had the depth of their faith challenged, quite literally, in a Faith Challenge. The implication was two-fold: 1) anyone seeking HIVab or STD testing must already have sinned, and 2) those who have Faith cannot get infected. I have seen vividly in the field many times how one's Christian belief and church allegiance can be challenged of peer educators and condom distributors, of the ways in which the boundaries between medical science and religion become blurred and how gender conservative ideals are fallen back upon in the breach. Bible-based signs and symbols, moreover, such as the number 666 and tropes of Hell, are readily deployed to oppose or scare off HIVab testing.

> *Globalizing discourses of risk don't describe so much as inscribe reality. They are in Papua New Guinea particularly difficult to fight against. In Kopi village, which is upriver from Kikori station, we encountered a situation in which fears arose one morning that the Mark of the Beast, the number 666, would appear at the site of venipuncture were study participants to test HIVab+. From one moment to the next, potential participants scurried from the opportunity to be counselled and tested for HIVab and also to be treated for STDs. Interestingly, at almost the precise time that this was happening to my IMR colleagues in Kopi village, I was at the Kopi base camp and was handed a facsimile transmission that consisted of a 'chain letter' – although this time, mass-faxed–announcing precisely the same rumour. It had, no less, said the letter-head, emanated from a church mission in San Diego, California. I never did establish which had happened first, but perhaps it doesn't matter ...*

Being agnostic, I have special sympathy for devoutly Christian friends and colleagues who yet oppose punitive and ineffective practices and policies about sexual matters. Those include condom disinformation, calls to return to the worship of the Cult of the Virgin Mary (e.g. Vinit 2004; discussed in Hermkens 2007), the mandating of premarital HIVab testing, calls to have students be tested for HIVab prior to receiving tuition subsidies, and the further criminalisation of homosexuality and prostitution. That some church leaders and churches are allowed to skirt health policies that clearly guarantee the right of clinic attendees to receive condoms and the knowledge of how to use them is not discussed in mainstream media circles, and I have been rebuked for these and similar infractions. When aid-post kits are returned *in toto* to provincial health offices by order of Catholic and evangelical Baptist church officials because they happen to carry condoms, stink is seldom raised. While the Catholic air carrier has the right not to carry alcohol and condoms, entire villages are denied lifesaving measures – and not just in the form of condoms. Not everyone in such villages, either, belongs to that denomination or agrees with the policy. Several public followers of the Bishop, for example, yet privately use and/or distribute condoms (author's fieldnotes, Vanimo, December 2005).

Christian doctrine-induced fear and stigma about sex and infection have further torqued 'traditional' sexual ideologies that were in many Papua New Guinean cultures already full of shame and have thus further hampered condom distribution and prevented its usage. The evangelical Catholic, Dr Thomas Vinit, then working for a resource extraction company in Gulf and Southern Highlands provinces, commended and supported the Eastern Highlands PAC and its chairman for taking in 2004 their 'bold stand' in decrying condom use and calling for a province-wide total ban on condoms. Dr Vinit also stood up for the right of the Prime Minister to quash the findings of the so-called Moti Report, which provided evidence of the Australian fugitive Julian Moti having been whisked out of Papua New Guinea on a Papua New Guinea Defense Force-provided jet to the Solomon Islands, where he became Attorney-General. Mr Moti was wanted at the time in Australia on child-sex charges involving rape of a 13-year-old girl in Vanuatu. PAC members sponsored an 'AIDS Awareness' booth at the 2004 Goroka Show replete with hand-drawn diagrams of condom porosity and homespun wisdom regarding their links to promiscuity. Many religious leaders, heads of women's groups and at least three provincial governors supported his and other calls by way of letters sent to the editors of newspapers. Near this time Dr Vinit claimed that condoms had only 'encouraged' the spread of STDs and hastened HIV transmission and later began in public and cyber-space to preach for a return to the worship of the Cult of the Virgin Mary (Vinit 2004). The question remains: what does the Virgin Mary have to teach us?

The IMR, the NHASP and the authors of other nationwide and smaller studies (e.g. Levy 2005, 2006) have found consistently that coming to sexual knowledge and practice from within a religious tradition that eschews frank talk of body parts and functions and that isn't mindful of or realistic about imbalanced gender relations and uncontrollable sexual desires leads to more unprotected sex and to ineffective transmission risk assessments. I mentioned above the findings from some US-based studies. Similar findings have been reported in Brazil (Paiva 2007[2004]). Similar situations have been described for Fiji. The Australian National University-based researcher Miliakere Kaitani found during conduct of her study of the sexual practices and ideologies of Fijian males aged 25 and younger that the sexual health education to which they had access was poor and seemed to have had little if any effect on reducing risk or inducing more consensual and healthful sexual acts (Kaitani 2003). Although subject to Christian moral code formation and shame-induction as regards sexual matters, these Fijian males had commenced their sexual lives earlier than had non-believers and exhibited greater numbers of sexual partners, lifetime, and a higher frequency of sexual partner change. Kaitani also found that religious gatherings provided the milieu for multiple, concurrent sexual networking, just as has been found in Papua New Guinea and Indonesian Papua. In the Republic of the Marshall Islands, a team of three Japanese researchers studying students from the 9th to 12th grades found 'increasing the knowledge of high school students in the Marshall Islands may improve their health risk behavior', partly because, for religious and cultural reasons, they had been exposed to so little (Suzuki et al. 2006: 143). Religious and public health officials, however, are more apt to blame nightclubs, drinking and prostitution than marriage, husbands and fellowship crusades. Few church leaders have been willing to criticise the policies of their churches or the politicians from their own denominations: 'we the health educators have failed in influencing the decision-makers in this country, both at government and church levels. Many of them still hide behind reasons such as it is against our religion, culture or tradition to talk about these sensitive issues' (Bouten 1996: 226).

Anti-condom rhetoric harms the national response. It is entrenched deeply on a cognitive level and seems impervious to critique on evidentiary grounds. The NACS correctly gave much credit to Papua New Guinea's mainline churches for their efforts in strengthening the national response, but also noted that 'their position on the use of condoms or "just turning a blind eye" to condom distribution and not moving beyond awareness to addressing behaviour change by promoting abstinence and being faithful have little relevance to a large number of [women who] have no control over the behaviour of their partners' (NACS 2008: 65–6). For example, findings that 72% and 68% of unmarried male and female youth, respectively, in Port Moresby's settlements are already sexually active (NACS 2008: 26) show that church-sponsored abstinence-fidelity programmes risk irrelevance of focus (see also Smith 2004). Unfortunately, the behavioural fruits of anti-condom rhetoric tend to justify it. If condoms occasionally break or otherwise don't work properly, that is partly due to the ways in which they are stored, allowed to expire and not demonstrated properly to clients by health workers. Many men, for example, have the mistaken belief that the condom must be unrolled first and pulled open, and so find them difficult to apply. I met in three years only one female health worker who would say publicly that she uses condoms and did actually show people how to apply, use and dispose of them. Because condoms are thrown away and burned in front of others, they are said to be for 'high-risk', 'bad' people. 'Bad' people are forced, in notable cases by policemen in Port Moresby and Lae, to swallow them. In a three-district-wide study Catherine Levy found (2006: 12) that 'some women are embarrassed to say that they know about condoms, lest they should be judged'. Others believe condom usage to be incompatible with Christian faith, that justification is provided in scripture regarding adultery, lust and skin disease. The books of Isaiah and Leviticus, for example, guide safe sex-related exhortations on the radio from health offices and during 'HIV/AIDS Awareness' sessions conducted by religious leaders. Zenner and Russell (2005) have written of similar situations facing those in Vanuatu who would like to use condoms but for the way they've been constructed. Even Ministry of Health officials see them as being only for casual sex and that they make their users promiscuous.

Many Pacific islanders thus don't use condoms even though they should (to the extent their intimate partners are infected) because they have been told repeatedly that 'good' people don't. For the same reason but from a different vantage point, those who are socially scorned as 'bad' people (e.g. sex workers) also don't use them when they should so as to appear 'good' or at least better. Women in the Guam sex industry also appear to be rather selective in their choice, holding some men to be 'suspicious' but who, if they offer enough money, will be allowed to forego condom usage (Workman *et al.* 2001). The effects of the condom disinformation campaign have to be examined, therefore, not just in terms of whether people do or don't use them but also in terms of with whom (or not) they'll use them. If they were asked 'is using condoms consistently a good way to prevent HIV transmission?', probably 90% of Papua New Guineans would nowadays answer 'yes'. If they were asked, however, 'were you to use condoms for sex, how many should you use?' most would answer 'two' – or more. If asked on the street, with whom should a man use a condom?, and they were offered several possibilities, most men would pick 'sex worker' but probably none of them would say 'wife'. Lepani's critique of the HRSS is quite apt: 'To affect normative use of condoms and increase people's ability to put HIV awareness into action, it is important that the language of interventions moves away from negative notions of sexual risk to positive representations of consensual sexual relations and healthy sexual practice' (2004: 7; see also 2008b).

Anti-condom rhetoric also enables and sustains sex-negative attitudes. Ironically, the Human Life International's own web-site pages, which Bishop Bonivento endorsed, that were devoted to an alleged condom exposé warn away readers who may be 'vulnerable' to its own words! The Bishop's condemnation of masturbation and other forms of safer sex are well-known locally, but his audience includes readers elsewhere who are exposed to print media. He has claimed that sexual health education regarding masturbation is 'abusive'. He cited in his 2001 Pastoral Letter the following example of sexual health advice provided to Catholic school students in Swaziland as being a form of brainwashing:

> You and your partner can give each other sexual pleasure just by touching each other's sex parts. In this way, your sex parts don't come into contact with your partner's sex parts, so you don't risk getting infected. We call this non-penetrative sex, because the penis does not penetrate, or go into, the vagina. (Bonivento 2001b: 34, n. 76, quoting Matjila John, *The Macmillan AIDS Awareness Program*, Teachers Guide, 1994, pp. 21–2)

The Bishop's condemnation of this kind of forward-thinking advice for especially younger people only justifies more unsafe (that is to say, condomless but penetrative) sex. Anti-condom rhetoric helps to produce 'faithful' girlfriends and housewives who, by doing precisely what their boyfriends, husbands, families, and church and public health officials tell them to do – trust their spouse, be fruitful and multiply, and for God's sake, don't use condoms – get infected anyway. This result has been used against them – infection is seen as something they brought on themselves. Either way, the best they can hope for is 'innocent victim' status via condomless sex.

Ideological struggles in and over condoms and sex, sin and illness, are extremely and perhaps even increasingly fierce. Dr Vinit has argued that AusAID funding of condoms is tacit support for prostitution, as have Bishop Bonivento and other religious leaders argued in other ways and contexts. Even in a newspaper article that was titled 'Use Condoms to Fight Virus' (Taime 2006: 7), the provincial coordinator of the Western Highlands HRSS told Papua New Guineans that, were they to repent and give their lives to God, 'they would avoid contracting the virus'. Letters to the editor, workshop convenings, press releases and other forums and media are filled with the best intended, most earnest prayers to a just and merciful God to help pull Papua New Guinea out of this looming nightmare. But yet ...

Conclusions

In summary, three kinds of objections seem to be fuelling the anti-condom rhetoric in Papua New Guinea. First, church leaders claim that condoms 'are not in the Bible', that they 'are against God's law', that they are 'anti-Christian'. One nun-counsellor in the highlands preaches against them (*'Gumi nogat pawa'* – 'condoms aren't effective'), and her Catholic physician colleague in the area tells female respondents not to use condoms with husbands, whom God himself, he said, had chosen for them (author's fieldnotes, Wabag, April, 2006). The fact that health centres, tinned fish and HIVab test counsellors aren't in the Bible either, when stated, usually leads rhetorically to appeals to the evils of lust and adultery, fornication and sinning. Assessment of condoms, consent and pleasure from a scriptural perspective is thus diverted. Goalpost-shifting helps no one.

Second, Christian objections to condoms often deploy 'two-bodies-must-become-one' rhetoric that might appear to be pro-sex, but that seems ambivalent about sexual pleasure anyway. Perhaps this is because it is so difficult to express erotic desire otherwise. On the one hand, sex is 'bad'. Community leaders in the Alaido district of West New Britain Province, for example, opposed condom distribution on the grounds that it was a waste of money. They thought money would be better spent teaching kids the 'Christian principles' that would dampen instead of arouse sexual excitement (NHASP 2005j: 28). Sex is seen as a precious resource to be preserved, channelled, nurtured and 'used' in the right way. On the other hand, most of us know that sex is good, or at least that it can be. Bishop Bonivento reflects official church doctrine when he writes of the 'reciprocal self-giving' nature of heterosexual intercourse, the unitive aspect of matrimony (2001b: 17).

'The Bible tells us to stay faithful when we get married, and so yes, the condom is anti-Christian. Also, the prostitutes use the condom, not the women who have good husbands. The Bible tells us that God will bless our marriage if we do so. Nothing must come between the wife and the husband. This rubber thing, it's anti-Christian because it comes between me and my husband. "You're my husband," I tell him, and so "you join your body to mine and we stay that way" ...What is this condom for? It is just a rubber thing, that's all. I don't want him making love to the condom, not to me' (Tari, April 7, 2006, translated from the Tok Pisin).

Trobriand islander sexual aesthetics value 'the reciprocal movement between partners during sexual intercourse that results in orgasm' (Lepani 2007b: 258). Perhaps, like the woman quoted at the outset of this chapter and the text box quote here suggest, wire-to-wire connectivity is precluded by a thin piece of rubber. This female health worker in the Tari Basin gave this answer to my question as to whether or not she considered condom usage to be anti-Christian. Research is urgently needed to examine decreased pleasure when condoms are used but that might be due to absent sexual lubricants or decreased or insufficient female sexual arousal. Condoms needn't rub women raw, dermally or aesthetically. The Trobriand island women who don't like the feeling of condoms inside them (Lepani 2007b: 258) have counterparts elsewhere (e.g. Hammar 1996a, 1999b; Hughes 1991, 2002) who worry that they will come off, go loose and lodge themselves inaccessibly in the vagina or uterus. The genitophobia that underwrites such worries has yet to be addressed in pro-sex, body-positive campaigns and messages.

Third, as I showed in detail above, opponents to condom usage assert that they are 'unsafe' in their alleged promotion of promiscuity and in their alleged degrees of porosity induced by manufacturing flaws that required that they be used in duplicate and triplicate. For religious leaders and many health officials, condoms aren't 'safe' in terms of prevention of STD or HIV transmission, but their users have come to fear bodily or reproductive harm to them accordingly (WHO 2001b: 34). This kind of rhetoric is often phrased in terms that are almost epistemological in nature. People seem to hold that an object can have only one inherent purpose or function, and when such objects can be shown to have multi-purposes, multi-functions, such as condoms, objections can conveniently be made to them in their entirety, that is, that condoms are 'bad' on both counts. In this way are roused especially Catholic Church and other conservative church elements to proclaim that, as Bishop Bevilacqua did in another context, 'it is not responsible action to use the devastating disease of AIDS as an excuse to promote artificial birth control' (quoted in Gamson 1990: 274). A prominent religious figure in the National Capital District PAC said that Papua New Guineans wouldn't have to 'adopt ungodly ways to win this battle' and wouldn't be 'threatened' by the growing spectre of AIDS (quoted in Gerawa 2006), implicitly accepting the HIV preventive properties of condoms. Perhaps to get away from such tacit admissions of the properties of condoms, Bishop Bonivento frequently uses phrasings such as 'contraceptives like condoms' and 'contraceptives especially condoms' and refers to as a form of pharisaism, the holding of condoms as being both contraceptive and STD preventive (Bonivento 2001b: 4, 5, 21).

Thus we have come to a complete log-jam in the national response. The Summary Report of the NHASP-sponsored social mapping study concluded on the basis of review of 19 individual reports that '50% of respondents mentioned condoms as a protection against the spread of HIV/AIDS [sic], while the remaining 50% argued that a total ban of condoms would have a preventive effect since condoms make people feel safe to have many partners' (2005g: 5). Only two choices are allowed currently, but those are on cognitive, behavioural and ideological levels mutually exclusive. Behind

Door Number One lies more sex, probably better sex, maybe even with more partners, and certainly better protected, but which would risk societal approbation and condemnation from scriptural perspectives and church and public health officials. Behind Door Number Two lies, for females anyway, the prescription to have fewer partners, maybe less sex, maybe not, and without any protection, but which would gain the approval of church and community. Biological death versus social leperhood. With tremendous respect I have in my heart for the depth of the terrible dilemma facing Papua New Guineas, I ask the following question in all seriousness: Truly, What Would Jesus Do? Is there a Door Number Three?

NOTES

1. The NAC has claimed on its web-site that 19,000,000 male condoms are available for distribution in 2007. If that is true, then it is an absolutely stunning achievement on a number of levels, including that it represents an increase from the 2,386,718 distributed in 2004 and the 3,517,279 given out in 2005 (NACS 2006a: 13–4). Is it a sufficient number, however? Assuming a 2007 population in Papua New Guinea of 5,500,000 and that 40% of those are age 15 and younger, that would leave about 60% of that number (3,300,000) being at all sexually active, that is, quite a few younger than 15 being active but also quite a few older folks who are no longer active. That leaves still fewer than six condoms annually for each sexually active Papua New Guinean. How many of those condoms will never leave the warehouse? How many of them will be hoarded by programme managers and provincial offices? How many of them will languish on the shelves of provincial hospitals, rural hospitals, health sub-centres and aid posts? Programme managers would do well to remember Lepani's warning that condoms are 'fetishized resources' (e.g. Lepani 2007b: 262).

2. I hasten to point out, however, that what are taken to be 'Christian' attitudes to sex and to condoms needn't necessarily be negative. Based upon long-term immersion in Trobriand island lifeways and immediately upon AIDS-related fieldwork she conducted from 2000–2003, Kathy Lepani has shown persuasively that 'Christian' remonstrations in the context of HIV awareness campaigns can be gentle, encouraging ones that lead the faithful toward bodily care and safety, toward thoughtful behaviour, but without the sex-negativity (2007b: 256). On another count, however, the political and especially funding sources of the abstinence movement and abstinence industry in the US from whence it comes is quite gluttonous; it comes greatly from the Massachusetts-based Gerard Health Foundation, headed by Raymond Ruddy, an intimate of the Bush White House, who received a $115,000,000 retirement package for stepping down from Maximus (Reynolds 2007).

3. http://www.w-cpc.org/sexuality/teensex.html .

4. http://www.dianedew.com/condom.htm .

5. http://www.epigee.org/pregnancy/birthcontrol.html .

6. http://www.epigee.org/guide/risks.html .

7. http://www.bchealthguide.org/kbase/topic/symptom/stdis/prevention.htm .

8. http://www.siecus.org/pubs/fact/fact0011.html .

9. http://www.britannica.com/eb/topic-131570/condom .

10. http://www.acdp.org.za/oldpress/CondomSafety19Mar03.htm .

11. http://www4.nau.edu/fronske/birthcontrol/cc_handouts/condom_ spermicidal_jelly.html .

12. http://healthydevil.studentaffairs.duke.edu/ .

13. http://www.uml.edu/student-services/counseling/mental_health_information/other_issues/ condom_use.html .

14. http://www.cha.state.md.us/edcp/factsheets/condom_m.html .

15. http://www.healthcentral.com/genital-herpes/prevention-8800-108_2.html .

16. http://www.healthcentral.com/genital-herpes/news-534496-105.html .

17. A Tokyo-based company now sells women's underwear that comes complete with Global Positioning System tracking device (http://www.forgetmenotpanties.com). Among the testimonials offered is one from a father who 'nearly had a heart attack' when his daughter hit puberty. He suggested that video camera devices somehow become part of the next version of this nauseating new technology.

18. http://216.146.213.75/Publications/Documentaries/video/AFRBroadbandLG.mov .

19. http://www.ashastd.org/hpv/hpv_learn_myths.cfm .

Part Two

What the experts (still) don't get

> Social theory in concert with sound ethnographic knowledge has the potential to completely reorient the understandings of ... social behaviour gained on the basis of a naïve empiricism. (Graham Fordham, *A New Look at Thai Aids*, 2005: 243)

A recurring theme throughout especially Chapters 3, 4 and 5 has been that ABC may be a great way to teach children the English alphabet, but not such a great way to teach adults, a safer and more pleasurable and consensual sexual practice. I have shown the legal, frequently compulsory nature of heterosexuality, marriage and sexual intercourse, and that such can disable the rights of women to consensual, pleasurable erotic expression. According to the author of several nationwide studies on family, violence and sexuality, '[t]he majority of adult women of PNG have been physically assaulted by their husbands, forced to have sex with them, or have been raped or sexually assaulted by other men' (Bradley 2000: 51). Hell, girls and women are beaten by husbands even *before* the marriage is consummated (e.g. Whiteman 1973: 161). Children are sexually violated by (mostly male) adults before they even get married (Darius 2004; Hammar 1996a, b, 1998a, b, c, 1999a, b; Help Resources 2005; Luluaki 2003; Zimmer-Tamakoshi 2004), just as they are elsewhere in the Pacific and around the world (Ali 2006; Hammar 2006a; Herbert 2007; Salomon and Hamelin 2008). The UNICEF-sponsored report on the extent of child sexual assault (CSA) and commercial sexual exploitation of children (CSEC) in the insular Pacific concluded that CSA and CSEC 'occur on a regular basis across all strata of Port Moresby society. Cases reported are believed to be the tip of the iceberg. Most rape cases presenting at the [Port Moresby General Hospital] are of girls under 18 years. There are about 1–2 cases of children per day, most occurring at home' (Help Resources 2005: 82). Given that condoms are associated by religious figures with sin and promiscuity (sometimes being dubbed 'Satan's Tools') and by epidemiologists and NGOs with 'high-risk' sex, many people would rather risk biological death than social censure (see also Wardlow 2007, 2008). On the level of policy, many organisations, especially those that are church-run, would rather avoid the facts of sexual practice than discuss them and hide or disavow the specifically religious source of much confusion about sexual matters. As for matters alphabetic, nothing could be simpler than ABC but that captures so little of the nature of sexual relations and gender inequalities. A high-ranking NACS official was quoted as saying that 'risky behaviour' was having multiple sex partners *and* being promiscuous (without defining either of the two or their relationship to one another). He then warned against having 'unprotected sexual encounters with strangers' (Per 2006: 5). This ignores the common infectiousness between spouses or other kinds of 'intimate' partners, again externalising risk.

Unfortunately, this linchpin of the national response, the ABC message, remains the mantra that politicians, preachers and health bodies and officials feel they must repeat, no matter how many times or in how many ways it has been revealed by empirical research to be inappropriate for Papua New Guinea. Among 10 Papua New Guinean research cadets who returned from an international AIDS conference in Colombo, Sri Lanka, two relayed the conclusion that ABC was ineffective because none of its constituent components spoke Truth to the Power of gender relations. 'Contributing factors which undermine abstinence include high levels of sexual violence against women and young girls, incest, and sex under the influence of alcohol and drugs', said Kritor Keleba, while Barbara Kepa contributed that 'negotiating safer sex in a marriage can be more difficult because it implies unfaithfulness and husbands may become angry and violent, raping their wives' (Drysdale 2007). ABC has been the focus of significant debate in African countries, Indonesia, Australia, the US and certainly Papua New Guinea. It has received a mixed report card, garnering both glowing reviews (that have subsequently been criticised severely) and failing grades (e.g. Brown 2006; J. Cohen 2005; S. Cohen 2004; van Kampen 2006; Parikh 2007; Ukuonzi and Epstein 2005) but that have then led to howls of protest. Bill Bowtell (2007: 5) has reviewed the history of attempts to implement ABC in many countries and concluded that 'HIV containment policies based on promotion of sexual abstinence, repressive drug control measures and limited or no access to condoms, honest information about sexuality or clean needles have demonstrably failed.' 'In some ways', noted one NHASP review, 'the basic ABC approach may have the effect of actually increasing women's risk' (2005b: 28). Nevertheless, this uncomfortable truth has yet to be taken on board by policy-makers. Neither have they yet quite grasped just how opaque can be local understandings of the meanings of HIV and AIDS. Leach, Gooey and Elaripe helpfully critiqued the progress made to date of meaningful involvement of people living with HIV and/or AIDS (2006). They note that while Papua New Guinea's HIV epidemic has for some time been 'generalised', and despite the fact that the incidence of new infections continues to rise, 'HIV is still not visible in PNG. The signs of the epidemic are certainly there, but people have not yet learned to recognise them' (2006: 11). The words of a rural-based politician that appeared at the outset of this book represent well even 'well-educated' understandings, and his understandings of condom use and efficacy have yet a long way to go.

To recap, previous chapters explored the behavioural influences upon, the policies about, the prevalence of and the ill health effects of sexually transmitted dis-ease in the insular Pacific. Chapter 2 looked at ethnological and other data in showing how 'traditional' forms of sexual networking can become commodified and commercialised as Europeans and European goods, sexual desires, instruments of rule and resource extractive economies are introduced. Those processes were shown to stigmatise sex and those who engage in it, and helped to explain why it was that mainstream epidemiological (mis)understandings of the infectiousness of 'prostitution' got a healthy, homegrown infusion of the same when HIV and AIDS arrived to Papua New Guinea in the mid-late 1980s. Chapters 3 and 4 examined the rising seroprevalence of HIV and the programmes and initiatives launched in recognition. I showed that those programmes and messages and kinds of discourse were responses to largely unforeseen social, economic and behavioural changes, but also to health crises already well known. New masculinities and femininities have burst Christian and 'culturally' prescribed gender roles and relations. I covered in Chapter 5 the cognitive and behavioural fall-out of such inabilities to inhabit contradictory roles and fulfil competing obligations in view of anti-condom rhetoric.

> *'Gather available qualitative and quantitative information via an initial stock-take of all surveillance studies, STI data, social and high risk mapping, and anthropological and other social research written about PNG, to generate an understanding of the bigger picture, and identify additional research needs to fill gaps within the surveillance system' (NACS 2007: 30).*

If there is a singular lesson of Chapters 3, 4 and 5, it is the dangers of missing or questionable databases and the inability or unwillingness to link the findings of those databases to the formulation and monitoring of the effects of the application of sound public health policy. Health officials, political bodies and community organisations alike have shown themselves to be unwilling to become familiar with and to translate relevant social science findings. Despite the undeniably 'intimate' location of the vast majority of transmission of HIV and STD, public health messages and models are pitched away from it, and no matter the evidentiary weight of in-depth, contextual, ethnographically informed assessments of transmissive risk. 'A great deal of social science research has been undertaken in the past into the social and cultural backgrounds of sexual beliefs and practices in PNG', wrote the author of a NHASP document. 'For instance', it continued, 'when it had a functioning medical anthropology section, the IMR produced considerable relevant research, including a national study of sexual and reproductive knowledge and behaviour. It is a pity that, so far, little use has been made of this wealth of knowledge' (NHASP 2003a: vii). Another NHASP review (NHASP 2005b: 17) noted that '[n]ot enough is known about this disturbing phenomenon [sexual abuse of boys], and research is urgently needed', even though this has been one of the most thoroughly researched topics in Melanesianist anthropology for the past 25 years! Recommendation #4 from the '2007 Estimation Report' appears in the text box above, and I don't know whether to scream or cry: scream at the persistent refusal of officials to acknowledge what social scientists have already learned; or cry at the great heaps of data not being put to good work. It is too late for an 'initial' stock-take.[1] I have shown that there is little room for evidence-based approaches and for ethnographic data that challenge assumptions about what 'good' sex is or who the 'bad' people are that one must avoid. Relevant data about ways in which Papua New Guineans construct risk in the face of confusing and contradictory information have been stubbornly ignored. Not *lacking*, as the NACS still has it in the text box below, but *ignored*.

In addition to the many other casualties mentioned to this point, there has yet to occur a serious consideration as to what is replacing condom usage (other than prayer).

> 'Research must provide information on risk behaviour, sexual networking, mobility and migrations and commercial/ transactional sexual activities and the impact of this risky behaviour on their wives/husbands or regular sex partners. Research into the cultural factors influencing HIV transmission and the social responses to it is lacking' (NACS 2008: 30).

Supercise Me

The vast majority of male prisoners at Bomana incise their foreskins. This operation is forbidden by prison rules, so it must be carried out in secret. (Adam Reed, Papua New Guinea's Last Place, 2003, p. 113)

An evangelist I interviewed in Wabag told me in some detail about how he and his best buddy had 'circumcised' each other when they were 13 or 14, he didn't know. He said they did it because of their interpretation of what they had heard of *tumbuna pasin*, traditional custom, since his village was Christian and so didn't do these things anymore – or at least not publicly. He told me that he remembered the advice his male relatives had given him previously when, about two decades later (three years ago), he graduated from a Christian leaders training seminar held down the road in Kudjip at the Nazarene Church-funded hospital. At the end of it, but in private, he helped to group-circumcise other students – about eight or nine of them, he said. His teachers had taught them that, by doing so, they could avoid AIDS. Condoms, he told me, were unsafe. They're filled with micropores, don't 'cha know? (Author's fieldnote, August, 2006)

Genital cutting is now 'widespread in all areas and promoted as a substitute for condom use'. (Carol Jenkins and Michael Alpers, 'Urbanization, Youth and Sexuality', 1996, p. 249)

Many hundreds of articles and books have been written about genital surgeries, practices, modifications and embellishments, from male circumcision to female infibulation, from vaginal douching and 'dry sex' to labial piercing and penile implantation. For a partial sampling of that literature and of how such practices influence current efforts at HIV prevention, see Aggleton (2007), Berer (2007a, b), Dowsett and Couch (2007), Hankins (2007) and Silverman (2004). A great many of those, at least those that are about male genitalia, concern Pacific islanders. Relevant cultural practices of Polynesians, Australian Aborigines and Melanesians have been documented extensively for over one hundred years, just as they have for Asian and Southeast Asian cultures for many hundreds of years more. In pre-contact Hawai'i, a 'blower' was designated by family and community for each baby boy so as to make the male infant's foreskin 'balloon' in preparation for later subincision at age six or seven: 'the penis was blown into daily starting from birth. The blowing was said to loosen and balloon the foreskin [and] continued daily … until … penile subincision takes place' (Diamond 1990: 430–1). One authority in 1927 quoted a Chinese explorer to Thailand in 1392 as having seen widely that 'the penis is slit for the insertion of jewels that indicate wealth and position' (quoted in Brown, Edwards and Moore 1988: 52). This and similar practices have been documented in hundreds of sources in thousands of settings, including those of plantation labor, incarceration, royal courts, criminal gangs, sex work and logging.

Genital cutting is a term perhaps preferable in that it covers a broad range of practices including circumcision proper and penile insertions. It is performed for myriad reasons and by all manner of parties, few if any of them disinterested. Melanesian cultures, practices and peoples feature commonly in these broad-ranging literatures. 'Penile incision is reported often in the New Guinea ethnography', said Donald Tuzin in his *The Voice of the Tambaran*, good portions of which are devoted to the issue of the hazing of young male initiates. Tuzin wrote compellingly of the 'dramatically staged assault on the penes of the novices' by (slightly tongue-in-cheek now) 'a savagely attired adult under conditions calculated to inspire maximum horror', culminating in the attack by a man dressed as a pig who delivers 'deep cutting strokes on their glans penis' (Tuzin 1980: 67, 66, 67, 71). Tuzin later described the Ilahita Arapesh male practice of urethral abuse and glans penis slashing as being almost autoerotic. It functioned as an emotive, inward, psychological confirmation by means of induced erection and a sort of therapeutic cleansing, of men's outward, social and economic power over women. Elsewhere he noted that in front of his new bride for the first and last time an adult Arapesh male slashes his penis to bleeding into a small dam of twigs and debris made by his bride in a small creek; when she bursts the dam and the blood is washed away, the couple pledge their love for each other and their promise of fidelity, 'praying to the ancestral spirits in the stream to grant their marriage fruitfulness and permanence' (Tuzin 1982: 330). Thus is (hetero)sexuality commenced properly. Gilbert Lewis also included provocative accounts of glans penis-bleeding in another Sepik river area culture in *Day of Shining Red* (Lewis 1980). This passage denotes the intimate, caring, intergenerational nature of male initiation:

Then he took Wowulden's penis, rolled back the foreskin and bored the *kuti's* point into the dorsum of the penis just above the glans. It was not rapidly done and he seemed to dig it well in and hold it there. Wowulden's whole body stiffened but held the position: he gave one brief moan. Saibuten withdrew the *kuti* and there were exclamations of approval, congratulation and satisfaction from the older men watching ... While this was happening, shouts and cries came from Tiflai (Wowulden's younger brother) who was resisting having his penis stabbed ... Other men ... then stabbed their own penises and the blood was smeared on sons of Wandi, Sakai, Selpak and Peikəp, and Tawo's grandson Wərmei. All the men present washed after this. Parku carefully washed his penis and gave water to Wowulden to wash his. They put hunting ash ... on Wowulden's wound. (1980: 78–9)

Philip Newman and David Boyd (Newman and Boyd 1982: 254), write that, following a period of the forced gagging and nose-bleeding of initiates, both being done to facilitate the purging of substances thought dangerous and polluting,

the glans penis of each initiate is cut. This bleeding is accomplished by several men lifting the youth off his feet and firmly holding him stomach up with his legs spread wide apart. The foreskin is held back with a split stick, and an incision is made on each side of the glans with a bamboo knife. He is then released to bleed into the stream.

By contrast, the Wogeo male of Milne Bay Province cuts at his own penis, but to effect the same cleansing result that later adds a spring to his step:

The technique of male menstruation is as follows. First the man catches a crayfish or crab and removes one of the claws, which he keeps wrapped up with ginger until it is required ... Then late in the afternoon he goes to a lonely beach, covers his head with a palm spathe, removes his clothing, and wades out till the water is up to his knees... When ready he pushes back the foreskin and hacks at the glans, first on the left side, then on the right ... He waits till the cut has begun to dry and the sea is no longer pink and then walks ashore. After wrapping the penis in leaves, he dresses and goes back to the village, where he enters the club. Here he remains for two or three days. Sexual intercourse is forbidden till the next new moon – the soreness, in any event, may take that long to wear off. (Hogbin 1970: 88–9)

Circumcision, subincision, supercision, superincision and the exceptionally rare circumincision (in which a cut is made around the base of the penis, and sometimes includes a flaying of the penile skin) have each been seen to be linked to complex notions of society, gender, sexuality, kinship and cosmology. John Layard's *Stone Men of Malekula* theorised tight links between ritualised homosexuality, political power, the fully exposed glans penis, extravagant bark penis-wrappers and the practice of circumincision (Layard 1942).

Owing to the appearance of HIV and AIDS in fact and in rumour, new cognitive models of medicine, risk and illness have surfaced in many Pacific island cultures and countries. Carol Jenkins noted that '[i]n the 1990s, numerous reports surfaced of young men [in Papua New Guinea] obtaining homemade circumcisions in the village, or circumcising themselves in small groups. As this often led to severe infections and was not an effective substitute for condom use as protection against HIV or other STIs, efforts were made to discourage this trend ... ' (Jenkins 2007: 40). Such expectations of lowered HIV transmission by way of genital cutting are probably linked to anti-condom sentiments espoused by religious leaders and health officials. They should acknowledge this and apologize to the women and men affected.

More than mere (mis)information and (dis)information is at work, however. The preference of males in many Australian Aboriginal groups for subincision has for many millennia (and in the minds of researchers, many decades) been linked to questions of reproduction and specifically male jealousy of female ability to menstruate. Older arguments had it that subincision among Australian Aboriginal males functioned as a sort of 'primitive fertility control' (Basedow 1927). Bruno Bettelheim quoted authorities such as Berndt and Fison, Warner and Howitt to the effect that subincision wounds in males resemble vaginas, 'and the blood coming from the cut (or from subsequent piercing) symbolized both the after-birth and menstruation' (1971[1954]: 175). Michael Allen analysed many of the same materials from North Vanuatu as had Layard and other data he collected more recently and concluded that 'I do not think that I am being unduly speculative in asserting that among the Small Islanders the generative and reproductive powers believed to reside in the penis and in semen are themselves directly modelled on the reproductive powers of women' (1993[1984]:119). M.F. Ashley-Montagu theorised in an essay published in an early issue of *Oceania* that Australian Aboriginal males subincised themselves and one another in mimic of the moiety-arranged social order and in multi-faceted envy of the kangaroo's bifid penis, an argument that sustained much commentary and many critiques for the next three decades (cf. Ashley-Montagu 1937; Singer and DeSole 1967). Penile supercision is still practised in Tahiti among some groups; Jeannette Mageo has interpreted it as a ritual designed to 'stir up fear' in adolescent males and then, to the extent they endure the ritual, to enable them to overcome it and thus speed themselves toward social manhood (1991: 14).

The distribution in Southeast Asian cultures of practices of penile insertions and cuttings and use of penile rings (sometimes so as to effect a form of male infibulation) has been surveyed by a number of scholars (e.g. Brown *et al.* 1988; Hull and Budiharsana 2001a, b; Lee 2006; Lee *et al.* 2002; see also Re/Search 1989). They and other researchers have uncovered similarly broad concerns of those who embellish or modify one's or another's genitalia with fertility, sexual access, social status, disease avoidance and an effective mimicking of the natural and animal worlds. The anthropologist Eric Silverman's in-depth exploration of these topics for Jewish, Muslim, Hindu and other males shows that, depending on context, historical epoch and relationships with dominant religions, circumcision (or its absence) and other forms of bodily modification or adornment can be an expression, positive or negative, of religious identity (Silverman 2004). A medieval female mystic is said by the historian Caroline Bynum to have wed Christ symbolically by way of the Holy Prepuce, that is, by putting it on her finger (Bynum 1987). Others pierce, insert things into and otherwise modify male

genitals to express occupational loyalty and rank. 'Pearling' is engaged in
by Japanese criminal gang members, each pearl inserted into the corpus
spongiosum marking one year spent behind bars but not ratting on one's
boss. Heather McDonald reported that she had had a yakuza gang member
boyfriend 'who had 13 pearls in there, and they weren't real small pearls,
either' (quoted in Re/Search 1989: 156). Similar practices can be engaged in
to mark sexual identity and fetishes and, through erotic piercing, to obtain
and maintain a 'modern' body (e.g. Buhrich 1983; Myers 1992) or to signify
women's comparatively high status in traditional Southeast Asian cultures
that mandated male foreskin infibulation (Siriratmongkhon 2002). Hull and
Budiharsana have documented extensive genital manipulations and surgeries
in Indonesia, the Philippines, Malaysia and Thailand that exhibit both traces
of historical contacts with Chinese traders and indigenous innovation in the
face of globalisation and socioeconomic change. 'The implanted objects',
they write, 'range from the very simple, e.g. ball bearings sewn under the
skin, to the elaborate, e.g. specially selected semi-precious stones, gold bar
(*palang*) or rings inserted through the glans. Recent research has found that
the use of such inserts is spreading among working class men in Southeast
Asia and Melanesia' (2001b: 63–4).

Although genital cutting practices of many kinds have been documented
for many Melanesian cultures, the question of the extent to which
circumcision is among them is still debated. Carol Jenkins has several times
pointed out that nowhere was it really 'traditional' in Papua New Guinea to
'circumcise', in the strictest sense of the term. A number of researchers have,
however, recently complicated things with new research findings. Terence
Hull and Meiwati Budiharsana include 'many groups in Eastern Indonesia
and Melanesia' (2001a: 2) in their designation of those cultures practicing
male circumcision. As if in reply to Jenkins' contention, Catherine Levy
and her VSO-sponsored team found that in the Ambunti and Raikos areas
of Madang and East Sepik provinces, penile foreskin was actually removed,
not just severed, in traditional practice (2005: 27), which would appear to
be circumcision, not just supercision. Nancy Sullivan and associates have
asserted that 'Madang people are renowned for their circumcision practices
in male initiation' (Sullivan *et al.* 2003: 39) and that Nobnob people in
particular had done so up until 2000 or so when the older men gave up
on the younger, whom they accused of being too soft and impure. Eric
Silverman also mentions that male circumcision was traditionally practised
in 'Melanesian' cultures (2004).

Wolfgang Kempf (2002: 63) has written about the Ngaing people of
Madang Province and the introduction of male supercision by health
orderlies in the wake of World War Two, which he argues helped the awkward
meshing of 'traditional' rituals of male initiation with first stabs at modernity.
Kempf shows that Ngaing males began to change their conception of their
place in the world upon digesting the events of the coming of first Lutheran
and then Catholic missionaries, and especially the coming of 'western' mores
and medicines in the wake of World War Two. Kempf notes that although the
Ngaing people of Yawing village (a pseudonym) had witnessed circumcisions
in European-sponsored hospitals during World War Two, supercision arrived

to the Ngaing in about 1950, on the advice of an Australian health worker. Several years later he notes that a Yawing NMO (Native Medical Orderly), who had himself been supercised elsewhere, brought the new custom to his home village for the first time and asserted his affinal ties to the peoples on the coast who had cut him. Conceiving of the foreskin already as 'dark', 'impure' and maternal blood-stained, and being impressed with biblical accounts of both circumcision and crucifixion, when they saw western medical orderlies begin to introduce the practice of supercision, ostensibly to treat, if not also prevent STDs, Ngaing took eagerly to the practice.

> Since being introduced some fifty years ago, this *incisio praeputii* has steadily grown in importance, as has its integration into the local structures of secret initiation rites of male adolescents. In Yawing the point is often made that the introduction of supercision has been rendered by the need to protect oneself against sexual diseases. Its adoption was legitimated with references to western-medical hygienic discourses and to the fact that whites themselves practiced circumcision. (Kempf 2002: 63)

Ngaing males are especially anxious to show their affinity with Christianity, and so find in the idea of circumcision and practice of supercision a literal marking of their covenant with God and local missionaries. Supercision allows Ngaing males to oppose European domination, to expand their conceptual and geographic place in the universe (whatever you do I can do at least as well) and to gain a further leg-up on despised persons – the unsupercised and the female. In functionally like manner, Reed's account of genital cutting in Port Moresby's Bomana prison suggests that supercision reconstitutes flagging gender identity: 'Being separated from women means being separated from a part of oneself' (2003: 115). Jenkins and Alpers found in their multi-site study of urban youth and gender that '[i]n all areas, young men are more closely bonded to each other than to young women or to parents. They are strongly subject to peer pressures and, in an atmosphere of violence and crime, need each other for protection' (1996: 249).

Anecdotal and other evidence has been reported throughout Papua New Guinea of men individually and in groups taking up this or that form of genital cutting for religious reasons and to avoid sickness. Sometimes it occurs with medically disastrous consequences (Jenkins and Alpers 1996; Greg Law, personal communication, 2004–6). While engaged in consultancy fieldwork in a remote area of Southern Highlands Province in April of 2006, I ran into a learned and well travelled man from a Huli-speaking village of the Tari Basin who had not only heard of the alleged relationship between 'circumcision' and 'AIDS risk', but also of a man whose name is virtually synonymous with these complicated debates: John Caldwell (alongside Robert Bailey, Daniel Halperin, Edward Green and others). He had learned of circumcision and circumincision when he was in Madang in the mid-1990s training to be a priest, and later came to perform supercisions on fellow students and catechists. Here is how he described his method (translated from the Tok Pisin, April, 2006):

When I am about to circumcise them ['circumcise' said in English] I have
them come to me and sit on a coconut-scraper [a stool sat upon while
scraping coconut meat] and I give them one, two betel-nut to chew. They
must continue to chew. Sometimes I mix it with the guava leaves. It's better
with the guava leaves. Then I take the Kobra [a flat-stick, often a tongue-
depressor or a popsicle-stick, soaked, softened and broken or bent into an
L-shape]. I take the Kobra and I pull his foreskin all the way out. I pull out
the foreskin and shove the Kobra into [under] the foreskin. That's the base. I
get the scalpel [obtained or purloined from local health centres] and I make
a cut along the Kobra with a stone [pounded sharply along the back of the
scalpel]. I fold the foreskin back and I tell him, I tell him, 'you spit the guava
leaves onto the wound', and I wrap it with bandage. And if I have Amoxi or
[methylated] spirits, I dose him with that ['dose' said in English].

This account squares with the procedure as it occurs in Bomana prison:

Cast in the gloom of a cell corner, a convict or remand inmate removes his
waistcloth and lies down naked on the concrete floor. Leaning over this
reclining figure, another prisoner, the 'doctor' (Dokta), spreads the man's legs
and grasps his penis in order to pull back the foreskin. He slips a wooden
spatula, usually stolen from the prison clinic, under the prepuce and in his
other hand lifts a razor blade. Careful to avoid any veins, the doctor rips
swiftly through the top of the foreskin. Blood, dark and thick, oozes from the
wound and is allowed to flow until it runs red and translucent and the lesion
is gripped. When the bleeding stops he releases hand pressure and lets the
torn skin drop to either side of the penis. There it curls and folds, and is left
to hang. (Reed 2003: 113–14)

Reed likens this form of surgery to remade rituals of male separation,
initiation and reincorporation, which have been analysed in great detail by
fieldworkers such as Gilbert Herdt, Deborah Gewertz, Fitz John Porter-Poole,
Donald Tuzin and many others. Other accounts suggest an analysis along the
lines of passage from liminal to adult status, such as this one drawn from a
Port Moresby settlement (translated by the author from Tok Pisin):

It's, it's like, when I go to [supercise] them, I tell them to come and sit down,
they'll remove their pants ... and [I'll cut] this foreskin here ... So, I'll put
the flat stick underneath; I've got a stick that we use to do this ... Okay, we
push the stick under the foreskin, then pull it down over the stick, flatten
the foreskin, and then cut it lengthwise ... Now there's two kinds of skin, one
is like plastic, that's his virginity. After you've cut it, it goes underneath the
glans penis, above it will be the head of the penis, and it'll be like a 'V' shape
(Hammar 2006b: 35).

Many Health Extension Officers (HEOs) and Community Health Workers
(CHWs) throughout the country also perform 'circumcisions' on male youth
(both proper and in a hygienic setting and also supercisions, informally).
Moreover, male health workers in at least two provincial capitals have been
called upon to perform other, far more dangerous and socially disruptive
procedures. While conducting fieldwork in Wewak and Vanimo I interviewed
many, many men and women who affirmed that penile supercision and even
injections were commonly employed to effect greater girth and length. This
snippet is drawn from the report that followed a fact-finding mission led to
Vanimo by a technical advisor to the NDoH:

During the visit it became obvious that the practice of performing the penile injections was being carried out by some untrained village and community men but also (and of considerable concern) by some health workers (both retired and still working). These health workers were either purchasing the products from across the border or were concocting their own preparations from medicinal and non-medicinal substances. It is apparent that these people are making a tidy additional income from charging for these practices and men who approach them for the 'service' have confidence that because they are getting the injections from either registered or retired health workers, that it is an acceptable procedure and not harmful. (quoted in Hammar 2006c: 17–8, used by permission of the author, obtained on 9 March 2006)

It is interesting to ponder the original source of and some of the reasons for the spread of information about and the newly invented meanings of such practices. One informal interviewee in Wabag (in April 2006), a young man, had made a lengthy and lengthwise incision of his foreskin, near the end thereof but not all the way, and then let it heal. After several weeks' worth of attempts to stretch and tug at the foreskin so as to lengthen it, he said, it left a permanent opening, through which he then poked the head of the penis. This left the bunched up foreskin to dangle permanently to one side, in essence, bunching up together both 'sides' of the foreskin, into which were then put one or two ball-bearings prior to sexual activity, which he then removed at completion of the sex act. He said that women thereby felt more sexual pleasure and he didn't any longer need to worry about AIDS. Surely this practice was not 'traditional', but it is interesting to note how similar it appears to be to a practice among the children of elite Javanese: '[t]he retained skin [following the foreskin incision] is tied in a "bundle" or left as a flap with a hole that can be used to occasionally attach horsehair or other stimulants prior to intercourse' (Hull and Budiharsana 2001a: 3). Adam Reed notes from the perspective of Bomana prison that '[t]he sliced prepuce, which hangs below the penis, is said to form a "double head" and thus improve sexual performance. Male prisoners boast that this enlargement makes them more desirable' (2003: 116). When I met a District

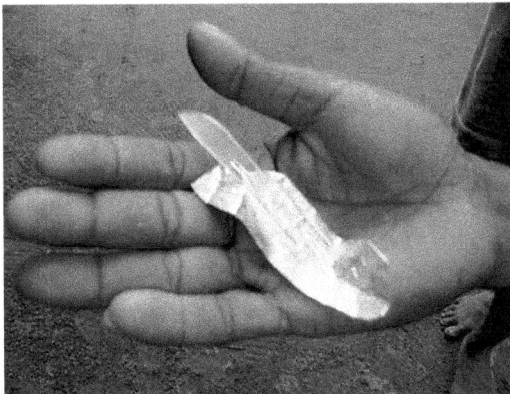

Purloined scalpel for use in male supercision

Disease Control Officer at a highlands administrative centre, he told me that he had 'heard from Headquarters' that condoms were particularly 'unsafe' and 'harmful' to men and women, but that 'circumcision' (by which he seemed to mean supercision) was an effective substitute. Because the local Assemblies of God pastor so opposed condom promotion on grounds of not wanting to induce promiscuity, and since he himself believed condoms to be riddled with manufacturing flaws, he became from that point engaged in informal 'AIDS prevention' along those lines: 'I've heard it said that if you'll just remove this little tag of skin, you'll be okay. AIDS can collect in that piece of skin' (translated from the Tok Pisin, author's fieldnotes, April 2006). The photo here is of the kind of purloined scalpel that is used.

Anywhere such practices are not engaged in under proper medical supervision and hygienic conditions there can be extremely serious bodily health consequences, including septic shock, excessive bleeding, urethral inflammation, gangrene necessitating surgical amputation and even mortality owing to tetanus and toxic shock. The clinical sequelae of such operations when performed under less than optimal conditions can be so serious that NGO- and mission-sponsored medical doctors have in Vanuatu, East Timor and Papua New Guinea been tapped to perform circumcisions in prison settings (Hull and Budiharsana 2001a). One such doctor writes of what he and his colleagues found when they visited a Papua New Guinea prison and also noted that the Secretary for Health was completely unaware of the practice of foreskin-slitting:

> Here we also came across numerous cases of self-inflicted, longitudinal lacerations of the foreskin, often gruesomely infected. We were told that this custom was traditionally practiced in one or two remote highland villages, but in Mt. Hag[e]n prison widespread belief is that it not only protects against AIDS and STDs, but also improves sexual performance. This belief and practice also extended to some staff. (Mulhern 2001: 4–5)

In Papua New Guinea male genital cuttings and modifications are engaged in now for all manner of reasons. 'It's in Every Corner Now: a nationwide study of HIV, AIDS and STDs' (Hammar 2006b) contains preliminary analysis of a large number of data from select field-sites that suggest the broad parameters of genital cutting behaviours and commonly shared experiences and feelings. Apart from a small number of men aged about 40 years-old or greater who may have been supercised when young as part of male initiation, most males are doing so in their teenage years or young adulthood. In rough order of frequency, they do it to please Self aesthetically by changing the appearance of the penis; to avoid HIV or STDs, partly by minimising contact with female genitalia; to follow the Bible or traditional teachings they missed out on for not having grown up in the village; to please Other sexually by increasing the size, girth or particular shape of the penis by auto-insertion of beads, seeds, stones and pearls; and to harm Other, by 'really busting the asses' of other male prisoners or to punish women deemed recalcitrant or sexually promiscuous. In addition, rubber-bands and petrol drum rings are commonly doubled and then wrapped around the penis to increase girth. Ball-bearings, balls formed from melted plastic, polished glass beads and marbles are among the other items inserted into the corpus spongiosum; the butt end of a toothbrush or the hard-plastic cap from a ballpoint pen is filed and sharpened for the purpose of opening a slit, the object(s) is(are) inserted and then the wound fastened with gauze bandages or cloth strips, sometimes sprinkled first with Amoxicillin or doused in saltwater. In addition, rope, wire, cassowary feathers and nylon stitches are sometimes inserted through an opening made in the skin on the ventral side of the penis.

Insofar as many of these practices are common elsewhere, many believe that they come ultimately from Filipino and Malaysian fishermen and loggers, although they clearly undergo local and sometimes ethnographically unique permutation. A newspaper reporter based in Bali posted to AIDS_ASIA@yahoogroups.com (10 September 2007) a story recounting that:

> Some fishermen also insert BB-sized, glass or plastic pellets into cuts in their penises for enhancement. The wound is sometimes still fresh when they make shore, but it doesn't stop them from hitting the bars lined with women in miniskirts. 'They don't have any self-esteem. They are ordered around by the company and the captain to do this and that', said Setiawan, who's researching the fishermen. 'Sex workers can give them their self-esteem back.'

In Vanimo, capital of West Sepik Province, which shares a border with Indonesian Papua, silicon and oils and other substances purchased from across the border at Wutung are rubbed onto or injected into the penis, either to delay ejaculation (in the case of Samsu, which is a penile anaesthetic), to increase penile length (as with Cobra and King Cobra – oil and tablets) or to enlarge the width of the penis (in the case of silicon injections). Different kinds of Spanish Fly are sold that men put surreptitiously into women's food and drink. Vaginal pessaries such as Madura stick and soaps such as Sari Sabun Kesed, both of which have tacking and astringent properties, are now sold in great quantities and resold in villages along the border to and past Vanimo into Wewak and even into the highlands. In Goroka, capital of Eastern Highlands Province, I was told by an as yet unmarried man home on leave from the Ok Tedi mine in Western Province that applications to the penis such as Cobra and penile insertions such as of ball-bearings and melted plastic beads enable them to please women sexually such that the vaginal excitement induced will 'go straight to their heart so they will not be able to forget you' (author's fieldnotes, August, 2006). Others say that such genital embellishments help them to punish sexual partners (as I heard during Daru-based fieldwork, 1990–2 and then again throughout the country, 2003–6; see also Reed 2003). A similar situation is described for the Solomon Islands, according to Buchanan-Aruwafu and Maebiru (2008), and for a similar range of reasons, from enhancing one's own or one's sexual partner's pleasure to hurting them sexually to enhancing erections and stamina. They note the use of *mabol, hos hea, raba, kat da skin* and *foget mi not*, in order, 1) insertions into the corpus spongiosum of polished bits of glass or ceramic (5% of males surveyed); 2) the tying of horse hairs through a ventral cut in the prepuce; 3) the wearing of petrol drum rings over the penis (together with *hos hea*, 34% of those surveyed); 4) circumcision; and 5) probably supercision, in which a small amount of prepuce is left behind.

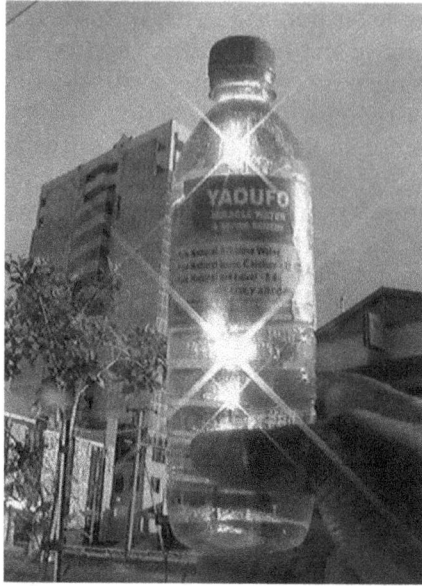

Yaoufo water

Apart from penile insertions and other forms of embellishment, the contemporary practice of supercision and other forms of genital cutting seems designed to help males avoid disease, which is unlike the case analysed by Romeo Lee for contemporary Philippines. He argues that Filipino male circumcision is a contemporary social phenomenon but that expresses desire to 'conform to a centuries-old tradition and to acquire, through that tradition, a range of masculine-related traits, capacities and opportunities' (Lee 2006: 232). Papua New Guinea has no such centuries-old tradition on which to base such contemporary practices. In one informal group setting in Wabag in April of 2006, younger unmarried males said things like *'nogut mi kisim sik nogut long dispela hap skin nogut, ya'* ('I don't want my foreskin to pick up AIDS/an STD'), *'mi harim olsem em bai abrusim sik'* ('I've heard that you'll avoid sickness that way'), *'mi wok long abrusim deti bilong ol meri, mipela ken kisim sik olsem'* ('I don't want to get infected with women's uncleanliness, 'cuz we can get sick that way') and *'gumi i no seif tumas, ol i pulap long liklik hul olsem na binatang sikAIDS i ken pas long yu'* ('condoms aren't very safe; they're so filled with little holes the virus can pass through and infect you').

Three aspects of male genital cutting pose immediate sexual and reproductive health risks to men and boys and to others. First, the unwanted clinical repercussions can be quite serious, ranging from infection and excessive blood loss to growing resistance to antibiotics to septic and even toxic shock, often necessitating hospitalisation and surgery. Second, to the extent wounds aren't fully healed when next they have sex, the degree of their infectiousness to others (if they happen to be suffering from an STD) is increased just as they are made more vulnerable to infected others through abrasions and open sores. Studies have shown that HIVab+ married men resume intercourse more quickly and unsafely following circumcision than

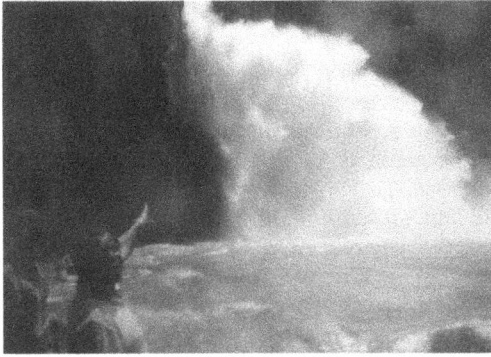

Waterfall where likeness of Jesus allegedly resides

do unmarried men also seropositive. Third, to the extent they are engaging in such practice as an alternative to condom use, they have been sadly misled by promoters of condom mis- and disinformation.

✳ ✳ ✳

In the three following chapters, I and my colleagues explore several issues that the acknowledged authorities seem still not to want to address straight-forwardly. I've made seven points here to focus our discussion. First, cultural politics around sexuality don't have to be so coddled and babied on grounds of 'culture' or religious sentiment. As frequently as it is asserted that messages 'must be put in culturally appropriate language' and delivered in 'culturally appropriate settings', doing so sometimes constitutes a new problem: not everything 'cultural' about sex is good or deserves equally respectful air-ing. Religious sentiments – or more personal or idiosyncratic ones that are couched in religious terms – sometimes need to be confronted more directly. There frequently appear sign-boards and notices placed in public places and health facilities promoting alleged cures for tuberculosis and AIDS, uterine cancer and infertility. One such features the 'Magnificent Yaoufo Water Fall and its healing waters', a bottle of which appears here, the brilliant reflecting indicating 'Divine Light', according to the web-site (http://www.healthre-form.com.pg/).

The *Post-Courier* carried a two-page, full-colour fold-out featuring on one side the promoter of the healing waters and on the other, a likeness of Jesus. The text underneath Him contains an arrow pointing to the waterfall and what is claimed to be 'A visible image of Christ looking out from the Water fall.' The water is bottled by those representing an organisation called 'Health Reform' led by Mr Amos Yali, who participated in the 10th annual National Health Expo. Their bottling and selling of the water constitutes 'proclaimation of a divine cure through Yaoufo water as divine remedy'. The anointed water 'has the power to fully revitalize and strengthen the body's immune system to stand against all forms of disease'. This particular ad stops short of claiming a cure for AIDS, though many similar advertisements are not so modest and do root their allegedly curative powers in Christian faith. The web-site claims that, without any side-effects whatsoever, 'Yaoufo

'"We tested HIV-positive in Nomvalo; the community health
worker there said we must come here". And the nurse said to
them, "You must go home and not come back until you get sick".
So now the two girls came back from the hospital empty-handed.
They were very confused. They went to their church to share with
their prophet what had happened to them. And at the church
they were told that if they pray they will get better. God will
make them better, not pills. That was when they began to deny
that they were HIV-positive. They started to visit this one – she
pointed to Nosiviwe – and told her that she must stop taking
ARVs and come and pray' (quoted in Steinberg 2008: 188).*

Miracle Water will completely eliminate every secondary infections' and
challenges the skeptical to have a 'CD4 or Viral Load Count' before and
after trying the 'Yaoufo Miracle Water Treatment. After 2 to 4 weeks time
you will be surprised with the result', because it 'cures all forms of illness
because it is God given' (http://www.healthreform.com.pg/). Seldom are
those proclamations challenged or disputed by health authorities. Indeed,
sometimes they actively endorse such products. The head of the Disease
Control Branch of the National Department of Health endorsed on
Department of Health letterhead an advertisement for the widely available
Bio-Normalizer, which he dubbed a potential 'panacea for most, may be all
of the medical conditions in this country' including HIV and other viral
infection (17 February 2004, p. 2, 1; copy in author's possession).

Second, as indicated by the text box quote, many things 'theological'
about sex and HIV and STD prevention messages are manifestly harmful.
Despite frequent protestations that 'Papua New Guinea is a predominantly
Christian country and that churches have an important role to play in the
national response', church leaders and doctrines can also preclude true
gender equality in the family and community more broadly. They also
collude in expectations that NGOs and private capital have that males
will represent 'the community' or 'public health' or 'government', such as
when oil exploration companies sponsor male corporate group junkets to
Port Moresby. Churches promote male sexual prerogative in relationships
and (especially by pretending to valorise) feminine submission. Appeals to
Christian ethics by way of slogans such as 'Follow God's Law' and 'ABC' or
Radio Doctor programmes that instruct in 'safe sex' by way of the Book of
Leviticus have restricted the clear presentation of factually correct, vitally
needed information about sexual and reproductive function and health.
Christian leaders promote sex-negative, anti-condom and homophobic
attitudes that blame the infected instead of looking at how (and sometimes
by whom) they became infected (AusAID 2005a; Bouten 1996; Cummings
2008; Dundon 2007; Eves and Butt 2008; Farmer 1996; Hammar 1998a;
Hauck et al. 2005; Jenkins 1996; Keck 2007; Luker 2004; McPherson 2008;
NHASP 2005b; Wardlow 2006a, b, 2007, 2008).

Third, the experts don't appreciate how much foreign researchers, NGOs and even national health officials bend over backwards so as not to inflame religious leaders and sensibilities around HIV and AIDS. They certainly don't comment upon how little Christian reciprocity is shown in the other direction. A new book published by the Asian Development Bank, *Cultures and Contexts Matter: understanding and preventing HIV in the Pacific*, features the work of two well-respected Melanesianist anthropologists, Holly Aruwafu-Buchanan and Carol Jenkins. Like its predecessor in some ways from more than a decade earlier (NSRRT and Jenkins 1994), it warns readers on the first page that some may find certain language offensive (the Censorship Board restricted the viewing of this earlier work only to medical personnel). Nevertheless, while this new work blocks out the 'F' word, which *isn't* going to hurt its readers, frequent mention is made (as it should be) of sex trafficking, sexual violence and non-consensual sex, which do hurt people. Are vulnerable people or Christian sensibilities being protected here? The NHASP review of the High Risk Settings Strategy (HRSS) noted that 'respectful' discussions with churches and their representatives worked best (NHASP 2006e: vii). Social scientists, however, complain (but only privately) of disrespectful and heavy-handed approaches taken by the NACS, NHASP and especially HRSS representatives and their employers and sponsors. Certainly, local people at said high-risk settings have complained of same. Workshop attendees, conference discussants and list-serv discussion members often introduce themselves as being 'devout Christians'. When they make homophobic comments and spread misinformation about HIV and AIDS and sexual matters, extremely little commentary ensues from sponsoring officials, whether national or expatriate, despite the presence of gay, lesbian and bisexual colleagues and stakeholders in the room or group. The NHASP review of Church Engagement in the national response included recommendations that there should be *more* 'Biblical and Theological input in the NACS Basic HIV and AIDS training program' and that *more* workshops therein should be facilitated by the short-term, NHASP-hired, expatriate Faith-based Advisor. Is there more in the Bible about HIV and AIDS that we haven't read yet? They recommended further that a Papua New Guinea national be trained to become a 'vision-keeper' by receiving *more* training in theology overseas (NHASP 2006c: 10, 11, v), not in HIV transmission dynamics, the principles of gender equality, the true efficacy of condom usage or the public health benefits of sex-positive attitudes. The review allowed mildly only that *some* (not *most*) *believed* (not *without a doubt, knew on multiple grounds*) that religious organisations had facilitated the decline of traditional practices and cultural values (2006c: 8). In its support for the Red Ribbon Churches Initiative, it pledged practical support for churches that 'help to prevent spread of the virus', but nowhere mentions condom usage or how and why to promote non-penetrative intercourse, masturbation, use of sex toys or the sharing of erotica and other safer-sex measures (2006c: 29). Neither does it highlight that the Churches Covenant is characterised by the same omissions and thus also fails to engage the condom disinformation campaign or the blatant homophobia of many of its leaders and followers. The otherwise remarkably progressive NAC document, *National Gender Policy and Plan on HIV and AIDS, 2006–2010*, only mentions the words 'Christian' and 'church' once each, suggesting in the former case that it wasn't Christian scriptures themselves that endorse female gender subordination, but rather, some 'interpretations' thereof (NAC 2006: 25). In other words, the experts don't seem to get the ill public health effects of such omissions and silences.

Fourth, the experts don't seem to understand how little the national response has been propelled by critical, reflexive thought upon itself. Little engagement in sociology of knowledge production means that few assumptions are ever questioned and that reflexive thought isn't allowed to enable substantial change to occur in midstream when that has been called for. The abuses of gender and sexual privilege (including in medical settings, in conduct of research studies, at religious gatherings and while carrying out outreach activities) have been sanitised in official reports or brushed aside in person (author's fieldnotes, 2003–6; Levy 2006: 6; NHASP 2003b: 49). As Kathy Lepani points out in a recent essay, '[t]he illusion of being above the problem holds serious consequences for gender power relations as the national response to HIV becomes more of an industry in PNG, and people vie for positions of authority and control in program activities'. Lepani points to several well known anecdotes involving the sexual shenanigans of HIV programme managers whose preachings contradict their behaviour while, ahem, 'raising awareness' (Lepani 2008b). The Help Resources report on child sexual abuse (CSA) and commercial sexual exploitation of children (CSEC) mentioned many such incidents, for example, that 'many of the young women informants in Port Moresby frequently listed NGO workers as being their most regular "clients"' (2005: 21). It noted also that Christian citizens defer to 'notions of male rights enshrined in contemporary assertions on what is PNG culture and of women's obligation to submit as is implied in Christian teachings' (2005: 96).

Fifth, there is the tendency to co-opt the work of other social scientists directly and indirectly. There is the tendency to repeat but without grasping the meaning or importance or longevity of social scientific findings and ethnographic insights about 'gender' now being a significant aspect to the HIV epidemic, as if it weren't all along and as if it weren't a pressing concern prior to HIV coming to Papua New Guinea. Not a day goes by in real time or cyber-space that a speech, press release or posting to AIDSTOK doesn't mention as if it were news, that ABC is inappropriate, that homophobia exists or that gender relations disempower women and girls. Reviews and policy statements sometimes contain ideas and data and even paragraphs that are lifted from one source without *proper* quotation or citation (e.g. NHASP 2006c: 7, 9; NACS 2008). The NACS, the NDoH and the NHASP have in the past several years 'got gender', and that is a good thing, but it doesn't seem to be out of deep philosophical training or sincere political activism so much as by its iteration at conferences and workshops. The NHASP-sponsored review of the Gender Impact Evaluation found that while many NHASP positions were filled by females, '[i]n NACS, the opposite situation prevails, with a preponderance of men in both senior and administrative positions. Women here did feel that their lack of numbers (and relative youth) meant that their contribution to decision making was limited' (NHASP 2005b: 20). This has led to a stilted, conservative take on sex and gender and that leads often to a perspective that totters between paternalistic (in both 'good' and bad ways) and alarmist takes on women's and girls' vulnerability. The vulnerability is assumed on biological grounds (not social) to be double, triple or even quadruple that of males.

To take another example, the NHASP review of the High-Risk Settings Strategy (HRSS) noted the drafting for Save the Children (in Papua New Guinea) of a 'Concept Paper' by a well-respected ethnographer about leadership roles proposed for them. Lepani's analysis and commentary (2004), however, which spoke just as fairly as firmly *against* the stigmatising language, debatable assumptions, overly narrow focus and even the name of the HRSS, are not at all reflected in the few lines devoted to the topics in her thorough critique (NHASP 2006e: 16). Quite to the contrary; she noted (personal communication, 23 May 2007) consternation at how her work was misrepresented. I have been told that at international conferences I have been quoted as saying that there are 'nine kinds of prostitutes', when in fact I have written of the multiple venues and labour forms of sexual networking (Hammar n.d.). Others who have written about the high costs to marriage, family, community and sexuality of resource extraction enclaves are interpreted as having pointed out where all the prostitutes are. The NHASP review notes correctly enough about one proposed HRS (high-risk setting) that people come and go at '*kakaruk maket*' all day long, but the language as regards sexual matters is quite telling: '[s]ex work has become a commercial activity, and women are no longer scared or ashamed of what they do, despite being concerned with the lack of privacy offered by the crowd. Once negotiations are made, the sex worker and client sneak out in search of a more secluded area where they have sex' (NHASP 2006e: 16). Substitute 'wife' for 'sex worker' and 'husband' for 'client', and that pretty much describes marital sexuality in a lot of households, too, even if one allows the 'sneak out' part. As well, sex became a commercial activity long ago, not recently, and I'm not sure that these women ought to be feeling ashamed, as is implied.

The three quotes in the text box on the next page are just a few of those I collected as I and my IMR colleagues worked just behind this or that visit made by the NHASP team anxious to set up an HRSS site. I strongly disagree with its proclamation *in advance of its establishment*; I am upset that it was pronounced with neither data nor context to support it, instead of being treated as the good empirical question it is. I am upset at the ease with which 'TSW' and 'MSM' were adopted by means of their introduction through foreign donors and consultants. This review (as with others) shows little theoretical grasp of the real constitution of risk in Papua New Guinea because it shows no familiarity with relevant findings from rural sociology, medical anthropology, ethnography and other qualitative forms of knowing. In terms of questions of epistemology, there has been an over-reliance upon KAP(B)-type approaches, said the anthropologist writer of another review, 'while more sophisticated studies that address the complexities of behaviour change are disregarded. This is despite the fact that KAP have largely been superseded by more perceptive and useful methodologies' (NHASP 2003a: 55). Neither did the review of the Social Marketing Evaluation Review critique the truth

'They didn't come to find out what the "hot-spots" were; they only told us' (local HRSS representative, Tabubil, November, 2005; author's field-notes, translated from the Tok Pisin).

'I told him we could take him to where the married women are having the sex without the condoms, and lots of drinking, at the officers' quarters and the Hotel, but he said to take him to the border [at Wutung] and to Karanas Pit Place because of all the condoms there. He likes those "hot-spots"' (local HRSS representative, Vanimo, January, 2006; author's field-notes, translated from the Tok Pisin)!

'As for me, I was very angry when they came to Red Scar and told us we were the high-risk people. We try to use those condoms when the highway drivers come' (Red Scar resident, Madang, April, 2006; author's field-notes, translated from the Tok Pisin).

content of the questions asked, but only the alleged knowledge bases of respondents (NHASP 2006h). The experts aren't grasping how much they're missing by refusing to commit to a sociology-of-their-own-knowledge.

Sixth, the experts haven't squarely acknowledged the extent to which the foreign, external nature of funding sources shapes the contours of a national response and influences the contents of programme initiatives. Before it was 'rebranded' (says the NACS web-site, which indicates once again the tension between substance and rhetoric about it) as Tingim Laip (i.e., Think Life), the HRSS absolved health bodies and officials from responsibility of promoting a more critical and reflexive approach. Ditto, for the sentinel surveillance sites that track along lines of ruling and authority (discipline, registration, ideology, governmentality) instead of along the empirical lines of infection (in companionate relationships, gender- and otherwise-imbalanced social relationships). The massive targeting of prostitution over the years absolves 'experts', politicians and programme managers from examining the demand side of the ledger. All available evidence shows that real transmissive risk lies in companionate relationships, but yet the national response continues to 'target' 'MSM', 'youth' and 'sex workers' who are alleged to *pose* risk to others while others such as Defence Force or health personnel are assumed to be *at risk* (AusAID 2005a: 2; NAC 2007; NHASP 2004: 15; WHO-NACS-NDoH 2000). This problem is evident elsewhere in the Pacific. Aliti Vunisea writes of Pacific seafarers as being vulnerable *to* infection as they travel to foreign ports (which is true, but they themselves become infected …), and treats them as relatively innocent babes in the woods when they hit port and are 'bombarded with sex workers and alcohol' (Vunisea 2005: 8). One article about the 'disciplined forces' and that correctly noted in its title 'Military Deemed as High Risk' (Kewa 2003) slipped rhetorically in the first sentence by referring to military forces being *at* high risk owing to the combined infectiousness of the women with whom they had sex, consensual or not, in single fashion or group, outside of marriage. As the following snippet from Help Resources shows, there are particular costs associated with such an approach that lets off the hook the perpetrators of sexual violence and targets instead their frequent victims:

> What is more worrying is that youth are a special target group and their vulnerability is closely linked to being rendered drunk and sexually aroused in the venues that 'host' commercial sex work, including CSEC. A more sophisticated approach is required to work in and around these venues rather than just providing condoms to the men [e.g. policemen and security guards] who opportunistically rape young sex workers, or adding condoms as freebies to performances that commodify girls. (Help Resources 2005: 22)

Seventh, it is extremely rare to encounter frank assessments by Australian observers of the risks to health, security or social relations that Australian presence constitutes in the form of soldiers, missionaries, businessmen, aid workers, miners, athletes, diplomats or the policemen who were brought in 2004 in the Enhanced Co-Operation Package to help unravel the culture of violence among their Papua New Guinean counterparts (Fowke 2006). To that extent, Wright (1959: 72–3) is among the striking exceptions for having noted half a century ago the 'sexual vices' and promiscuity of transient whites among the Maori in New Zealand. When a brothel/outcall service was in 1962 closed down by the authorities in Lae, it was noted that most of the infections that male customers had transmitted to local girls and women emanated originally from Sydney, and that the owner-operator was herself an Australian woman (Abbott 1962). August Kituai's *My Gun, My Brother* (1998), although it has been severely criticised by kiaps (Australian colonial-era patrol officers) on factual and other counts, shows something of the extent of Australian-introduced sexual networking and violence in context of patrolling and colonial pacification. Tour guides, government web-sites and other sources always warn travellers *to* Papua New Guinea of sexual and other interpersonal risk but not Papua New Guineans *about* those same travellers. The threat of Papua New Guineans to Australians featured prominently in the Four Corners programme 'Sick No Good', which was aired on Australian national television in August of 2006. This documentary insulted first by its title (which should have read *Sik Nogut*), thus abusing Papua New Guinea's most flavorful lingua franca – Tok Pisin – and second by its pronouncing a 'disaster', a 'Catastrophe on Australia's Doorstep' (Carney 2006; Cronau 2006). A recent review written for the North Queensland Department of Health noted with great pessimism the depth and breadth of health woes in this region and the continuing stress upon Australian financial resources in the form of Papua New Guineans opting to be treated not in Western Province but on Thursday island:

> As the financial crisis in PNG continues to worsen, the population in the Western Province continues to grow, and as infrastructure improves on the Australian side of the border, the number of visitations to the islands in the Torres Strait will continue to increase as people visit family, seek economic opportunities, food and health care. (Donaldson 2003: 3)

The report was filled with examples such as the following: '[i]n 1999 a PNG person with a mildly drug resistant strain of TB who was living with family on Erub (Darnley) infected 18 people on the island, some of whom travelled to the Cairns region before they were located' (Donaldson 2003: 12). A controversial piece by Miranda Tobias concluded that 'The Torres Strait has a very high prevalence of sexually transmitted diseases', and so, 'high HIV levels in Papua New Guinea could be of great concern for Australia. HIV/ AIDS is thus not only a humanitarian issue, but is becoming a health and security concern' (Tobias 2007: 14). Others have issued little-nuanced media releases and 'position papers' that construct Papua New Guinea as a regional security problem, whose putative 'hot-spots' need 'targeting'. Australian AIDS activists quickly and angrily denounced the comments made in April of 2007 by the Prime Minister John Howard regarding the possibility that HIVab+ asylum seekers should be granted access to Australia: 'My initial reaction is no [the HIVab+ should not be allowed in]. There may be some humanitarian considerations that could temper that in certain cases but prima facie – no.' Lost in the quick and angry condemnation was the fact that after the first 11,000 votes had been cast in a newspaper poll, a majority of Australians felt the same way (Hart 2007; *Sydney Morning Herald* 2007c). I don't think national health or political authorities yet realise the dangers of uncountered, uncontested xenophobia on the part of non-Papua New Guineans, whether Australian or from elsewhere in the insular Pacific.

✳ ✳ ✳

The purpose of the conversations in this second Part is therefore to bring even more fully into the light than in previous chapters the hidden assumptions and unasked questions of the national response. In particular we wish to investigate disjunctures between the considerable *rhetoric* in Papua New Guinea and other Asia-Pacific countries and cultures of HIV and AIDS, which can be quite progressive in tone and content and remarkably well-intended, and *the reality*, on the ground, as it were, which can be rather less so. Examples might include claims made by the government of a 100% condom usage policy but that are retracted almost as soon as they are uttered and that were never applied to marriage anyway. Legislation is formulated that alleges to protect the HIVab+ and punish those who hinder prevention efforts, but have successful test cases of such been mounted? The Acting Director of the NAC proclaimed as an example of the provisions of the HAMP Act being implemented that 'female sex workers feel comfortable to seek counselling or treatment by female medical/social work' (NACS 2008: 123), when the contrary has been documented far more often.

The following three chapters are designed therefore to encourage health professionals to think harder about health services delivery and why systems of them sometimes fail. We want to enable policy-makers to understand the likelihood that their programmes will succeed. We want to keep external donor country representatives from throwing away good money after bad. We want to show would-be researchers how they might investigate new topics ethnographically. We want to encourage programme managers and policy-makers to make better use of existing data. Along those lines I can reiterate here how frustrating it has been to deal with the seeming unwillingness of especially national authorities to grapple with alternative interpretations of the national response. For example, I wrote to the Acting Director of the NACS, Mr Romanus Pakure, and offered him and his colleagues the chance to read and respond, just as I have repeatedly to NACS media officials. I did so partly to try to understand better the court case that led to the temporary sacking of NACS officials and their eventual reinstatement on a legal technicality. It's not so much that the silence hurts personally as that yet another good opportunity has been wasted.

In Chapter 6 Sarah Hewat and I compare the national response to HIV and AIDS in Indonesian Papua with that in Papua New Guinea and more broadly throughout Indonesia (see also Richards 2004; Butt, Munro and Wong 2004; Butt, Numbery and Morin 2002a, b). I rely in Chapter 7 upon Dr Alison Murray's considerable experience and expertise in sex worker advocacy (see especially Murray 2001). We look at the role that NGOs and others might play (and some of the obstacles they might face) in attempting to foster a modern, Western sense of professional, individual identity and 'community' mobilisation in Papua New Guinea around sex work. Peer group mobilisation has its supporters and detractors, to be sure, but perhaps sexual networking in Papua New Guinea is, well, sufficiently different in ways that even the experts haven't yet grasped. Dr Mark Boyd reflects in Chapter 8 upon the tensions between biomedical and social scientific ways of knowing about HIVab serosurveillance and the roll-out of antiretroviral therapies (see Boyd *et al.* 2006). Among many other topics we discuss is the extent to which the extraordinary toxicity of such drugs was investigated before mandating their usage in clinical trials. Difficulties of medical licensure are implicated in this and other thorny problems. Combined with the fact of an absent consumer rights movement in Papua New Guinea and the already great stigma and fear that characterise such matters, antiretroviral therapy roll-out has been plagued by problems that deserve an airing alongside their notable successes.

In the Epilogue, Chapter 9, I try to pull together some of the ideas covered elsewhere in the book and that are brought out more clearly in the previous three chapters. I suggest that what needs to occur is not a more technical or biomedical 'fix' such as mass male circumcision or an effective HIV vaccine or even full-body condoms – however much we may wish for such simple fixes – but rather a change in the very social structures within which we fit and that give meaning and purpose to our lives. Marge Berer has asked pointedly whether, given a state of finite resources, 'is it ethical to suggest that certain countries prioritise an intervention that will (partially) protect only men in the next 10–20 years?' (2007b: 45; see also 2007a). Peter Aggleton concluded his thoughtful contribution to the HIV and male circumcision debates by noting that

> Both in academic journals and in the corridors of international HIV
> conferences, colleagues murmur that the time has come for 'biomedical
> prevention' – the roll-out of antiretroviral drugs to otherwise healthy
> populations of sex workers and other vulnerable groups ... But there are other
> forces at work. (Aggleton 2007: 20).

Indeed.

NOTES

1. The same can be said for the domestic and sexual violence research headed by Susan Toft under the Law Reform Commission (in 1986, and taken over by Christine Bradley in the early 1990s). It was revisited again in 2000, and despite all indications to that point and since then that the problem has worsened and deepened, the 54 recommendations that came from that research were shelved (NACS 2008: 55–6).

Chapter 6

Courting disaster

HIV and AIDS, secrets and sexscapes in Indonesian Papua

The romantic underground

> However, 'ABC' approaches to HIV/AIDS prevention … are premised on a
> unitary and highly idealized Western construction of the marital relationship.
> The social science literature often refers to this as companionate marriage,
> where marriage is expected to be a person's primary source of emotional
> gratification and marital sexual fidelity is a key symbol of this intense
> emotional bond … The literature on ABC approaches to HIV/AIDS prevention
> rarely acknowledges that the marital relationship may not be universally
> conceptualized as companionate in accordance with an idealized Western
> model or that there may be competing economic and ideological pressures on
> men that minimize the value and practicability of marital fidelity. (Wardlow
> 2007: 1006)

LH: Lawrence Hammar
SH: Sarah Hewat

I have invited my anthropologist colleague Sarah Hewat of the University of
Melbourne to discuss with me HIV- and AIDS- related numbers, responses,
behaviours, ideas and policies across the border to the west. No matter what
terminology we use, we're going to inflame some and confuse some others,
but here goes: commonly referred to as West Papua, but previously as Irian
Jaya and Irian Barat, in 2003 a Jakarta-led decree split the province of Papua
into three. Today, for complex reasons, only two provinces, Papua and West
Papua, which comprises the Bird's Head Peninsula, are recognised by the
provincial government. For the sake of simplicity, in this chapter these two
Papuas will be referred to as 'Indonesian Papua'.

Anyway, Sarah's ethnographic setting in the Manokwari area of Papua's
south-eastern corner involved intimate human concerns such as marital life
and courtship strategies, public health concerns and sexual networking, and
certainly HIV and AIDS. In 2004 she published a fine essay in the *Papua New*

Guinea Medical Journal, 'God's Curse and Hysteria: women's narratives of AIDS in Manokwari, West Papua' (Richards 2004), based upon focus-group interviews she conducted with devout, often quite well-educated Christian women, many of them being wives of civil servants and quite active in women's groups. She argued in that essay that HIV is often understood in Manokwari as being spread by willful, that is to say, sinful human activity, but that AIDS itself somehow 'comes from' God. She wrote also that only three female informants 'distinguished between HIV and AIDS', seeming to suggest that they were variations of each other, each and both together becoming important parts of a 'clustered set of symptoms' (2004: 77). In that and in many other issues I find much that is similar between Indonesian Papua and Papua New Guinea, despite differences of scale, religion, sovereignty and politics. Moreover, as is the case in Papua New Guinea, but perhaps even more so, it seems that ethnographic data and sociological insights have no place yet in state policies about HIV and AIDS, and that officials there show even less interest in them than do their counterparts in Papua New Guinea. Her fieldwork in Manokwari is extremely relevant to what is happening in Papua New Guinea, and she joins a long and growing list of social scientific investigators of the special risks of love, faith, courtship and marriage (see also Hirsch and Wardlow 2006; Nyanzi *et al.* 2007[2004]; Paiva 2007[2004]; Parikh 2007; Smith 2004; Wardlow 2007).

✳ ✳ ✳

LH: Tell me, Sarah, what it was like working with devoutly Christian women in Papua over such sensitive and contentious issues as sexuality and disease, love and courtship.

SH: I did not go to Manokwari with the intent of studying love and sex, and at first it was hard to find evidence that women expended much energy caring about such matters. After quite a few months in the field, however, I became aware that both romantic love and sex were topics of grave concern, and that the silence was because it was seen as improper to discuss them. In mixed-age groups of women, and never if children are present, sex is discussed indirectly and in a passive/aggressive, joking manner that targets individuals. In the company of same-sex peers, on the other hand, sex can be talked about candidly, so long as it is referred to in a general and not a specific way. So private is information about one's sexuality that not even one's closest friend or relative can ever know about one's sexual exploits, lest they be tempted to expose one through gossip. Interestingly, young women came to enjoy confiding in me, alone in my room, as they knew it was a space that had no eavesdroppers or interruptions. I am convinced it was my status as non-gossipy Westerner that gave me access to rich data about emerging sexual cultures in Manokwari. Over two years of fieldwork I built trust with young women in the way that one builds trust with anyone: through generosity, confidentiality, openness, sharing meals, keeping a sense of humour and maintaining a sense of mutual self-disclosure.

Being a Westerner counted for a great deal in my investigation into issues of a sexual nature. Local Papuans see the West as a place of sexual debauchery or, depending on one's moral position, a locus of tolerance towards sexual orientations and expression. My teenage friends especially admired Western liberal attitudes towards sexuality and lamented what they saw as sexual hypocrisy in their hometown. Unlike other parts of Papua in which I have lived, such as in Wamena where Dani people, for complex reasons, strive to keep their illnesses secret, disease is not a sensitive subject in Manokwari. Friends talked openly about their aches, nausea and dizziness, eagerly sought the counsel of doctors, and freely consumed medicine. Yet when symptoms were of a sexual nature, the shame associated with sex eclipsed the general openness about illness, so that diseases transmitted through sex became as taboo as sex itself. Not surprisingly, women seemingly afflicted with STDs are reluctant to visit doctors for fear of potentially invasive treatments and of having to sit through a moral diatribe; they also have no faith in medical confidentiality. Even when women suffered horrendous pain associated with pelvic inflammatory disease, which is extremely and unsurprisingly common in Manokwari, they would rather turn deathly pale and keel over, motionless for extended periods, than seek medical help. I encouraged a few women in this condition to see a local gynaecologist, and when they finally did, they found the experience not so bad as they were expecting. 'He had lots of housewives in the waiting room and very modern technologies,' one women explained, 'and so he did not even need me to take off my pants. He just put some cold jelly on my stomach and rubbed a camera over it and watched my infection on a computer. One injection later and I was told to go.' However, this suspiciously ineffective consultation highlights just how much more there is to the problem of sexual health than the inability to talk openly about sex. I can only guess that giving an injection was a kind of compromise in the face of widespread local resistance to taking complete courses of antibiotics.

LH: Well, that might be a difference with Papua New Guinea, where 'Amoxi' is the first, last and middle recourse, and where it's freely available on the street-corner, in tradestores, in one or two departure lounges and through friends. There may also be similarities though, in that perhaps oral doses or injections of antibiotics, say, in the case of a real or suspected STD, are not just tolerated but actually welcomed because they are 'broad spectrum', and they in a sense obviate a full genital inspection. The doctor above seems to be so 'modern' that he doesn't even need to touch the (female) patient, which is perhaps just as welcomed by her. Papua New Guinean patients seem to get a raw deal from doctors and public health officials, in that they are accused of understanding cause and effect, sign and symptom, in vague and nondescript ways, but how much is ever explained to them in the detail warranted?

On another note, your analysis in 'God's Curse and Hysteria' provides an interesting foil for comparison on a number of points.

First, HIV and AIDS are in Papua New Guinea conceptually separated about as often by villagers as by health officials, which is to say not very often. Several similar constructions include 'HIV/AIDS', 'HIV/AIDS virus', 'sikHIV/AIDS' and the like. By contrast, the civil servants and their wives with whom you worked demarcate the two, but not so much in terms of cause and effect as in terms of moral or theological sources. Not surprisingly, cognitive mayhem ensues: many fear something that is physically impossible – 'catching' AIDS (not 'being infected with HIV') and not by engaging in a particular sexual act but by inhabiting a 'mode' of transmission (being promiscuous) but which they deny in themselves. That's a real problem in Papua New Guinea: public health messages disable that sharper sense of transmissive risk for people who just can't imagine themselves to be at risk or to be already infected; or they suggest that HIV 'belongs' in fleeting sexual encounters even though condoms are used.

Second, Christianity is decidedly a minority religion in Indonesia, although what I take to be Christian moral/sexual codes are still deployed to construct and disseminate understandings of AIDS.

Third, seemingly quite like many Papua New Guineans, your Manokwari hosts and informants seemed to have been both disdainful of but also titillated by the literal, visual spectre of AIDS in the bodies of sufferers. Leslie Butt, too, has written interestingly of the first 'AIDS Open House' held in 2001 in the provincial capital of Jayapura. She writes that the over-complicated diagrams and explanations of AIDS and HIV were greatly

> overshadowed by enormous blown-up images of grotesquely deformed
> black bodies suffering from AIDS-related complications. An enormous
> display on STDs other than AIDS captured the most attention. Enlarged
> close-up photographs of diseased sex organs were posted around an area
> where attendees could test their knowledge of STDs and drug treatments.
> The sole condom booth was tucked away at the rear of the hall, staffed by a
> uniformed health worker who blushed crimson whenever anyone approached
> her booth. (Butt 2005: 428)

This public display of disease and genitalia doesn't seem to be the case in the Papua New Guinea I know. I think Papua New Guineans already 'know' (or think they know) what AIDS 'looks like' because they modelled their conceptions of AIDS sufferers from visual material well before they gained any direct, personal knowledge. What role does the visual currently play in risk assessment or understandings of transmission dynamics in Manokwari?

SH: It is true that in Manokwari, as with the rest of Papua, understandings of the disease syndrome are not biomedically nuanced. Instead, there is a deep concern that there is something 'out there', something deadly nasty that in no certain way may come 'in here'. As people do whenever they are confronted with an abstractly hostile force, Papuans are struggling to use whatever information comes their way to make sense of this new thing they call *sakit AIDS* and to help prevent them from becoming infected. Local reasoning in Manokwari, but also in other Papuan towns, goes something like this: people who have 'free sex' ...

LH: That is to say, without obligation?

SH: Yes, but that is of secondary importance. 'Free sex' here refers to indiscriminate and mindless shagging that is more about quantity than the quality of sexual encounters. The local slang synonymous with free sex is BNS or *'baku naik sembarang'*, which can loosely be translated as meaning 'getting on top of anyone'. Such promiscuity can lead, it is thought and said, to *sakit AIDS*, but then again, it's also considered possible to catch 'it' from objects such as toilet seats, from sharing plates and stuff like that. So, it's best if you are not promiscuous but that if you do have sex with someone, look really closely to make sure that they don't have sores like the ones that people with *sakit AIDS* get. In fact, even if you are just hanging out with friends, you should be really mindful of what kind of people they are because if they are secretly 'naughty' then you may catch *sakit AIDS* from them. In the context of locally available information, such as the anti-AIDS posters that are misleading, biased media reports, local gossip and government-sponsored AIDS information sessions, these beliefs are certainly not illogical.

LH: I've got two responses to that. First, you're pointing out for West Papua what I think is true across the border too, namely, that it's not that, or not *just* that rural villagers are being illogical in their association of contagion with HIV and AIDS, but that the premises are wrong or at least inconsistent and that they trickle down from 'above'; they don't just emerge out of rural ignorance or something, which is what NGOs and programme managers and health officials always assume. There are so many mixed messages: there's no medicine, there's a new medicine; don't have sex, do have it (but with the right person); use a condom, but they're not really safe, so go ahead and use a couple at a time. No wonder there's so much cognitive mayhem.

Second, the thing that has so fascinated me about gender relations and sexuality in post-colonial Indonesia is that sex sort of is and sort of isn't 'bad', for lack of a better word; that purity (chastity, maidenhood, covering up the body and so on) is sort of sexy, even eroticised, even despite sex being 'naughty' and even though loss of virginity would be for an unmarried young woman quite damaging to her socially. I wonder whether that plays into the alternating repulsion/titillation that people feel towards people suffering from AIDS. That's something you've found for West Papua that I don't think is true about Papua New Guinea.

SH: At first I was confronted by the conflation of *sakit AIDS* with gruesome bodily suffering and even the relish with which people spoke of this topic. Yet on second thoughts, it did not seem out of place to fetishize the surface, because outward appearances have a special place in local disease histories and also in pre-contact medical beliefs. The idea that one can avoid infection by relying on one's better judgment is based on the resilient cultural assumption that good health is a result of good morality, which is often gauged by the condition of one's skin.

LH: Well, any Papua New Guinean reading this is certainly going to appreciate the similarity! 'Skin' is literal and dermal, genital and sexual, and metaphorical and moral – and a million other things.

SH: This explanation makes sense considering that contagious diseases that have clear symptoms have a long history in Papua, and are still the most common form of illness across the province. In light of Papuan experiences of illness, socially based ideas of health and the quality of local information about HIV and AIDS, focusing on the visual over the invisible, the social over the cellular, and the symptomatic over the asymptomatic, will persist for some time to come.

LH: Fair enough. That seems true with regard to Papua New Guinea, too.

SH: Regarding your point about Christian moral codes informing local responses, I would suggest that the ABC model, as locally applied, is not only filtered through Christian frameworks but also through other dominant traditions and institutions such as Islam, the State and *Adat* (customary law). In the case of the latter, despite the variety of sexualities in pre-contact Papua, such historical practices are considered, when they are known about, as instances of 'bad' tradition and are erased in favour of the view that the monogamous nuclear family is the true and proud Papuan way.

LH: That's also the way in which health officials and politicians in Papua New Guinea deal with ritualised homosexuality, too, very much so. Or *don't* deal with it.

SH: Authorities in these secular, religious and traditional domains all share the moral outlook that A and B, which neatly translate to '*abstinens*' and '*baku setia*' (loyalty), are of higher priority than condoms, which are to be used, if at all, as a last resort if you are so deranged that you cannot uphold righteous sex. Whilst there is a convergence of moral ideologies of these dominant institutions, they espouse this message in different ways and vary in their methods of policing and channelling youth sexuality. Condom availability is not a priority for any church or state programme; but punishment for transgressing sexual boundaries, through forced bride-price payments or demands for compensation, public shaming through expulsion from one's Church or being fired from work, make sure that A and B are kept strongly on the public agenda by the powers-that-be.

✳ ✳ ✳

LH: I wonder if you could tell us a little bit about what you're wrestling with in the Ph.D. dissertation you're writing, beginning with the meaning of your great title: *The Romantic Underground: Expectations and Anger Amongst a Coastal Papuan Community.*

SH: My thesis is about the emergence of courtship in Manokwari, where marrying for love is eulogised but where there is very little tolerance by parents and community members for young men and women getting to know one other. I am interested in exploring how women with ancestral links to the Cenderawasih Bay Islands negotiate this space, how they manage the tensions inside this 'cultural contradiction'. In places in which the desire for romantic courtship and marriages that are based on love are relatively recent phenomenon, public 'dating' is rarely socially acceptable. It reeks of unrestrained sexuality and so opposes the moral parameters imposed by neo-traditional structures, by churches and by the State. Such tension can be creatively mediated, such as in many parts of Asia where the 'arranged meeting' has become an institution. It has been documented elsewhere in Indonesia by Linda Rae Bennett in her recent book, *Women, Islam and Modernity: single women, sexuality and reproductive health in contemporary Indonesia* (2007) and by Leslie Butt in several essays, especially '"Lipstick Girls" and "Fallen Women": AIDS and conspiratorial thinking in Papua, Indonesia' (2005, see also 2008), based upon her fieldwork in Wamena. I found that the strength of desire compels the women in my study to delve into a kind of underground scene of romantic courtship and sexual activity. When exposed through pregnancy or by infection with an STD or simply via rumour, the discrepancy between expectations and reality leads to an eruption of anger and sometimes even violent punishment.

LH: Whose anger? Punishment of whom, by whom?

SH: It all depends on the case, but teachers and relatives, your own or your lovers', most often get angry with 'naughty' teenagers. The former will give them a harsh, moralising lecture and/or suspend and even expel them from school. Adults who are overly concerned and even beat teenagers for suspected sexual immorality tend to be men's wives who want to teach the schoolgirl who seduced their husband a lesson, a family member of one's lover who is outraged that their 'child' was seduced, or one's own parents or senior relatives who, depending on their hot-headedness and penchant for violence, will also single out and beat a 'child' to re-establish family authority after a sexual transgression.

My thesis then explores the ways in which the conservative ethos is at odds with the sexual lives of young people. It explores youth culture and sexual subcultures, and it examines the kinds of violence and suffering that can follow from illegitimate sex, as well as the motivations for a number of practices that clash with the expectation of one's family as well as of Church, State and *Adat* authorities.

LH: Papua New Guinea is similar, with excessive shows of moral force in support of chastity and fidelity that have no grounding in either social-structure or political-economy. How would you characterise that portion of the rhetoric aimed at sexuality, secrecy and the body in Indonesian Papua? Whose sexualities? Whose bodies? How secret are those secrets? What kinds of effects are felt in HIV intervention programmes?

SH: We must be careful with generalising, because sexual rhetoric varies between regions based on such factors as length of exposure to modernising influences, the configuration of pre-contact sexual cultures and the resilience of these traditions. Nonetheless, it is fair to say that new ideas about sexuality from churches, schools and the media have had an impact upon most of the out- of-the-way-places. The idea that the body is a temple that should be used with utmost modesty within monogamous nuclear marriage, and preferably behind the walls of a parents-only bedroom, is core to modern messages. And if the number of pre-schoolers watching television, attending church with their parents, and beginning their education in subjects such as 'moral philosophy' (*pancasila*) is anything to go by, such ideals must at some level be colonising consciousness.

If we take as axiomatic the Sapir-Whorf hypothesis that language constructs reality, then the adoption of Bahasa as the *lingua franca* in even the most remote villages suggests that conservative Malay ideas about sex and the body are conditioning new patterns of thought. For instance, the word for genitals, '*kemaluan*' or 'embarrassment', and the word for vagina, '*liang peranakan*' or 'womb hole', both yield specific ways of thinking about the body, the former being moral and the latter functional.

LH: No different in Papua New Guinea's *lingua franca*, Tok Pisin, where vagina is rendered in many ways, but among them, '*sem bilong yu*' ('your shame') and '*ples nogut*' ('bad place'), and in more functional terms as '*maket*' (a money-maker), '*rot bilong pikinini*' ('birth canal') and also '*rot bilong pik*', meaning to imply the trade partners a man will gain through his wife to her brother and her other male relatives.

SH: Rhetoric about good sex being socially 'useful' sex means that only married people are considered suitable for such activity, and this belief is enshrined in certain practices such as contraception only being available to married people, and hotels ruling, although rarely enforcing, that to book a double room one needs to produce a marriage certificate.

In provincial cities such as are found in Papua, the conservative ethos surrounding sex and the body is even more palpable. Girls in large Indonesian cities are known to dress in miniskirts and singlet tops and even with an Islamic *jilbab*, but in Papua dress codes are more formal and it is considered bad taste to show too much arm or leg. While sexual activity can be assumed in the context of marriage, it can never be spoken of outside this institution and there are plenty of unpleasant consequences for those who dare transgress the normative boundaries. This ensures that sexual secrets remain very secret indeed, and in Manokwari I found not only that girls speak to no one about their sexual endeavours, but also that many girls may even be in denial about their sexual practices. Such shame translates into low sexual confidence that would affect the terms on which sex takes place, and no doubt impacts on the risks young women take, in that it would leave many vulnerable to kinds of sex they do not like. Shame would also affect the attention a woman gives to her body: its relative pleasure during sex, in interpreting the signs of an STD and whether bodily signs warrant a trip to the doctor. What is true of findings about gay men who are in the closet about their sexuality is also true of many women in my study: when people are deeply shamed about their sexuality and can barely admit to themselves that they are sexual creatures and sexually active, they are less likely to take control of their sexual health. When the discrepancy between beliefs and behaviour is so great, the likelihood of using condoms is minimal. Having a condom, after all, implies prior planning of a sexual act that in turn implies awareness and acceptance of oneself as a sexually active subject.

LH: Well, we certainly can't have that.

* * *

LH: In ways similar to the sentiments expressed by Christian leaders and led in Papua New Guinea, it seems that Indonesian authorities are only too pleased that AIDS has come along and lent its considerable metaphorical power in religious and even community, ostensibly secular, settings. Naomi McPherson, for example, has written of rural West New Britain Province that

> From the Christian perspective, one can only blame oneself for choosing to engage in immoral, sinful behavior and punishment does not rest with the community but with God, who, for example, punishes sexual transgressors by giving them *sik*AIDS. Even though they have been punished, a stigma is attached to known sinners; people with AIDS are stigmatised not only for their evident sinning but also for having brought *sik*AIDS into the community. (McPherson 2008: 231)

In Indonesian Papua, has the wholesale rearrangement of sexuality been attempted in the name of HIV and AIDS? Do you think it would have continued to occur despite their appearance, I mean, for example, to expedite the aims of *transmigrasi* or aid the mission of nation-building?

SH: I get the feeling that in Papua New Guinea there is a great deal more discourse on HIV and AIDS than in Indonesian Papua, where other concerns, mostly to do with dramatic changes at the political level, are dominating collective emotions. In Indonesian Papua people are concerned with the rising rates of HIV, but as the predicted epidemic is still in its early stages, these rates are just that: statistics that have not yet been felt in the embodied sense of suffering, of caring for or even of burying loved ones who have died. Of greater and more real danger to most Papuans, and especially women, is the fear of being exposed as 'naughty' (*nakal*). No teenager wants to shame his or her family and possibly drag them through the ordeal of seeking justice in *Adat* courts or at the police station. Church leaders, teachers and other moralising officials still prefer to manipulate the fear of slipping outside the 'good girl/boy/woman/man' category and so, when *sakit AIDS* is evoked, it is usually as a lesser and more distant danger alongside other possible dangers. Health workers will just as likely evoke the fear of malaria, pregnancy or *masuk angin* for overly mobile young people as they will invoke *sakit AIDS*. *Masuk angin* literally means 'entering winds', a humoral-based illness of Malay origins said to be caused by winds entering the body. Church leaders, for their part, are prone to drop the term *sakit AIDS* into their list of Armageddon-like scenarios when giving a sermon on the consequences of giving in to modern temptations.

In this sense, *sakit AIDS* is evoked as a threat but rarely exclusively, since that lack of experience with the disease syndrome, the higher priority of avoiding shame, and the belief that in the end you can avoid *sakit AIDS* by having sex with healthy-looking people, reduces its coercive power and lessens its discursive weight. As Paul Farmer found in his longitudinal

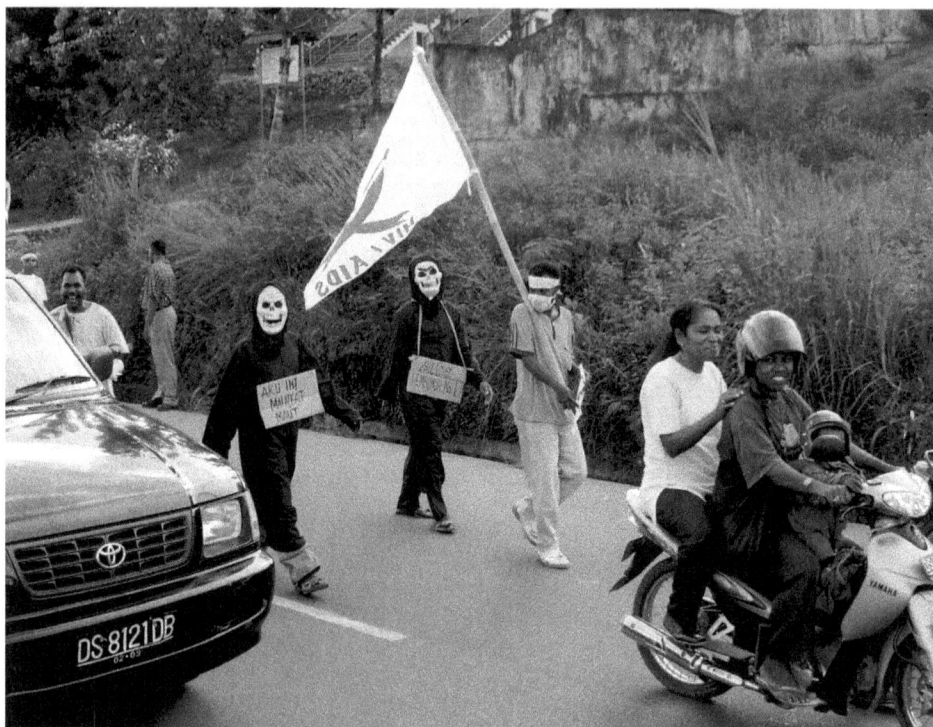

GKI theology school cares about HIV/AIDS

research in Haiti, as HIV comes to have its impacts upon people's lives, the meanings and symbolic potency of HIV and AIDS can alter; indeed, I am detecting elements of this already in Manokwari. In 2006 a gathering joined the initiative of a group called 'GKI theology school cares about HIV/AIDS', who held a gentle street protest with some, as we can see in the picture, dressed as death angels (*malaikat maut*) and others holding placards that read '*stop sex bebas*' or '*stop BNS: Baku Naik Sebarang*'. This is a somewhat scurrilous term that means 'to get on top randomly'.

It is likely that this group, as with all good university fringe groups, has the potential to morph into a mainstream movement. But even if it did, AIDS would not have the power to contribute to the 'wholesale rearrangement of sexuality', for the simple reason that sex, in its 'useful' guise inside monogamous marriage, was rearranged decades ago by the Church in the name of salvation and by the State in the name of progress.

LH: Okay, so that's two ways in which such discourses were already in progress before the arrival of HIV and AIDS. Now that they (and discourse about them) have arrived, however, I wonder whether this doesn't raise other questions about the ways in which people understand transmissive risks in the context of attempts at Christian salvation or in the name of nation-building. I mean, in-migrating Indonesians seem in official documents not to pose risks to one another or to indigenous Papuans, just as I have highlighted elsewhere in this book that elite national males and expatriate males are not 'targeted' by any public health campaigns or slogans. I'm thinking out loud that perhaps that's because no one really wants to implicate the social identities involved in sexual networking, for example, 'politician', 'step-father', 'teacher' and the like. I think that it remains too difficult to confront squarely the privileges of gender, class, political power and ruling, and so instead policy-makers and public health messages target the female persons who engage in it. The work of our friend Leslie Butt and several other colleagues has shown that Papuans aren't engaging in commercial sex with Indonesians in the context of the dense social and other obligations that otherwise give meaning to sexual networking. She and others have shown that gift-giving expectations have been affected and that sex 'takes place outside of valued cultural norms' and that AIDS-related interventions ostensibly designed to help Papuans can end up 'favouring Indonesians' (Butt, Numbery and Morin 2002b: 31 and 45). What is it about changing norms of sex, Sarah, especially around gifts, court-ship expectations, marriage and reciprocity, that have implications for HIV transmission and its prevention?

SH: It is found, in diverse areas of the world, that when women identify as sex workers, and notwithstanding the power discrepancies with 'clients', they are more likely to use condoms. This rule of thumb, while also true for Papua, is complicated by the evidence that although Papuan women may accept money or goods for sex with men from a number of ethnic categories, it is usually only with Indonesian men that they will recognise the commercial nature of such a transaction. Papuans, on the other hand, are involved in dense sexual networks that are characterised by emotional involvement and generalised reciprocity with multiple sexual partners that in local terms are called 'friends'.

LH: Just like in Papua New Guinea, with '*koap poro*' ('fuck buddies') on the one hand, who may be more or less 'regular' partners, and, on the other hand, those to whom women refer as 'boyfriends', with whom they might have shared a single sexual encounter. It's about the money, certainly not the sex; it's about keeping the material skids greased and a belief in love that keeps them trying.

SH: In this context, sexual transactions for money or goods are more likely to be interpreted by the values of the gift economy and not by the market economy. Sex is therefore rarely cognised as commercial, and so condoms are rarely used. The upshot here is that anti-AIDS messages inadvertently favour straight-haired Indonesians for pro-condom messages, and are more likely to resonate in relationships between Papuan women and Indonesian men.

 Aside from this economic explanation, the use of condoms is complicated by socio-emotional factors. Women with whom I spoke said that using condoms with 'friends' is synonymous with accusing a lover of being dirty and diseased, whereas to have a lover suggest the use of condoms with one is synonymous with one being called promiscuous and a slut. While it's never nice to be thought of as polluted, it's much worse to be considered a slut, for when a woman tips over into 'slut' territory it is harder to 'catch' a good man. At a deeper level, there is something existential at play with aversion to condoms in the context of romantic passions. Whenever relationships fall more into the imaginative realm of the romantic, in the sense that it is the pleasure of the company that in itself motivates, then trust becomes an issue. No matter how illusory, the need to feel as though one is the 'one and only', even if just for the moment, seems to be inherent to the logic of romance and positions condoms as a natural metaphor for the blocking, the interruption of trust. Amongst heterosexual intimates, the desire to avoid pregnancy may override the need to prove trust, and yet in many parts of Papua where it is thought babies are made from serial intercourse with just the one person, this is less likely. Unfortunately, this belief can raise the idea that having sex with multiple partners is 'safer'.

LH: All of that sounds most Papua New Guinean, Sarah, and it's been hinted at by Kathy Lepani, by me, by Carol Jenkins, by Holly Wardlow and by a number of other fieldworkers. I think that this is where we need to consider frankly the disadvantages, the negative public health consequences of the lack of sexual and reproductive health education. It is too easy to blame such cognitive dissonance and condom disinformation on powerful bishops or relative educational gaps (that is, the presumption that if students just stayed in school longer, they'd learn healthier attitudes to these things). It makes more sense to me to imagine just how 'sticky' gender-conservative mainstream public health messages and campaigns have been since about 1990. We need to do the intellectual genealogy-type work of tracing when, by whom and, especially, how consistently, risk has been externalised away from the (ideal) norms of faithful monogamy and how sex-negative those messages, implicitly and explicitly, have been.

The intellectual genealogy of such is lengthy. One of the books I used to see pretty often in Papua New Guinea that just sickens me every time I pick it up is *Christian Marriage and Family Life*, by a male author, Ian Malins (1987), but despite this I know that his model is quite popular. One of the headings I remember is 'Submission: thy name is wife', and it informs the reader that God planned it so that women come under men's leadership, supporting them and helping and not opposing them ... no matter what, and even if they're beating the shit outta you (e.g. Bradley 1998 and 2000; Macintyre 1998). The Law Reform Commission's own report, for instance, found that 'the majority of rural Papua New Guineans, especially of males, appeared to be in favour of wife-beating' (Bradley 1998: 353). Malins said, further, that 'The wife's part in keeping the marriage strong is for her to submit to her husband. Even if your husband is harsh and unkind, the teaching of submission still applies' (1987: 67). Another book that I've seen a fair number of times in guest-houses and second-hand clothing shops (where second-hand books are sometimes sold) is called *One Woman's Liberation*. It reminds its readers that 'Pat and I consider the girls' knowledge of Satan part of their sex education', and that the temptation 'to misuse any of God's gifts ... *comes from the devil*' (Boone 1972: 92). Fair enough: the author's pop-star husband *did* go to Vegas, and 25 years later he *did* record the mildly rough-leather, *In a Metal Mood* (Boone 1997). Yet and still, this kind of Satan-Made-Me-Do-It attitude does not well prepare a person in this day and age (even in 1972, when Pat Boone's wife published her autobiography, let alone 35 years later) to understand his or her body, to come to one's sexual desire under one's own steam, to know enough about sexually transmitted pathogens so as to avoid them. As the author herself says (Boone 1972: 97), 'I don't like things I don't understand.' Indeed.

✳ ✳ ✳

LH: There seems to be inordinate management of rhetoric about HIV transmission, rather than of the vectors themselves. The HIVab seroprevalence of indigenous Papuans is touted frequently in Indonesian mass media and in international health circles as being, at least until recently, double, triple or even quadruple the level in the remainder of Indonesia (for example, *Jakarta Post* 2007a). Not surprisingly, the 'knowledge' of Papuans of such matters is held to be correspondingly low, with one newspaper story titled: 'Half in Indonesia's remote Papua province unaware of HIV/AIDS' (*Jakarta Post* 2007b). Just like lots of similar claims made in Papua New Guinean newspapers and press releases, the claim is absurd logically and otherwise, but it is also accompanied by the further claim that HIVab seroprevalence is said to be 15-times higher than the rest of the nation. How does the *Jakarta Post* get away with such outlandish claims? Do indigenous Papuans ever fight back? Is there any attempt at truth in reporting in Indonesian popular media?

SH: Firstly, newspapers everywhere get away with outlandish claims, especially when journalists believe their claims are grounded in 'facts'. In Indonesia statistics are a very weak kind of 'fact', yet the media and the government obscure this truth with a near obsession with statistics. The need to report numbers is, no doubt, born from the need to feel some mastery over the HIV problem and to feel that at least something is being done about it. Personally, I have always felt suspicious of the claim that Papua has many, many more HIV and AIDS cases than any other part of the archipelago, where the 'fault lines' are just as plentiful and intense as in Papua. How can the prevalence of HIV in Papua so vastly exceed that in Bali, a worldwide destination for sex tourism? How can it greatly surpass cases of HIV in Java, the Indonesian island that has the greatest number of intravenous drug users and absolute poor? The inferior quality of health surveillance across the country, not to mention other factors that prevent reliable enumeration, suggest that an adequate epidemiological map of HIV cannot be tabulated for Papua.

In light of this, while the generation of statistics may allude to trends, more than anything else it should be seen as a politically motivated activity. Some clues to the quality of this motivation are found in the sweeping generalisations of media reports whereby Papuans are depicted as highly sexed, lacking in morals and ignorant. As you say, it is absurd to suggest that some dreadful disease afflicts Papuans to such an extent and that they don't even know about it. In dominant discourse the stress is on what Papuans lack – they lack straight hair, they lack rice-cultivating technologies, they lack sexual restraint and they lack awareness. What they do have is never explored. Some of the other things determining what they lack, for

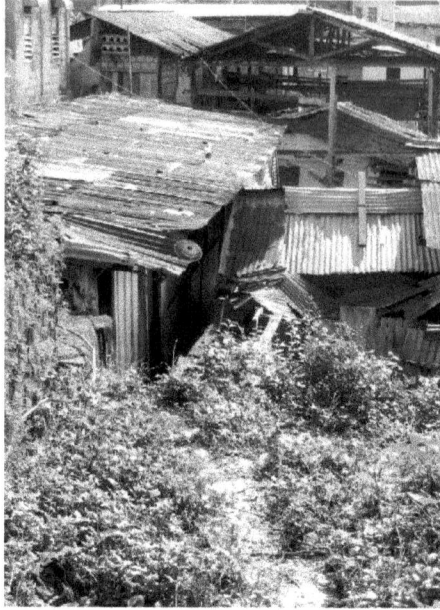

Jayapura brothel

example, access to employment, decent health care and education, are also not explored. So, yes, the national media always report on HIV in Papua in a simplistic manner that blames Papuans for the spread of HIV and that reinforces the national view of *'Papua bodoh'* – stupid Papuans. Papuans, for their part, feel resentment about generalised racism and disadvantage, but no, they have not been known to fight a libelous media article or to sue the Health Department for statistical slander.

LH: In the past three years, especially as I've worked on Daru and along the north-west coast of Papua New Guinea I've found that many Papua New Guineans blame Indonesian Papua, and especially its provincial capital and administrative centre, Jayapura and Merauke, for infections now being reported in villages and provincial capitals along the border. More than anything, there is the suggestion that they are kind of Sodom and Gomorrah for Papua New Guineans, repulsive and titillating simultaneously, blasphemous and irresistible. From what I was told, the rude brothel depicted here, although staffed by Javanese and Balinese women, serves an almost wholly Papua New Guinean clientele. Tellingly, it sits underneath the Papua New Guinea consulate in Jayapura, but on the other side of the hill, down a long, winding stone staircase and then bush track. While on leave from my work in Vanimo I was directed by two health officials to this and to two other brothels, one rude and informal, the other spiff and state-regulated, and they said more or less the same thing, that these brothels served a significant cross-border trade.

I guess my question is what Jayapura (or Merauke) means for non-Papuan Indonesians in terms of risk and pleasure. Is it considered just one big red-light district? Can non-Papuan Indonesians hold simultaneously the notions that Papuan sex workers are the ones to be feared, on the one hand, but also that the abstemious, Islamic Indonesian male body is, or at least appears to be so in Jayapura, a promiscuous one? Do Papuan or non-Papuan Indonesian men find Papua New Guinean women alluring in any way relevant to HIV and AIDS?

SH: I would imagine that in Papua New Guinea, Jayapura would represent cheap, anonymous and abundant sexual opportunities, while as far as non-Papuan Indonesians are concerned, Jayapura is just another Indonesian provincial town where you can get cheap, anonymous and abundant sex. If Papuan towns were scaled according to their 'red light' quality, Jayapura would in no way be at the top. I would imagine that we could measure this hypothetical scale by the proximity of the centre of town to the town's main brothel. On this continuum Sorong, a town on the tip of the Bird's Head where oil mining is the dominant industry, would be at the 'Sexual Mecca' end of the continuum as its main brothel is located in the centre of town. Manokwari, on the other hand, would probably be at the other end of the continuum for it takes several hours to drive to the main brothel. Jayapura would be located somewhere between the two poles since its main brothel lies along the road connecting the town with its satellite city, Sentani. By 'main' brothel I mean what is known in Indonesia as *lokalisasi*. Unlike the makeshift brothel in this picture, *lokalisasi* run under government supervision and are considered the 'top end', as the product is women from other areas of Indonesia who are renowned for their paler skin. These women are not only considered more beautiful but, due to visits by doctors who, I was told, give the workers regular antibiotic injections, are thought to be relatively free of STDs.

LH: That raises the issue of the political-economy of sex, doesn't it, the different venues and 'labour forms' of sexual networking, and how the providers and purchasers of sexual services find each other and all of the other players and agents involved. All of the cities, towns and administrative centres in Papua New Guinea, and in addition, the rural enclaves, have sex industries, and like everywhere else, it involves taxi-cab drivers, policemen, local businessmen, security guards and the like. What's it like across the border?

SH: It is difficult to know exactly how many people make up the sex industry in Papua, but the industry can be divided into two broad structures, each with two main forms. The first kind is of the organised variety, whereby women, who have usually been trafficked through debt bondage, provide sex in indoor venues for the financial gain of people other than themselves. One form of organised sex is *lokalisasi*; the other form, which is more common, runs out of different venues: karaoke bars, discotheques, massage parlours, cafes and private brothels like the one in the above picture. While women in *lokalisasi* cannot refuse sex with a client, rules about whether a woman is obliged to provide sex for a client in these other venues varies and so, too, do the work and living conditions. While workers in *lokalisasi* are under heavy surveillance, women in other locations may have more freedom to travel outside, although usually chaperoned. Whether they want to go out, given the murderous rage many feel towards migrant sex workers in Papua, is another matter.

LH: Ditto, Papua New Guinea.

SH: In their report on the trafficking of women and girls in fifteen provinces of Indonesia, the ICMC and Solidarity Center report that women who work in organised prostitution in Papua have usually fallen prey to recruiting agents who make good money from trafficking females for the sex industry in Papua. In this scheme young women, mostly from Sulawesi but also from parts of East Nusa Tenggara and Java, are approached with the offer of a well-paid job in Papua, perhaps in a supermarket or restaurant or as the manager of a karaoke bar. Upon arrival these women discover that there is no job as promised and that, to pay back the money they borrowed to get there as well as the ongoing costs of boarding in the brothel, they must provide sex for clients. Those tend to be Indonesian and Papuan men who earn a regular wage. Due to its economic growth and the beliefs that Papua is job-rich and that indigenous Papuans do not want to work, non Papuan young women are gullible to such a promise.

LH: There's a good example of the tribal/ethnic/racial cleavages in sex industries that I've written about (Hammar n.d., 1996a and b).

SH: Solidarity International found that many women in such establishments are high-school graduates and even hold degrees. They suggest that, being already aspiring, such highly educated women may be more vulnerable to job deception because of the sense that they are deserving and are qualified for such 'good' work. Aside from the perceptions of provincial prosperity making deception easier, the growing trend of sex trafficking to Papua is facilitated by other factors. For one, domestic and foreign boats and ships make regular visits to Papuan ports for cargos of minerals and timber, just as do Indonesian and Malaysian ones to Vanimo and Wewak and Madang. Not only does this offer ease of access for trafficking women, it underscores that geographical isolation and reliance on boats and air transport makes it harder for women to escape. The shifting population of sailors and other visitors, as well as migrants and a class of Papuans who have prospered, contribute to a highly skewed sex ratio in the province, the highest in Indonesia, and generates a strong demand for commercial sex. Add to this the demonstrated lack of will of most government officials in Papua to recognise that there is something wrong with trafficking women in the province, or that it even exists.

In the other major form I mentioned, sex takes place in what Leslie Butt has referred to as 'open sex sites' – temporary shelters, or outdoors. This labour form of sexual networking, which in reality is a complex constellation of forms can, again following Leslie's lead (see Butt, Numbery and Morin 2002a), be broken into two types, 'secret sex' and 'street sex'. These forms differ from one another in terms of emotional involvement, quality of sexual pleasure and degree of financial calculation. Secret sex takes place in a clandestine manner between Papuans of a similar cultural group and is typically motivated by felt affection and the pursuit of mutual pleasure. Secret sex can be understood in economic terms because a woman likes to receive gifts or money from her lover, but this is understood through cultural understandings of exchange relations. For Papuan women, the ethnic profile of a sex partner is significant insofar as having sex with foreigners, either in the sense of being outside one's tribal group or with straight-haired Indonesians, seems to be a critical moment in the transition from having 'secret sex' to having 'street sex'. Street sex, which is engaged in by Papuans and Indonesians, more approximates 'prostitution' insofar as payment is clearly negotiated and is less intimate. Street sex promotes more commercialised relationships. Street sex costs a great deal less than brothel-based sex and may be 'managed' by middlemen or else the workers may arrange the sexual transaction themselves. Both men and women, Papuan and Indonesian, perform street sex, although the latter tend to work from a fixed location such as a *warung* (food stall), selling tea and soft drinks as a base. The numbers of *waria* (transsexuals) are rising on the streets of urban Papua, and while they are more often Indonesian, Papuan *waria* are an emerging trend.

LH: I'd say the same thing about Port Moresby and Lae, and Aly Murray has written similarly (2001) about what she calls 'New Emerging Sexualities' in Indonesia and elsewhere.

SH: In terms of freedom of movement, the ability to indulge themselves by buying fashionable clothes and cheap cosmetics, the choices they have in what to eat and drink, and even where to live (many lived in groups in boarding houses), street-based sex workers are better off than their venue-based sisters. Yet by not being confined to the employers' premises, street-sex workers are consistently finding themselves in situations of high risk for violence, unprotected sex and sickness due to unsanitary conditions.

This leads into your second question. Brothels like the one in the picture, and Papuan women who work off the streets, are thought less clean than those in the *lokalisasi*, and yet the fact that Muslim migrant men still patronise Papuans suggests that they either truly believe they can avoid infection (most likely by inspecting her physical condition), or will take the risk to get bargain sex, or there are less rational psychic forces involved. I remember once reading that in Northern Thailand men interpret risky sex through Buddhist notions of destiny and through the framework of their other great passion, gambling (see Fordham 2005). Even when they knew they stood a good chance of contracting HIV in town, the writer argued that these men enjoyed patronising sex workers not only for the immediate pleasure they brought but for their value as the ultimate thrill of all – testing and tempting fate. I am not saying that this is the case with non-Papuan men who patronise non-regulated sex workers in Papuan cities, just that it would be worthwhile to investigate further the motivations and understandings of such men.

With regards to your last question, while the brothels in Jayapura may arouse men from Papua New Guinea, I cannot say the reverse is true; for even when we take into account the seemingly pan-human eroticisation of difference, this tends to be offset by the increasingly hegemonic ideals of beauty in Indonesia, not to mention the lower cost of sex in Indonesia. In Indonesia beauty is scaled according to the straightness of hair, the paleness of skin and the ability to adorn oneself with feminine accoutrements such as hair clips, clippy-clop heels and lipstick. To put it bluntly, the dark-skinned, frizzy-haired appearance of Melanesians gives them less market value, and in Papua New Guinea, where women are less likely to 'do' modern beauty, this is especially so. It is disturbing to see just how hegemonic, in the sense of infused consciousness, this aesthetic ideal has become in Papua, where hair is kept either short, slicked back or chemically straightened and where faces, especially on the Sabbath, are heavily powdered.

✳ ✳ ✳

LH: Leslie Butt has taken conspiracy theory in Indonesian Papua to be more of an accurate, detailed, even pragmatic reflection of Papuan lived experience under Indonesian rule than one of magical thinking or merely 'incorrect' understandings of what's 'really' happening (Butt 2005). By looking at tropes of 'lipstick girls' and 'fallen women' in HIV epidemiology she examines closely the 'inconsistencies and disjunctures' that 'evolve from and echo conspiratorial strategies of governance in the province' (2005: 414). Much in the same way, Karen Kroeger has argued that rumours are 'more than just wrong or incomplete information; they are socially constructed, performed and interpreted narratives, a reflection of beliefs about the way the world works in a particular place and time' (Kroeger 2003: 243). Stuart Kirsch in *Reverse Anthropology* takes Yonggom discourses of sorcery seriously to reveal indigenous indictments of environmental damage and the duplicity of mega-corporations (Kirsch 2006). There seems to be a revitalisation of anthropological interest in such matters, in rumour and especially in conspiracy theory, especially so in context of HIV and AIDS. What do state- and military-level authorities in Indonesia think about such conspiracy theories? Does it have any implications for public health, say, in treatment regimes, clinic attendance or condom usage? Are there any such examples ongoing in Manokwari?

SH: I don't know what state and military authorities think of conspiracy theories. I would guess, though, that they would hover between not caring about such triviality and using these so-called 'irrational beliefs' to justify their notion that the grassroots are silly, even stupid. It is more likely, however, that those locally referred to as 'big people' (*orang besar*) would not be aware of the socio-political beliefs of those referred to as 'little people' (*orang kecil*). Because modern hierarchies in Papua have followed Malay lines, it is considered disrespectful to bother a big person with what would be seen as the gossip of little people.

As conspiracy theory thrives in conditions of great social upheaval, weak civil society and vast discrepancies in power and wealth, it is inevitable that in Papua, HIV and AIDS will feed off uncertainties and the gaps in information. Unfortunately, this piecing together of an HIV narrative using the available evidence and through a personalised framework of attribution has the effect of creating a more virus-friendly environment. In Manokwari the conspiratorial view that sex workers brought HIV into Papua gives rise to the socially harmful view that risk can be demarcated on moral lines. If pathogens run along the axis of social goodness then it follows that all you have to do, to avoid illness, is be good.

LH: Or at least have sex with them. That is so true in PNG, too. Anna-Karina Hermkens writes of her research in Madang and Port Moresby among devoutly Catholic women that 'people strongly believe in God's power to safeguard them against HIV infection. This indicates a belief in God as protector of those who have strong faith and lead a good Christian life. At the same time, it reflects a belief that those who have AIDS have called down misfortune on themselves through immoral behaviour' (Hermkens 2007: 6).

SH: In a contradictory vein but equally valid is the belief that AIDS is contagious, which is impossible, although HIV is infectious. This misinformation or attitude can compromise the care provided by health workers. One told me that when a person comes to a hospital with *sakit AIDS* they have to lock them up in a small room adjacent to the main building, push their meals under the door and call someone to take them away to Jakarta where they know what to do with them. Fear of 'catching' *sakit AIDS* has given rise to rumours about evil people, such as certain taxi drivers who have sought to infect people who ride with them. I was even told about a male paramedic (*mantri*) who was spreading infection with his syringe and so, thankfully, was murdered. Although it is not clear whether the *mantri* had filled his syringe with blood containing pathogens or was using a dirty needle, stories like this are damaging of trust in health workers. The power of this rumour, however, is nowhere near the conspiratorial potential of a recent news report that the Health Department in Papua has received a proposal for inserting or implanting micro-chips into the bodies of people with HIV. The details of the story, such as the fact that it was only a suggestion (albeit a perverse one), will be lost on many Papuans. Instead, they will likely fixate on the themes of technological power and state control as they refract through older conspiratorial ideas about the ability of computers to perform superhuman feats and the common belief that government-sponsored family planning is a means of sterilising Papuans. Significantly, the fear of branding and surveillance to which this rumour gives rise could further fuel the belief that health professionals cannot be trusted and that clinics should be avoided. In other words, this rumour could erode trust in medical clinics, which would pose a major obstacle to any future anti-HIV initiatives.

✳ ✳ ✳

LH: I wanted next to talk about the border between the two countries and, more specifically, the road from Vanimo to Jayapura. Borders are funny things. Even to say that this one is porous on a good day is to say too much. This photo, snapped in Jayapura at the beach of embarkation and disembarkation,

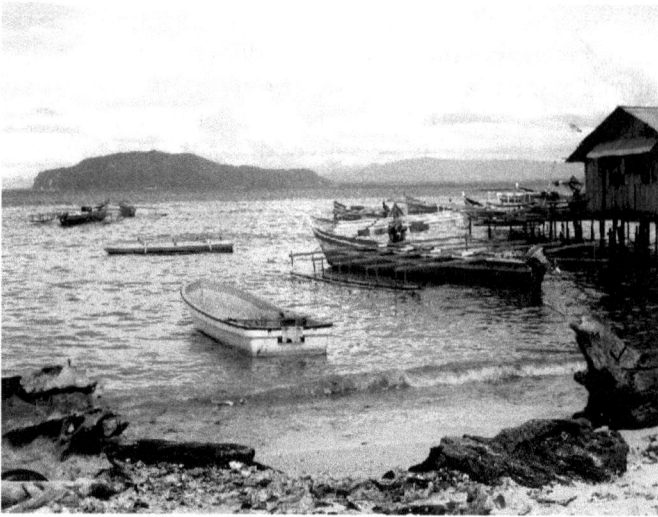

Jayapura disembarkation

looks eastward back across to Papua New Guinea, whose border is approached and crossed many hundreds of times each day. Doug Porter's comments about another border are very much apropos here, in noting that '[t]he nexus of HIV transmission across this territory is a metaphor for the globalisation of investment, trade, and cultural identity' (1997: 213). In this case, Papua New Guineans can get a TBC card signifying their cultural identity (and rights) as a Traditional Border Crosser, shop to their heart's content in Jayapura, and come home to resell the products they've purchased. That includes the por-nographic videos, the sex toys and the love-potions that are illegal in Papua New Guinea and the 'feminine hygiene' products that are perhaps harmful, the soaps, the vaginal pessaries and whatnot. What is it that non-Papuan Indonesians want in Papua New Guinea and from Papua New Guineans?

SH: As I have pointed out, Papua New Guinean women hold little allure for Indonesian men and so, as far as Indonesian Papuans and other Indonesians are concerned, Papua New Guinea has come to be seen as a trading opportu-nity. Although I haven't been on the road from Jayapura to Vanimo since it opened up, I am told that people exchange goods at the border. Commodity flows are heavier from Indonesia, where drum whisky and Asian-made prod-ucts can be sold at inflated prices in Papua New Guinea, although there are instances of the reverse, as with trading in the very popular snack of Papua New Guinea-made Twisties. Papua New Guinea has a market for different grades of cocoa and vanilla, whereas in Indonesia this produce has a low blanket value, meaning, that such products all fetch the one price regardless of quality. Indonesian Papua's superior quality vanilla and cocoa tend to get traded at the border. When I have asked Indonesian Papuans in Vanimo of their motivation for being there, most respond by saying: to escape boredom, to scratch the itch of curiosity and to enjoy a change of scenery. While these reasons have particular cultural meanings, at the core, a trip to Papua New Guinea offers Indonesian Papuans what people generally get out of travelling.

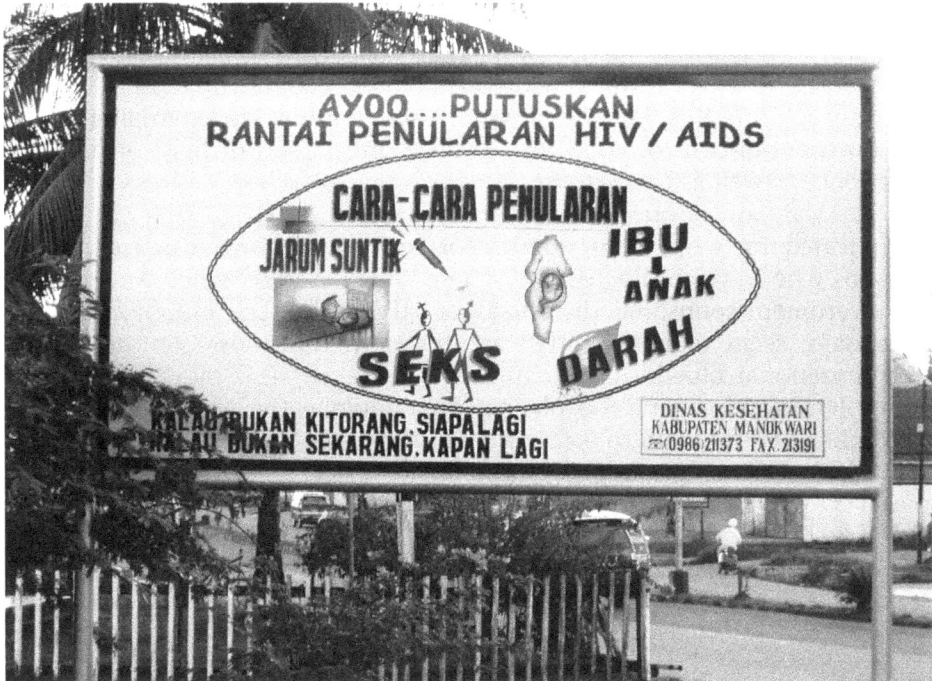

Avoid AIDS

LH: One of Leslie Butt's co-authored papers, 'The Smokescreen of Culture' (Butt, Numbery and Morin 2002a) is insightful about the unwillingness of organisations to examine their pronouncements about 'risk' and 'target groups' more critically. This is especially so when women and girls in prostitution or who themselves more freely sell their sexual labour are compared to this seeming catch-all, teflon-coated category of 'housewives'. It seems to me that the Indonesian government-bureaucratic regime has done all too much to externalise risk, projecting it generally eastwards, toward Papua, and downwards at the same time, toward disaffected youth, drug users and especially the dreaded 'sex workers'. Could you reflect a moment on the forms that externalisation of risk takes in Indonesia and perhaps why this might be so? What function does the 'housewife' body play in intervention language and programmes?

SH: I have already mentioned that, using a statistical sleight of hand, blame has throughout Indonesia been pushed eastwards towards Papua, whilst within Papua, blame has been pushed downwards and in recent years, scapegoating categories have alternated from sex workers to wayward youth. When *sakit AIDS* first emerged, media reports gave rise to the understanding that foreigners, in particular Thai fishermen, had brought HIV to Papua; and that sex workers in the brothels the fishermen frequented and elsewhere were 'spreading' *sakit AIDS*. Already a despised category in the minds of Papuans and Malays, sex workers were an easy target for blame. Throughout the 1990s 'good' women were known to stage protests outside certain brothels, whilst the government focused their interventions on 'cleaning up' *lokalisasi*. Some may say the belief that the doctor makes regular visits to *lokalisasi* is behind the decrease in anger towards sex workers for spreading HIV, and men have certainly told me this, but the province-wide, nationwide externalisation of risk onto out-of-control youth can best be understood in light of personal experience as well as the *zeitgeist*.

The standard moral binaries that underpin scapegoating are being complicated by a growing number of real, well-known cases of 'good' Papuans who have contracted HIV. These same binaries, which were central to government-sponsored discourses of HIV and AIDS, especially in the early days, seem to have shifted as official rhetoric now conforms more to international blueprints. For instance, there are now more posters and pamphlets, which are still the materials that underlay the dominant approach to combat HIV, that aim to communicate all the modes of HIV transmission. While promoting biomedical truths may be an improvement on older messages, such truths are lost through vague, muddled, overcrowded and ultimately, misleading graphics, as these photographs depict. By presenting a multitude of scenarios in which one may contract HIV, transmission is seemingly democratised. Combined with the fewer degrees of separation between the infected and uninfected, this sense that it could happen to anyone has seen Indonesian Papuans turn their emotional energies inwards, from hating the fallen women 'out there' to exhibiting greater concern for morality within one's community.

Although there is now more UNAIDS-like literature in circulation, Suharto era-type graphics are still abundant and can resonate with the heightened concern for the morality of one's own. For instance, in Manokwari there are two nearly identical billboards (depicted here), one with a figure dangling from ropes over a steaming pot that reads 'save the young generation from the dangers of drugs', and the other with a figure also strung up in ropes with the words 'save the young generation from HIV AIDS'. The fact that one mentions drugs and the other AIDS is less important here than what they share: the message that drugs and AIDS are much the same things: they have the same 'causes', a lack of care; and the same fate, death; and because they threaten youth, it is up to everyone to guide young people in the right direction.

This shift in blame from outsiders to insiders and the central position of morality in contemporary discourse can be understood in light of the socio-political changes in Papua that have occurred at the end of the previous and at the beginning of this new millenium. The push for democracy has seen ethnic pride, or *Papuanisasi*, find its voice on the streets and through the proliferating print media. The concern for Papuan identity and morality is evident in recent vernacular expressions about HIV and AIDS. The AIDS poster that has served in so many venues (see: http://www.papuaweb.org/dlib/tema/hiv-aids/plaket.pdf), which many theology school protestors were holding during their demonstration, shows seven young people who could easily have been plucked off Jayapura's streets, all dressed up, but with skin tones and hairstyles and clothing styles that reflect broad characteristics of Papuan ethnicity. The text 'we are Papuans together'

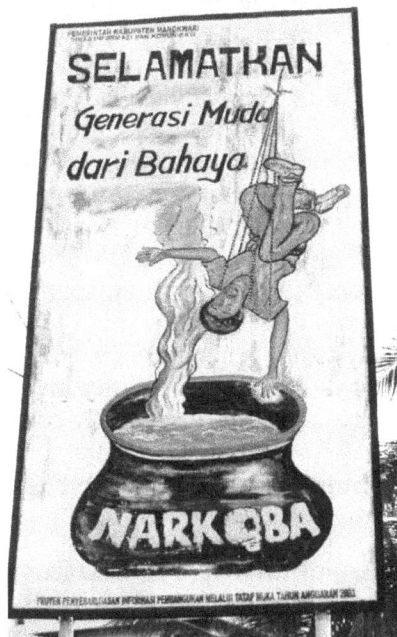

Save the Young Generation From the Dangers of Drugs

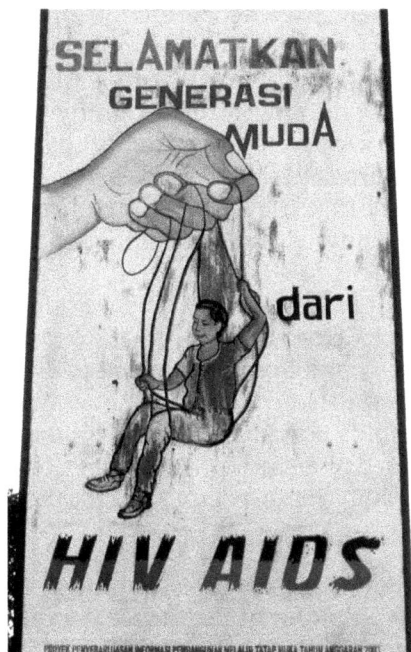

Save the Young Generation From HIV AIDS

highlights how Papuan unity and pride has become the dominant idiom in attempts to push the message of vigilance in the face of HIV and AIDS. The implementation of Special Autonomy in Papua has influenced the drawing of new administrative regencies and seen an increasing number of Papuans enter the middle and upper echelons of the civil service. Indeed, it can be said that the regional government, from the governor and mayors (*bupati*) down, is now orchestrated by an elite class of Papuans and that this Papuanisation of the government has had the effect of blurring the boundaries between friend and foe. This state of affairs is symbolically projected onto the social body: HIV is no longer simply 'out there' as 'the enemy', but rather, may be amongst us, may even be one of us.

LH: A newspaper article published on 5 May in the *Jakarta Post* (2007a) was titled 'Impact of High-risk Sexual Behavior Knocks on the Doors of Nation's Families'. It quotes the national AIDS Commission secretary, Nafsiah Mboi, as hand-wringing over the apparently rising number of housewives being infected with HIV, if not yet beginning en masse to suffer from AIDS. More to the point, it shows a prevalence figure that exceeds that of 'sex workers'. The statistic thrown out was '43 percent of HIV infections in Papua occurred among women who were not sex workers'. Where does this sharp division come from, and what do those numbers mean in the sense of ideology and history?

SH: We must first understand that in Indonesia the *ibu rummah tangga* or 'housewife' is a category that has emerged from concerns about the role of women in the construction of a modern nation. At the level of the state, being a housewife is the only legitimate category of womanhood and should come, ideally, many years past menarche, after receiving a full state education, plus after formal training in 'women's crafts' (*ketrampilan wanita*) such as cooking, sewing, beauty, hygiene and etiquette. Despite these modern requirements, housewives are expected not to be individualised, in the sense that they must remain loyal to the tasks of servicing, containing the sexuality of and strengthening the moral foundations of their nuclear family. This role is considered so important because the morally sound nuclear family is considered the keystone for the development of national prosperity. Considering its place in history and its symbolic potency, any woman who does not follow this trajectory is considered 'less developed' (*kurang maju*) or 'simple' (*sederhana*) or else a 'WTS' (prostitute). A WTS, or as the acronym unfolds, a woman without morals (*wanita tuna susila*), is mythologically construed as a kind of vixen who not only wastes her reproductive potential, but through her predatory approach to men, undermines the reproductive basis of marriage.

LH: Yeah, that's been common in Papua New Guinea newspapers and from the pulpit for at least three decades. 'Pamuks on the rise' was how one newspaper editorial titled it. This sounds also like what Holly Wardlow says about so-called *pasindia meri* in the Tari Basin of Southern Highlands Province who, by refusing any longer to remain 'under the legs' of men and by protesting their own previous victimisation, truncate the exchange networks in which their male relatives and would-be husbands attempt to enmesh them.

SH: By overestimating agency and underestimating economic and other constraints, Indonesians such as Nafsiah, who is the National AIDS Commission Secretary, not to mention most Papuans, can justify where their sympathy for HIV infections lies. But now that reproductively viable women are seen to be at risk, the moral logic of epidemiology no longer makes sense. Much like Australia in the 1980s, the awareness that 'good women' are also at risk of HIV forces Indonesians, who were slow to recognise HIV in their country, to accept that there really is an HIV problem and that greater resources will need to be mobilised to tackle it. Unfortunately, the same assumptions that eulogise housewives and so motivate concern for HIV are the same ones that block effective intervention. If it is impolite, even taboo, to imply that people other than married couples may be having sex, and if married people in their need to keep up the appearance of monogamy do not need advice about HIV, thank-you-very-much, then what can be done other than employing the least threatening technique, that of designing brochures and posters for a no-name audience?

LH: It seems as if absolute and percent numbers get bandied about pretty easily in Indonesia, and that incidence and prevalence are also frequently confused. The alleged recent increases claimed in the newspaper story, however, seem to have already been evident from 2002 to 2004, but that's hard to say, since the health officials seem to be counting infected individuals ('housewives' on the one hand, and 'sex workers' on the other) as opposed to assessing percentages infected, checking those against incidence of new infections and what might be some of the relative risks involved. Talk to me about 'counting' in terms of Indonesian epidemiology. I'd want to know, for example, whether in any kind of nationwide study or setting those who test HIVab- also get enumerated. Chapters 3 and 4 are filled with examples of ways in which shoddy use of sometimes dubious data are blunting the efficacy of the national response.

SH: As I have mentioned above, the generation of statistics, no matter how weak their validity and reliability, creates a role for authorities and makes them feel as though they are doing something. There are many reasons for the poor quality of quantitative data on HIV in Papua, beginning with the paucity of sampling groups. Secondly, the nuances of the disease syndrome are little understood in Papua and so misdiagnosis would be likely. Thirdly, despite posters that urge them to do so, Papuans will not go out of their way to get an 'AIDS test' (which ought to be called an HIVab test); given the levels of community stigma toward people living with AIDS, why would they want to know their HIVab status? Testing that is done by urban hospitals, providing they are not waiting for a shipment of testing materials, may be done as a matter of course when they visit the doctor for other reasons. Testing tends to be done without the patient's consent, for it is considered distasteful for a doctor to talk about such matters, and at the same time it is considered rude to question a doctor. The distance of many rural villagers from urban hospitals and the cost of consultation fees and medicine also preclude large numbers of Papuans. Aside from the real problems of non-representative samples, minimal resources for surveillance and the lack of motivation of health personnel ensure that all health statistics in Indonesia should be taken with a grain of salt. While the National Epidemiology Network has identified four factors as enabling HIV to spread – low use of condoms, a large sex industry, high rates of male migration and mobility, and a high incidence of other STDs – there is little concern with the configurations of desire and texture of sexual cultures, which is arguably the kind of knowledge needed to assess impacts on the epidemic more accurately and to design better, more appropriate, intervention strategies.

LH: That, too, sounds a lot like Papua New Guinea. The article went on to quote Nafsiah as asserting that, in 2002, six of every ten Indonesian men having sex with sex workers (a number thought to be somewhere between seven and nine million) were married. What does that figure mean, and if true, why is there so much extra-marital sex? Does it surprise you?

SH: I have to say again, I have little faith in the truth of statistics produced in Indonesia, but if we take this finding as indicating a trend such that Indonesian men are engaging *increasingly* in extra-marital sex, then yes, I am not surprised at all. Why do men engage in so much extra-marital sex? This demands a complex answer, but simply put: because they can. It may be unpopular to think so, but it strikes me that, in general, men are geared towards sexual rapaciousness and, notwithstanding exceptions, social structures and cultural expectations keep sexual licentiousness in check. In Indonesia the strength of the Madonna/Whore archetypes and other patriarchal features, such as the monitoring of female mobility and the anti-divorce ethos, ensure that men can get away with extra-marital sex in a way that women cannot. This is not to say that there is not variation in levels of desire amongst men, or that women are not sexually voracious, because they certainly can be, but the higher moral expectations and surveillance of women and the energy-sapping tasks of bearing and nurturing children, which fill up so many reproductive years, can deter or offset what is seen as illicit sexual activity for women.

Moreover, the lack of financial care for, or social tolerance of, women outside marriage ensures that wives, especially when they are financially dependent, will be wary of protesting their husbands' extramarital liaisons. Common philosophies that stress marriage to be a duty that is endured would no doubt act as a support for under-resourced women who need to withstand infidelity. Islamic and Melanesian cultures both have histories of polygyny, and even where this is no longer practised, knowledge of alternative sexual arrangements would act as a haunting reminder that monogamy is, after all, relative. Last but not least, bedding women, in ways that have been little explored, is a source of prestige between Papuan men in provincial towns. Considering that Melanesians once held extra-marital sex, with notable exceptions, to be highly taboo and even punishable by death, this promiscuity-as-status-template development is curious, and I hope to explore it further as I analyse the fruits of my Ph.D. research.

LH: Nafsiah goes on to say that 'And we cannot just ignore the fact that the remaining 40 percent are single males that will be married one day. What will happen to their future wives if these men have been unknowingly infected?' Why doesn't she seem to care about all the infected non-housewives? This strikes me as all too common in Papua New Guinea, where sexually *active* young women get no pity, but where sexual *vulnerable* ones get heaps.

SH: Nafsiah is the voice of national consciousness. Her matter-of-factness about single men and how they *will* be married one day reveals the truth about choice in Indonesia and offers us insight into the national logic of gendered morality. Her revelations about the chain of transmission, from males who have been 'unknowingly infected', presumably by sex workers, to their wives and thence to their children reflects widespread assumptions about the moral nature of transmission. Wherever marital status determines whether one 'deserves' to have HIV, sex workers will be at the deserving end, wives will be on the opposite pole, and men, who may sit on either end, can ultimately be redeemed through the role of husband.

LH: With redemption being possible for sex workers in marriage?

SH: Yes. Most sex workers hope that marrying a decent man will redeem them, financially as much as morally, but the longer a woman is involved in transactional sex, amongst other complex factors, the less likely are her chances are of such redemption. I guess the impact of the epidemic on house-wives is Nafsiah's main concern because it is housewives who most saliently uphold good, productive *and* reproductive femininity. Housewives, after children, are the most innocent of social categories, for they are seen as coming into marriage as virgins and transferring the obedience they have had to parents to their husbands. Like I have said, they are pivotal to reproducing the nation and so their well-being is of utmost concern. Women who are neither housewives nor sex workers are off the epidemiological radar altogether, or else they are counted as children.

LH: Yeah, that's what I was saying above about Papua New Guinea. Nafsiah really encouraged the use of female condoms, too. Do you think that female condoms make a viable preventive measure in Indonesia? What are some of the social and ideological forces working against them? What do Christian housewives married to civil servants say about condoms?

SH: For men in Manokwari at least, condoms are seen as a nuisance, distracting from the full pleasure of intercourse. Women, knowing where men stand on this issue, would not dare challenge them over their perceived 'right' to not use condoms. That no man has to justify his position on 'logical' grounds, such as that 'condoms are not 100% effective', as is found all across Papua New Guinea, simply reeks of male privilege and underscores the patriarchal social structure in Manokwari. The hypothetical scenario of a civil servant's wife wanting to negotiate for condom use on the grounds of family planning would not get very far, for contraception is seen as women's business and family planning clinics are patronised and led by women. The fact is, when women are dependent on men's earnings, as housewives are, or if they want to keep their marriage, then they are unable to 'Just Say "No"'.

There are other factors that militate against condom use, and I have touched on many when I discussed sexual networking, but one factor that deserves further mention is the motivation for women to avoid being considered a slut, or '*perempuan nakal*'. To have sex before marriage is to negotiate the tricky act of being sexual while not appearing sexualised, and to this end, asking for a condom is to be sexually assertive, and having a condom handy is evidence that one premeditated the sex act. As a caveat, although moral expectations and economic dependence tend to rule out the use of condoms, I have known of exceptions to this rule in relationships that conform to a more Western mode of courtship in which the couple is committed and trust one another and use condoms because they are 'not ready' for children. Not unlike couples in Western countries, the use of condoms in this context is justified on the basis of life planning, and so no mention need be made of avoiding disease.

LH: That sounds a lot like Joshua Gamson's argument in 'Rubber Wars' (Gamson 1990). The Nafsiah article went on to claim more than 193,000 cases of AIDS had been reported throughout the country, but that is obviously incorrect. Jakarta topped the list with 26,805 reported cases, followed by Papua with 21,487 cases, East Java with 15,699 cases and West Java with

14,341 cases. I know that there are 32 provinces, but still, do these numbers add up? Is the author confusing HIV with AIDS here? The article concluded with some rather striking figures from the world of intravenous drug users (IDUs) in Indonesia, claiming that 12,780 of the 93,420 women partners of IDUs were 'infected with HIV/AIDS[sic]', so roughly 15%. Are any of those 'housewives'? Do housewives 'count' in any meaningful way in Indonesian epidemiology?

SH: Well, no, in terms of epidemiology, but obviously, yes, in terms of discourses of religion, the State, and nation-building. I want to comment, however, on another interesting issue that your question raises: the possibility of intravenous transmission in Papua. Unlike in Indonesian mega-cities, IDUs are a rare phenomenon in Papua and substance abuse tends to be experienced through alcohol, solvent-sniffing and, to a much lesser extent, the smoking of marijuana and ingestion of Ecstasy. There is, however, the real threat that HIV may be transmitted intravenously because of the pan-Papuan love of medical injections, or *suntik*. I will not discuss the complex reasons for this, but rather, point out that the Papuan belief that a *suntik* is 'strong' medicine has implications for the spread of HIV since during subcutaneous treatments the virus can be introduced directly into the bloodstream. During the time I lived in Manokwari, Jayapura and Wamena, so central were injections to biomedical treatment that locals thought there would be no point in visiting a doctor or nurse if one was not given a *suntik*. With similar effect, in Manokwari, the dominant Papuan group (from the Cenderawasih Bay Islands) will demand to be put on a glucose drip in the first instance of feeling faint or dizzy, and regardless of how well they have been eating or drinking. Indeed, it struck me that how many IV-drip bags one takes in is a source for bragging.

LH: Well, the residents of a turn-of-the-century montane sanatorium in Thomas Mann's *The Magic Mountain* used to carry around in their breast-pocket (should anyone wish to look at) their chest x-rays confirming diagnoses of their tuberculosis. Interestingly, Mann's character representing the Dutch colonial holdings in Indonesia is named Herr Pieperkorn!

SH: Of course, all this would pose a health risk if clinics were well resourced and health workers were rigorous in their hygiene procedures, but they are not, and lip service is paid to hygiene rituals whilst poverty works against the belief that needles should be used once and thrown away.

LH: One question open for discussion here and elsewhere is that of the geographic locus of intervention efforts, specifically, where should the bulk of counselling, testing and treatment services that are relevant to HIV and AIDS occur? One good review of these issues by James Shelton and Nomi Fuchs, and not based on any intimate knowledge of Papua New Guinea, struck a rather pessimistic view of a clinic-based approach:

> In our view, the health clinic is generally a weak platform to bring about
> the behavior change so vital to HIV prevention. First, the fragility of typical
> clinical services is a serious constraint. Counselling for clinical health services

is notoriously weak, continuation rates are poor, and contact with women is intermittent. Moreover, typical family planning clients are older aged married women, who are generally the least likely to transmit HIV and are poorly empowered to negotiate condom use. (Shelton and Fuchs 2004: 13)

Would you care to comment on their formulation in context of what you have observed in Indonesian Papua?

SH: What Shelton and Fuchs note can certainly be extended to the situation in Indonesian Papua. The capacity of government health services is weak right across the province, but especially so in remote locations where health supplies are erratic, where accountability is opaque and where staff spend so much time chasing up their often late wages in administrative centres. In remote regions it is not uncommon for the local health nurse, the *mantri*, not to be at the clinic, for he is often involved in money-spinning home visits as a kind of freelance pluralistic medicine healer.

LH: Again, very similar to Papua New Guinea.

SH: It should also be mentioned that formal health settings in Indonesia, including Papua, are infused with a hierarchical and pedagogic ethos that is anathema to genuine trust and effective counselling. These constraints of logistics, not to mention the diversity of cultural understandings that Papuans bring into biomedical settings, ensures that macro-level planning to combat the spread of HIV will be fraught with difficulties. Shelton and Fuchs' comment that family planning services usually treat older married women is especially true in Indonesia, where birth control is only legally available to married people. There is also the problem of who patronises clinics, and Shelton and Fuchs' comment that family planning services usually treat older married women is especially true in Indonesia, where birth control is only legally available to married people.

In a constructive vein, establishing what would be a viable platform for HIV-related interventions would demand asking questions about local structures and power dynamics. How is the community divided, and in what forums do they mobilise themselves? Which NGOs operate in the area, and what are they like? How many churches are there, and is their sense of social justice more Old or New Testament? Do *Adat* organisations exist, and are their approaches at least a bit liberal and secular? It is more likely though that young people will not be comfortable talking about sex in any institutional context, and so it would be better to educate youth on sexual health and condom usage in small peer-based groups. In terms of communicating productive messages about HIV, I would highly recommend the use of Papuan drama groups, as my Papuan friends have all loved the tapes of performances by Ni Vanuatu's drama group, Wan Smolbag. After a lifetime of Javanese and foreign soap operas and films, people marvel at how similar are the people and their problems in these productions, and as any good development practitioner knows, true participation and entertainment are the best ingredients for bringing about a change in consciousness.

LH: I'm intrigued what you say, Sarah, about differentiating between the health related messages of the Old versus New Testament. What do you mean?

SH: As I see it, churches can be divided into those that model themselves on a forgiving and tolerant Jesus, and those that imagine Christianity in more punitive terms, and this affects how they communicate about HIV and AIDS. Whether they are the 'eye-for-an-eye' or 'turn-the-other-cheek' kind of Church seems to depend more on the quality of their leader than on what denomination the Church is. Having said that, certain kinds of ego are attracted to certain denominations in Papua, and by far the most compassionate Church representatives I have met are Catholic nuns. In a conference on HIV in Papua, leaders of several denominations were present, but it was the nuns who were sitting close to, and even holding the hands of, Papuans who were HIVab positive or also suffering from AIDS.

* * *

LH: Despite Papua New Guinea being an independent country and Indonesian Papua being a province ruled from somewhere else, a point of similarity in both locales seems to be the inability of health officials and bodies to formulate and present clearly a set of factually correct, effective public health messages and promotions. Leslie Butt and her colleagues concluded upon completion of a study of knowledge, attitudes and practices that '[t]he biggest barrier to awareness and HIV/AIDS prevention in Papua is the lack of relevant information presented in an appropriate fashion' (Butt, Morin and Numbery 2002b: 55). Elsewhere (Butt, Numbery and Morin 2002a), she and her colleagues have argued that effective intervention in Indonesian Papua must grapple not so much with culture as with its reification, not just with individual acts of a sexual nature (for example, the ethnic and racial intricacies of sexual networking in myriad locales), but also with the fact and the structure of Indonesian rule there and its effect on sexual practice, specifically harassment, rape and other forms of sexual violence. Taking a somewhat opposite tack, Heather Young Leslie has argued in 'Producing *What* in the Transition?: health messaging and cultural constructions of health in Tonga' (Leslie 2002: 297) that 'culture is stronger than health promotion dictums'. What I appreciate about her paper is that she has written cogently about culture but without falling into the easy trap of assuming that culture is an obstacle as such. Could you reflect a little bit on that in terms of HIV transmission in Indonesian Papua, especially in the Manokwari region? How would you conceive of or rank the importance of culture, on the one hand, and social-structure and history, on the other, meaning to incorporate *transmigrasi,* militarism, a raging civil war, and so on? Is there a better way of enlisting culture for progressive movements of intervention?

SH: In Indonesian Papua, simply implementing the ABC model will, as it has in countless other areas, lead development practitioners to distraction as they puzzle over why people would want to ignore such an important message and persist in tempting death. In the conservative political climate of today, Papuans are selling sexual services and intimate access to their bodies for a number of reasons that have absolutely nothing to do with imputed promiscuity. They do so because they have no other way to make money, or because they are trying to avoid or are coping with gendered violence, or because they are seeking sexual activity without shaming one's family. Given these facts, prioritising the avoidance of HIV is either an unaffordable luxury or is seen as being a far less dangerous option than other hazards that go into negotiating sexual desire.

Let me try to tease out some of the ideological and structural conditions that are altering the sexscape of Papua in a way that has implications for HIV transmission. Across Papua, there is an increasingly wide gap between the onset of menarche and the expected age of marriage, which means that fewer Papuans are willing to wait for marriage to commence sexual activity. This is especially the case in the rapidly expanding towns, where the possibility of mobility, privacy and mobile-phone networks allows one to pursue sexual adventures with greater ease and anonymity. In this context, and with greater sexual mingling with people outside one's own cultural group, sexual subcultures are flourishing like never before. A robust theme in my research is how the saturation of sexual imagery in the environments of youth, from advertisements to pornography, makes their 'appetite rise' (*nafsu naik*), which in turn makes them want to act out what they see, especially when they drink alcohol, which makes them especially 'brave'. I would add to this mix the role of changing ideals of marriage, from love-made to arranged, on the sexualisation of Papuan culture. Marrying for love requires getting to know someone, which in turn requires intimacy. Sex, being the most intimate of experiences, is then an essential element in the mythic logic of romance. Another powerful factor contributing to new sexual cultures, and one that I want to explore in my thesis, is the emotive power of boredom, which is palpable in any Papuan town and which gives rise to a kind of yearning. As money is hard to come by, and traditional experiences for being or remaining liminal have eroded, sex has become a form of free entertainment and an avenue for oceanic oneness all rolled into one.

Clashing with these 'pulls' are a series of 'pushes' that make for very choppy seas. For different reasons and in different ways, State, Church and *Adat* each promote a vigorous regime of bodily discipline, and the powers invested in their corresponding institutions allow them to punish would-be transgressors against ideals and practices of monogamous married sex. In this new world with the need for thrills, for money and for obtaining and maintaining modern identities, any attempts to stamp out sexual desire will only push it underground, and in its invisibility, HIV will flourish. While the topic of sexual violence in Papua has rarely been an object of study, we are safe to assume that given the taboo nature of sex and the patriarchal social structures, rape of various kinds would not be uncommon, and especially when women enter taboo spaces and times, like all-night parties and even just walking around on the streets after nine o'clock. Marriage itself, regardless of recent laws that recognise the possibility of rape within marriage, is seen as a permanent signal of 'yes', and again, forced sex within marriage is a complex and sensitive topic that has not been investigated in Papua.

LH: Well, that's one difference with Papua New Guinea, where such has been studied by government and academic researcher, NGO and community organisation alike.

SH: Yes, I would love to see more cutting-edge research in Indonesian Papua of the kind that has been done in Papua New Guinea. In towns where money is needed, Papuans find themselves at an unfair disadvantage in the labour market vis-à-vis straight-haired migrants, and this, combined with the need for money and the lack of land, skills, capital or commodities, produces conditions ripe for Papuans to fall back on selling the one resource that they do have: their bodies. The increasing number of Papuans who are top civil servants is bringing about a new phenomenon of Papuan-style 'sugar daddies', which is another theme I am exploring in my thesis. The state's *dwi fungsi* policy, whereby the armed forces are given the role of policing internal as well as foreign threats has led to a heavy military presence in secessionist, threatening provinces such as Papua. In town this manifests as a shifting population of single, virile, macho (*jagoan*) soldiers who spend much of their time hunting for sex whilst battalions in remote regions, with similar sexual appetites, hunt in ways that are less accountable. In particular, murder, rape, torture and other kinds of violence are most common around the Freeport copper-mine in the south, where the army is paid to 'protect' the mine, and along the border, where soldiers patrol to 'remove' guerrilla elements.

Given that risky behaviour and HIV transmission are so deeply entwined with social-structures it is hard to imagine how culture can be enlisted for progressive intervention. The linking of AIDS prevention to cultural identity and ethnic pride are the vernacular ways in which culture is being used to combat AIDS and so, given this lead, the idiom of physical and cultural well-being would be an appropriate one on which to base future messages about HIV prevention and care of people living with HIV and AIDS. However, as long as the conservative sexual ethos and the corresponding denial of sexual behaviour exist, the A and B components of the ABC message will predominate. Inversely, condoms will be accepted as an option to further the interests of Papuan pride only when young people, and especially women, are more empowered in their decision-making. As many others have noted, the real answers to halting the epidemic lie in addressing the root causes of age and gender inequalities such as the global inequities in wealth and the failure of democratic participation in civil societies. While 'structure' is hugely important it is also possible that 'practice' theorists are right in suggesting that historical change is an outcome of the dialectical pressures of agency and structure. To this end, culturally appropriate and accurate messages delivered through local drama groups about HIV stress that it is a threat to the reproduction of Papuans. Combined with more direct experience of people contracting HIV, this may just alter Papuan feelings about and relationships to condom usage. I would hope that this change, in turn, will have just as positive an impact upon the mainstream sexual culture.

LH: On that last point, that's sort of what Kathy Lepani is arguing in her several essays about the reception by Trobriand islanders of HIV and AIDS messages: 'we better do something, otherwise we're not going to be able to reproduce our way of life'.

I want to pick up on another angle of what you just said: in Papua New Guinea, by contrast, diplomats, soldiers, policemen and security guards are extremely sexually active, but they could be argued to stand proxy for and represent capital more than they represent the state. I would probably argue that they tend to be put to the service of furthering economic interests in resource extraction, entertainment and commerce more than in consolidating the interests of the state, and when it comes to sexual matters, they're not there by and large to see to it that existing laws aren't being broken. As well, they tend to get pulled away by resource extraction companies who can afford them, instead of being forced to toil in an under-resourced police station that has no petrol for police vehicles that may have been already crashed by a previous police chief. I remember seeing this in the Kikori area; while a young girl had been terribly traumatised, first, by her own father, then was raped by security guards at a base camp, the police who could have, should have done something had been hired privately by a logging giant in the area. In any event, even by conservative estimates (e.g. AusAID 2005a: 2) the 'national response' in Papua New Guinea to HIV and AIDS is at least 90% external donor country-funded, and Australia provides roughly 95% of that. Thus, HIV transmission and prevention and AIDS care and treatment are being approached in many ways indirectly, yet forcefully, by means of or in terms of what Australians think about Papua New Guineans.

Given that so much of yours and Leslie's work in Papua deals with what Indonesian elites and government functionaries know or think they know about Papuans, this invites comparison of the effects of varying kinds and degrees of state-level input and control over the intimate realms of sexuality, family, fertility and health. If I play Devil's Advocate for a moment, I will assert that a certain 'managed transmission' of HIV is occurring in both locales, but perhaps for quite different reasons. For example, in Papua New Guinea, I am certainly not alone in pointing out that the Papua New Guinean nationals operating at a high level in the NDoH, the NACS and the NHASP have not forcefully opposed anti-condom rhetoric. Quite to the contrary, one doctor from within the former staunchly opposes them, another surveillance officer believes in the power of prayer to remove HIV from the body, and yet another promotes a 'Bio-energizer' that targets HIV. Even the ones who oppose the opposition, so to speak, do so rather blandly, in my opinion. An external research outfit, for example, Marketsearch, has noted the soft-pedaling over the years of the national response, which has harped more upon abstinence, fidelity and stigma than upon structural factors like health services collapse and political corruption which determine transmission or that preclude its prevention. 'The condom issue has been further clouded', they said, by a distinct antipathy from some faith-based organisations whose lobbying and anti-publicity has not been effectively confronted. The political will and commitment to the promotion of condoms is questionable.

The small-change target also acknowledges the strong opposition to strong condom-promotion campaigns among Church and other leaders that exists in PNG that indeed has hampered the development and running of frank/open condom promotion campaigns. (NHASP 2006i: 7, quoting, first, Marketsearch, and, second, another NHASP document from 2005)

What are the Indonesian government and private business interests willing to tolerate in terms of policies and practices that don't prevent HIV transmission, and that perhaps hasten its spread?

SH: If by 'managed transmission' you mean that there are certain structures and policies that facilitate the transmission of HIV, then yes, the structural and ideological context of Indonesian Papua, as my last answer demonstrates, is managing HIV transmission very well. Yet because I consider genocide to be an organised and willful process, I would never suggest that this 'managed transmission' of HIV is genocidal. The increasingly Papuanised bureaucracy and other officials are, I believe, operating on socialised assumptions about how to enact modernity, and so the sluggish government are simply following decades-old utilitarian codes of conduct. To this end, pro-marriage rules, such as that one must be married to get a free sack of monthly rice, and that contraception is only available when one is married, are so hegemonic that people would not question how they contribute to de-legitimatizing alternative sexual arrangements. So, too, it is not questioned why contraception that assumes a long-term relationship, such as temporary sterilisation, is promoted over one-fuck options like condoms. Business in Indonesian Papua is mostly of the resource extraction kind. As it has been shown in countless other areas in the developing world, sex work is often the economic solution for people who have drifted to projects only to find few opportunities for employment, and in Indonesian Papua, the employment tends to go to straight-haired Indonesians. It should be recognised, however, that sex work more than piggybacks onto resource extraction, and companies more than 'tolerate' its presence for, quite frankly, sex work is good for business, the business of the government, the business of companies as well as of pimps. Local governments, for their part, regard the adult entertainment sector as not only supporting the growth of business but as being a significant revenue earner itself. The giant gold and copper mine P.T. Freeport near Timika, the Papuan town that has the highest concentration of *lokalisasi*, provides an example of the fact that business is implicated in the Papuan sex trade. By paying the military for 'protection' the mine encourages a large military presence and in remote postings, where the military benefit materially from illegal activity, resource extraction, protection rackets and brokering the sex trade are huge revenue earners. The interests of sex workers are all too often conflated with the interests of the company, for not only do sexual services make for 'happy workers', they can also be used as a resource for the company to broker deals, including with local men who are known to be plied with alcohol and sex before being asked to sign away their land. In Papua, sex is also used as a currency for bartering eaglewood (*gaharu*). This prized resin is sourced by traders, soldiers, private businessmen and Papuans themselves, who bring migrant sex workers along, and in the case of Papuan men, their wives to trade for eaglewood. It is reported that one kilogram of eaglewood is worth about three to five days of sex. Lastly, I just want to say that the Wild-West ethos that has for decades dominated Indonesia's last frontier is only becoming more intense in the era of Special Autonomy. Would-be entrepreneurs no longer have to go through official and legal channels in Jakarta which, I might add, have become more stringent with the recent success in International Conservation laws, for they can gain access to business permits for the right fee from any local official. Since the right to dig, chop and trawl anywhere one likes has become easier, this can only spell danger in terms of HIV transmission.

LH: Thank you so very much, Sarah, for having done this extremely important fieldwork. I look forward to seeing *The Romantic Underground* sometime soon. I hope that we can work together to make social scientific works about HIV and AIDS in Indonesian Papua more palatable to policy makers and opinion leaders.

Chapter 7

'What do they expect – angels with dirty faces?'

Sexual identities and networking in Papua New Guinea

Subject: positions

> The sex trade for foreigners profits from domestic configurations of kinship, heterosexuality, and gender in which male sexual activity is a natural entitlement, and, other things being equal, men are considered senior (phi) and treated with deference. The integral role of intimate realms in modern market venues belies the common image of global capitalism as neutral and homogeneous. (Ara Wilson, *The Intimate Economies of Bangkok*, 2004, p. 190)

> Sexual minority 'third sex' Pacific communities go under a variety of different names: Fa'afafine (Samoa), Mahu (Hawaii), Fakaleiti (Tonga), Whakawahine (Aotearoa), 'Akava'ine (Cook Is), Vaka sa lewa lewa (Fiji), Rae rae (Tahiti) and Fiafifine (Niue). (AIDS Foundation of New Zealand posting on AIDSTOK, 22 October 2007)

> See him over there? He's my cousin. He is an 'MSM'. (22-year-old 'contract wife' of an Australian construction supervisor, Port Moresby, August 2006, translated from the Tok Pisin)

> When I have sex, I feel alright again. (35-year-old married man, Mt. Hagen, April, 2006, translated from the Tok Pisin)

LH: Lawrence Hammar
AM: Alison Murray

The study of gender relations and sexual identities in New Guinea has come a long way from the classic works of Bronislau Malinowski and Margaret Mead, of Mervyn Meggitt and Marie Reay, of Hortense Powdermaker and Paula Brown, of Laurent Serpenti and Jan van Baal. These and many other fieldworkers, ranging from Ruth Craig to Edwin Cook, Annette Weiner to Robert Glasse, Denise O'Brien to Karl Heider, worked in New Guinea highlands and islands settings on both sides of the border that Papua New Guinea now shares with Indonesia. Their fieldwork was conducted often during time periods of rapid socioeconomic change and in places marked by religious fervour and conversion. Chris Gregory has shown that in portions of the central highlands, up to 25% of the adult male population moved (more or less permanently) to coastal areas for work on plantations and in shipping and domestic labor (Gregory 1982: 194). The essays and monographs of members of this 'first wave' of prominent anthropologists laid down local ideas about fertility, marriage and sexuality (or their negation) in laudable detail and with a mind to controlled comparison. Mervyn Meggitt pointed out nearly four decades ago, for example, that nowhere in the highlands region could one find 'matrilineal descent systems or extensive *de facto* matrifiliation' (as one does, for example, in the Massim region) and that prescriptive marriage systems were rare if they could be found at all (Meggitt 1969: 3, 5). As well, he invited approach to the 'question of the extent to which the highlanders' complicated attitudes towards sexual pollution, which vary greatly from one society to another, condition or are conditioned by their domiciliary patterns' (1969: 15). The methods these anthropologists used in the field were based on intensive immersion in local lifeways and economies, sometimes of a repeated, longer-term sort such that they could distinguish with experience and empirical evidence between prescriptive rules about this or that and actual social practice. They had sometimes also, however, to take a sort of 'salvage' approach to sexual matters not easily spoken of in the open, for example, gender-based, sexualised punishment of females or the ritualised forms of homosexual and heterosexual copulation that had been prohibited by missionaries and colonial administrators.

Owing to prudishness in anthropology and the recent appearance in urban settlements and rural areas of relative poverty, most of these works neglected really to link social process to sexual intercourse. No works in this earlier generation of which I am aware analyse the structure and function of sex industries, for example, despite their clear existence at this time, and few even link sexual networking *per se* to historical forces. The third of Mervyn Meggitt's famous dictums about many Papua New Guinea highland men (the first two being that 'we marry the people we fight' and 'blood is our argument') is that they tend in terms of sexual practice to fall into either the 'prudes' or 'lechers' category (1964). Meggitt's typology was useful in bringing to bear variables of agricultural productivity and human fertility on analyses of gender relations and social life more generally. Nevertheless, his schema entailed little in the way of broader historical and economic forces acting upon sexual identity and practice, apart from the environmental and agricultural influences which in these earlier monographs seemed almost to determine sexual practice. In the Mae Enga region, that would have included European patrolling, gold-field exploration, attempts to 'pacify' local populations and the coming of Christian doctrines, missions and missionaries.

Although she later contributed several provocative typologies of gender, geography, exchange and sexuality, Shirley Lindenbaum's 1972 essay, 'Sorcerers, Ghosts and Polluting Women' moved beyond structural models of group exchange to consider the importance of bodily fluids and body parts in building structural models of gender. She theorised that highlanders were 'telling us something' about their understandings of human, animal and agricultural fertility insofar as they engaged in sexual intercourse in, at or away from sites of agricultural productivity and animal fecundity (Lindenbaum 1972). Hortense Powdermaker's Lesu hosts were similarly telling her something when they conveyed to her the local term, *malis lotin*, that Lesu women used for the lovers they took extra-maritally: 'husband/ bush' (Powdermaker 1971[1933]: 244). Neither Powdermaker's ethnography, *Life in Lesu*, nor Lindenbaum's model, however, bear many traces of recent changes that had swept across the areas of now Eastern Highlands and New Ireland provinces, just as above with Meggitt's Mae Enga, but also cash-cropping, immunisation and vaccination campaigns and eventually highway construction. Powdermaker says that marital forms had changed greatly in New Ireland with the coming of the Europeans but that the extent of extra-marital sexual activities hadn't changed (1971[1933]: 228). This is a claim difficult to square with other claims and data she presents, for example, regarding the prohibition by missions and colonial authorities of ritualised promiscuous intercourse at the cessation of inter-village feasting (1971[1933]: 130; see also Crawford 1981; Knauft 1993). As well, women who were the second and subsequent wives of men who had to cut them loose owing to mission prohibitions of their practice of polygyny often found themselves needing to step up receipt of payments made by men of *tsera* used as tokens to recognise the gift of and reciprocity entailed in sexual intercourse. Although written in context of neither the Mae Enga, Powdermaker's Lesu nor the Fore among whom Lindenbaum worked (nor even of heterosexuality), Gilbert Herdt's remark is *a propos*: 'It is difficult for us to adequately gauge the tremendous toll that Western agents and missionaries have taken on [sexual] practices, including their suppression by force' (1993b: xvi). Frederick Errington notes (1974: 84) that a youngish informant of 35 was 'shocked when I asked him about this practice' (ritualised fellatio performed by young boys on old men), and who said that 'he had never seen nor heard of such a custom'. Similar alarms have been raised in public, on the Internet and in newspapers by native sons and daughters angered by or ashamed of *reports* (whether or not they are true) of ritualised male homosexuality occurring 'traditionally' among the Gogodala, the Marawaka and especially as it has been imputed to several Sepik River groups. This last issue has been raised in classrooms and seminars, including methods-training workshops I have led. I note, however, that no such alarms are ever raised at imputations of 'MSM', who seem to function rhetorically quite well to pick up the slack.1

In all fairness, albeit from other contexts altogether and even different geographic or cultural areas, some of those same Western agents, social processes and missionaries have expanded and offered new opportunities for local sexual practice. Those have not always been 'good' or particularly healthy ones, of course, such as regarding the ideals and practices of love and romance that heighten risk of STD transmission and that alienate them further geographically from natal groups and emotionally in terms of elopement and failed sister-exchange and other bride-wealth-related expectations (e.g. Hewat 2008; Hirsch and Wardlow 2006; Richards 2004; Zimmer-Tamakoshi

1993b). Nevertheless, sexual matters have been cracked open to previously unheard of degrees of scrutiny and commentary around issues of money, sexual violence, employment, education and certainly HIV and AIDS. Just below, my friend and colleague Alison Murray mentions the phenomenon of 'contract marriages', short-term but extremely affective, primarily sexual relationships that may entail particular STD and HIV transmissive risks.[2] One of Powdermaker's many fascinating sexual history case studies was of a woman, Kawitti, who had stayed on in Rabaul, now capital of East New Britain Province, to which she had come with her copra plantation-working husband. Upon becoming widowed, she enjoyed many lovers, just as she had pre-maritally. The list of her paramours included a white man who 'paid her "plenty"' (Powdermaker 1971[1933]: 282, n. 1). Malinowski, too, writes in *The Sexual Lives of Savages* that an important chief in the Trobriand islands frequently 'prostitutes his wives to white men' (1929: 323)

For a couple of hundred years or more European observers have written of the apparent ubiquity of the provision of sexual services in Pacific island communities, on the one hand, but also of distinct *types* and *meanings* that sexual service provision takes, on the other. Those include 'hospitality' prostitution, 'war-captive' prostitution, 'wife-lending', and so on. Sometimes 'prostitution' didn't have a name or even involve sex, for example, the 'village harlotry' theorised by Geza Roheim (1940, 1946) or the payments made by females to males who can prove sexual self control, as in aboriginal Nagovisi, on Bougainville (Nash 1981, 1987), or the gifts given between sweethearts but specifically in recognition *of* sex (Malinowski 1929; Pospisil 1963; Powdermaker 1971[1933]). Historical accounts written by or about the crews of captains Wallis, Bougainville, Cook and Bligh suggest that new forms of sexual networking were introduced but that didn't necessarily require or even imply cash exchanges (or at least not to both parties). Nails, clothing, fresh (and eventually frozen) fish, other foods, shell valuables and other finery, favours, fatherhood, transportation, vanilla and coffee beans and seedlings, names and semen are just a few of the things and behaviours that have in the Pacific been observed historically to be traded for sex (Chappell 1992; Hammar 1992, 1996a, b; Mageo 1998; Snow and Waine 1979). Nowadays those include transportation, employment, access to telephones, extension of credit and the like. Nancy Sullivan and her colleagues (2003: 37) note the 'desperate and recent shift from bartering for food to bartering for sex' in context of the developments and depredations of intensive fishing industries.

These kinds of remarks about and practices regarding sexual networking (see also Hammar 1998a) are difficult to square with those of prior fieldworkers who asserted a rather more restricted, perhaps even more prudish attitude to sex. Margaret Mead remarked about the Arapesh that sex for them was not seriously conceived of outside the marital bond, that the 'sudden stirring of desire that must be satisfied quickly' does not occur to them (1963: 99). Hers mirror the remarks of Karl Heider about Grand Valley Dani sexuality having allegedly a 'low-energy' to it, that sex 'does not hold much interest for them' (1976a: 189), that 'all Grand Valley Dani' observe a five-year period post-partum of sexual abstinence (1976b: 68). Powdermaker comments about there being really only one sexual position, that 'rape by a native is unknown', and that 'sexual perversion scarcely exists' (1971[1933]: 241, n. 1, 245, 277). Readers of *Pigs, Pearlshells, and Women: marriage in the New Guinea highlands*, the preeminent collection at the time of theory of social structure in New Guinea, will find hardly mention and no discussion of sexual desire or practice. Edward Schieffelin notes that Kaluli newlyweds might take a couple of months before they have sex together, which seems designed not to facilitate pleasure or better spousal communication so much as to transfer smoked meats and cement affinal ties, and that, when not looking to procreate, 'Kaluli avoid sex, lest a man dissipate his energy' (1976: 121–2, 124).

Such comments are sometimes difficult to swallow without knowing more about fieldwork style, community relations and publishing trends, but sometimes they can appear ahistorical or be flatly contradicted by other facts. Leslie Butt (Butt 2008; Butt and Munro 2007), Sarah Hewat (2008), Jeffrey Clark (1997), Jenny Hughes (Clark and Hughes 1995), Sarah Richards (2004), Holly Wardlow (2007) and others have studied 'states of desire' and the impact of money, travel, colonialism and modernisation on indigenous modes of sexual conduct. Butt and Munro (2007: 586) have written about the social effects of recent upsurge in 'unregulated sexuality of young men and women' in Indonesian Papua; young people look fondly upon the new opportunities for sexual assignations that their elders find particularly troubling insofar as it accompanies 'the rapid influx of Indonesian settlers'. Raymond Kelly analysed with great skill some of the sociodemographic and sociomedical determinants of changes that had occurred in the Etoro marital system. In only a few decades, he showed, whereas pre-pubescent girls were once normally married to males twice their age, men came normatively to marry widows instead (Kelly 1980: 171). To cite only four texts at my fingertips, Bruce Knauft's *South Coast New Guinea Cultures* (1993), the two editions of Gilbert Herdt's *Ritualized Homosexuality in Melanesia* (1993[1984]), the Richard Marksbury-edited *The Business of Marriage: transformations in Oceanic matrimony* (1993), and the volume edited by Lenore Manderson and Margaret Jolly, *Sites of Desire/Economies of Pleasure* (1997) have led to massive reworkings of Western understandings of gender relations and sexual identity and practice in the insular Pacific. 'Prudes' has come more to mean the personality types of Western observers of Pacific sexual agents than of Pacific islanders themselves, and 'Lechers', the expatriate males who populate karaoke lounges, nightclubs and go-go bars in Port Moresby, Bangkok and Jayapura. When they make sexual assignations there they are 'telling us something' about the pace of migration, the influence of Western modes of sexual commerce and the reach of globalising forces.

Still less well developed, however, have been studies of the commercialisation and commoditisation of sexual acts and identities. Some sources discuss the emergence of infectious diseases in terms of the emergence of sex industries, for instance, in the Commonwealth of the Northern Marianas Islands (Yamada 1998), in Guam (Workman, Hill and Pinhey 2001), or in the Torres Straits region (Sissons 1976, 1977), but not the sex industries themselves. Other valuable texts discuss the eroticisation of countries and culture areas and important historical moments broadly, for example, Hawai'i (Bailey and Farber 1992), Polynesia (Jolly 1997) or Thailand (Manderson 1997), but without necessarily plumbing very deeply their intimate ties with kinship, marriage, residence and other obligations of the social-structure (see Hammar 2007c). The vast majority of treatises about prostitution and sexual networking in the contemporary Pacific, although often rich in estimates of the number of imported brothel workers or of the estimated prevalence of their STDs, can be accordingly quite poor regarding the routes by which they arrived and the dynamics of their transmission. Many discussions of the introduction of foreign women and girls into forms of sexual toil refer little to the mechanisms and other persons (male and female) and states and companies by and through which they thrived and reproduced. Owing to the complex politics of nationalism ('that which is now bad was foreign-brought') and of evangelical Christianity ('that which is good came from missionaries'), few wish to talk frankly about the sometimes quite ugly social facts of sexual commerce and exploitation in 'traditional' cultures, as I showed in Chapter 2.

Nowhere is this more evident than in the ways in which national responses to HIV and AIDS deal with the epidemiological questions raised by commercialised sexual networking. Examples drawn from the Pacific make evident that health officials and politicians and even researchers often either *overlook* the question of female agency altogether, preferring instead to promote the victim slot that robs females of choice and manipulation and victimises them further, or *presume* it without interrogating the actors, data sources and contexts involved.3 Caroline Ralston notes that for Polynesian history, 'the use of terms such as "prostitution," "promiscuity," and "debauchery" to describe the behaviour of Polynesian women' reveals more about (male) European subjects than (female) Polynesian objects (1988: 77). Even when Hawaiian women began to exchange sexual services for 'a range of highly desired goods of western manufacture', she argues, it neither constituted prostitution categorically nor was stigmatised locally (1988: 77). Voluminous evidence to the contrary (Chappell 1992) doesn't seem to have budged this position much. Powdermaker states just as firmly as Ralston that the 'extra-marital intercourse for payment' in which Lesu women engaged can in no way be considered the 'prostitution of our civilization', that Lesu women who failed to receive *tsera* from lovers would lose prestige and status (1971[1933: 245]). Siusiua Lafitani seems also to want to take the sting out of the term 'prostitution' in application to Tonga by defining it as involving those non-married women who have non-marital sex for money, pleasure, food and other material resources. She points to American soldiers after the Second World War who provided food and cash in exchange for sex with loaned wives and daughters and unmarried women, thus involving them simply in '*reciprocity*' (1998: 79). This leaves open the questions of the agency of Tongan men in pimping their wives and daughters but also of the one-sidedness of the exchange: what were American soldiers *loaning* in exchange? Making love to the Americans, she argues, was an aspect of Tongan women's attempts to win social capital and gain prestige locally insofar as Americans connoted wealth and overseas status (1998: 79). Ralston implies in two publications (1988, 1992) that prostitution did not exist in the

Pacific prior to European contact, that female sexuality was never deployed by husbands or male relatives without their consent, that sexual aspects of polygyny were never exploitive, and that, had it occurred or been evident on contact with Europeans, 'prostitution' would have been evidence of female agency anyway. Powdermaker, too, argues that payments of *tsera* were for Lesu women not payments for sex 'any more than the marriage price is a payment for the bride' (1971[1933]: 244). Ralston argues that whatever it was that Europeans glossed as prostitution was actually the struggle of Pacific islander commoners, specifically female, to improve their status, to maneuver socially, not only by the gifts of material goods they amassed, but literally, by insemination, commensality and other forms of intimate contact with Europeans. Sahlins notes that Hawaiian women who had babies by Cook's crew put the umbilical cords in the nooks and crannies of the ships before the fathers left (Sahlins, cited in Chappell 1992: 134). That's all good and well for that side of the ledger, but probably few European males (and only rarely) shared such sanguine feelings about such transactions.

This important issue is complicated further because of how partial is the evidence, how non-comparable can sometimes be the linguistic utterances and how great can be the cultural and intellectual divides of perspective and interest. Imputing prostitution where it does not exist can be racist and ethnocentric, as Ralston and Lafitani and many others rightfully point out. Putting it necessarily beyond the pale of Pacific islander women and communities, however, isn't necessarily any less shortsighted. Chappell notes that while the androcentrism of historical documents (say, about shipboard relations in the eighteenth and nineteenth centuries between Europeans and Pacific islanders) gets in the way, so has the 'decolonisation' of historiography. The historiographic movement from ships to beaches (Chappell 1992: 131) constitutes a humongous geographic and philosophic shift that has probably exaggerated female agency and obscured the social structures within which female sexual services were (you take your pick) peddled, purchased, bartered, given, sold, shared and stolen. The recent shift back again to ships (this time, fingering fishing vessels from Asian countries that dock in Pacific island ports and whose sailors who mess with local girls and women) represents not so much the continuing decolonisation of scholarship as the diseasification, for lack of a better term, of contemporary concerns over sexual matters, the omnipresent threat now that HIV and AIDS pose to fragile countries, territories and cultures in the Pacific.

The pendulum seems to swing harder and harder, exaggerating female agency, but then neglecting the question altogether; interpreting sexual networking as all sale and purchase, but then as all exchange and mutuality; reciprocity versus exploitation; female choice versus husbandly prerogative. Given the intimate connections between prostitution and STD epidemics, sometimes empirically real enough but always rhetorical, these debates are extremely relevant to today's struggles against HIV and AIDS. Nowhere could that be clearer than with regards to the prominence of prostitution and related persons, locations and behaviours in the HRSS and related strategies. Prostitution has always borne a heavy rhetorical burden in terms of public health, but also more recently in terms of epidemiology. An explanation was offered long ago by historian Jeffrey Sissons regarding the hydraulic view of sexuality that guided British and then Australian colonial policies about it that is extremely relevant to today's debates in Papua New Guinea. His definition would need to substitute only a few derogatory nouns for 'Japanese' and 'housewives' for 'Caucasian' to be wholly applicable to contemporary debates over the legalisation of prostitution in state-regulated brothels (Hammar n.d.). As he explained (1977: 479),

> he [the colonial administrator] considered that a certain level of prostitution must be tolerated. In particular he felt that in the sugar districts there must be outlets for the sexual passions of the kanakas and that it was less revolting and degrading if these were satisfied by Japanese rather than by Caucasian women.

Let's Talk About Sex

Like Chapter 6, but with different topics, this chapter converses with another colleague, Dr Alison Murray. Aly has conducted and written about ethnographic research and activism throughout the Asia-Pacific region from different vantage points and subject positions, including the 1991 publication of her Ph.D. dissertation, *No Money, No Honey: A Study of Street Traders and Prostitutes in Jakarta* (Murray 1991), and her lively collection of essays, *Pink Fits: Sex, Subcultures and Discourses in the Asia-Pacific* (2001). This latter is useful particularly in theorising what she calls 'New Emerging Sexualities' that appropriate 'both traditional and Western elements in the urban context' (Murray 2001:35; see also Hammar 2007c), but also for interrogating the utility of concepts of Peers and Queers across time and cultural space.

This applies to 'FSW' and 'MSM' identities in surveillance programmes as they have been discussed in previous chapters. That rates of HIV infection in sex workers can be zero, as is the case often in context of legal prostitution in the US, and that it can be lower amongst sex workers than amongst non- in Southeast Asian settings (Murray 2001:113) is another way in which Aly's work resonates with the present one. Hers, mine and that of others cannot fail to address thorny questions of representation. Gare *et al.* (2005), for example, found that none of the 211 women they claim to have self-identified as 'FSW' in an outreach project in Eastern Highlands Province had tested HIVab+. Apart from the debatable accuracy of the claim that all 211 had held up their hands to say 'I am a Female Sex Worker', their finding of zero prevalence of HIVab hasn't been registered in either national or international circles regarding *the* infectedness of 'prostitutes'. I showed in Chapter 4 that, as often as not, such estimates (e.g. that of 17%) come to take categorical form.

LH: Aly, as I left Papua New Guinea in August of 2006 and passed briefly through Sydney, sharing a couple of beers with you on Coogee Beach, I began to imagine a productive conversation with you about what you have called New Emerging Sexualities. You've got under your belt so much relevant and compelling experience, having conducted fieldwork in Australia and Indonesia and written so widely about sexual practice there and in other Asian and Pacific countries. Plus, you've done so much as an activist in

Sydney and elsewhere around gay, lesbian and sex worker issues and causes. You've written more provocatively than anyone I know about sexual identity construction and maintenance.

AM: Thanks, Lawrence, I think. It's taken me so long to get back to these topics, after working with a sex worker network in Papua New Guinea in 2006 and all of the highs and lows that entailed. What you have said as an introduction is the background to Papua New Guinea's apparent sexual dysfunction, and the impossibility or at least difficulties of definition, generalisation or comparison with other areas of the Asia-Pacific. Studying anthropology at Oxford in 1980, you could be sure that Papua New Guinea would be represented by every kind of gender and sexual set-up possible, Malinowski and Mead and all those great characters talking about free-love festivals, gay initiation, bride-price and bride-wealth, measuring humans on a scale of pigs. Colonialism, central government and Christian missionaries conspired to eliminate all the fun stuff and sex for trade, but they haven't succeeded completely: and once HIV is acknowledged, then all that non-conforming sex needs to be acknowledged, too. You've written forcefully about the blinkered and dogmatic views prevailing in Papua New Guinea, often where religious morality is being inserted as a universal solution before the actual issues have even been partly understood.

LH: Yeah, ABC just shuts it down, doesn't it?, even before you crank it up.

AM: Yes, it's just brilliant, really: what could be more inappropriate for Papua New Guinea than to tell everyone to just abstain from sex? ... but I am no expert on Papua New Guinea, any more than I am on Indonesia, and I have lived and worked in Indonesia for many more years. My contribution, however, tries to combine academic, anthropological training and practice, with my own life in sex work and with living in slums and settlements. Given that 'objectivity' is no longer such a primary criterion in research, such that my work gets dismissed out of hand, and also because of the urgency of the AIDS pandemic in Papua New Guinea, hopefully something useful will come from our discussion.

LH: Aly, believe me, I picked you for a reason! Actually, for many reasons. Much of what you write about the importation and reception of Western discourses of sexual identity is ringing true in Papua New Guinea. For example, 'I am an MSM' is how some young Papuan men introduce themselves to expatriate health authorities in context of potential workshop attendance and outreach activities. I'm wondering about thoughts you might have in regards to Papua New Guinea and the emergence of so-called 'MSM' identities, those of allegedly 'self-identified' 'FSW', members of 'high-risk' groups and the like. Are those what you take to be 'New Emerging Sexualities'?

AM: Well, just a couple of quick comments first on 'What the Experts Don't Get'. The 'experts' are the top-down people and policy makers and elitist academics speaking their own jargon, but we've been part of that ourselves, haven't we? Perhaps by acknowledging that, we can have a stronger position from which to critique others. It's a tricky balance, which I'm still trying to achieve, to work outside the box and challenge the imposed doctrine, without becoming so much of an outsider that your efforts just get blown off. I'm as frustrated as you are with 'naïve empiricism' and the underrating and ignoring of qualitative work. Statistics get used to make arguments sound solid and factual, when there can be so many interpretations and potentials for manipulation. I mean, in Sydney there has been a recent rise in HIV infections that sounds startling from the headline figures and leads to hair-pulling, funding and more campaigns, but the numbers of people involved are tiny in comparison to Papua New Guinea, and the infection rate is also so much lower, so there is a sub-text there about the measurement of the value of life itself. Your quote about Papua New Guinea where 2% became 20% and no one noticed, or dodgy extrapolated totals of PLWHA in India that lurch from 5 million to 2.5 million overnight – you just wouldn't get reports like that about Australians.

LH: Yeah, and the same thing seems to have happened, as I discussed in Chapter 6 with Sarah Hewat, with regards to Indonesian Papua. Figures of seroprevalence there are attributed to indigenous Papuans that are outlandish in their presumption and never attributed to Indonesians, even where intravenous drug-use is common.

AM: I'd say that it's an example of the massive shock-and-awe numbers that've been wheeled out to kick-start Western concerns for and funding of the Third World amorphous masses for HIV prevention campaigns. Once someone starts actually counting, however, and insofar as the real numbers bear no relation to the estimate, then they just show even more poignantly how these experts aren't thinking in human terms at all, so much as putting forth variations on disaster-for-profit capitalism.

Getting back to your question, yes, NES (New Emerging Sexualities) can imply the kind of categories being created by the discourses about HIV and AIDS, as in MSM, FSW and the way that affected people respond to those labels, buzz-words and funding conveniences and/or relate them to their own sexual experiences. NES wasn't supposed to be an acronym or any kind of rigid category, but you can't really keep people from running with what you've put out there. NES was originally a bit of a piss-take on Sukarno's New Emerging Forces (NEFOS), and in my discussions it is no more or less than the more visible and fluid sexualities being seen in Indonesia from the early 1980s. In Australia the AIDS-era was starting, but so also were feminist and gay movements giving the nod to sexuality being linked to self-identity. When I was coming out then, it was very scary: there was really only one lesbian bar in town, where the women seemed to be trying to be as ugly and unfriendly as they could. I now think that because there was no template for homosexual interaction, everyone was just as scared as everyone else. It's hard enough to feel different without getting the brush-off from your few 'peers'. It can still be scary for a young dyke now, but there's been the emergence of identities, peer groups, spaces and places. And along with other academics looking at the Asia-Pacific, such as Dennis Altman, it seems clear that metropolitan centres such as Bangkok and Jakarta have similarities to Sydney and San Francisco as much as to their own hinterlands. In other words, global, urban similarities across cultures have developed, although being 'different' in Tasikmalaya, on Daru or in the backblocks of Minto is about as hard as it's ever been.

This immediately raises the question of distinguishing between the identity that is developed among members of a sexually marginalised group and an imposed label that is then adopted, such as MSM or FSW. The current top-down imposition of HIV terminology is trying to get rid of the 'high-risk' group concept, having realised that it creates and reproduces stigma, but the ideas have stuck because that's where the funding has come in. The national strategy sponsored by the NACS moved to 'High Risk Settings' and became even more disastrous 'cuz of drawing attention to 'hot-spots' that could have been quietly introduced to harm minimisation. By labelling those places as high risk, people stay away, self-appointed leaders condemn them and the owners and managers get mad at the HIV organisations, or they even get shut down, like what happened in Mt. Hagen at KK Paradise, sending sex workers and others further away from what pathetic information and support networks there may have been.4 The next brainwave was to replace HRSS with 'Tingim Laip' (Think About Life), which is sufficiently inoffensive as to be meaningless.

Risk group labels have stuck, and the jargon is a bit of a conundrum and I don't like using it, but anyway, I am here, with the excuse of convenience. You've got women not wanting to be known as FSW in their communities and so not coming to programmes, and you've got non-FSW coming to programmes because they know that there's benefits in doing so ...

LH: Yep, and it's just as true of MSM who aren't (Yeka *et al.* 2006) and of drug-users who don't or at least who don't talk about it without the cash incentive (Draus *et al.* 2005: 184) – just to qualify for the twenty bucks.

AM: and you've got sex workers preferring to be represented by non-peers at the moment because they trust those women to speak for them until they themselves are confident to 'come out'. In organising a network of Papua New Guinean sex workers, which I'll talk about later, we really tried to create safe spaces and emphasise the importance of peer education, but in the end we were pushed to get quick results and accept a couple of non-peers to represent FSW groups because it was clearly what the FSW wanted. And it's what I've argued before, that FSW are not 'empowered', that they need all the help they can get from supportive people in more advantaged positions, as long as those people then have an understanding of the need to pass on particular skills, for FSW to replace them. This is, of course, common 'best-practice' behaviour for expatriate inputs and roles, but I don't know how much it happens in real time, when it means someone is signing away their own job, and appears to those more advantaged people to be downgrading the 'qualifications' that maintain their privilege.

I think it can also be problematic, the way some NGOs and INGOs run programmes that are supposed to represent several sexual minorities who may not have anything in common and may not feel represented. The Poro Sapot Project, for example, is run by Save the Children (in Papua New Guinea), for FSW *and* MSM. The MSM identity in Papua New Guinea is very small, even though there may be lots of male-to-male sex happening. It's hard to say 'how many' MSM there are, owing to difficulties of communication and lack of funding and support for them. So this creates a lot of problems, because where men *do* identify as MSM they can be further stigmatised, and more than likely will be sex-working. So why not just combine sex workers of all genders, as I'll describe how we tried to do in the network?

At first the MSM from NGOs didn't want to talk about sex work and seemed to have a higher status within the NGOs than FSW (who were a far more numerous group), and this created problems for us, too. For a start, there's the 'sheer male privilege'.

LH: Now I know how you use that term.

AM: Then you've got expat MSM running HIV projects all over the place, but you don't have any expat FSW doing the same thing. So the FSW talk about how funerals for MSM dying of AIDS get paid for by the project, and the more frequent FSW AIDS deaths are left in the morgue. The MSM staff (not FSW) at Poro Sapot Project expected to be the chosen FSW representatives, once they perceived some benefits in that, so they didn't even bother to come to sex worker decision-making forums. So when they weren't chosen, and when out-there Hanuabadan, HIVab+, sex workers *were*, I got abused over it.

LH: Male sexual privilege, thy coat has many colours …

AM: A gigantic problem, of course, with applying the term 'FSW' to a group in the same way as 'MSM' is applied as a shorthand for connotations of identity and sexuality increasingly attached to the label, is that FSW is not an identity related to sexuality, if it's even an identity at all. It's the 'gay pride' model being applied all over HIV projects, because that was where the early ideas and successes were, but it hasn't really been challenged in non-Western/non-gay contexts. I'm talking a bit about gay and lesbian issues here because of the HIV impetus and the MSM projects, but the links to sex work are tenuous, as I'm trying to emphasise, for HIV *affects* lesbians, who work in disproportionate numbers in HIV projects, far more than it *infects* lesbians.

LH: Yes, that point was made in all manner of ways and sources beginning at least as early as the early 1990s, at least for the US. Books such as *AIDS: the women* and others lauded the disproportionate caring burden shouldered by lesbians but were also somewhat disturbed by it, if only because straight folks and gay men didn't seem to return the favour much. I wonder if that's going to happen in Papua New Guinea, too.

AM: Another point about NES is that Papua New Guinea is changing fast, and a range of gendered and sexualised ways of being are now coming in contact like never before. It wasn't just white people discovering the highlands, but also the coastal people.

LH: Good point; the carriers, the coastal peoples who became the constabulary force.

AM: Yes, the vast range of sex/gender models arose in an incredibly rugged environment where different cultures had little contact – and hence the hundreds of mutually unintelligible and antagonistic language groups in such a small geographic area. So, for example, you hear about gang-rapes or *lainap* where no one got involved to prevent them because the women were not from the same local area and had no *wantoks* and so no one cared. It seemed to me that FSW are at the forefront of change, being very mobile and often from mixed backgrounds, with their children being even more mixed: I kept seeing sex workers changing the rules a bit because they do link to several different *wantoks* in ways that are important for HIV projects. So for instance, when meetings are held in Port Moresby and you go around and ask sex workers where they're from, they don't say Three-Mile or Waigani, but Morobe/Enga, that is, they note their parents' background. And they travel between the coast and highlands, up and down the Highlands Highway, and to the economic enclaves like HKL Kainantu (Highlands Kainantu, Ltd.). A lot of coastal women had actually married highlands men and then regretted it or split up over cultural differences. At the national forum it was a bit like a microcosm of Papua New Guinea's problems and potential solutions.

Many sex workers in Australia and Indonesia are fluid in their sexuality, so I was interested to talk to FSW in Papua New Guinea about lesbian practice. Loads of them had stories to tell about themselves or friends, and although women are generally affectionate in a homosocial sense, there is quite a lot of behaviour going on in clubs that goes beyond that. One fascinating thing was how confronted the expatriates and experts seemed to be by this line of inquiry. I think that's because there are so many closeted gay men in international HIV projects, who have had real problems with stigma and threats related to the illegality of homosexuality in Papua New Guinea. Because of that, they were confused about fundamental differences between gay male and lesbian issues, and how lesbian practice mostly slips under the radar. I heard some stories of women being beaten by their husbands for having sex with other women, but then I heard so many stories of women being beaten by their husbands that it was hard to tell if the sex with women was seen as a particularly bad thing.

LH: A former Deputy Prime Minister, Dr Allan Marat, opened a Christian men's network by arguing that it is in fact gay men and lesbians who cause straight men to become alcoholics and wife-beaters (see John 2003) ...

AM: Well, that's just lovely. Anyway, as in most places, I found the sex workers themselves far more open-minded about sexual matters than the experts creating projects for them. We felt very safe out and about in settlements and 'hot-spots', taking advice from local sex workers about what to do, when to leave and so on, as opposed to some experts who are happy to get paid well to supposedly save sex workers from HIV, but who define 'high risk' for themselves as straying beyond the barbed-wire compound and barbeque circuit. Am I cynical? Yes, very.

✳ ✳ ✳

LH: When we last met I was obsessing over the Final Report I had to write (Hammar 2006b). This presented the lowlights and highlights of our nation-wide study, summarising the grim results of the clinical portions of the study and speaking as truthfully as I could to the gruelling nature of the study on a more personal level. We travelled to 11 field-sites in 10 provinces in screening well over 3,000 clients for five STDs (or markers thereof) and found just a staggering *at-all* infected rate, especially if you count multiple infections. Having worked a bit in Papua New Guinea, you wouldn't be shocked to learn that sexual networking is ubiquitous and that people's knowledge of their own body's anatomy and sexual function and of the signs and symptoms of STDs is, shall we say, sub-optimal. Having worked also in Indonesia, do these rates seem at all comparable to urban settings with which you are familiar? Is frank discussion of these matters discouraged, too, and is there evidence of condom disinformation campaigns?

AM: Yes, I saw you gruelling away last in Wewak, as I recall. Papua New Guinea does have extraordinarily high STD rates as far as we can know, with the extraordinary difficulty of finding out those rates. Your introduction hints at all the disparate pre-colonialist and pre-capitalist sexual cultures that have come into contact with each other, into contact with Christian dogma in various forms and degrees of extreme inappropriateness, and discovered the potential to commodify sex along with everything else in a cash economy. Meanwhile there are no locally applicable and acceptable guidelines for how to deal with all this social and sexual networking, mangling and sharing of viruses.

Indonesia has a very structured family planning network that goes right down to the neighbourhood unit, enabled by the tight administration set up by the wartime Japanese occupation. That's one reason urban Indonesia has nothing like the kind of STD/HIV rates found in Papua New Guinea, but it's another very complicated country. When we're already struggling with the imposition of inappropriate Western concepts in HIV programmes in Papua New Guinea, I'm a bit dubious about adding another layer of confusion by trying to compare it with Indonesia. Even in Indonesian Papua, where you would expect similarities with the Melanesian cultures, I think it would be dangerous to go down that path. Jayapura is more like an Asian city than Papua New Guinea, with Javanese domination and transmigration adding very different elements to sexual understandings and practices.

People are always saying, why don't you target the clients, how can sex worker projects work? The thing is that sex workers are the most knowledgeable about sex and have the best reasons to protect themselves, so once relevant information is available, you often find the lower rates of infection that you mentioned earlier. Papua New Guineans in general often have little idea about their own bodies, about clinical signs and symptoms or sexual function and physiology, so they're naturally reluctant to attend clinics and end up suffering with symptoms of rough sex and STDs along with quack cures, which can make them worse. Even though 'sex worker' is not really an identity along the lines that western activists would want, it is a lot more like an identity than 'client'. Clients can be any kind of men, and the significance of their role in passing infections to their wives and families is precisely why they don't want to be identified. Clients range from the guys hanging around darts- and cards-playing and drinking spots looking to barter whatever they have, to workers on payday, to every kind of office big-shot on up to politicians and big businessmen. And HIV programme managers and Christian leaders. You're right, that it is marriages and 'companionate relationships' that are a huge factor in transmission, but in practical terms it's a hard one for prevention and education when there is so much denial and the rhetoric is so far removed from reality. Even if clients are up to steam on HIV, it doesn't mean they will practice safe sex – I've seen plenty of doctors and the like in Australia who will try it on without a condom when they should know better, and some NGO workers, including gay men, are notorious in countries like Papua New Guinea. So even if you educate clients, you still have to make sure that sex workers have the knowledge and ability to insist on safe sex. They are great educators for the community. As I said before, being so mobile, moving and marrying between the highlands and the coast, puts them in a good position to 'spread the word' as it were: a reversal of the idea that sex workers spread disease.

Having said all that, I was sometimes left profoundly unimpressed by the education being passed on by peer educators.

LH: Aly, you're not alone, and that goes for nurses and trainers and all the rest, although there are sterling exceptions to that. Anna Golang, Jenny Jerry and Ross Hutton from Oil Search Limited are doing great things in Moro, for example. Nevertheless, I've said it many times before, that there doesn't seem to be much attention paid to content.

AM: I'm not sure what kind of quality control there is behind the training courses that they do to get the free T-shirt and cap. Not that I'm dissing the T-shirts: the status earned by doing a course and obtaining such a symbol as a T-shirt can be a big deal for members of extremely marginalised groups, and self-confidence is very important for insisting on safe sex. The peer educators I talked to had trouble reconciling ABC (Abstinence, Be Faithful, Condoms as a last resort but preferably follow Christ) with the realities of sex work. ABC is so not about supporting and training sex workers to support each other to work safely with condoms. It's saying that what sex workers do is wrong, but doesn't give them any alternatives to support themselves and dependents. Not surprisingly, they also had trouble explaining or distinguishing HIV from AIDS, and struggled to answer common questions about 'black-magic' causing, curing or generally over-riding anything to do with HIV. I also heard a sex worker peer educator telling a bunch of policemen that praying hard enough would cure HIV, and I know you've got hundreds of similarly wacky stories, Lawrence. I'll get back to some of the problems with peer education in terms of the sex worker network. The magnitude of the task of HIV prevention is so overwhelming in Papua New Guinea that there is really nothing else to do but get on with it.

LH: Yeah, Mark Boyd has dubbed this 'building the boat while you're sailing it'. I'll play Devil's Advocate, however, in saying that Papua New Guinea finds itself in this position precisely because so little effort has been paid to programme content, to addressing the anti-condom rhetoric, to confronting Church-related stigma, and so on.

AM: While my time there has been limited and necessarily structured around existing projects, I'm acutely aware of how little of the population is in meaningful contact with any project, good or bad. Whenever our friends took us to a settlement off the beaten track, there was either no idea about HIV, or ideas that were quite frighteningly wrong. I'm not sure why the HIV training is so lame, or the level of basic knowledge so low, but I'd hazard the following few suggestions. When we talked to sex workers about checking clients for STDs, it was a very novel concept, as in general I don't think there's too much removing of clothes and observing of the genital areas. The Christian influence limits sex education on top of limited education in general, so HIV education has a pretty stony field to work on. Tok Pisin doesn't have a great vocabulary for discussing sex, HIV or AIDS, and with information being passed on orally there's endless potential for confusion and misinformation. Those things together create chaos, hysteria, folk devils and moral panics around HIV and sex workers, while challenging incorrect ideas means taking on all kinds of received wisdom way beyond the sexual transmission of infections. And by the way, 'sub-optimal' is a very polite way to say someone doesn't know their arse-grass from their fanny pack.

LH: Okay, you're right: I was being charitable. I've been thinking a lot about your experiences in and between Australia and Papua New Guinea with the Scarlet Alliance and Save the Children (in Papua New Guinea), two organisations that have in some ways been really ahead of the curve. You are to be congratulated for helping to put together the first-ever national sex workers' conference in Port Moresby in April of 2006. I'm sure that you've got a lot to get off your chest, too, in that so little seems to have come from that, and after such enormous effort on your part. In a nutshell, what happened, and why?

AM: Okay, I had to expect that one. My involvement in Papua New Guinea goes back to the early–mid 1990s when the Institute of Medical Research did a national survey of sex and reproduction, which showed an awful lot of sex and reproduction going on, and early efforts were being made to prevent HIV transmission. The Transex project focused on sex workers plus transport workers, security guards, stevedores and the like in Port Moresby and along the Highlands Highway: it was probably way ahead of mainstream attitudes at the time, and it did lay a lot of groundwork for future projects and fostered the first publicly acknowledged sex worker organisation, the Henao Sisters, named after Henao street where their house was located.

Transex has since been praised for Best Practice by UNAIDS (but does the praise still count if it's written by the project's manager?), although back then the funding agencies weren't exactly banging on the whores' doors to keep it going. A handful of women who had become involved stayed with it through various incarnations and umbrellas, including the NAC and the YWCA and the Slavos, I mean Salvos, whose philosophies ranged from basket-weaving to, well, exploitative basket-weaving.

LH: Let's not forget their important work in 'homosexual conversion', too!

AM: I don't know much about that, mate; I'm just going on what I know about one particular project where participants' money was appropriated, 'cuz I've also seen and heard of FBOs doing very useful and well-received work elsewhere. Anyway, this project ended up in the seemingly inappropriate arms of Save the Children (in Papua New Guinea). It's easy to be cynical about the strange bedfellows created by combining massive funding for HIV with NGOs set up for very different purposes, and I have queried the motives of some groups I've been involved with, but as you've said, Save the Children's HIV work in Papua New Guinea has been way ahead of the curve. The Poro Sapot Project (which means friends supporting each other) includes peer education, condom distribution and drop-in centres for MSM and FSW in Port Moresby, Lae, Goroka and Kainantu, which are, respectively the nation's capital and several key points on the Highlands Highway.

Poro Sapot Project was clearly the best partner for Scarlet Alliance, which is based in Sydney and which is Australia's national sex worker rights organisation, since they wanted funding to set up an equivalent Papua New Guinean national organisation. A model existed with the Australian HIV positive people's group (NAPWA) assisting an equivalent in Papua New Guinea (Igat Hope, which means There's Hope). It was to be funded by a relatively small amount of money and was to be a relatively small project, with big implications. It isn't easy for sex workers to get funding in Australia, one reason being the old chestnut that activists are their own worst enemies. For instance, the New South Wales government set out in the late 1980s to fund a sex worker organisation to combat AIDS, but ended up blaming intransigent conflict between the two main groups when funding a new group under the wing of the AIDS Council. This created complications that reverberate to this day. So, to my knowledge the Papua New Guinea initiative was the first stand-alone funding given to a sex worker group.5 And that funding was complicated because Scarlet Alliance was unfunded: an immediate problem arose between the executive's obvious desire to create an office and jobs in Sydney to run Scarlet Alliance as a whole, and my belief, as the initial project officer, that the project should be run mainly in Papua New Guinea for and by the Papua New Guinean sex workers. Scarlet Alliance management didn't think they could do the work in Papua New Guinea without a strong Aussie base, while I was ranting about what's been called 'boomerang aid', where Australian 'aid' to Papua New Guinea ends up benefiting Australian companies and consultants. That was the main difference of opinion as I saw it, that we were being rushed to keep the Papua New Guinea end of things minimal, rather than do the best we could do.

Anyway, we ended up having thousands of sex workers from all areas, ages and genders become interested and express their motivation to get involved in a sex worker network that would respond not only to HIV but also to issues of rights and advocacy on the other issues facing sex workers, like violence, 'sheer male privilege', stigma and discrimination, dealing with the police in a confused legal environment (see especially Amnesty International 2006; Stewart 2004), coping with kids and family breakdowns. So many of these issues are subtly or completely different from those faced by sex workers in Australia, such as dramas over bride-price and polygamy, moving to your husband's village and being abandoned there, the wantok system overall, alcohol and distilled 'steam' being the main drug of choice, bartering, the frequency of individual and pack-rape, illiteracy and extreme poverty and evangelical Christianity. And on the health side, which needs to be rammed home to outside funding agencies, a barely functioning hospital system, unavailable treatments, ubiquitous malaria, tuberculosis and other tropical diseases.

LH: Aly, you mentioned 'thousands of sex workers from all areas, ages and genders'. In a way that would be helpful for office-bound health officials and NGO programme managers in Port Moresby, what would you tell them of the character of sex industries throughout Papua New Guinea?

AM: There didn't seem at the start to be a very good understanding of how commodified sex happens in Papua New Guinea. Sex workers have been 'othered' in the HIV discourse because of the initial 'high risk group'/infectious vector stuff. That just stigmatises people and pushes them away from information and support, making the whole process take that much longer. It's when sex workers are seen as people with rights and strong individuals who have something to say that changes happen. There're a few Asian brothel start-ups in Papua New Guinea, but I don't know about talking about 'sex industries' when it's mostly independent women and some men, and not so many pimps and middle-managers. For HIV projects, that makes it essential to get involved with the peer networks and respecting the sex workers' rights, 'cuz on the plus side they will go around 'gate-keepers' and make it happen.

This isn't the place to get into the whole debacle, but on the plus side, just about every GO, NGO and FBO we approached came onside to support the network, we had a very successful national meeting and a network called Friends Frangipani was established that has a constitution and peer-based leadership. As you said, things have slowed right down, but I think there's a profile for Frangipani now within Papua New Guinea.

LH: So you say. I can't get information from anyone as to what's happening and, like the folks at NACS, they haven't ever replied to any of my e-mail messages.

AM: There have been some staff turnover issues. I just get the occasional news from or about the sex workers involved that they are still in touch and interested in the HIV programmes, and that policy-makers do know about them.

Anyway, back then, with so many sex workers getting involved, and given how tight were our time limits, it was hard to develop decision-making procedures and avoid jealousies over leadership positions and representation at meetings around the country and overseas. There was a level of jealousy and gossip and back-stabbing that I was naïve to think we could rise above. Overall, I was trying to avoid the kind of elitism I've seen develop in many contexts in the region, where there is funding for a marginalised group to send a representative to a conference, on a scholarship or whatever, but it ends up being the same person picked over and over again. That person acquires knowledge, contacts, language skills and appropriate jargon so that they become increasingly the obvious and repeated choice. Unfortunately, this can also result in that person becoming more comfortable and increasingly lauded in the international HIV scene while at the same time becoming more distanced from and actually less representative of the group for whom he or she is supposed to be speaking. In Papua New Guinea it's so clear that knowledge means power, and once having obtained knowledge there is little incentive to share it. It was also hard to extend the project into a representative 'national' network, as the link with Poro Sapot Project made their centres the main game. The relationship between Poro Sapot Project and Scarlet Alliance was not thrashed out from the start, and it wasn't always clear whether people were involved because they represented sex workers or because they worked for Poro Sapot Project. Another thing I have often observed is that, given the ultra-low status of sex workers, 'peers' who have completed training courses and then become peer educators or 'volunteers' (another tricky concept in societies based on reciprocal exchange) or staff tend to identify as HIV educators or any other likely job title, and actively avoid discussion of sex work, even though working with sex workers as peers is supposedly the reason they have joined the NGO. And NGOs provide ID cards, another extremely valuable commodity. Having management be based in Sydney and expect to get instant results in Papua New Guinea via the Internet and use of credit cards added unnecessary layers of hassle to the stuff-ups that happen anyway. When I had to contact Sydney it was tempting to pass on messages like 'tell 'em this is a Third World country' and 'what do they expect: angels with dirty faces?'

I was just so impressed with all the sex workers who made it to Goroka, where the meeting was held, mostly by public motor vehicle, and all happily piled in together with us in a very basic guesthouse (that was also very cold for most of the coastal crew). The camaraderie and sustained commitment was amazing. We'd been warned about people sticking with *wantoks* and not co-operating in something 'national': there was a bit of that (those Wewak women do things differently, for sure!) but commonalities were stronger, including between 'FSW' and 'MSM'. We'd been warned about Christian protests, too, and the meltdown possibilities of plonking down thirty 'out' sex workers in a sleepy part of Goroka. The guesthouse was run by Seventh Day Adventists and when we all left they came to the airport and cried;

the community was puzzled at first but then so supportive that the leaders asked to have an HIV *toksave* (presentation) put on for them. It went so well that it really made me think about what sex workers can teach the rest of society, and not just about HIV or sex in general. The last day of the meeting was a public forum attended by GO, NGO and FBO people, and our gang spontaneously improvised a little play about safe sex. It was in the fantastic Raun-Raun theatre building, there were prayers, there were trannies and women dancing, there was a *mumu* (an earth-oven feast), there were sex workers standing up and having their issues discussed, and there were politicians and big fellahs saying nice things. It felt like a good day.

And then ... we got everyone back home, I went back to Sydney, differences became irreconcilable, and that was the end of it for me. When people are starting with nothing to lose, I tend to think it's a good plan to leave them alone, if the best you are going to do is to offer something, and then take it away.

∗ ∗ ∗

LH: I enjoyed reading your second book, Aly, the deliciously titled *Pink Fits* (Murray 2001; see also Hammar 2007b). I found so much about your critique of the Indonesian national response to AIDS throughout the 1990s to be relevant to what's happening in Papua New Guinea. You showed that the assumption of HIV programmes is that (especially male) bourgeois sexual prerogative and norms must at all costs be protected. In his new collection of essays, too, *A New Look at Thai Aids* (2005), another anthropologist, Graham Fordham, argues on the basis of his long experience in Thailand that what he calls the 'normative AIDS paradigm' was designed not so much to prevent HIV transmission as to protect state, religious and especially bureaucratic sensibilities. Just like in Papua New Guinea, HIV transmission risks were pronounced into being, iterated, cited and reiterated well before any empirically verifiable transmission dynamics could be ascertained. That recalls the assumptions of the HRSS about which I've written previously. You and he both showed that globalisation isn't just the profusion across borders of signs and symbols that induce consumer lust or that enable and support the emergence of what you called New Emerging Sexualities. You showed clearly that in globalisation are found also the cognitive frameworks by which people (mis)understand new threats, both viral and social. Could you talk a bit about how Indonesians perceived and talked about such threats in the 1990s?

AM: This is very important, Lawrence, and I don't think I've got the space here to say much more than I did in *Pink Fits*: I actually wanted to call it *Loose Lips (Pink Fits)*, because the discourses around HIV and sexuality can be so shonky, so jargon-laden and just so plain manipulative. But I've got a lot of mates doing a great job in Indonesia, whereas I haven't been very actively involved there in the last few years, so I'm not wanting to sound too superficial. Not that that has ever stopped me from putting in my two cents' worth! Indonesia certainly went through the same kind of initial response to HIV, with the externally conjured and 'othered' risk group of gay men, especially foreign gay men, becoming an obvious target for fear and loathing. When more adequate information became available showing that infections were mostly occurring through straight sex, then sex workers became the focus. And then in the last ten years there has been a massive increase in injecting drug use in Indonesia, with inevitable results for HIV because that's a vastly more efficient way of sharing viruses than sex. HIV projects have struggled to catch up with IDU issues, beyond a proliferation of expensive cold-turkey farms that rich and worried parents can pay for. When I visited Kerobokan jail in Bali two years ago they had set up a methadone programme, which seemed quite unusually sensible, given the profusion of drugs inside Indonesia's prisons. I can't help mentioning that Kerobokan's chief has been busted since then, for dealing a profusion of drugs inside the prison.

The NGOs I'd been involved with during the Soeharto dictatorship took a radical left-wing stance and tended to dismiss sexuality and HIV as being concerns that only the bourgeoisie would have the luxury to discuss: post-Soeharto, it's become much more *de rigeur* for alternative-type NGOs to run HIV projects. Gay organisations were among the first, and they still have a key role in HIV in Indonesia. They almost invariably involve transexuals or *banci*, who are very visible and who are sort of accepted (there's quite a lot of literature on the subject, tracing cultural origins and so on). *Banci* performances and entertainment have been a popular part of HIV awareness campaigns, so there are ways that Indonesia has moved beyond global stereotypes and developed more locally specific programmes. Elizabeth Pisani has written quite perceptively about HIV funding narratives in Indonesia.

LH: I'd love to see that happen in Papua New Guinea, but I think that's another fall-out of the almost wholly external donor-funded nature of the national response. The best that I see happening on the local level tends to be around issues of care, not so much around communication of factual information or prevention in the first place.

AM: I'm thinking also of peer-based work with the young male 'guides' or gigolos in Bali, Lombok and other tourist areas. Overall though, there is the same issue as in Papua New Guinea, that HIV affects everyone in a general-ised pandemic, so it's not good enough to focus on small groups. Funding projects in Bali is great for avoiding tricky cultural and religious, that is to say Muslim sensibilities, and it looks good for maintaining the tourist dollar and confidence in the face of unfortunate ugly diseases, but it's a bit of a finger in the dyke approach to the flood.

LH: As it were. And as you showed for Indonesia, the models and expecta-tions about membership in putative 'risk groups' that constitute Papua New Guinea's 'normative AIDS paradigm' stigmatises the already stigmatised. Unlike Indonesia, however, there appears to be little in the way of a consum-er, feminist, gay or sex workers movement, and so it seems to produce rhetor-ics of risk that are even more off-kilter. It's weird, how much is presumed and pronounced in the name of sex but with so little empirical evidence. The intractable nature of the ABC approach is another example, as are the many references to 'African'-style HIV epidemics that threaten Papua New Guinea.

Like Indonesia and Thailand, the profusion of NGOs and INGOs, CBOs, GOs and FBOs devoted in one or another way to these important issues is pretty impressive. Nevertheless, it just seems that, from our perspectives as activists, researchers and anthropologists, they keep getting things having to do with sex horribly wrong. Why do you think that is? Why can't policy-makers keep it real when it comes to sex?

AM: I think we've started to answer that already, in that these organisations have an interest in maintaining a fantasy about sex that conspires against keeping it real. If your spiritual leader disapproves of condoms, then it limits your policy options. Likewise, if your government wants to talk only about Thatcherite nuclear family units. The Bush-Howard era was so reactionary, and there was not much scope for talking about sex beyond affective, monogamous, heterosexual relationships. There's an assumption of male domination, but not much acknowledgment of women's role in bartering sex for cash or favours, or ultimately having the controlling role in fertility. (I could put a plug in here for my next book, *Drawing Blood*, which is going to be a reading of tattooing practice in some pre-capitalist, pre-Christian societies, to show that male awe at female fertility, as represented by bleeding, is the defining feature of the culture). You've mentioned genital cutting and 'male menstruation' earlier'.

It was important to me in working with the Papua New Guinea sex workers that I wasn't using incomprehensible language, but I also became acutely aware that their own language and ideas are affected by their involvement with organisations, government bodies and churches. Like the inability to think outside ABC: if it doesn't fit, can we just add letters? How about D for **D**ecrease clients, E and F and onwards to alphabetical lunacy? And I'll get on to 'basket-weaving' as a mentality. As I was talking about with the 'elite' representatives of marginalised groups, there are so many sex workers in Papua New Guinea, yet various funded groups seem to compete to work with the same people, mutter darkly about 'poaching', and are so secretive and suspicious of one another that the same wheels are invented over and over again. 'Peer educators' are treated differently at each place in terms of payment, transport, smokes and betel-nut, before we even get started on what peer means …

LH: Go ahead, let me get you started on what 'peer' means!, or on what it *doesn't* mean. How is that different than in, say, Australia?

AM: As I've tried to say, there's confusion around 'peer' in general, about whether it can be an identity in the way the gay community has used it, how 'peer' will get ditched in favour of 'health educator' or anything similar because of the discrimination that goes with sex work (and less so in Papua New Guinea), but in Australia I'd rather come out as gay than a sex worker – and I'd get more support for it. Sex worker peer networks do exist, generally around a local place of work, so it's definitely possible to extend that commonality of interest. The group I was most involved with in Australia, the Queer & Esoteric Workers' Union, got a very mixed bunch of sex workers together and active. The thing is that the commonalities are around sex worker rights, violence, cops, gender issues, where HIV is related but not the priority. I'm like a lot of activists who've worked in HIV mostly because that's where the funding is, to get things happening around rights. And what that means in practice varies radically between a rich country like Australia and an impoverished one like Papua New Guinea: the rhetoric is there about HIV being a development issue but then it still gets isolated out away from the bigger picture. The Millennium Development Goals talk about HIV, but that's not what people see on the ground: no one dies of HIV, they are still dying of tuberculosis, pneumonia and malaria, supposedly treatable diseases that may or may not be related to HIV infection. External funding agencies just don't seem to acknowledge, in their imported projects, what kind of lives and priorities and sex the majority of Papua New Guineans have.

This isn't particularly on-message, but I get upset constantly by the entrenched hierarchies that rank over-paid expatriates (and experts) over underpaid nationals over downtrodden peers and volunteers. All manner of double standards are then applied. It's horrible to stay at such fancy hotels as the Crowne Plaza and Coral Seas' joints where your local friends can't come in without you, where they get told to take off hats and change thongs but you don't.

LH: But Aly, it's such an efficient way of spending money on Leadership Forums!

AM: Mmm ... Apart from Poro Sapot Project, most organisations have links to a church, and most of their dealings with sex workers are variations on the basket-weaving mentality. Sex workers are seen as victims who need 'retraining', usually in some kind of domestic skill like cooking or basket- or *bilum*-making, that is, things that most women already do.

LH: I'm betting that few Papua New Guinean health officials are familiar with the Magdalen Societies of modern Europe or of the gender relations encoded therein, but that's what such impulses remind me of. They're training them in essence to become wives (or better wives), when that's what's gotten them into trouble in the first place!

AM: Umm ... I have no idea about Magdalen Societies either. Meanwhile, as a new organisation in Papua New Guinea, the veteran peers came and sussed us out, sometimes with little basket-weaving funding proposals they'd prepared earlier. They were more than happy to ditch them in favour of what we were doing, though. It's not hard to explain that domestic skills are just lovely but can't bring in the income needed to support kids, which is why you're doing sex work in the first place. Fine, do some training in the down-time, learn English, but don't give up your night job!

Personally, I think the churches have been a disaster overall for Papua New Guinea, but they are not going to go away, so the only thing is to work with them – you could call it harm minimisation. I think some of your references to Christianity are over-generalised – some of the FBOs I've met aren't so bad, and it must be possible to get some of them to support condoms and for practical reasons to acknowledge extra-marital sex. Pretty much all the sex workers follow some kind of church. Meetings always start and finish with prayers, and anyone will be happy to lead them. When I've stayed with sex workers I've woken up to find them mumbling their way through the Bible, the only book they have. It must be terrible to feel like your religion condemns you for the stuff you have to do just to survive and feed your kids. It's a recipe for low self-esteem, which then militates against safe practices and making informed choices. I'd like to see you discuss the need to confront religious doctrine a bit more productively, for example, by deconstructing the megalithic enemy into a whole range of interpretations, from open-minded to completely raving bonkers.

LH: Fair enough, and since first reading your words I've made some changes, but I have to say that even the most open-minded still blocks any attention being paid to male sexual prerogative *per se* and tends to believe that marriage is the solution instead of the problem, which, I'm sorry, is just way off the mark.

AM: Well maybe, but I just don't see much debate about male privilege inside Papua New Guinea, and women are helping to perpetuate it, like the way you see mothers letting their little boys boss and hit them. Right-field reactionaries have been allowed to dominate in Papua New Guinea, but I don't think it has to be like that. However much I disagree from the outside and get upset about extreme quotes and letters to the editor, nothing's going to change from my criticisms alone. One of the planks of the sex work project was getting on side with religious people, like the Anglican Bishop and some of the Baptists, for instance, and getting them to support a more pro-sex outlook. And naming and shaming the loonies to make it clear they don't represent all Christians – even with my limited understanding of religion, I reckon there's a good case to be made using the same Bible, to make them back off. Like you say, the funding agencies bend over backwards to accommodate Christians but maybe they would be more discerning if different opinions among the churches were out in the open. It's in the interests of churches, since they are all in competition for the same flock, to accept sex workers as part of the community, and in the interests of sex workers to feel part of the church community and eventually have their own say.

LH: Well, a couple of reactions, Aly. First, I don't disagree with your characterisations about mine, I mean, about perhaps painting with an overly broad stroke, but I wonder whether you could summarise your impressions of these characteristic differences between denominations you found. For example, you've mentioned but not gone into any detail what might be differences in policy and practice between Seventh Day Adventists, Anglicans or Baptists on matters of sex, condoms, HIV and AIDS. If anything, what some representatives have said is that ABC is too liberal! I mean, even the Anglican Bishop has okayed condom usage really only for *extra*-marital sex, not for unprotected sex *per se*, that is, between spouses, and we don't need to discuss what some of Catholic leaders or Pentecostal officials say and do about condoms, homosexuality, prostitution and the like. In three years I just didn't encounter many progressive ideas or practices from Catholics, SDA or Baptists. Quite to the contrary. I think it's too easy to cut the Christian churches slack *in this specific regard* about sex-positive, safer sex initiatives.

Second, you have talked about the 'sex work' concept being misapplied in a Papua New Guinea context, about the 'different' nature of sexuality and sexual networking in Papua New Guinea and their implications for HIV and STD prevention campaigns. I'd like to know how you'd expand upon that here, especially in terms of to what extent health bodies and officials understand anything of that.

AM: Yeah, there are differences. Sex worker activists in the West define sex work as a choice, but the 'choice' of sex work in impoverished countries is made from a very different set of options. And there are huge differences between notions of choice, and what a branch of feminists and their hangers-on label as coercion and trafficking and patriarchal oppression and so on. In Papua New Guinea we had a lot of debate as to what to even call sex work because the concept is so slippery and a lot of women are drifting in and out of survival sex work and sex for favours. Some NGO workers were coming around to just translating the English as *seks wok*, but it's never exactly clear how that's understood. One flier we translated painstakingly was taken home by another NGO worker and came back the next day with all the *seks wokas* changed to *pamuks*, which is extremely pejorative. Most Tok Pisin terms like that are very degrading, sexist and horrible. Like *tu kina bus meri*, meaning a woman who will do it in the bush for 2 kina or the price of a beer, and that's a more acceptable one: I've got a page full of terms for female sex workers. There's no welfare, a lot of poverty and a lot of women who have dependent children. At the same time churches are imposing their moral standards and there is all the harmful, intrusive gossip. There's a high level of awareness of sex work but with very negative connotations.

LH: I was struck also by the argument that Kathy Lepani made in her ASAO conference presentation a few years ago, '"Still in the process of knowing": making sense of HIV and AIDS in the Trobriand Islands' (Lepani 2004). Her opening claim was that 'In the Trobriands, the "process of knowing" about the epidemic requires people to reconcile the fear of impending sickness and death with sexual practices largely viewed and experienced as life-affirming, pleasurable expressions of sociality'. I was struck partly because such sex-positive affirmations are so rarely encountered in Papua New Guinea. How might that compare to some of the places you've worked in Indonesia?

AM: I was also struck by Kathy's work because it is so rare in Papua New Guinea to hear sex talked about as being pleasurable for all parties. In most discussions about sex work you'd never know that what was being traded was enjoyable, at least for the client, like your opening quote that links the sex trade in Thailand to both global capitalism and male domination. Is it all just a grim patriarchal power trip? So why would men in Papua New Guinea ever pay for sex, if they can just impose it?

LH: Or if sex is so terrible and evil and morally distasteful and dangerous. Above all, policy makers seem unable to imagine that prostitution and marriage are, among many, many other things, linked dialectically. Women are prostituted in marriage, by husbands and other male relatives, but in prostitution of various forms women also find lovers, boyfriends and husbands. I mean, go pool-side or bar-side in 10 of Port Moresby's finer hotels on most afternoons and you'll see this in action. Other scholars and activists have written quite perceptively about these dynamics elsewhere in the Pacific. Siusiua Lafitani (1998: 81), for example, has written that 'Sex for cash has increasingly become the main goal to be pursued ... in the marketplace, though some prostitutes end up falling in love with foreigners and joining them abroad in a marriage relationship.'

AM: Right. There is a huge difference between non-consensual sex and a bartered agreement between adults, while the line between sex work and affective relationships can be very blurry, with sex workers 'giving it away' to someone they like, and women who would never call themselves sex workers marrying purely for acquired wealth and status: it's all very subjective, and maybe that's why policy-makers have a hard time with it all. As you point out, it is not uncommon for sex workers to find lovers or husbands from their clients. Settling for one man might be a calculated economic move, or not. In Jakarta, where the competition over rich expatriates could be fierce, some of the (to me, anyway) most attractive girls would end up marrying someone like the bouncer because he was just the one they loved.

When HIV comes into the picture, there are also the cognitive struggles women undergo between sex/pleasure/money/other benefits *now*, versus HIV/sickness/death *later*. For a survival sex worker, that means feeding herself and her kids now, versus the possibility of HIV acquired through a sexual transaction. It's pretty much a no-brainer (but which some 'experts' don't get), to prioritise the immediate threat of starvation and/or violence, over the future, which is hazy at best. HIV is hard to understand, and the Grim Reaper-style shock campaigns have been tempered with antiretroviral combinations that appear to make HIV more like a treatable chronic infection than a death sentence, as well as the quack medicines and black magic stories all over Papua New Guinea that not many people would be brave enough to dismiss. Arguments that HIV is some kind of colonialist-capitalist plot are not too hard to sell either, compared with the complications of 'safe' and 'safer' sex, 'window-periods', and a collection of more-or-less life-threatening, formerly obscure diseases that a virus will eventually make you susceptible to. Or like I said, if you're dying of something like TB in a crappy health system, is it worth knowing or caring if you also have HIV? Will that just bring pointing fingers and ostracism?

The main message in Papua New Guinea, encouraged by the Bush-era anti-prostitution stance, is ABC: get rid of the problem (sex) by pretending it doesn't happen. Your use of 'sexual networking' is much more realistic, although to me it has some echoes of 'contact tracing'. While most people are probably aware that the person they are having sex with is also having and/or has had sex all over the place, they don't really want to know, and the other person doesn't really want to tell – that ad in Australia in which a couple are in bed and then the screen widens to a sea of beds and a caption reads something like 'who are you really sleeping with?' – wasn't terribly successful. You couldn't even begin to try something like that in Papua New Guinea. We all have some degree of performance anxiety about sex even when it's a profession, and the ghosts of other partners in the room don't help at all.

Sexual networking is a good term though, because it can cover the whole variety of sex within and outside affective relationships, sex for pleasure and sex having a transactable value, and different values being attached to sex depending on the gender and sexual identity of those involved. And just about any of these kinds of sexual networking can involve some kind of sex work if you move beyond simplistic definitions. That is, virtually any of the inequalities of power, wealth, pleasure and sex drive, age and whatever other distinctions can be variously compensated for. (I think I'm now reacting to over-simplifications by over-complicating!) You comment that HIV literature has been unable to see the dialectical link between prostitution and marriage, and there is a big problem with focusing on monogamous heterosexual marriage as the gold standard which, if followed, will save us all from HIV. I have a strange admiration for faith-based projects in Papua New Guinea doggedly plugging that line in the midst of such a rampantly sexual environment.

LH: Yes, that is strange! Don't tell me that you're suffering from cognitive dissonance, too?!

AM: Well, I wouldn't know. I *would* suggest, however, from my argument before, that there is more of a continuum than a dialectic between prostitution and marriage, with the Madonna/Whore dichotomy having more of a symbolic importance for social and religious structures. It's divide-and-rule applied to women to maintain the status quo. Good women blame the bad women for their husband's infidelities, so women police themselves. Shit, you even get the good whores blaming the bad whores for their regular client's infidelities.

LH: Yeah, I don't disagree, and I employ the notion of a continuum in most of my writings about these matters. I should be more clear when I'm talking specifically about the rhetoric (as opposed to empirical facts) of social life, including of HIV prevention campaign messages, that is, that don't look at the sociological factors at work that push especially women back and forth across that divide. I don't disagree with your point about the continuum, obviously, but the fact of a continuum (of, in this case, forms of sexual networking) doesn't to my mind disqualify there also being a dialectical relationship at work between (forms of) marriage and (forms of) prostitution. What I mean is that, although it is obviously true in empirical, behavioural fact, the notion of a continuum of sexual networking would never be accepted by religious leaders and health officials in Papua New Guinea. That would never happen because that would focus on the nitty-gritty of sex (that is, increasingly safer or pleasurable sexual acts or forms of transactions) instead of on its moral attributes (in which there is only 'good' or 'bad' sex, marriage or prostitution).

AM: One more point that should be emphasised from this discussion is that the most common inequality being traded off in sex is that between male and female. Arranged marriages have been found more long-lasting than 'love matches', possibly because the trade-offs, such as fertility against status, are clear from the beginning. In parts of Java and the Papua New Guinea highlands where polygamy is still practised it's even easier to see how men use 'ownership' of women to ensure paternity and acquire status (plus being perceived to benefit from the pleasure of readily available sex). This is in contrast with how a woman who has many partners is viewed: there will be connotations of 'prostitution' whether or not there is any financial gain. Women are easily commodified in a way that men are not, MSM and Bali gigolos notwithstanding.

Just in terms of that continuum, I'd like to make a bit of a distinction with Australia, where sex work has a more 'professionalised' image, propagated by sex worker rights groups, of sex work as being a job that has regulations and standards. There are survival sex workers who fall into cracks in the (currently pretty cracked) system; but in Papua New Guinea there is, to coin a phrase, more crack than system. Sex work in Papua New Guinea is not so isolated from other parts of life such as other relationships and the having and rearing of kids. Aussie sex workers form affective relationships with clients, too, but in Papua New Guinea and Indonesia there's probably more acknowledgment that a rich client who becomes a regular partner or husband is desirable and can even be literally life-saving. Sex has a value to be traded. That may take the form of cash, beer, favours, or credits towards a longer term pay-off, such as when a woman becomes an expat's 'contract wife', a fairly exclusive sexual property for the term of a work contract.

LH: That's true in Papua New Guinea, too, definitely, but sometimes the length of the contract is two weeks or two months or whatever, and the woman may be the 'exclusive' sexual property of a man only as long as he is around, which is to say, potentially of several guys simultaneously, if she can get away with it. It's so weird, that especially national health bodies and officials have been so silent about this, since Port Moresby, Lae, Madang and Mt. Hagen examples are so very easy to find. They're even easier to find, however, at enclaves of resource extraction, in Moro, in Tabubil, and so on.

AM: This kind of credit arrangement rarely has clear rules, and I have seen many relationships end up in tears because the woman's expectations have not been made sufficiently clear: she has acted like a dutiful in-love girlfriend while tallying up a grand total in her head, and then been ditched for a younger model and left with nothing.

LH: *Hello...* plain-old marriage in the US!

AM: In such a case, however, the man is not then held to blame; more likely, the women involved will fight it out amongst themselves in best divide-and-rule fashion! I'm trying to emphasise sex worker peer groups and awareness of them, but there is always the other side, of individual competition, hierarchies between groups, racism and every kind of divisive behaviour found among marginalised groups (including sex worker activists) under pressure from social stigma and/or impoverishment. People in Papua New Guinea are having sex all over the shop, and making policy more real means accepting that and starting in on the discrimination and basic causes of poverty that militate against all that sex being safer.

NOTES

1. I acknowledge the request from an anonymous review that I remove any mention of ritualised homosexuality among Sepik river cultures, but I believe that I have been misunderstood on the point. My point was not at all whether or not imputations of such to them had a ring of truth, and I didn't say so, but rather, to question the all-too-quick acceptance of 'MSM' despite denying 'traditional' homosexuality among Sepik river groups. In any event, Christine Stewart's provocative new essay, for example, 'Men Behaving Badly: sodomy cases in the Colonial Courts of Papua New Guinea' (2008) mentions ethnographers, patrol officers and circuit court judges who noted that male–male sexual contact was, for example, 'contrary to the customs of the people of the Sepik District', but that it did in fact happen, especially in view of the special dictates of plantation labour economies. Another colonial authority, she writes, 'conceded that homosexuality was a product of the "abnormal conditions" of the labour lines' (Stewart 2008: 83) and yet another, four decades later, expressed his concern about the 'unnatural vice' frequently reported in context of labour line conditions (2008: 83).

2. The third of the four opening epigraphs comes from one such, a young woman whom I met in a Port Moresby hotel infamous for expatriate male/Papuan female couplings and who was the 'wife' of a 'fly-in/fly-out' contractor for five to six weeks in a row but who then also lived in the apartment of an expatriate pilot for Air Niugini to whom she belonged when he was in town on break.

3. It is difficult for commentators nowadays to admit to *already sexually transacted women* in Pacific communities prior to European contact, whether in or toward marriage or in and following ritualised copulation. Few wish to tangle with the complexities of gendered language, behavior and motivation that occurred aboard many thousands of ships in the eighteenth and nineteenth centuries, much less upon the beaches and in the domiciles of Pacific islanders. The sexual desires of male expatriates in the twentieth and twenty-first centuries remain blank slates in epidemiological terms (see Chapters 3 and 4), and conference convenors and workshop attendees seem not to want to think about them. To examine reflexively the sexual double standards at work in Christian doctrine and practice that aid and abet such is even more difficult nowadays, especially for those who, in their capacity as health or religious officials, must stump for ABC and other faith-based initiatives. To allow critically that there is a political-economy to sex, that prostitution comes from somewhere or something within social-structure, not just externally, that contemporary 'prostitutes' don't simply suffer from some kind of moral taint, has proven almost impossible in public discourse in contemporary Papua New Guinea.

4. There was for a couple of years a video parlor attached to this particular guest house and '*kai ba*' (fast-food joint). When I interviewed the owner, a South Korean expatriate whose family was from North Korea, she told me that K8.50/hour was paid to rent video and room, and females were available in the foyer. The video parlor was shut down when bribes were not paid to police chiefs, according to the owner, but according to Murray here, who has spoken with other informants, it was shut down owing to its being labelled as a 'high-risk' setting and ultimately to its being stigmatised by Christian groups and representatives.

5. Ruta Fiti-Sinclair was funded some time ago, in about 1993 or thereabouts, to conduct fieldwork amongst and to try to foment a sense of identity and community between sex workers (she called them 'prostitutes') in Port Moresby, although only one very brief publication resulted therefrom (see Fiti-Sinclair 1996).

Chapter 8

'Trust me, I'm a doctor'

Side effects, adverse events and other problems of HAART in PNG

Adverse events and side effects

PNG is a resource poor country and so shouldn't put too much into HIV/ AIDS treatment, especially the antiretroviral medications. I don't think the PNG government should put even a single toea into HIV drugs. They should be saved only for HIV infections that health workers get on the job. And we should pour the money [we save thereby] into education. If you have a situation where no ARVs are available, then people will be more careful about sex. (Medical doctor in Papua New Guinea, Personal communication, 17 July 2007)

LH: Lawrence Hammar
MB: Mark Boyd

I first became interested in the work of Mark Boyd and his colleagues in Australia and Thailand upon reading a proposal he put in service of a Masters degree he was pursuing in Health and International Development. His proposal drew attention to the limited usefulness of 'awareness'-heavy interventions in HIV programmes, the kinds that were covered in Chapters 3 and 4. I remember him warning of the dangers of assuming that biomedical, pharmaceutical understandings of disease and its prevention would win the day in Papua New Guinea without also attending to issues of the sexual culture. He was addressing problems of HIV and AIDS, in other words, not just in terms of intervening in immune system function, but more fundamentally, in attempts to heal harmful, damaging social relations and the symptoms of HIV infection, whatever those may be. Mark has for some years been involved in clinical trials of the antiretroviral therapies whose recent 'scaling-up' has become a national priority in Papua New Guinea.

Their economic, social and medical costs in 'resource-limited settings' (RLS) alongside their penchant for enabling the development of resistance to them are extremely serious issues to consider. Neither has really garnered all that much public discussion in Papua New Guinea, however, nor of their not inconsiderable toxicity. The nausea and weight loss they can cause, the diarrhoea and anaemia that can accompany antiretroviral therapies, are dubbed 'side effects' and 'adverse events', which raise many clinical issues and beg questions of language and cognition, too. Nina Etkin published an essay some time ago, '"Side Effects": cultural constructions and reinterpretations of Western pharmaceuticals' (Etkin 1992), that is extremely relevant here. Asha Persson (2004) has recently written quite cogently about lipodystrophy in 'Incorporating Pharmakon: HIV, medicine and body shape change' that affects many who go on antiretrovirals and that has some interesting gender-distinct manifestations, too. Mark's points below about the individual bodily suffering of both HIV and of the antiretrovirals designed to minimise their impact underscore a larger point, too, regarding the remarkable differences of scale between countries that are posed by HIV and AIDS. Two of his colleagues in Australia, David Wilkinson and Greg Dore, note that the suffering in a single district of South Africa outstrips that in the entirety of Australia, which remains far less vulnerable and has drastically more resources to throw at the problem (Wilkinson and Dore 2000: 279).

✳ ✳ ✳

LH: Mark, a recent paper by you and your colleagues (Boyd et al. 2006) reported on the results of conduct of a randomised, controlled trial (an RCT) of HIV medicines. It looked at the effects of two different combinations of antiretroviral therapies. One regimen of ritonavir-boosted saquinavir (that comes in tablet and in soft-gel form and in a hard-gel capsule form, which is used in 200-mg potency, as Invirase® and Fortovase®), which is an HIV-protease inhibitor, and efavirenz (brand names Sustiva® and Stocrin®), which is a non-nucleoside analogue reverse transcriptase inhibitor (NNRTI), was given with, and those same drugs were given without enfuvirtide, which is an HIV-fusion inhibitor. You concluded that 'relatively simple antiretroviral combination regimens, when used at maximal efficiency, may exert sufficient potency for the optimal treatment of chronic HIV infection' (Boyd et al. 2006: 1322). I'm wondering whether at this point you could say more about this particular study. What's so special about enfuvirtide for Papua New Guinea? What's reasonable to assume would be 'optimal treatment' there? How simple are the treatment regimens for patients to adhere to and physicians to monitor closely? What happens under markedly less than optimal conditions?

MB: In some ways this is perhaps the least useful study to discuss. Firstly, enfuvirtide is an antiretroviral agent licensed for use in what is termed 'late' or 'deep salvage' situations. That is to say that it is used to improve the chances of patients to respond to therapy when they have been exposed to all other classes of antiretroviral therapies (ART) and have for one reason or another failed them. Or perhaps it is fairer to say that the therapy has failed the patient.

LH: I wasn't going to say anything! Well, actually, I was, but you picked up on it already. The language of the medical sciences (e.g. 'child delivery', IRIS, 'AIDS virus', 'peri-menopausal', 'coital debut', 'reservoirs of infection' and the like) can sometimes get social scientists in a snit over the ways it can hide power relations, medicalise normal human bodily function and oversimplify disease causation. Labels are powerful things.

MB: Yes, labels are powerful things, and the notion of 'failure' is a good example of the way in which the construction of the language suggests that the patient is at fault, that is, has 'failed the therapy'. This is unhelpful because it is well known that taking medication on a regular basis is challenging and difficult, and particularly so when, as you pointed out, the therapy is associated with toxic effects. Anyway, having said that, enfuvirtide is a very useful agent in this situation, but it is also an expensive and complicated agent to manufacture. Also, because of the fact that it has to be injected, not swallowed, and that it has been licensed for deep salvage situations only, it is not a drug that has wide application as yet in settings outside the developed world.

However, your question about 'optimal treatment' is quite relevant and does to an extent flow from our conclusion to the study you mentioned regarding the optimal management of HIV-infection. Let's start with that study and that conclusion. The rationale for the conduct of that study was that it was biologically plausible that the more viral targets you hit with the various types (or classes) of ART, the more potent the therapy might be. The study compared the use of a ritonavir-boosted protease-inhibitor and a non-nucleoside analogue reverse transcriptase inhibitor.

LH: That's a mouthful.

MB: Protease inhibitors (PIs) target the viral process through which the virus comes to adopt its mature, three-dimensional shape prior to escaping from the human cell and going on to infect other cells. One of the problems with the PIs in the early combination ART days (1996–2000) was that they required frequent dosing in order to maintain an adequate amount of the drug in the body to provide continuous antiviral activity against HIV. This meant dosing three times daily, and it has been known for a long time (from other chronic disease states such as hypertension) that a dosing schedule that includes a lunch time dose is always difficult for patients to adhere to – they forget to bring the tablet, forget to take the dose because they are busy and/or distracted, or sometimes may not want to bring it to work for confidentiality reasons. To make matters worse, the drugs at that time came with various dosing restrictions such as having to be taken apart from eating food, as food adversely affected drug absorption. The answer to this problem came ironically in the form of using a low dose of an early PI called ritonavir, which profoundly affects the metabolism of the other PIs in the liver and thereby maintains adequate drug levels in the body with less frequent dosing (typically, 'ritonavir-boosted PIs' or 'boosted PIs' or 'bPIs' need to be taken either twice or just once per day) and without food restrictions. Non-nucleoside analogue reverse transcriptase inhibitors (or NNRTIs) are those agents that change the confirmation of the reverse transcriptase enzyme, thereby inhibiting viral replication …

LH: Sort of pushing them into a cul-de-sac, a dead-end?

MB: Well no, this 'cul-de-sac'-type strategy is how the nucleoside analogue reverse transcriptase inhibitors (NRTIs) work; these agents are dummy forms of the natural nucleotides that are used by the reverse transcriptase enzyme to reproduce itself. They are not quite the same though, and when these NRTIs become incorporated into the growing HIV chain, replication is terminated (the 'cul-de-sac' in your metaphor). The *non*-nucleoside analogue reverse transcriptase inhibitors (NNRTIs) work away from the active catalytic site and bind the reverse transcriptase enzyme itself in such a way that the enzyme undergoes a conformational change which renders its activity inefficient. In any case, all these agents act to impede the replication of the virus in the body and thereby bring down the HIV load. What we found was that the characteristics of the viral decline in plasma following initiation of therapy with either one of those regimens was similar. What that means is that the addition of an agent that targeted a separate mechanism of the process of HIV replication (for example, the enfuvirtide targeting the fusion of the virus with the human cellular membrane) didn't seem to make any difference to the rate of decline in the amount of virus in the plasma. So we therefore concluded that combinations of conventional agents may inhibit viral replication to an extent that might not be greatly improved by adding extra drug classes.

LH: Okay, I follow you, but you mentioned plasma and also therapy. Did you do this experiment *in vitro* or *in vivo*?

MB: Yeah, we did this study in HIV-infected Thai patients, that is, it was a clinical study and not a laboratory experiment conducted *in vitro*. The reason that we frequently discuss findings in plasma in such studies is that we routinely draw blood (plasma is the component of blood that remains once you have removed the blood cells) from patients in order to quantify how much viral replication is occurring, as well as assess other biochemical and cellular indicators of organ health such as liver enzymes, electrolyte balance and the amount of red blood cells.

Anyway, to answer your question about optimal treatment and simplicity more directly, both in terms of adherence and monitoring, the first thing to say is that treatment regimens have become substantially simpler and more tolerable over the 11 years that we have had what we call 'potent combination ART' (sometimes also referred to as 'highly active antiretroviral therapy', or HAART). At the advent of the potent combination ART era …

LH: Sorry, which was roughly when?

MB: ... since 1996; at that time the regimens were frequently complex and not very much fun for the patient. They were associated with various restrictions (for example, certain medications had to be taken with or without food), they involved high pill burdens (usually >10 tablets per day) and they were associated with substantial adverse events (such as nausea, loose stools, vomiting, headache, lethargy, changes in body fat morphology, dyslipidaemia, glucose intolerance and more). This should be contrasted with the situation now in both developed- and developing-country settings in which the pill burden for first-line ART can be as few as one tablet taken daily. There are few restrictions to consider, and there seems to be reasonable tolerance, too. So the short answer is that contemporary treatment regimens, particularly first-line regimens, are not that tough to adhere to.

LH: That's absolutely great news for Papua New Guinea then, right?

MB: Well, it's good news for everybody, including people in resource-limited settings like those in Papua New Guinea. In general, and in varied settings, the experience has been that if patients understand what the medicines are for, if they are given reasonable explanations of the expected adverse effects, and if they have reasonable support (both in the community and in the clinic) the majority do well, at least in the short-term (by which I mean the first couple of years). There is an extensive literature now from both developed- and developing-world settings suggesting that of all patients who were started on a standard first-line regimen, somewhere around 60% to 80% of patients will have had an optimal response after one year (which is defined as an 'undetectable' amount of HIV RNA in their plasma). In terms of medium- to long-term outcomes we don't have enough evidence yet to judge, but if one extrapolates from the experience in developed countries, the attrition rates over the following three or four years are relatively small, such that one might still expect 50% of all patients to be experiencing sustained success on their first-line ART. These medium-term data should be appearing from some of the sites in the developing world that some time ago commenced with ART roll-out programmes.

LH: Okay, I follow you, but isn't that a big 'if', to 'extrapolate from the experience in developed countries'? I mean, what will this mean to someone getting treatment from an STD clinic in Mt. Hagen but who lives two hours away or to someone from an inaccessible rural enclave or an urban settlement-dweller in Port Moresby or Lae? From what I've read, the bulk of ART patients and candidates in Papua New Guinea barely have two toea to rub together, many have little hope of good nutrition and probably most have to suffer through less than hygienic living conditions, including access to clean water. I'm just throwing out those scenarios because others have raised them as possible impediments to the expansion of the antiretroviral programme to rural areas.

MB: Well, yes, that is a fair comment. However, given that the data suggest that ART access programmes in many diverse settings in developing countries, many in quite poor countries, achieve similar outcomes to those in developed countries, I think it is reasonable to believe that the medium-term outcomes will also be similar to those seen in resource-rich settings. This is particularly the case as much of the attrition in ART programmes (in rich and poor countries alike) occurs in the first year, often within the first six months, as patients adjust to being on therapy, deal with early side-effects and other adversities such as immune reconstitution phenomena. Once you are over that 'hump', so to speak, things often settle down and follow-up becomes relatively routine.

Anyway, from the point-of-view of clinical monitoring, the serious adverse events associated with the standard first-line regimens are in general reasonably well understood by clinicians. The public health approach to ART monitoring and the ART guidelines that have been adopted by the WHO have promoted a simple, standardised approach to clinical monitoring, including what to do in situations in which ART toxicity is suspected.

So, the short answer to your question about the use of combination ART in less than optimal settings, by which I take it you mean the performance of such programmes in resource-limited settings where health infrastructure is often weak ...

LH: I do.

MB: ... is that they have performed exceptionally well.

However, it is important to acknowledge that they haven't been without their problems. There are data, for instance, from ART programmes in Southern African countries that are quite worrying. They suggest a lot of early mortality in patients who have been diagnosed with AIDS and who commence ART but with very low CD4 counts (by that I mean <50 cells/μL). Left completely untreated for their AIDS-related infections, they are predicted to be dead within six months. Unfortunately, the exact cause of this early and unexpected attrition is incompletely understood, but it almost certainly relates to the high morbidity associated with severe HIV-induced immunodeficiency prior to commencing ART.

LH: That sounds tautologous to me, if you accept the HIV-is-the-sole-and-sufficient-cause-of-AIDS scenario: HIV infection produces the diagnoses of AIDS at commencement of ART and which is due to severe HIV-induced immunodeficiency prior to commencing ART. How does one disentangle the varied effects of HIV and ART, both of which are 'toxic', for lack of a better term?

MB: Well yes, if not tautologous then certainly paradoxical. However, these paradoxical reactions to the introduction of therapy have been described before the advent of HIV and combination ART. In the therapy of tuberculosis, for instance, there is an extensive literature describing the phenomenon of an apparent 'worsening' of the disease after anti-TB therapy has been initiated (for instance, the appearance of large, painful, swollen lymph nodes where such didn't exist pre-treatment). What this represents is not in fact a worsening of the disease process but a manifestation of an improved immune response to the presence of TB as a consequence of therapy. If therapy is continued, such patients generally do very well in the long term, meaning full and complete cure in the case of TB.

However, whatever the cause, what seems clear is that these outcomes could be avoided if patients were identified before they developed late-stage HIV disease as reflected by an AIDS diagnosis and/or a very low CD4 count. This is partly what has inspired the WHO to call recently for a modified approach to HIVab testing in order that we might identify HIV-infected people before they reach such a precarious stage of ill health and can offer them therapy at a time before it is associated with excessive risks. In this modified approach the conventional 'opt-in' testing strategy (in which HIVab testing only occurs with the explicit consent of the individual following appropriate counselling) is changed to one of 'opt-out', in which the expectation is that an HIVab test will be done unless that person specifically asks that it not be done).

In parallel with this there is a new focus on the benefits of earlier introduction of ART in all settings as we begin to understand that uncontrolled HIV-infection may be related to various adverse outcomes that had been previously attributed to the adverse effects of ART. Fortunately, an important study conducted by the SMART Study Group (2006) was published in the *New England Journal of Medicine*.

LH: Do tell. I'd like your opinion about this because when I read it I saw an immediate application to the situation in Papua New Guinea. I was glad that you said these study findings seemed paradoxical, because the first couple of times through I was all confused about simultaneous increase of one risk and seeming non-decrease but of another risk. It turns out they were talking about risks to the patient of unhindered HIV infection during planned periods of HIV treatment interruption, on the one hand, compared to the risks of taking ART continuously, on the other. The SMART Study Group assigned for 16 months a sample of 5,472 patients who were HIVab+ to two arms of a study. Half of them went into the 'drug conservation' arm, where they received 'episodic', that is, planned but intermittent therapy, and the other half were put into the constant, 'viral suppression' arm. They called this study 'CD4+ Count: guided interruption of antiretroviral treatment' and monitored all clinical outcomes of interest including death, new AIDS diagnoses as well as important outcomes such as heart attacks, liver and kidney disease and quality of life. Therefore, the study very deliberately investigated morbidity (illness) and mortality (death) outcomes and not what are called 'surrogate markers' (such as CD4, HIV RNA) of these ultimate outcomes. This is why the study was so large – the largest trial ever done in HIV, by the way – because the events are relatively rare in the era of effective combination ART, in order to study them, one needs to enroll thousands of people. More than double the number of people died of 'opportunistic disease or death from any cause', they said, in the 'drug conservation' arm (120 people) than in the 'viral suppression' arm (47 people). Death as measured in person-years was one-third as frequent in the latter (1.3 per 100 person-years) as in the former (3.3). The authors concluded that this was due to increases in the viral load with consequent lowering of the CD4 count. Anyway, is that the conclusion you would draw with regards to Papua New Guinea? Does that take the heat off of some criticisms of the toxicity of ART, or just focus it on a particular kind of clinical patient? How should 'risks' and 'benefits' be described to potential clients?

MB: Well, I don't think that one can conclude from this that it pertains only to a particular kind of patient. The SMART study was conducted in various countries and settings around the world so the results should be fairly generalisable. What the results suggest is that some of the adversities that we have observed over the past decade of combination ART may have more to do with HIV itself than we previously thought. Until these results were published there was a broad consensus that many of the 'morbidities' (illnesses) we were seeing were a direct result of the drugs. It is fascinating that in fact so many of us (and I include myself here) may have got it so wrong. I say 'may' because the SMART study was not designed to answer this question. That is, can we say that heart attacks, liver disease and kidney disease are a result of antiretrovirals or of HIV infection or of some combination of them? Accordingly, there are plans to interrogate this finding more directly by conducting another large RCT, a random, controlled trial.

LH: Yeah, that's emerged as an issue in Papua New Guinea, definitely. Five of the first cohort of people to go on antiretrovirals through the Heduru Clinic died, one of a heart attack secondary to anaemia (NHASP 2005a: 10).

MB: From the point of view of how to describe risks and benefits to potential clients the short answer is to do it honestly and openly in simple language that can be readily understood and allow time for questions. One needs to include as much information as possible without overwhelming the patient with detail. Finally, one needs to explain that if the patient is having experiences that they are concerned about and that might be related to the medication, then they should seek review or at minimum contact the treatment centre (if possible) to discuss what to do.

✳ ✳ ✳

LH: You're now once again based in Sydney with the National Centre in HIV Epidemiology and Clinical Research (NCHECR), one of three such national centres in Australia. What does NCHECR do that the other two research centres don't, and which of their activities and programmes and research interests are relevant to the national response in Papua New Guinea to HIV and AIDS?

MB: At NCHECR we are focused, as our name suggests, on the clinical and epidemiological aspects of HIV infection. The NCHECR is split into seven programmes, some of which are clinical, some of which are epidemiological and some of which are a mix of both. I work in the Therapeutic and Vaccine Research Program (TVRP) which, again as suggested by the name, is a clinically focused programme. Therefore, we concentrate on the assessment and use of ART and vaccines.

In terms of Papua New Guinea a good example of the kind of NCHECR activity that has direct relevance is the HEMI study, an AusAID-sponsored modelling project in which a couple of NCHECR personnel participated, and that attempted to predict the course of HIV infection in Papua New Guinea, Timor Leste and Indonesia based around a number of varying assumptions regarding specific HIV interventions and their intensity.

LH: That's the one that John Kaldor helped to write.

MB: Right, and Matthew Law, who is the head of the Database and Statistics Program at NCHECR, also contributed. From the point-of-view of the TVRP we understand that the implementation of ART in Papua New Guinea is going to be a substantial challenge. However, given that the general consensus is that the current HIV prevalence across PNG is ~3% …

LH: I hate to burst your bubble, Mark, and I certainly don't disagree with you, but the recent consensus was pushed downwards to be 1.28%, and that was among 15–49 year-olds! I'll get back to that.

MB: … there is an imperative for broadening access to care including ART. Papua New Guinea presents a set of unique challenges including its geography and rudimentary health-care infrastructure, to name only two. However, implementation of ART has been shown possible in very poor countries of sub-Saharan Africa that have characteristics similar to the situation in Papua New Guinea, and therefore we know it can be done. Having said that, in order to ensure success any effort to assist Papua New Guinea in its ART roll-out would require a fully considered and well supported partnership. Where an organisation like NCHECR could contribute would be in helping to build the capacity of Papua New Guinea to monitor what is happening, for example, how effective it is in terms of data collection and analysis. The NCHECR could augment the clinical expertise of healthcare personnel, too, through education and training. Ultimately, the NCHECR could help augment the capacity of Papua New Guinean personnel to reflect critically on the ART roll-out and thereby ask questions about how it might be refined or altered to fit the local situation better. We'd like to help them ask relevant research questions, develop ways to answer them through the process of converting an idea into a clinical trial protocol, and then executing the protocol through good research practice.

LH: Sounds great, Mark, and that fits with lots of government documentation about particularly clinical research needs. I'm just curious: what would be a couple of those 'relevant research questions' you're thinking of, and what is it about the antiretroviral roll-out that needs critical reflection? I mean, if it hasn't happened by now, how come?

MB: Well, you may well be surprised to hear this but in fact a lot of very simple issues in the management of HIV-infection are not at all well understood, even in areas of high levels of technological development and human welfare. For instance, we have a pretty good idea of what combination therapy to offer patients up front (that is, 'first-line therapy'), but once that therapy fails we really don't know what is the next optimal regimen. In the developed world this hasn't mattered so much as you have various drugs and drug-classes to choose from, so your chance of success as measured in terms of viral suppression is relatively good. Nevertheless, in resource-limited settings in which there is less choice and one is trying to provide clear, simple messages about what to do, we just don't have the evidence to guide people confidently. Even the question of what the optimal approach is to monitoring the patients after they have commenced ART is simply not known. In developed countries patients come on average every three months and undergo an entire battery of tests including measurement of immune cells, red cells, organ function and viral load. How necessary this all is, and what difference it makes to ultimate outcomes like death and illness, we simply do not know.

✳ ✳ ✳

LH: Mark, you've been involved in issues of HIV clinical medicine since at least the early 1990s, when Australia's HIV epidemiology was perhaps most clearly patterned and sharply focused. How would you describe Australia's HIV epidemiology now? Do you think its national response has been successful, and if so, why? Is any of that relevant to strengthening Papua New Guinea's national response?

MB: My understanding (as a non-epidemiologist) is that the Australian epidemic remains fairly focused on or confined to men who have sex with men. There is a smattering of migrants across the country, particularly those from high HIV-prevalence countries, who have been found to be HIVab+, but this remains a small minority. Australia, fortunately, implemented harm-reduction strategies to protect the intravenous drug-use/ing (IDU) community …

LH: Protecting those that are most vulnerable; what a concept!

MB: … yeah, I know, and we have subsequently never seen IDU as a major risk factor for HIV-infection. There has been an increase over the past five or so years, however, from around 500 newly diagnosed HIV infections to over 1,000 newly diagnosed HIV infections. The best estimate is that most of that increase is due to an apparent increase in unprotected sex amongst MSM. The reasons for this are debated and are probably multiple. So, yes, I think Australia's HIV-prevention programme has been successful, although what the recent rise in notifications tells us is that success can be reversed and must be maintained through sustained efforts.

How might this be relevant to PNG's experience? For that you need to look at the elements of the early Australian response, but off the cuff I'd single out several elements that certainly were and that probably remain crucial, beginning with political engagement, commitment and leadership and bipartisan support.

LH: That seems finally to have kicked into gear in Papua New Guinea, after too many years of denial. I mean, it took Ronald Reagan five years, into his second term of office, before he uttered the word 'AIDS' in public in the US.

MB: Yes, the great fortune for Australia, in direct comparison to the US, was that we had just elected a progressive, inclusive government with some very well educated and imaginative ministers, one of whom, Neal Blewett, understood quickly the implications of the HIV epidemic for the community and was active in supporting important interventions. So, one message is that a critical arm of an effective response is that there has to be a real and significant political will. There has to be meaningful engagement with Persons Living With HIV or AIDS (PLWHA), too, and making them key stakeholders at all levels, including that of policy discussions. Once again, the involvement of PLWHA has been a mainstay of the Australian response to HIV.

LH: I'm glad to hear you say that.

MB: There must be a frank and unambiguous prevention campaign targeted at particular community risk-groups but with an education campaign targeted at the community in general. We've talked a bit about treatment already, so there's got to be support for the development of treatment and access to it once it becomes available through the government health insurance scheme. There have got to be anti-discrimination and anti-stigma laws, and I'd like to see followed the human rights approach that was taken to HIVab testing and care, which meant that those undergoing testing did so in the absence of fear or prejudice. In order to effect a successful response in Papua New Guinea, these same elements are likely to be necessary inclusions.

LH: Yeah, that's what everything I've read has said about how successful the Australian national response has been. Papua New Guinea has anti-discrimination laws on the books in the form of the HAMP Act of 2003, which followed from HIV and AIDS Management Protection bills that were debated in the House of Parliament. There haven't been many prosecutions, however, so far as I'm aware, whether of cases of people being buried alive or companies using HIVab seropositivity to exclude potential employees or even parliamentarians brought to justice for knowingly infecting their multiple wives.

✳ ✳ ✳

LH: Much of your work now seems to involve the clinical treatment of HIV, the conduct of pharmaceutical trials and the study of immune system function, especially in Thailand, where you've coordinated studies involving the efficacy of one or another drug in the HAART arsenal. I'd like us to examine what has already transpired in Papua New Guinea regarding their 'roll-out' since 2003 under the auspices of the so-called '3x5' programme. As I understand things, but which is based on very little published information, it doesn't seem to have been too terribly successful for the first couple of years and it doesn't seem to have been preceded by any investigation or assumption-questioning. Again, I could be wrong about that, but I've read everything I could get my hands on, and there just doesn't seem to have been much public discussion beyond those few items I mentioned in Chapter 4.

I worry about the levels of resistance to antiretrovirals that have been induced by a combination of biological interactions, patient decisions to discontinue such treatment regimens and/or a less than perfect monitoring of patient adherence to treatment. What would you say about these issues as they came up in Thailand that might be relevant in a Papua New Guinea context? In particular, do you think that Papua New Guinea has between its national and expatriate personnel and healthcare infrastructure the technical expertise so as *in a mass way* to monitor viral load of people on antiretrovirals? I'm worried, too, about the effect of immune system reconstitution that physicians call attention to (e.g. McBride and Bradford 2004; Murdoch *et al.* 2007) that can then lead to outbreak of long-dormant infections. I'm certain that that's going to make people think that the antiretrovirals are what's causing the, say, herpes zoster or genital herpes outbreaks or diarrhoea or weight loss. Did that put further stress on Thai health workers then to treat those long-dormant, now-emergent infections?

MB: Firstly, you should understand that I went to work in a specific research institute (HIV-NAT) that was set up as a model of HIV-research in the region and backed by powerful institutions – the Thai Red Cross AIDS Research Centre, the NCHECR and the IATEC (the International Antiviral Therapy Evaluation Centre, which is like an NCHECR of the Netherlands). I worked amongst a group of highly qualified individuals, from Thailand and overseas, who had broad experience in the management of HIV infection. Therefore, it's not as if I was out 'in the field' working in a setting in which HIV infection was considered a kind of feared 'unknown'. We also offered HIV-infected Thai patients entry into carefully considered randomised controlled trials (RCTs) in which all those who enrolled were offered active treatment (we never offered placebos). The great majority did extremely well.

LH: Very quickly, what do you mean by 'great majority', and 'extremely well' in terms of what?

MB: Well to give you a specific example of a study for which I was directly responsible, of 61 patients who had failed various combinations of NRTIs and who then commenced a combination of a boosted-PI and an NNRTI, 49 of them were receiving the same ART regimen four years after entering this trial, and 42 of those 49 had an undetectable viral load (defined as <50 copies/ml of plasma) and were in generally good health.

Your concerns about the development of drug resistance have always been present and were voiced loudly by many at the time that the feasibility of widespread access to care in the developing world was being debated. At HIV-NAT we certainly saw the development of drug resistance as well as episodes of what has come to be called the 'immune-reconstitution inflammatory syndrome' ('IRIS') or 'immune reconstitution disease' (IRD). Nevertheless, these phenomena were relatively uncommon and didn't detract from the overwhelming success of the majority of participants and the programme in general. The outcomes of patients in the HIV-NAT cohort have been reported by Chris Duncombe and colleagues in an article published in *AIDS* (Duncombe *et al.* 2005). Clearly, when one sets up an HIV treatment and care service the education of health-care workers about issues such as drug resistance and IRIS figure prominently. Once they are educated about the occurrence of such phenomena and are given strategies (for instance, written protocols) for how to approach their investigation and management, these complications do not seem to be such a big deal but come to be just another part of what to expect in an HIV treatment and care programme.

As to your worries about monitoring capacity and so on, these are concerns shared by many across the global ART roll-out programme. In fact HIV viral load monitoring is done in very few programmes in developing countries as a result of the expense and the need for the appropriate technical capacity and infrastructure. Even monitoring of CD4 T-cells is available in only a few programmes.

LH: Yeah, Evelyn Lavu and colleagues have a nice paper in the *Papua New Guinea Medical Journal* (Lavu *et al.* 2004) that discusses use of lymphocyte counters as something of a workaround in resource-limited settings where it's not possible to conduct expensive virological tests.

MB: Whether such monitoring is absolutely necessary is, oddly enough, not really known. In the developed world these tools have been introduced as the technologies have become available on the assumption that, for instance, HIV viral load monitoring, measurement of CD4 T-cell count and the testing of antiretroviral resistance should contribute to the success of programmes. In fact, only the question of the utility of resistance testing has been tested in randomised controlled trials, and if you believe Bernard Hirschel (from Geneva, Switzerland), who gave a presentation on this topic last month at the IAS conference in Sydney, the jury is still out on whether resistance testing is genuinely useful.

LH: Do tell. How does one test testing? What did Hirschel say in his presentation that might be relevant to a Papua New Guinea setting?

MB: Well, it's straightforward enough. The best way to test a test is randomly to assign patients to monitoring with that test or with 'standard of care', that is, everything being the same as the other arm minus the test under interrogation. You then choose a primary endpoint of study. For example, in the case of resistance testing it could be something like rates of 'success' after a defined time period (typically one year) on the subsequent drug regimen that has been chosen in the control 'standard of care' arm on the basis of a patient history, a clinical examination and analysis of standard lab test results, and in the experimental arm on the basis of the same plus the drug resistance test. What we know, and Bernard nicely summarised this in July at the conference, is that despite what might seem 'obvious' to many, that is, that resistance testing should increase the patient's chance of being prescribed a successful regimen, the few studies that have been conducted doing precisely this haven't generally been able convincingly to demonstrate that.

✳ ✳ ✳

LH: Extending the key insights of Jacques Derrida over two decades ago, Asha Persson (2004) has argued that Westerners no longer appreciate the original meaning of the Greek *pharmakon*. Persson analysed rich contextual data obtained from her study of the iatrogenesis of lipodystrophy and lipoatrophy in those taking various combinations of antiretroviral drugs. She demonstrates that this inherently ambivalent term, *pharmakon*, one that originally linked medicinal cure to poisonous toxin, has emerged one-sidedly over the centuries, top-heavily, to mean only the former, not the latter. This development has fetishized viral entities further, has hidden iatrogenesis ever more, and has spawned the curious notion in the biomedical sciences and in culture more generally of 'side effects' (Etkin 1992). For example, Zidovudine (AZT) was originally designed to kill cancer cells and was in fact taken off the US market for doing too good a job thereof (Arno and Feiden 1992), which is to say, killing cancer cells so effectively it killed their hosts. Now the ill effects that people suffer when they take antiretrovirals (despite all the good they can do many takers) are dubbed 'side effects', no matter how consistently people suffer them or how much prescriptions must shift in 'trial-and-error' fashion to keep up with the body's wisdom. It kinda ticks me off when such people who don't go on them in the first place (perhaps because they've already heard too much about them) are dubbed something like 'ART-naïve' or that when they start and then go off them they are said not to comply well, to have 'failed' at treatment adherence, and so on. That doesn't seem fair. It remains an open question as to how well or poorly Papua New Guineans are tolerating their extreme toxicity, what shapes 'non-adherence' will take, and what treatment gaps will mean in terms of the development of resistance to antiretrovirals. I'd like to see a lot more public discussion of these issues.

MB: Lawrence, your interest in the toxicity or 'adverse events' associated with ART' is shared by me and the NCHECR in general, as well as by many in the world of HIV care and research. However, before I take this issue on let me correct a couple of elements in your question.

LH: Fair enough.

MB: Firstly, you misunderstand the term 'HIV naïve'; by this is meant simply those HIV-infected patients who have not yet been exposed to ART; it is in no way a criticism of PLWHA or their ability to adhere to therapy. The other aspect of your question worth exploring a little is the notion of medicine versus toxin. As a medical student I remember being taught that medicines are substances but that are toxins if given in the wrong dose, and in general, my impression is that the medical profession is acutely aware of this. For instance, in general hospital practice there are many useful drugs that, if given in the wrong dose, are toxic and dangerous, for example, morphine, digoxin (which is a derivative of digitalis or 'foxglove', a well known poison) or aminoglycoside antibiotics, to name only a few. In the US and Australia there has been an increased focus on the toxicity of medicines recently as it is becoming understood that many hospital admissions are prolonged as a result of iatrogenesis. This is not only inadequate but costly.

In reference to iatrogenesis and AZT you are quite right that AZT was originally a drug investigated for use as an anti-cancer agent. In the scramble to find some product that could halt or at least delay the inexorable decline associated with HIV infection, AZT was shown in the late 1980s to have an effect. In the early days it was used at a relatively high-dose, and was associated with toxicity to the bone marrow in particular, manifesting particularly as low levels of hemoglobin, as well as sometimes of the white cells and platelets (all of which are produced in the bone marrow). It was also toxic to muscle, and the phenomenon of 'AZT buttocks' (representing muscle wasting of the gluteal muscles) was well known within the PLWHA and medical communities. AZT is still in use, however, and nowadays we have learnt that it can be effectively used as part of combination ART at lower (and therefore better tolerated) doses; while we still see anaemia from time to time we very rarely see muscle toxicity. This is in fact a good example of that poison/medicine nexus we discussed above.

The final thing to say is that I'm not sure that the debate regarding lipodystrophy (LD) has fetished the virus. If anything the entire debate has clearly highlighted the potential toxicity of antiretrovirals and concentrated the HIV treatment community on trying to find the balance between unnecessary iatrogenesis and not allowing PLWHA to develop a dangerous level of immunodeficiency. As a result, in combination with evidence coming from studies of cohorts who begin therapy with higher as opposed to lower CD4 counts (say, >500 as opposed to <200), the approach over the past five years or so has been to hold off commencing ART for as long as possible without allowing patients to run into trouble.

Ironically, and as referred to above, we are now developing an appreciation that with some of the newer ART agents that have developed since concern began to be expressed about LD appear to be associated with less iatrogenesis. There is also an emerging consensus such that some of the 'adverse events', the supposed iatrogenesis (with ART causing patient morbidity and mortality), may be instead yet another manifestation of HIV replication. As a result of these parallel developments we may well see a move towards earlier intervention with ART, although many would prefer to see this approach tested in a randomised controlled trial before widespread implementation. This is a hot topic of debate at the moment.

LH: Why is that, why is 'side effects' not used in favour of 'adverse events', or why is 'side effects' used at all, since they are in fact quite central to what the drugs do, right?

MB: In fact we and others do refer to these effects as either adverse effects or, more commonly 'toxicity' or 'toxic effects', which makes the meaning plain, I hope. What I and others find disturbing is that this aspect (toxicity) of ART tends to be downplayed somewhat in the ART roll-out language. Some even seem unwilling to discuss it publicly. As an example, in February, 2005

I acted as a clinical preceptor to a PEPFAR-sponsored HIV treatment and care programme in a sub-Saharan Africa country.

LH: As with many other things, I must apologize for being American! *Mea culpa, mea culpa, mea maxima culpa.* PEPFAR stands for the 'President's Emergency Plan For AIDS Relief', and it's been a staggeringly costly programme – US$15,000,000,000 – designed under the G.W. Bush administration to target 15 countries hard-hit by HIV, mostly being in sub-Saharan Africa and the Caribbean. Among many other things, it has helped to propel ineffective, abstinence-only sex education programmes, to further conservative sexual ethics and to strangle many other more progressive initiatives regarding condom promotion, distribution and usage.

MB: Well yes, there are certainly aspects of the PEPFAR programme that appear to have been driven more by political considerations than by evidence of what is effective. In fact your own Institute of Medicine, in reviewing the performance of PEPFAR earlier this year, made direct criticisms of these aspects and advised that they should be reviewed with an eye to the prevention evidence base. Having said that, there are elements of the PEPFAR programme which I and others commend and support, and primary amongst these are the implementation of not only access to HIV treatment and care services but the creation of an infrastructure around it that plans for the long-term sustainability of the effort.

Anyhow, getting back to the ART toxicity issue, toward the end of my four weeks at the PEPFAR programme I reviewed three young women in succession who were on first-line ART consisting of nevirapine/stavudine/lamivudine with what the medical teams found to be a mysterious syndrome, but which to me clearly represented three slightly varied manifestations of 'mitochondrial toxicity' of the nucleoside components of the ART (which we explored in that *Journal of Infectious Disease* article I sent you [Boyd et al. 2006]). I found this observation disturbing and suggested that it warranted a small write-up or some kind of letter to a journal in order at least to 'flag' this to other programmes and clinicians. At the very least I wanted to say that, if this was being seen widely in programmes elsewhere, then we needed to think about lobbying for a safer NNRTI component, which is now widely available in the rich world. This syndrome seems to be associated with what are termed the 'thymidine-analogue' NNRTI drugs such as stavudine (d4T) and zidovudine (AZT). There is good evidence to suggest that if these drugs are replaced with non-thymidine analogue NNRTIs such as abacavir and tenotovir, this syndrome does not occur. Unfortunately, this suggestion seemed to be met by the PEPFAR team with a degree of coolness I didn't really comprehend. I heard nothing further, and dropped it after trying to pursue it a couple of times.

Actually, since that time there has been a flow of evidence that demonstrated clearly that young, overweight, sub-Saharan African females in particular were prone to this ta-NRTI toxicity, and in fact the newly released update of the WHO Guidelines for Management of HIV-Infection in Adults and Adolescents has recommended a transition from the preferential use of d4T and AZT to safer non ta-NRTIs such as tenofovir.

LH: Well, please don't take it personally, and I know it wasn't anti-Australian sentiment talking, so what do you think was up with that, without going into gory details?

MB: Well, I suppose that there were probably a few issues at play. This particular programme was still relatively new and had just begun getting patients on therapy. Perhaps there was a fear that if it started making a lot of noise about the potential toxicity of the chosen regimens this would threaten the roll-out as a whole or entail a complete rethinking of which drugs should be offered, and thereby considerable delays. This is always a delicate balance, and in many ways you can understand that if policy makers are too cautious and want to consider every new bit of evidence or programmatic hiccough there is a risk of becoming paralysed and doing nothing, and doing nothing in this context means people dying.

Another disturbing aspect for us is that PEPFAR does not support research of any kind within its programme.

LH: I didn't know that.

MB: The Global Fund for AIDS, Tuberculosis and Malaria (GFATM) does allow for up to 10% of its grants to be spent on integrated research activities (or 'operational research'). But they're pretty underutilised, according to Michel Kazatchkine, Executive Director of the GFATM, who spoke in July of 2007 at the IAS Conference in Sydney. That probably reflects the fact that the writing teams for these GFATM grants infrequently include researchers.

LH: Man, that's so true on so many levels.

MB: Yes, we see this as a missed opportunity to learn from the process of the roll-out (and thereby improve it). People from the WHO, UNAIDS and the World Bank said the same thing at the IAS conference. I participated in the writing of a declaration (called the 'The Sydney Declaration') that was announced at the conference and published in a special IAS Conference edition of *The Lancet* (July 2007). The Declaration calls for 10% of such funds to be dedicated to research so that we can learn from and improve on what we are doing. I believe explicitly in the need to continue and refine the roll-out of ART, as well as to plan now for the needs of PLWHA for whom first-line therapy fails (see Boyd and Cooper 2007). I also believe that, given the reasonable concern about using ART in 'new' populations (such as Papua New Guinea), we need to be extra vigilant about 'toxicity' (as well as its efficacy, of course). We need therefore to conduct ethical, community-inclusive, participatory and collaborative research to help countries like Papua New Guinea find out what works best for Papua New Guineans.

LH: Your comments now make a lot more sense to me. You once sent me a presentation that you gave in Bangkok at the Symposium on HIV Medicine (Boyd 2007). I was intrigued by a lot of your findings although not surprised by some of your recommendations regarding the need for more clinical research. Now I realise better where some of your concerns come from. You called for more clinical research but in a sense of a markedly different kind. I've told you this before – and you seemed to respond sympathetically to me saying that – sometimes social scientific and biomedical ways of knowing about and working on HIV and AIDS and STDs and condoms and what-not seem almost to be incommensurable languages, not even just different dialects. The second slide in your presentation, for example, acknowledged potential conflicts of interest in terms of you having been sponsored by Merck, Roche, Tibotec, Gilead, BMS and GSK biopharmaceutical companies. I *wish* I'd been sponsored! What kinds of conflicts ensued in real-life situations in the field that you faced in Thailand? Are those kinds of conflicts happening in Papua New Guinea, for example, with regards to pressures exerted by those who either sell antiretrovirals or otherwise enable the ART roll-out? Are they being addressed?

MB: The PowerPoint presentation I sent you was something I delivered in Bangkok in January at a regional annual symposium run by HIV-NAT, the HIV Netherlands Australia Thai Research Collaboration, where I worked from 2000–4. HIV-NAT initiatives have been addressing the gap between the WHO 'resource-limited' guidelines about the use of PIs (protease inhibitors) as second-line agents and their price, which makes them virtually inaccessible. You may well have been observing the current furor about this issue between Big Pharma and the governments of Thailand and Brazil (see Biehl 2007). They have both announced the issue of compulsory licenses consistent with the Doha Declaration of the WTO, the World Trade Organization. This declaration restated that while all nations who are signatories to the WTO must respect the trade-related aspects of property rights (TRIPS), countries were at liberty to issue compulsory licenses in situations in which the general public health is judged to necessitate such action. In practical issues, what this has meant is that countries threaten the compulsory licensing scheme and this leads to negotiations and eventually price reductions from Big Pharma. Brazil, for example, is the only middle-income country that has a substantial HIV-prevalence and that offers PLWHA access to a state-subsidised, free ART programme. However, the recent argument with Abbott (the manufacturers of a product known as 'Kaletra') was not resolved, and both Thailand and Brazil issued compulsory licenses for the production of Kaletra by a third-party (as outlined in TRIPS). My understanding is that the Brazilians have come subsequently to an amicable agreement with Abbott and they are not ordering generic manufacture under the compulsory license. However, as far as I am aware Thailand is pushing on with the compulsory licensing. Abbott subsequently threatened to withhold registration of all new medicines in Thailand (and particularly their new 'heat-stable' form of ritonavir called 'Aluvia') and also pulled out of funding any pharmaceutical research.

I'm glad that you asked about Conflict of Interest (CoI) declarations, because I try to make a point of stating these at the outset of any presentation I give or articles I write. Either way, I try to let people know that I do deal with Big Pharma, sometimes in a paid capacity as an adviser. While I hope that I remain impartial in my decision making despite this, studies have demonstrated that CoI can influence the decision-making of doctors. This whole issue is in the spotlight at the moment in the wake of recent controversies over the safety of rofecoxib and other drugs and revelations that some FDA committees have included a number of individuals who have received funding from the company whose product is being considered for licensing.

LH: Well, I think that we could say fairly that this is a problem not restricted to HIV medicine, but yeah, I think that Arno and Feiden's *Against All Odds: the story of AIDS drug development, politics and profits* (1992) oughta be required reading every year.

MB: This has led to a perception of potential bias and perhaps a lack of concentration on the potential toxicity of some agents. In terms of whether I think this CoI has led me to conflicts in choosing one product over another 'in the field', I don't believe so, but then as stated above, it is possible that I am incapable of making an adequate judgment.

LH: Fair enough.

MB: The guidelines in Papua New Guinea are being developed with reference to the WHO guidelines, so I don't imagine that CoIs are relevant there.

LH: Unless, of course, CoIs are insinuated in the WHO, too ... I mean, there was a big flap recently as UNAIDS was called out by James Chin for allegedly inflating HIVab seroprevalence to justify funding surges.

MB: Ultimately, the WHO guidelines are informed by the best evidence available, and while some of the evidence is gathered from trials funded by Pharma (and could therefore be claimed to represent a certain bias), others are not. CoI tends to be more of a problem in developed countries in which there is intense competition in the ART market, particularly for the products included in the 'recommended for inclusion in first-line ART' category and in which Big Pharma has a greater product margin than that available in settings of resource limited settings such as Papua New Guinea, where they generally elect or are forced to sell 'at cost' if they are to gain a share of the market.

LH: So, let's say that you've been contracted by the Papua New Guinea Department of Health or, say, a huge NGO that has clinical expertise and technical capacity in Papua New Guinea, to make recommendations about recommended daily dosage and other aspects of treatment regimen, what would you say?

MB: I should start by saying that people from the Burnet Institute in Melbourne are already engaged in Papua New Guinea in offering their expertise and technical capacity to the ART roll-out programme. However, for the sake of general argument, let me say that there are a few strategies that might show some promise in making the current set of recommended agents and combinations better tolerated. The first issue is selection of NRTI agents. The first set of guidelines issued by the WHO for limited resource settings (the 2004 edition) recommended the use of the thymidine analogues as part of the first-line regimen, and particularly stavudine (d4T) because it is very cheap. Stavudine, however, has been closely linked to the disfiguring and stigmatising syndrome known as lipodystrophy (and most particularly the lipoatrophy component, which is to say, fat-wasting), and as a result its use has fallen out of favour in developed countries in which newer generation agents are readily available. The newer edition of the WHO guidelines (2006) has recommended not to use thymidine analogues if at all possible, and to use agents such as tenofovir instead. This is fine, but as discussed above, the cost-differential remains substantial and it seems likely that governments in RLS will continue to favour the cheaper regimens as it means they can offer access to therapy to four times more people. This is not unreasonable given that access to therapy means saving lives, whereas switching to a more expensive regimen means denying the widest possible access. Another recent finding is that lower doses than those routinely recommended of d4T and possibly even AZT retain potency and may be associated with less toxicity. The WHO has recently recommended the use of lower doses of d4T (30-mg bid max rather than 40-mg bid). Whether this will result in less neuropathy or lactic acidosis syndromes or lipodystrophy is not known, but it may.

Incidentally, this is exactly the sort of issue where clinical research can really help provide to a solid and reliable answer – we would like to see this sort of issue answered through the implementation of an RCT that could be conducted within one or preferably a number of ART roll-out programmes. That is, we want to see whether the result is consistent across a range of programmes, countries and groups. In addition, there is evidence that dose reductions of a number of agents within the HIV-protease inhibitor and NNRTI classes may retain antiretroviral potency and possibly lead to greater tolerability and perhaps even reduced toxicity. In some of the Phase II studies conducted in the development of other drugs, dose-ranging studies were done involving fairly small numbers of patients to look for the optimal dose. Optimal is in this sense defined as delivering maximal efficacy in reducing viral load but also resulting in minimal toxicity. In some cases, the dose that is taken to Phase III-levels of clinical research, which is to say larger, more complicated studies involving human cohorts may be slightly higher than the lowest possible dose required for efficacy but which nevertheless appears well tolerated. Therefore, it is possible that lower doses of various agents may retain potency and possibly offer reduced toxicity. This may be the case in particularly different populations, such as those in Asia and Africa.

What's a little difficult for me to understand as a researcher is the apparent reticence of the large funding agencies to condone and fund research, although I'm sure that there are many factors. One possibility is that the agencies are concerned about not wanting to appear to treat people in developing countries 'like guinea pigs'. The irony is that without well designed, thoughtful and well executed research this is precisely what we could end up doing.

LH: Well, yeah, and it wouldn't take us an hour to find references to 60 deeply ethically flawed studies involving HIV. I don't doubt that the experience recently in Senegal, Thailand and elsewhere regarding the studies of antiretrovirals and women in sex work has something to do with it. I'm curious, too, about your comment regarding 'particularly different populations': do you mean that there are bodily differences that make a difference, so to speak, when it comes to using HIV medicines across populations?

MB: Well, there may well be. We know, for instance, that African people are more likely to experience toxicity from the NNRTI drug efavirenz because of differences in the enzyme responsible for its metabolism. Conversely, we know that African people are less likely to experience the abacavir hypersensitivity reaction because of a lower carriage rate of a particular cell marker that predicts its likely occurrence.

LH: Okay, interesting. As for some of the ethical dimensions that this research raises, I see a lot of that rhetoric as being right-thinking but not well-intended. Maybe that's because of what I've seen in the five years I've spent living and working in Papua New Guinea, but for all kinds of reasons I see a lot of challenges ahead with regards to research ethics, and when I've mentioned such issues, I've been many times brushed aside. Plus, without there being any kind of well-developed consumer movement or body of public health advocates in Papua New Guinea, I don't see the great likelihood of there being that kind of ethical protection. Some of the NHASP reviews about clinical research issues (e.g. 2005a, d, f) would certainly give one pause in this regard, and although improvements have allegedly been made in the research approval process through the Research Advisory Committee, or at least people say that there have been certain kinds of progress made, I still wonder what kinds of checks and balances are in place to ensure that research is conducted both ethically but that also answers the questions that need to be asked. I guess that I'm suggesting that you need some kind of sociology-of-knowledge perspective on institutional arrangements and funding streams and especially on research epistemology before you even roll-out the clinical research itself. My comments are motivated by some really serious struggles even in the social sciences about research ethics in conduct of research not in one's own country. In public forums I've heard anthropologists, for example, questioning the importation of Eurocentric understandings of what 'confidentiality' is or means and whether some absolute moral stances are being misplaced. For example, Wendy Armstrong reports from Vanuatu that radio broadcasts regarding STD infections and need for follow-up treatment included the names of the infected: '[t]hen the announcer would read out a list of names of those who should attend for either follow up treatment or a check up! This apparent lack of sensitivity to the rights of individuals was accepted as the norm … ' (Armstrong 1996: 61). She writes painfully of her 'professional values' being 'constantly challenged' and at coming to the realisation sometimes that breaking confidentiality was best (1996: 61, 63).

MB: Well, by contrast, I would see your concerns as well intended but not right-thinking. In my experience people are usually involved in clinical research because they believe that things can be done better. In addition, human research has been guided since the mid-twentieth century by the tenets of the Geneva Convention and declarations since then have enunciated, defined and refined the ethical principles of human research. In Australia, for instance, there is now in circulation a newly revised national statement on ethical conduct in human research which runs to 102 pages and that is taken very seriously by all engaged in human research, from the conduct of street surveys all the way to the testing of medical interventions. All research conducted under the auspices of the NCHECR is reviewed by a Human Research Ethics Committee comprised of diverse members of the academic and general community whose responsibility it is to protect the research subjects.

Now all that isn't to say that all research is perfect and that perhaps in places without a tradition of the conduct of human research (and perhaps Papua New Guinea is one of those places) unethical research doesn't take place. However, part of what an institution like the NCHECR (or the Burnet Institute or other institutions from the developed world) offers in partnership with institutions in Papua New Guinea is to bring a rich experience and tradition of ethical and appropriately reviewed clinical research conduct to collaborative research programmes conducted at the highest level. So in that sense we see the exercise as capacity-building at many levels. However, given the urgency of the situation, I don't agree with your inference that we should take a cautious step-by-step approach. The situation is such that, and I recently saw this quote with regard to the ART roll-out, we have to build the boat as we sail.

LH: We may have to agree to disagree about that one, although of course we're both in favour of research being conducted of the highest ethical standards and that is most relevant to the research questions at hand. I've just finished reading *Medical Apartheid*, by Harriet Washington (Washington 2007), and it shows clearly not only that ethically flawed research traditions didn't magically or even incrementally slowly cease so much as they were stopped and outed by activists, but also that those tendencies are still there, especially as regards variables of class privilege, ethnicity, race and gender.

MB: …which is why we would encourage active participation by PLWHA including, for instance, the formation of Community Advisory Boards so that we could get input about what research the local PLWHA themselves would like to see done. I appreciate that PLWHA and community activism is probably underdeveloped in Papua New Guinea and similar countries of the region, but this is where the experience of places like NCHECR and the various PLWHA organisations in Australia could be helpful.

LH: Absolutely, and I can't agree with you enough. You may not be aware of the study I mentioned at the outset of Chapter 3, or perhaps of the terrible costs incurred when expatriate researchers come to Papua New Guinea and usually engage in rather extractive research instead of participatory. At the

Alleged spiritual cure for AIDS advertised in hospital

very least researcher aims and goals can be easily misunderstood (such as HIVab testing but that is confused with malaria or that appears to be testing for 'quality' of blood and so forth). At the very most, research participants can have their identities revealed in cases where confidentiality is not protected (that was certainly a nationwide problem the IMR study uncovered), and if I say that it happens frequently throughout the country I want to hasten to point out that improvements surely seem to have been made in this regard. Building the boat as we're sailing, pushing the bus we're riding in – whichever metaphor you wish to choose – I can understand the imperative, I can. Nevertheless, just imagine, knowing what you know about Papua New Guinea, trying to conduct an RCT that involved male circumcision or a female microbicide. Again, I'm not against research, but perhaps just overly sensitive to its conceptualisation and operationalisation wherever sexual matters, health services delivery and religious faith are concerned.

Anyway, I asked that question above because the phrase that you had used in your presentation and published article, 'when used at maximal efficiency', has special meaning in Papua New Guinea and perhaps in many other RLSs. I have raised in other chapters in this book some of the issues that I think are relevant to what is likely to become a primarily clinical, technical, pharmaceutical national response to HIV and AIDS. I have mentioned, for example, something of the tangled history of punitive attitudes to clinic attendance, the existence in former times of venereal Lock Hospitals and especially the recent appearance of so-called 'bush medicines' and 'prayer healings', special mushroom potions, 'bio-normalisers' and so on. All of those factors and perhaps the final two more especially, will surely dampen antiretroviral efficacy. The digital reproduction here, for example, is of a flier posted by the Revival Centres of PNG Fellowship that graced the Appointments Desk in the Heduru Clinic of the Port Moresby General Hospital, where the bulk of people receiving ART go for registration, medicine, counselling and support. This flier promises a cure for 'HIV/AIDS' in implementation of 'what the bible directs in Acts 2:38, John 3: 3–5, and Mark 16: 17'. Mark, are there comparable notices and public discourses in Thailand around promises of AIDS cures? Graham Fordham seems to suggest that there are, in his *A New Look at Thai Aids* (2005). When I look closely at the trajectory of, first, announcement of cure, then its coverage in local media sources, then the appearance of testimonies from makers and users of bush medicine, and so on, it begins to look eerily similar to the situation in Papua New Guinea except on one count: the greater literacy of Thai populations, and the greater degree in Papua New Guinea of oral, visual presentations.

MB: There probably are, although the analogous example that was promoted during my stay in Thailand was the promotion of a potion named V-1. Unfortunately, the history of snake-oil and snake-oil salespeople is long and sorry, and, despite the fact that the relationship between HIV-infection and AIDS is probably better established than, for example, the relationship between the mycobacterium tubercle and tuberculosis, there are plenty of people prepared to capitalize on the fear of the infection and the natural desire of people to wish for a simple and affordable cure.

LH: Yeah, you're probably right. That raises all kinds of other issues to me. Among them is the issue of medical licensure and the formal and informal endorsement (and forgings of same) by prominent health workers of some of these bush medicines, mushroom potions and so on. Gosh, I feel so bad for some of these doctors whose names and good reputations have been used fraudulently in stumping for some of these alleged medicines, but in all fairness, many seem quite earnestly to believe in them.

For reasons that ought by now to be clear, Papua New Guineans who are HIVab+ tend to be diagnosed rather late in their infections, they tend to be immuno-compromised in myriad ways having nothing to do with HIV, they tend to have poor nutrition and to suffer from residential and cultural dislocation. In addition, and for all manner of complicated reasons, they tend not to be monitored clinically in ways they might in Australia or the US. Even participation in clinical trials, which occurs millions of times each year in those countries, is a relatively new thing in Papua New Guinea. Isn't that going to present humongous problems of clinical 'adherence'? Won't that also disable somewhat the impulse that doctors should have to treat patient attitudes to clinics and doctors and medicine a bit more sympathetically? I'm wondering whether there are parallels that you may draw between this situation in Papua New Guinea and what you likely saw in the years you lived and worked in Thailand. Graham Fordham (2005), for example, has written very perceptively about the structure of popular discourse around so-called 'folk medicines' alleged to cure AIDS or to remove HIV from the body. Care to comment?

MB: Well, the short answer to your question is yes, rolling-out an ART access programme in Papua New Guinea will be no simple task. It will involve learning by doing (i.e., 'building the ship as we sail') and necessarily involve education of healthcare workers, patients and the broader community. We'll need to develop and mobilise a community of PLWHA as collaborators and colleagues. We'll need to deal with and educate those who purvey snake-oil (well intentioned or not), too, and endeavour to secure political leadership and support. It will of course be tremendously complex and demand the abil-

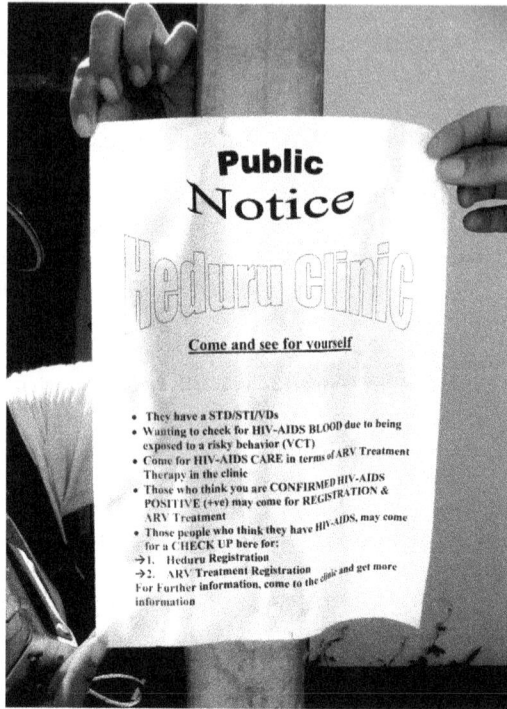

Public notice outside STD clinic

ity to adapt and to be open to a certain degree of failure ... and much more ... but when all is said and done, should we just all stay at home and forget it? Absolutely not.

LH: I agree with you wholeheartedly, Mark. I feel also, however, that to accomplish those things people are going to have to step on some toes and get in one another's face a bit more. I mean, it just seems that everyone's always so polite about even life and death issues. I see this happening on both sides of the ledgers. I've written in previous chapters how external donors and foreign consultants and NGOs seem to have this kind of hands-off attitude when it comes to the specific content and intent of programmes and messages, especially so as not to appear to offend Christian sensibilities or muddy the funding streams. STD clinics, for example, routinely feature posters and depictions of Jesus and Mary and other religious injunctions about sin and immorality, but nobody'll say squat. External reviewers will say that policies are 'probably' being abridged, that laws 'might' be being broken, that anti-condom rhetoric 'may' be working against the best interests of the national response, but yet it sits there.

But I see the same thing happening on the other side, that there doesn't seem to be much protest by Papua New Guineans of things that must rankle them, for example, salary differentials, housing provisions, sexual identity proclamations, and the privileges of class, skin colour and ethnicity. I mean, I think that what we need is a lot more fighting, a lot more people standing up and saying 'Enough is enough!' Just as an example, another flier posted outside the clinic to advertise its services is reproduced digitally here. It solicits 'Those who think you are CONFIRMED HIV-AIDS POSITIVE (+ve)' and those who 'have a STD/STI/VDs' to register for enrollment in a clinical programme. By itself, the notice's scary, confusing language – 'Wanting to check for HIV-AIDS BLOOD due to being exposed to a risky behavior (VCT)' – would definitely keep me away! It also implies that seeking voluntary counselling and testing is a risky behaviour! But none of the health officials I brought this to did anything other than roll their eyes as if to say 'what can you do?' We social scientists, well, most of us, care an awful lot about language, and I'm just curious how you feel about precision in language, for example, use of phrases such as 'HIV/AIDS', 'AIDS Test', 'AIDS Positive' and the like. 'Roll-out' is another one that doesn't seem to give anyone but us pause, and I still think that 'naïve' is a poor word choice when it comes to ARTs! 'Roll-out' sounds like a carpet sample, not the incredibly lengthy process it is, fraught with unbelievably complex politics. Carpets, by contrast, tend to roll-out pretty smoothly. Any thoughts about this? Are there parallels with Thailand that are worth mentioning?

MB: I arrived in Thailand at a time when the Thai HIV-epidemic was at a relatively mature phase, in a country that had been prepared, a little like Australia before it, to confront the problem head-on with substantial political backing. Therefore I am not qualified to make comparisons with the early phase of the epidemic, and Thailand and Papua New Guinea have many significant differences that might make comparisons dangerous and perhaps even unhelpful. Having said that I agree that the language in which public health messages and advertising of services are promulgated is important and needs to be carefully designed. This is another example in which the Australian HIV response model may be useful, as representatives of all stakeholders, from PLWHA to government health officials, were consulted in order to get this right. As a result of such consultation the agreed response varied between general awareness messages targeting the wider community to much franker and explicit messages targeted at specific high-risk groups.

LH: Mark, in the Thailand trial that you reported in your 2006 article, you noted that 'poor antiretroviral adherence in the past year' was sufficient to exclude potential participants. What were some of the reasons why in Thailand clinical attendance can be less than sterling? What can be done about that?

MB: This is a fairly standard exclusion criterion for most research trials. In general our experience at HIV-NAT is that patients adhered extremely well, not only to clinic visits, but to the therapy. One of the key factors for the long-term success of antiretroviral regimens is that patients must take their medication according to a strict schedule, and preferably take every single dose as prescribed. This is something that is emphasised in clinics, and the great majority of patients achieve this or something very close to it. However, some people do not achieve this, and part of the responsibility of the healthcare workers involved in patient care is to detect this (which involves developing an open and trusting relationship between patients and the clinic staff), to explore the reasons (which may be many and complex), and to find strategies to improve the adherence. One of the strongest predictors of poor adherence to a regimen or clinic visit schedule is poor adherence in the past. Therefore, when we consider people attending clinic who express interest in enrolling in a clinical trial, we have to consider a documented history of previous poor adherence as a reason to refuse enrolment.

LH: That sounds like a lot of paperwork! Right there is one of the challenges noted by academic researchers and NACS and NHASP reviews alike.

MB: Yeah, so we've got to look at prior clinic attendance. This is for a number of reasons – we know from bitter experience that patients who adhere poorly to ART end up with an HIV-mutant strain that becomes relatively or completely resistant to the particular ART combination they are taking, which further disadvantages that patient in the future. What that does is instantly to narrow that person's future ART options. Trial enrolment is thus based on statistical estimates of the numbers of patients required to prove a particular hypothesis or other, and patients who fail to adhere to the study protocol reduce the power of studies to test the hypothesis. The existence of clinical trials and other kinds of studies may open an opportunity for patients to gain access to a drug that may be particularly beneficial and that may not be otherwise available. Therefore, we try to enroll patients who we feel are likely to take the therapy as prescribed in order to gain maximum benefit.

In terms of 'what can be done about optimal adherence', the answer is to maintain communication with PLWHA receiving ART about their experiences and in particular any adverse events that may impede their desire or capacity to take their treatment as recommended. In many cases there are various strategies that can be employed to improve things up to and including changing therapy.

LH: In the conclusions to your Bangkok presentation, you mentioned several things that I'd like you to expand upon here if you would. You said, for example, that there is an 'urgent need for access to HIV-protease inhibitors in resource-poor settings'. Okay, I'll bite: I'll play Devil's Advocate and say that, although Papua New Guinea probably fits most people's definition of a 'resource-poor setting', the cat is already, as it were, out of the bag and that some of the careful, more cautious steps weren't taken some years ago to wrest the absolute maximum out of what ART can potentially do for Papua New Guineans. Again, I'm just playing Devil's Advocate, so hear me out. Personally, I think that it's too late to do maximum good with minimal harm because of the ways in which the programmes were mandated for Papua New Guinea and because of how immodest were the goals and aims. I think that lots of people, including doctors, would agree that many have been made sick and perhaps hastened to their death by the extraordinary toxicity of antiretrovirals, that the chances are good for interrupted and disrupted supply chains (the former Minister of Health said so himself on national television) and possible emergence on the black-market. I'm worried that any subsidisation now is only prolonging the inevitable, such as you mentioned above with regards to the development of fast-mutating, highly resistant strains of HIV that then narrow a patient's antiretroviral options. Some of the NHASP reviews that I've touched on in previous chapters present information about this, but very much between-the-lines, and I've had several medical doctors grumble to me privately that not enough is being done to publicise, if only with other doctors, the real 'side effects', if you will, to many Papua New Guineans and even to other programme planners, for example, of heart attacks, lipodystrophy, weight loss and anaemia. I'd say also that although prices for such are going likely to keep coming down, they're still going to be beyond the means of average Papua New Guineans if they have to be paid for on a monthly basis. Brazil, by contrast, makes ART available to many tens of thousands of citizens for free. If I were feeling especially cynical, I'd say also that every kina and dollar spent on treatment (which is unquestionably needed) is nevertheless a kina and a dollar not spent on prevention. Again, I'm playing Devil's Advocate here, but how would you respond? Also, how does treatment itself impact upon transmission and the prevention thereof, or rather, how is it hoped to work?

MB: Well, there are many issues there that you have touched on, all of which have been voiced in other contexts in the past. Let me begin with the notion that ART has in fact hastened peoples' demise. As I referred to much earlier in our discussion there is an element of truth in this, which can be seen in the results of a number of programmes in sub-Saharan Africa (e.g. from Zambia, Malawi and South Africa). As I explained, there has been a disturbing problem of very late stage HIV-infected patients enrolling in HIV treatment access programmes but dying within the first six months.

LH: That's right, and some of the NHASP reviews and other documents hint particularly at patients being lost in the shuffle, developing terrible anaemia, suffering heart attacks and what not. Helen Epstein's book, *The Invisible Cure* (2007) also contains several compelling examples of ethically suspect ART trials.

MB: Now as I explained earlier, the precise reasons for this are unknown, but likely stem from the profound immunodeficient state in which the patients enter the programme and commence their therapy. It is in fact unlikely that the deaths are a direct result of the toxicity of the antiretrovirals themselves, but in some cases are, paradoxically, an indirect result of their very effectiveness and potency in suppressing HIV-replication. In other words, at least a proportion of these premature deaths result from a profound return to immunocompetence as HIV replication is suppressed and the immune system redevelops a capacity to respond to other pathogens. These reactions can be dramatic and life-threatening.

LH: Yeah, the immune system reconstitution to which McBride and Bradford (2004) called. That's such a weird paradox. I wish that it could be communicated more broadly.

MB: In countries in sub-Saharan Africa, the most common immune reconstitution reaction is associated with tuberculosis. Some of the other deaths are likely to be a result of unrecognised infections at the commencement of ART (once again TB is common) that once again paradoxically and dramatically worsen as a result of the profound inflammatory reaction once people develop greater immune competence following introduction of ART. I remember one particular case that I had in that 61-patient study I referred to earlier. This guy had failed NRTI combination therapy for some time and had a very low CD4 count. He had been losing weight and had had a low-grade fever for a few weeks, but all this was explicable on the basis of his poorly controlled HIV-infection. In this study we actually looked pretty hard for evidence of TB in all the enrolling patients, including doing a chest X-ray and a TB skin test (the Mantoux Test). His chest x-ray was normal and his skin test was negative. Within a fortnight of starting the therapy he presented with florid TB, and in retrospect he clearly had TB when we did all the tests. Unfortunately, because of his profound immunodeficiency he just wasn't reacting to the presence of the TB, and hence the negative tests. This sort of syndrome is a major clinical problem, and as I indicated above the answer probably lies in identifying and treating PLWHA at an earlier stage, which in itself entails the reconceptualisation of testing strategies so they can be identified in a timely fashion.

LH: Yeah, and which is a real problem in Papua New Guinea given the ways in which the majority of the HIVab+ learn of their status and how late in their diagnosis they present.

MB: The prevention-versus-treatment argument has been played out for many years. The general consensus over the past five years is that prevention and treatment is not a zero-sum game, and that in fact the two elements are synergistic. What, for instance, is the incentive to undergo voluntary counselling and testing (VCT) for HIVab if a 'positive' result means nothing other than the knowledge that you will prematurely die and possibly become the object of fear and loathing in your own community, even perhaps your own family, without the hope of treatment?

LH: Good point.

MB: On the other hand, if VCT is linked to a treatment programme that has counselling, education and support, as well as help in finding ways to offer similar testing to your wife and family, then chances are that such testing may become more attractive. I think one of the most powerful texts that I have read dealing with this issue and the false dichotomy between prevention and treatment is contained within the autobiography of the South African Judge Edwin Cameron, called *Witness to AIDS* (Cameron 2005). I highly recommend it, as he deals cogently with many of the issues we've raised here.

In answer to your last question about the impact of treatment on prevention, there is some evidence that widespread treatment might itself act as a form of HIV prevention. This has a certain common-sense ring to it, but there is a body of evidence as well as a number of biological considerations that suggests that it may not really work in practice and therefore we must be very cautious about adopting this argument as a reason for introducing treatment itself.

LH: Yeah, I can remember your colleague Susan Kippax, Director of the National Centre in HIV Social Research (NCHSR), arguing in an editorial a few years ago that point, that is, regarding the unexamined assumption that more testing and more counselling and even more HIV medicines are necessarily and inherently good things.

MB: In summary, the evidence that treatment acts as prevention is in my opinion weak, which isn't to say that it might not be true, only that we need to test the hypothesis more thoroughly in the first instance, that is, do the research.

LH: Fair enough, and/but you've called attention to some of the institutional and technical stumbling blocks to doing precisely that great research that is most needed.

You also mentioned that there is a great potential for the use of lower doses of currently approved HIV-protease inhibitors, but that clinical research is needed first to address these questions. Thinking about RLSs generally but perhaps North Queensland, the Torres Straits and Papua New Guinea more specifically, and perhaps thinking ahead to the future of other countries in the region, such as the Solomon Islands, what shape should or would that clinical research take? Who ought to conduct it? What are the major questions that ought to be addressed, and by means of what kinds of methods and instruments should they be asked?

MB: Any research involving, for instance, the use of lower doses of ART agents would have to be conducted according to a process of consultative and inclusive discussions of, in the first instance, the research question itself, and then the shape of the research protocol designed to address it. We would ultimately hope that such a question could be answered through a collaborative research network that included not only Papua New Guinea but other parts of the Asia-Pacific (and even beyond), so that the effort of mounting such a trial could produce the maximal benefit for the maximum number across a broad range of populations. The trial standards would have to be of the highest quality, both in terms of the public health impact of the research question, the ethical standards of the human research, the quality of the trial conduct and patient care, down to the data collection and analysis, interpretation, reporting and public dissemination of the results. By conducting such a trial in as many developing regions and countries as possible, the results could be seen to be 'generalisable' and therefore when it comes to converting these results into guidelines and implementation, the various powers-that-be (e.g. WHO, UNAIDS, GFATM) can be satisfied that the findings are robust and reliable across a number of contexts and populations. For that reason major stakeholders such as WHO, UNAIDS and others would optimally be consulted early on in the process so that they could contribute to and review the research question and trial protocol before implementation.

In terms of who should take responsibility for the conduct of such a trial the answer is that it should be ultimately owned by the community in which it is being conducted but collaboratively run with key input from key stakeholders including the local PLWHA and research community(ies). Agencies in support would include developed world institutions such as NCHECR, which could lend their expertise and experience to the optimal design and conduct of the study.

LH: I'm sympathetic, but yet I would point out that civil societies are not yet that well developed in Papua New Guinea and that there don't seem (yet) to be sufficiently powerful or well-organised collections of HIV and AIDS advocates, including those who are on ART.

MB: The questions that should be addressed would again have to be determined primarily by researchers from the communities from whom the study subjects were to be drawn, with support from advisory partners with a proven track record in conducting appropriate clinical research in developing country contexts. One obvious example of a research question that has already been discussed in various forums is the question of what to do when first-line therapy fails.

✳ ✳ ✳

LH: Let me return to something I said about you at the outset, about the contentions in your proposal regarding interventions in sexual culture that were not necessarily just pharmaceutical or even clinical. What did you mean by that? How do those go over with some of your other colleagues in epidemiology and clinical medicine?

MB: I imagine that I was drawing attention to those structural determinants of HIV-infection that the biomedical disciplines tend to either forget or ignore. By this I mean that the vulnerability to becoming infected with HIV in Papua New Guinea involves a potent mix of structural circumstances: poverty, illiteracy, cultural and linguistic diversity, difficult geography, low status of women and widespread gender-based discrimination and violence, ignorance of sexually transmitted diseases (and also transmission routes and risks of HIV), internal migration, weak national government authority, poor governance, familial disruption, cultural breakdown and flagging, uneven economic development. Because those working in the biomedical sphere are not usually formally taught about these proximal determinants of disease, and because many biomedical workers are relatively conservative, politically …

LH: No!

MB: the attitude is generally that the responsibility to intervene to amend these determinants belongs to others (e.g. government) and therefore the focus of the biomedical community is only on the 'distal' context of individual HIV transmission and treatment. However, it seems to me that unless members of the biomedical community always keep in mind the proximal determinants of infection and support efforts to ameliorate them, our bio-medical interventions will likely not be as effective as they could be.

LH: Yeah, but I think that's because of something far more fundamentally wrong with how the incredible complexities of disease causation are over-simplified in this age of AIDS. I think that in many cases it's wrongheaded to blame for the eventual deaths of struggling, suffering people, only a virus and nothing more. I don't see why it is so difficult to accept that she had acquired immune deficiency syndrome, whether or not she was ever tested for HIVab. More and more researchers, too, are calling attention to the fact that lots of vaginal discharge is caused by wife-beating. According to some experts, for example, a majority of women suffering from vaginal and cervical complaints – especially discharge – is now thought not to be due to viruses and bacteria, that is, are not due to STDs (e.g. Lush *et al*. 2003; Sloan *et al*. 2000). What I mean is, why can't wife-beating and psychosocial distress and anxiety – or stigma, for that matter – be both proximate and ultimate at the same time? What if I said that HIV is only the symptom of a cause far more fundamental, located on the level of social-structure, of inequalities between persons and groups of them, that HIV has in a cruel way done us a service in revealing that? That's what I meant above several times when referring to the fetishization of HIV.

MB: Well, I'd have to say that you were starting to sound a lot like Thabo Mbeki. There is absolutely no doubt that structural influences play a pro-foundly important role in magnifying HIV risk and determining transmis-sion. This is why countries such as Australia can have a 0.1% HIV prevalence and countries such as Zimbabwe can have prevalence 200-fold higher that. Having said that, there is also absolutely no doubt that HIV exists, is the cause of AIDS, and that it requires specific and urgent intervention to reduce transmission risk as well as offer treatment to those already infected.

LH: Yeah, I'm not denying the existence of either HIV or AIDS, although anyone who asks any questions about anything gets dubbed an 'AIDS denial-ist', for example, the Robert Gallo group in response to a long article by the science writer, Celia Farber, or the vitriolic response to well-intended, com-peting models of AIDS causation by members of the so-called Perth Group. It's weird. Anyway, a recent article by Evelyn Lavu and her colleagues in Port Moresby (Lavu *et al*. 2004) said that '11% of those who were diagnosed with AIDS were consistently HIV-antibody-negative by serology' (2004: 37). Their remarks join those of many others around the world. Care to comment?

MB: I think what this probably indicates is that there are a number of people who may 'look like they have AIDS' in the sense that they fulfil one or more of the criteria established by the WHO for a diagnosis of AIDS (called, according to WHO criteria, 'Clinical Stage 4 HIV disease'), but who are found on testing not to be HIV-infected, and who therefore cannot by definition have AIDS. How can this be? Well, the criteria that define AIDS (Stage 4 disease) are a set of conditions that are associated with severe immunodeficiency, but are by no means exclusively seen in immunodeficiency secondary to

HIV-infection. Therefore, malnourished patients or patients who have an undiagnosed tumour or other chronic illness or infection (e.g. tuberculosis) may be suspected to have AIDS (most commonly on the basis of 'unexplained wasting', but on testing are found not to be infected with HIV). If this were to occur in a developed country with a government-subsidised universal health system like Australia, the next step would be to search for those other possible causes and refer such patients on to one specialist or another. Eventually, another cause is found. In a resource poor country such as Papua New Guinea, one that has weak health infrastructure and little capacity for complicated investigation, I imagine what might happen is that in the presence of an apparent 'AIDS' diagnosis but an absence of a positive HIV-antibody test and, say, the basic exclusion of another likely cause such as TB, the patient gets sent away and either presents later when the diagnosis has become manifest or simply dies without a diagnosis.

LH: Thanks, Mark. I appreciate your candour and for sharing so much of the aims and work of you and your colleagues. We've got a lot of work ahead of us, haven't we?

Chapter 9

Epilogue

The sickness in society

Risky social structures

> Just as everyone seems to have his or her own definition of 'structure' and 'violence', so too does the term "structural violence" cause epistemological jitters in our ranks ... An anthropology that tallies the body count must of course look at the dead and those left for dead. (Paul Farmer, 'An Anthropology of Structural Violence', 2004, p. 307)

> As much as humans in various societies, whether urban or folk, are capable of empathy, kindness, even love and as much as they sometimes achieve astounding mastery of the challenges posed by their environments, they are also capable of maintaining beliefs, values, and social institutions that result in senseless cruelty, needless suffering, and monumental folly in their relations among themselves ... (Robert Edgerton, *Sick Societies*, 1992, p. 15)

This epigraph from Robert Edgerton's controversial and still compelling book, *Sick Societies: challenging the myth of primitive harmony*, expresses well my thoughts about sex-repressive countries such as Indonesia, the US and Papua New Guinea in which sex industries and sexual violence also flourish. Good social scientists pay proper attention to both macro- and micro-levels of analysis, not overlooking, for example, the importance of deforestation and debt structure but also giving proper due to the properties of bacteria, viruses and protozoa to sicken and kill. An increasing number of social scientists are coming to locate the ultimate (if not also proximate) causes of sickness and death on the level of social-structure. We can only wait for our sisters and brothers in the biomedical sciences. In *Sick Societies* Edgerton puts his finger squarely upon wife-beating, child abuse, sexual assault, elderly neglect, ethnic bigotry and other forms of interpersonal violence. Endemic misery, he concludes, alongside extreme levels of morbidity and rising levels of mortality, results from social-structures having gone awry – not genes, not climate and certainly not God. The stories I begin to tell in the text boxes below in the section entitled 'In the Company of Men' show that 'disease' is social, too, not necessarily viral or bacterial, and that the cure is therefore also social justice and human rights, not just a new antibiotic or antiretroviral, although those have their place. Any fieldworker who studies such topics as have been covered in this book has easily several score similar stories to tell.

The logical conclusion to this book's argument is that if one is fully committed to the kind of holism for which many anthropologists have been arguing for a century or more, then the entire globe – people, viruses, atmosphere, animals, bacteria and ecosystems together – composes a living, breathing and sensitive entity that is vulnerable at many points but also amenable to healing. J.E. Lovelock put forward this thesis with great elegance and persuasion with the publication first in 1979 of his path-breaking book, *Gaia* (Lovelock 1987). Many have joined the chorus, from cultural ecologists to shamans to environmental biologists, in theorising the ill health effects of our world on the wane, as Levi-Strauss put it some time ago. We are now each and collectively carrying a 'body burden' that is simply too heavy, in the words of Sandra Steingraber (1997), a prominent theorist of environmental causes of cancer. Steingraber followed in the footsteps of Rachel Carson's *Silent Spring* (Carson 1962). That some are bearing far more than others, as anthropologists such as Nancy Scheper-Hughes and Paul Farmer have theorised (Farmer 2004; Scheper-Hughes 1994), reminds us of the ways in which AIDS *is* the social body in addition to appearing on and in bodies. Women shouldn't have to exchange sexual services just in order to eat, depicted here in the form of a styrofoam container of 'take-away' food and a used condom. It was taken in a rural enclave setting's *tu kina bus ples* (outdoor prostitution locale), and there are many more just like it.

Many indigenous peoples have come to similar conclusions (and well before Lovelock, obviously) about the social causation of illness, suggesting that we be wary of taking overly narrow approaches to health and welfare, that we be careful about the dangers to individual and public health of fetishizing the microscopic level of protozoa, bacteria and viruses. Interpersonal violence and social relations in disarray play their part, too, though they have been shown to be just as difficult to get rid of as mutating viruses. Good health and ill, that is, sickness and cure, immune system function and dysfunction – both can come from or be precluded by social *relations*,

> 'there is no technical shortcut to the social transformation needed in how men and women confront and act on their own sexuality and in sexual relationships. Safer sex is a frame of mind, and a way of thinking and relating to others sexually, and it is only safer sex that will defeat the epidemics of HIV and other STIs' (Berer 2007b: 47).

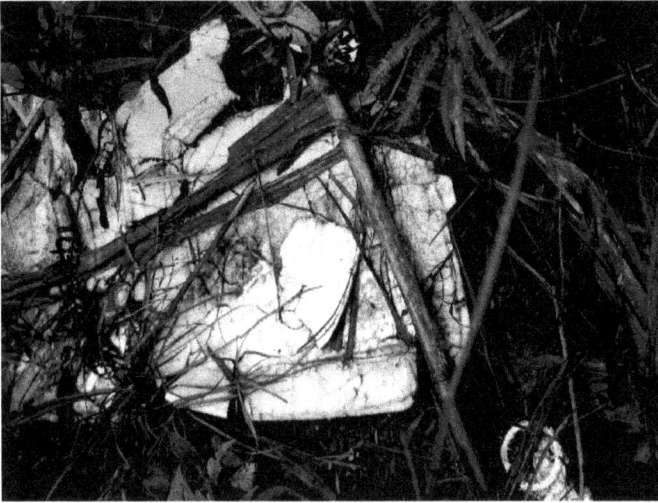

Sex for food: takeaway food container and used condom

just as they can from microscopically small *entities*. From this position, the choices that researchers, medical workers and policy-makers make regarding the assessment of disease causation – whether of microbes, social systems, environmental assaults, or world systems – are to a certain extent arbitrary. Biomedical practitioners could incorporate analytic levels other than that of microbes and thus expand and enrich their models of disease causation.

This is not going to be easy. In the mid–late nineteenth century the tenets of germ theory gradually began to be accepted. Waves of consensus began to consolidate at the turn of the twentieth century with Paul Ehrlich's discovery of the (for a time) magic bullets of Salvarsan and neo-Salvarsan and with other clinical, experimental successes in isolating the smallest etiological agent of infectious and communicable disease. Such occurred again in post-World War Two with discoveries of antibiotics and the mass production of new (for a time) magic bullets of penicillin and sulpha drug derivatives. Microbe-level models of disease causation gained more advocates in recent years with the coming of AIDS and with discoveries in the 1980s of two major types of HIV and in the past year with two new types of retrovirus, HTLV-III and HTLV-IV. New understandings of cervical cancer, Kaposi sarcoma, stomach ulcers and hepatitis were made possible by discovery of Human Papilloma Virus and Hepatitis C Virus, that some bacteria were more stubborn than previously suspected and that some skin cancers were sexually transmissible. These and many other issues and illnesses were sampled by Frank Ryan in his *Virus X* (Ryan 1997) and by a large handful of medical science writers such as Laurie Garrett (2005). The careful reader will see in the bibliographic notes to their books an apparent explosion occurring throughout the 1990s of attributions to microbes of causation of increasing human suffering. With regards specifically to disease causation, correspondingly little attention was paid to ecological breakdown and gender violence, to poverty and malnutrition, to cultural dislocation and to civil war, to wife-beating and sexual molestation.

I take from Lovelock's book the idea that the 'Gaia' hypothesis of a pulsating, responsive entity comprising many interlocking parts and vulnerable by threat to any of them is fundamentally about the ill effects of harmful social relations, of social-structure gone awry. In quite sobering fashion Ryan suggests that

> viruses have, through the empirics of evolution, become unwitting
> knights of nature, armed by evolution for furious genomic attack against
> her transgressors [I approve of the perhaps unwitting gendered imagery].
> Although not primarily designed to attack humanity, human exploitation
> and invasion of every ecological sphere has directed that aggression our way.
> (Ryan 1997: 320)

I want to take Ryan's suggested pushing outward of aggression toward the environment, and turn it around. I want us to begin to take seriously the aggression that is implicit in the operation of discombobulated, contradictory social-structures. In theorising disease causation I want also to look closely at what makes 'youth' vulnerable, at what makes marriage a double-edged sword, at why the already despised are blamed further and sexual transgressors punished even more. Robert Edgerton is one of the relatively few anthropologists in the past several decades to have modelled human suffering in terms of the very analytical level – social-structure – about which anthropologists are supposed to know the most. I think that we've lost track of many insights that an older, or slightly older medical anthropology once had for us and that are still relevant today, for example, about iatrogeny and the pathogenic effects of structural violence (e.g. Fabrega and Silver 1972; Glick 1977[1967]; Janzen 1978; Lewis 1975; Lindenbaum 1979; Mullings 1984). Franz Fanon, for example, the revolutionary psychotherapist, wrote compellingly in several critical texts about the bodily sickening effects of racism. In *Black Skins, White Masks*, for example, he wrote '[a] normal Negro child, having grown up within a normal family, will become abnormal on the slightest contact with the White world' (1967: 143). Two anthropologists who aren't well known for their contributions to medical anthropology, S.F. Nadel and Claude Levi-Strauss, have nevertheless each shown that there are lots of so-called medicines that don't have much to do with illness, or at least not with *curing* it so much as with *causing* it or curing the diseases that the healer has himself or herself caused (Nadel 1954: 132; Levi-Strauss 1963). The possibility of iatrogenic disease was warned against long ago by Hippocrates ('First, physician, do no harm'), but it comes in many forms, for example, in STDs that resist antibiotics, in the extreme toxicity of antiretroviral therapies and most recently in the incubation in medical settings and increasing strength of so-called 'superbugs'. Recent quasi-ethnographies and other critical explorations have shown the threat to individual, community and public health that are posed by overmedication, by overly narrow models of disease causation and especially the stubborn refusal of allopathic physicians to admit to iatrogenesis of disease and illness. This is most painfully obvious in works such as Ann Fadiman's *The Spirit Catches You and You Fall Down* (Fadiman 1998) and Peter Kramer's *Listening to Prozac* (Kramer 1993).

Unfortunately, we've almost completely lost sight of an older medical anthropology that insisted not just upon the social origins of disease but upon its social manifestation, too. An instructive dictum was Gilbert Lewis' demonstration that for the Gnau of Papua New Guinea, 'medicine' is inseparable from 'economics' and 'religion,' that illness provokes re-examination of social relations, not searches for microbial pathogens (Lewis 1975). Lewis' conclusion recalls a similar finding of Fabrega and Silver for Zinacantecos of Mexico, that whereas notions of illness, disease and their causation are 'logically separated in the scientific system, [they are] fused and condensed in Zinacantan' (Fabrega and Silver 1972: 93). When an individual becomes ill, they write, there begins 'a process that involves both individuals and various operations of the social system. We could depict the illness graphically as a pattern that extends across space and time … ' (1972: 89). They found that illness and disease for Zinacantecos are 'bound up in the processes of social control … A real illness … is an affliction that may affect one's body; but it is also a reflection of how the social system functions … [I]llness and bodily states may be seen as part of the social machinery that implements norms' (1972: 91). There is no shortage of other examples that could be cited from Pacific island countries and cultures, of course, just as for Western European ones. Maggie Cummings, for example, noted a kind of cognitive dissonance among ni-Vanuatu similar to what I showed in Chapter 4 as regards epidemiological models of risk and in Chapter 5 as regards condom efficacy. After noting that the study of 547 pregnant women aged 15–46 who were attending the First-Visit Antenatal Clinic at the Vila Central Hospital revealed a 25% prevalence figure for at least one of the four STDs for which they were tested (chlamydia, gonorrhea, trichomonas and syphilis), ni-Vanuatans nevertheless believed that AIDS was only a distant, future threat, 'and then only through being introduced by foreigners' (Cummings 2008: 143). Seemingly absent there was a consideration of what this figure implied (and these, mind you, were pregnant women, allegedly those at lowest risk) about social-structure and the imbalanced state of gender relations. What Cummings wrote about Vanuatu can stand for many other Pacific island countries and cultures. Ni-Vanuatu seem to hold two contradictory propositions simultaneously: that there is a 'slowly ticking time bomb' afoot, but that Vanuatu is still a 'safe place' because the threat to it came largely from the outside, from the future, from foreigners. Sadly, the resolution of these two contradictions has resulted in a strengthening of the very social structures that sicken them, which is to say, male privilege in all things sexual, Christian church-inspired sexual repression and female subservience (Cummings 2008: 143–4). Painfully, the National Council of Chiefs decided to ban female trousers-wearing, with the support of youth and women's groups, housewives and religious leaders. One is entitled to ask whether wearing Mother Hubbard-style dresses protects ni-Vanuatu women from STDs or HIV any better than do trousers. Cummings shows for Vanuatu what I have showed for Papua New Guinea: 'those who are most vulnerable are those who are stigmatized by that society's sexual culture' (Cummings 2008: 148). Just as in Papua New Guinea, as I showed in detail in Chapter 5, shame about their bodies, fuelled by both *kastom* and Christianity, secrecy about sexual matters and the purposeful forgoing of condom use is sickening and killing them.

The model of disease causation of both Zinacantecos and ni-Vanuatu calls to mind Leonard Glick's still useful little essay published in *Ethnology* in 1967, 'Medicine as an Ethnographic Category.' Glick drove home the point that when it comes to sickness and suffering, what ethnographers ought to be doing is *nailing down the state of power relations*, from whence and from whom they emanate. 'Where power resides,' he noted, 'in a particular sociocultural system is a question for the ethnographer to answer' (Glick 1977[1967]: 60). He allowed that 'power' may take different forms in different social systems, and that some communities might not even have a word for it. Still, the ethnographer's job is to find the loci of power, how they are mobilised, and what bodily effects varying amounts of power can have upon people who are placed differently in the social system. In the example presented by contemporary Papua New Guinea such as I have analysed here, this would include males versus females and certainly the land- and resource-rich and -poor, but also, in view of the policies and programmes I have critiqued, those who seem to adhere to and those who clearly transgress the norms of sexual ethics. Glick's essay is important also for arguing that while the causes of disease might (or might not) be invisible (thus allowing for microbial causes, for example), never are they impersonal. 'Illnesses are caused by *agents* who in some way bring their powers to bear against their victims ... who act not indifferently but in response to consciously perceived personal motives' (Glick 1977[1967]: 62). Glick reminded us that while there were multiple kinds of disease causation (personal and instrumental, sorcery, demonic beings, and so on), the most extensive explanations in most medical systems are reserved for 'such considerations as social and political competition, intra-familial disputes, quarrels, conflicts, and crimes' (Glick 1977[1967]: 68). Leith Mullings writes of the same processes at work in urban Ghana, where 'natural' diseases vied with those 'supernatural' and 'spiritual' in origin (Mullings 1984).

As Victor Turner argued in several of his works on the Ndembu, as Fabrega and Silver have remarked in their studies of sickness in Mexico, or Paul Farmer about HIV in Haiti or tuberculosis in the former Soviet Union, as Shirley Lindenbaum argued in *Kuru Sorcery* regarding the Fore of the New Guinea highlands – the list goes on and on – illness as socially caused and experienced, not microbially, refers to the tears, knots, rents and barren spots in the social-structure. Illness as a social phenomenon exists also at the level of gender and familial relations and at the level of the lineage, clan and community, problems in or with which weigh heavily upon organs and tissues, muscles and nerves. Abigail Harrison has written perceptively about a particular kind of contradiction in the social structures of rural South Africans that puts young men but especially women at markedly higher risk of infection with HIV and STDs. This is, after all, an area in which HIVab seroprevalence in young women is among the highest in the world. The case she analyses is of gender role norms and expectations that girls and young women *prove virginity* ... by engaging in sexual intercourse, most often unsafely, without benefit of condom use (Harrison 2008). Having sex to prove virginity is a bit like lighting a match to see whether or not it works. Unlike a spent match, however, a no-longer-virginal female in rural South Africa can face social stigmas and devaluation. 'None of the women had initiated sexual activity in their relationships,' writes Harrison, and moreover, 'most said they were not prepared or ready for their first intercourse.' Not surprisingly, 'none of the young men mentioned the importance of having a girlfriend who continued to preserve her virginity, nor did any of the men or their girlfriends mention virginity as desirable for themselves' (2008: 184). This is an example of what Roy Willis has referred to in his study of healing in Tanzania as being 'injurious communication among human beings' (Willis, quoted in Landy 1983: 220). Arthur Kleinman and his associates from the People's Republic of China began two decades ago to imagine the etiology of the suffering of people during the Great Leap Forward and the Cultural Revolution not by appeals to microbes but by moving up to the level of social relations. The chronic pains, lassitude, depression, headaches, anxieties, soul loss, wandering gonads and many other disorders that many tens of millions of Chinese people suffered were caused by stressful social relations, joining the other illnesses they suffered owing to parasites and protozoa and environmental poisons. Stressful social relations in the form of struggles to achieve, maintain, or resist attempts to mandate ideological purity *are* dis-ease. The omnipresent fear of what was going to happen to oneself, to one's family and to one's colleagues and friends under extreme political and social distress *is* dis-ease. As women's group leaders and writers of letters to the editor point out frequently, women and girls in contemporary Papua New Guinea live in a kind of prison, subject near constantly to degrees of terror, sometimes low-level, sometimes not. More recently, Kleinman has argued that the 'body becomes a mediator between individual and collective experience', that depression can be 'recast as a relationship between person and society' (Kleinman 1995: 11). Allen Feldman has argued that '[s]ocial structure itself can be telescoped in the violent act or the latter's interpretive reception' (Feldman 1999: 4).

Along with Kleinman, Lindenbaum, Farmer and others, I believe that this element needs to be wed better to 'physician'-centred models of disease causation, or what Willis calls the 'doctor theory'. Other examples in this vein might include the disturbing and controversial work of the Australian psychiatrist, John Cawte, who devoted his attention to one particularly desperate and unhealthy Australian Aboriginal group. One needn't accept his Malthusian *and* Hobbesian conclusions about stress being a sort of ecological adaptation to scarce and dwindling resources in order to appreciate his larger point: such stresses are felt on and in the body as the literal embodiment of stressful social relations. It was not microbes that caused their disease so much as that disease took the form of paranoia, fighting, homicide, mental disorders and wife-stealing (Cawte 1978). That pathology took heavily gendered forms, for example, in terms of STD transmission and in terms of wife- as opposed to husband-beating, is a telltale sign of a social-structure gone awry. Willis' comment captures nicely my feeling that dis-ease is located on the level of social-structure:

> In modern Western societies, however, it appears to be the case that
> scientific paradigms (for example, in physics) can exist in flat contradiction
> of corresponding social paradigms and there is an absence of shared

cosmological assumptions which might serve to integrate these disparate areas of knowledge and experience. (Willis, quoted in Landy 1983: 220)

From this perspective the appearance in Pacific bodies of the signs and symptoms of gonorrhea, syphilis and Donovanosis and now of AIDS-related illnesses is singly and collectively demonstrating ruptures in the social fabric. The transmission of HIV and the embodied suffering of AIDS are challenging the dermal, immunological and other defences we have to infection, just as they are revealing to us the weak links in our social-structure especially around sexual and political matters. These bodily eruptions are expressing to us, if we will only see them, the contours of the fact of and behavioural expressions of sexual expectations that spring from culture, religion and society. There are, for example, expectations that privilege 'intercourse', that expect it to be vaginal and preferably unhindered by condoms, that it not be preceded by examinations of or discussions about possibly infected genitalia, that it not implicate male privilege in other realms. In even a clinical sense STDs are suffered, thought about and treated quite differently in terms of gender and marital status (Hammar 2004b). Gonorrhea and chlamydia, syphilis and genital herpes may manifest on and in individual human bodies and body parts, but they also constitute signs in a larger Social Body (Scheper-Hughes 1994).

Appearing in the form of lesions, infertility, discharge, odours and pain, they also and more importantly signal and mediate relations between those bodies. Relatively speaking, we might for comparative purposes note for starters that such signs and symptoms do not appear very much to hinder the sexual practice of males, but greatly shape, perhaps even overdetermine the social and familial expectations of females. This is packing one kind of STD upon another. The sexually transmitted dis-ease of which I am thinking takes the form of stigmatisation, for example, the cultural branding of women as witches or the breaking of confidentiality in an ANC setting. It includes symbolic violence in the form of consignment to a 'high-risk' group and being branded sexual transgressors or blamed for one's own vulnerability. It can inhere in marital dissolution following apparent female infertility, which spells vastly different outcomes for male and female. Certainly it includes physical battering and rape, sexual molestation and harassment. These in turn help to explain why the presentation of physical symptoms is so often and so starkly patterned by gender, for example, in terms of late or inconsistent clinic attendance and what many medical practitioners, well meaning or not, have dubbed 'naïve' adherence to antiretrovirals, as we discussed in Chapter 8. These gender and gendered differences go right to the heart of one of the significant accomplishments in Papua New Guinea, the application of principles of the syndromic management of putative STDs.

This approach is technically sound for individual treatment of some syndromes, such as male urethral discharge. Unfortunately, syndromic management of vaginal discharge–the most common syndrome in the family planning context–appears technically unsound against cervical STIs and not programmatically feasible in such settings [references omitted]. Relatively few women in general maternal-child health settings who have a vaginal discharge actually have gonorrhea or chlamydia, while many with those same diseases have no discharge. (Shelton and Fuchs 2004: 14)

An influential review that preceded that of Shelton and Fuchs was that of Nancy Sloan and colleagues (Sloan *et al.* 2000). They found that a majority of cases found in women of vaginal discharge syndrome were not due to what are generally accepted to be STDs. Among many other questions that their conclusion begs is what causes those discharges and why female are not comparable to male discharges. Another large study conducted in the slums of New Delhi found clinical evidence of an abnormal vaginal discharge in nearly 95% of the women, infection rates of cervicitis of over 36%, of cervical erosion of almost 44%, and pelvic inflammatory disease affecting more than one-quarter of them (Garg *et al.* 2001: 82). Fewer than 60% of those found to be suffering from abnormal discharge were found to be infected (Garg *et al.* 2001: 90). Little notice of these issues has been aired in Papua New Guinea and that have been informed by non-clinical data and ethnographic insights, for example, that women apparently uninfected with STDs but who suffer from chronic vaginal and cervical discharges are often regularly assaulted by their 'intimate' partners. Pummelling fists and harmful social relations, in other words, not microbes, cause this kind of sexually transmitted dis-ease. Lindenbaum closes her account of *Kuru Sorcery* also with her finger squarely upon the level of social relations:

> In a masterly illusion projected by an egalitarian ethic, the dispossessed [Fore women and girls] are characterized as a threat [to Fore men and boys], a casuistic line of argument we share with the Fore. People in marginal positions are portrayed as a danger to the establishment ... A society stratified as little as the Fore [or as much] shows individual men and women living in relationships of mutual aid and as parasite and host [see Hammar 1989] ... Disease symptoms, like sorcery accusations, signal a corrective response, an attempted reassertion of dominance by the protesting host. (Lindenbaum 1979:146)

With these ideas firmly in place, it is time to ratchet up the argument. It may be true that the theoretical currents that connect these kinds of arguments from two and three decades ago (e.g. 'primitive' medicine or ethnoscience) with those of today (e.g. in critical medical anthropology, political economy of health, and radical phenomenology) may appear a bit murky. Still, it is virtually a truism now to say that pathogens and diseases, blame and illness, track along the 'fault-lines' of society, as Lindenbaum and others have been asserting for some time now. Given the data I presented and critiqued in Chapters 3, 4 and 5, it is clear enough that Papua New Guinea in the midst of HIV and AIDS epidemics is yet another case showing that the embodied suffering of AIDS and the added burdens of caring for others suffering from it have starkly patterned gender dynamics to them. Transmission of and infection with HIV (not to say also the many other STDs) are therefore unsurprisingly telling of the sociology of vulnerability. To make the point of my book more explicitly, I assert that those fault-lines are also manifestations of disease. I am not going to argue with those who still wish to see the cause of *kuru* amongst the Fore people as being first, last and middle the prion theorised and then isolated by Stanley Prusiner, that is, something so small you'd need an electron microscope to see it. I would argue, however, with those who exaggerated the more exotic transmission routes – endocannibalism – at the expense of those a lot less so – in this case, heavily gendered corpse-handling norms and practices that exposed women far more than men to contamination. In like manner, sexual networking exposes women differently than men to physical violence, legal punishment, societal approbation and pathogens and brings with it different constellations of pleasure and rewards.

In the company of men

> Within the great hall the men and women gathered together, and at times the dancing ceased and the place was plunged in darkness. Then from the far end of the building a man cried out, 'I am Aibaro, and these are my wives'. With them on either side of him he started to walk down the hall holding their hands until they were dragged from him by other men. Others followed, each announcing his name and bringing his womenfolk, until there had been a general interchange of wives. Then the fires were allowed to burn brightly for a time to give light for dance and song but during the night the whole ceremony was repeated several times with all present participating. At dawn the dancing stopped and the women streamed out from the great place and went to their clan houses or *moto* [houses] to rest, and for some hours the village was unnaturally quiet. (Benjamin Butcher, *My Friends, the New Guinea Headhunters*, 1964, pp. 174–5)

In Enga Province, I sat down in an antenatal clinic to conduct a scheduled interview with, in this case, a pregnant 16 year-old. Being new to the project and wanting to minimize likely cross-gender, cross-race and cross-generation dynamics, I went slowly and carefully. My young interviewee was experiencing her first-ever medical encounter (to check on the health of the fetus growing inside her) and seemed greatly uncomfortable. In addition to unbearable stomach pains and chronic headaches, when she unwound the thin rags wrapped around her hands, I learned that she was missing five and a half digits between her two hands. A week prior as she marketed garden foods with her mother a young male corporate group grabbed her, pressed her hands to the ground, and chopped off with a bush-knife as many fingers as they could get in two blows. Another male corporate group had previously done the same to one of 'theirs'. She is now minus two fully functional hands, and the 'husband' who recently impregnated her has already taken off. Pregnant, 16, disfigured, near mute, unmarried and no longer virginal. Any bets on her future?

As I and three collaborators have shown in the sections and chapters above, it is largely individual and corporate bodies of men who perpetrate the vast majority of physical, economic and especially sexual violence in Papua New Guinea, just as in the US. Petty and not-so-petty graft, theft and malfeasance also dampen educational opportunities for everyone. The gutting of health service delivery systems has compromised the public health even further. Risk has been projected onto the especially vulnerable members of the population, which is to say disaffected youth, the non-heterosexual, and the women, girls and boys consigned to toil in sex industries to support themselves and family. No wealthy businessmen have been strapped down and had their reproductive organs ripped out with fiery hooks to force confessions of having 'sent AIDS' throughout the village as have women (Haley 2008). No Australian construction workers or Malaysian fishermen *per se* have been targeted in HIV transmission prevention campaigns as have their female sex partners. No potential tourists or aid workers are warned away on web-site postings of having sex with members of parliament or with their professional sex partners. No security guards, soldiers or policemen have been paraded in front of onlookers and forced to swallow condoms as proof of *their* sexual transgressions as have women and girls. In fact, the sexual transgressions perpetrated by the powers-that-be in Papua New Guinea are only rarely reported. And it's not that they happen infrequently or that they aren't otherwise well-known. For example, the Second Round of BSS (Behavioural Science Survey) found that almost half of policemen surveyed had admitted to raping females, that 40% of truck drivers had done so, and that 18.4% of Ramu Sugar plantation workers and 27.3% of Lae transport industry workers had done so (NACS 2008: 25). Here is one rare published exception, from a member of the 'disciplined' forces:

> The public is against us and I don't want to be beaten up in the night clubs. You mean pay for sex? That is quite new to me. I f*** for nothing, why pay? I'm telling you the facts. Policemen f*** like nobody's business. How many times we bring girls into this single barracks, they never demand money. That's correct, we do group sex too. Well, you know the system yourself, brother boy! Policeman can f*** at anytime, any place … There are certain girls that we know of. They are regular faces to policemen, and we f*** them whenever we meet them and that is when group sex comes in. We call them 'public toilets'. Whenever we feel like f***ing, we go looking for them. As soon we spot them, we tell them to climb into the car or van. If they refuse, we use force to get them in. We always bash them up, so they know our ways. We pick them up any place – streets, outside the clubs, any place. Yes, sometimes we bash them up and order them to get into the car. Well, where will they go and report or lay complaints? Every policeman and policewoman in town knows them very well. Nowadays, they don't come to the police station because they know very well that their reports won't be heard. (Jenkins 2007: 55–6)

Sexually transmitted dis-ease, its most recent incarnation being the signs and symptoms of HIV, is sociological in the patterns of its causation and its embodiment. It is evident also in print, for example, in the euphemistic use

> *One morning in Lae, capital of Morobe Province, we lit out
> to a residential compound at which our friends/clients would
> receive test results, post-test counselling and treatment. En
> route, we per chance spotted at a male clubhouse four young
> women we had met days previous, and so we pulled into the
> Lae Football Association compound, chewed betel-nut with
> them and gave back promised photos. Because confidentiality
> is a must and because privacy is virtually nil, we offered to
> take them to a more 'neutral' place for the purpose of post-test
> counselling and provision of test results and treatment. Resident
> and visiting men began circling about us, however, began
> nosing into 'our' business and claiming 'compensation'. 'Mipela
> maritim em' ('we married her', 'she's married to one of us'),
> they said, in claiming compensation of them (a male corporate
> group bound by sex, blood, and alcohol) by us for having
> 'used', for having spilled/taken the blood of one of 'theirs'.*

of language to disseminate sexual health information and the inhibition even to use the real words of sexual violence.

Despite considerable rhetoric to the contrary, threats to good sexual and reproductive health, not also to say good health-inducing and pleasurable, consensual sex, are not by and large external to Papua New Guinea. They are homegrown, for the most part. In order to 'break the silence' surrounding sexual assault and violence in families and communities, UNICEF Pacific carried out in 2004 and 2005 five country-wide studies, involving Fiji, Kiribati, Papua New Guinea, Solomon Islands and Vanuatu. Their findings were clear and consistent:

> Each of the five studies confirms that in each country children are sexually
> abused by family members and neighbours and, to varying degrees, that
> child prostitution, child pornography, early marriage, child sex tourism
> and trafficking (for sexual purposes) occur. Perpetrators of the abuse and
> exploitation are overwhelmingly males and typically men with resources
> or other power in the community. The studies also reveal that, contrary to
> popular belief, the perpetrators of sexual abuse and sexual exploitation of
> children are also overwhelmingly men from the local community. While the
> report does highlight some incidence of sexual abuse and sexual exploitation
> committed by foreign tourists and foreign workers in the Pacific, children are
> most at risk in their homes and communities and with people they know and
> trust. (UNICEF, UNESCAP and ECPAT 2006: ix)

When the WHO examined experience among Samoan females aged 15–49 of physical and sexual violence, they found that 46% had suffered it by intimate partners and that most felt that they didn't have the right to refuse sex. Moreover, more than one-third of them who had experienced coitarche (first vaginal intercourse) prior to age 15 said that it had been forced (WHO 2005).

So, what kind of 'corrective response' must we muster in the face of AIDS? Can we do so without expressing further 'our' dominance? In 'AIDS and the Social Body', Nancy Scheper-Hughes quoted from her own monograph, *Death Without Weeping*, to the effect that 'If we cannot begin to think about social institutions and practices in moral or ethical terms, then anthropology strikes me as quite weak and useless' (1994: 991). From the vantage point of a different culture area – Thailand, in this case – the anthropologist Graham Fordham also takes extreme issue with a soft and flabby anthropology as regards HIV and AIDS. Its practitioners, he argues, often from a 'comfortably disengaged academic perspective' about sexual matters (2005: 241), collude with HIV prevention programme managers who believe that their charges 'are unable and unwilling to think about serious issues unless the subject is made exciting through the addition of games' (2005: 246). 'Enough', he says: 'it is high time that anthropologists act to reclaim their space, to reconstitute anthropology as a potentially uncomfortable, critically reflexive and socially engaged discipline – grounded in fieldwork and a strong sense of culture and of social theory' (2005: 247).

My agreement with their stances and with their specific points raises many new questions. First, how can anthropologists begin to do this without further abusing members of their host community? I know that this book is not going to go over well in Papua New Guinea, regardless of its truth content. I know that protests Christian in source will arise but that will attempt to sidetrack the challenges ahead of us. How can anthropologists speak out without adding to the already dense colonial, paternalist overlay that members of our host communities continue to struggle against? Whose set(s) of morals and ethics does one adopt while investigating phenomena such as I have explored here? Does one collect, obtain, or even invent particular kinds of ethnographic data so as to be able to bring them to bear on issues more global in scope, such as the many AIDS epidemics or the painful facts of sexual networking and violence? Or is it the other way round? Am I, in a sense, bringing my own personal, idiosyncratic, Eurocentric understanding of prostitution, social justice and disease causation into the field so as to convince Papua New Guineans of the error(s) of their ways? After all, is that not what morals and ethics are for? Alternatively, perhaps I am bringing my concerns as a located human being to bear upon sets of problem that appear to be, if not yet universal, at least globalizing.

When I began to write, first, my Ph.D. dissertation, about 20 years ago, and then this book 24 months ago, I did not know yet what precisely I was going to say. Fairly fresh out of three and a half years spent in the field (but still *in* it in important senses) many aspects of contemporary life in Papua New Guinea greatly displeased me, just as others of the contemporary US make me ashamed to be here. In conduct of Ph.D. research on Daru long ago I became particularly disturbed at what I took then (and now) to be male violence towards females, particularly of the alcoholic and sexual sort. As I have gotten deeper and deeper into it, I have been progressively more angered by the obvious mismatch between the empirical facts of risk and infection, on the one hand, and the policies and programmes devoted to them, on the other. What I saw, heard about, and otherwise have for five years experienced is real enough – outdoor, bush prostitution-style locales do exist and they express precisely the scope of male (sexual) privilege most ignored by religious and community leaders. Risk is clearly enough externalised by public health messages. Staggering quantities of money have been spent on structure and ideology that haven't a chance to work on the mass level hoped for. Condoms are expiring on the shelf and are subject to extraordinary myth-making. Sexually transmitted dis-ease presents such a significant health and social problems that one might call it ubiquitous. Statistical modelling of the HIV epidemics is logically and otherwise dubious. Unfortunately, none of these are an organic part of the national response; none of them have been allowed yet to inform a sociology-of-knowledge production and dissemination that might long ago have better guided concerned policy-makers, physicians and community leaders and led.

The independent review of progress made to date against Millennium Goals for the national response to HIV and AIDS in Papua New Guinea had this to say:

Effective leadership, good quality partnership, and clear and transparent systems of communication are central to an effective HIV response. Interviews with key stakeholders during the present visit and during the initial visit made by the IRG team leader in April 2007 raise questions about the authority and leadership offered by NAC, and about the ability and capacity of the Secretariat to take on the role of coordinating the national response. With respect to NAC, stakeholders raised questions concerning lack of strategic vision and discussion, the appropriateness of its present membership, the frequent process of substitution by key Council members, and the endorsement of actions after rather than before the event. NAC is perceived as having ignored the urgent requirement for effective political leadership in a rapidly expanding epidemic. It is seen as having failed to generate a multi-sectoral response which is locally owned and managed through NACS. Finally, it is seen as having failed to provide the necessary

Yeah, I know: patients don't normally demand compensation from their doctors upon receiving treatment – they pay for the privilege – but we've received similar such demands at several other field-sites. As well, the female in question was not more than 15 years-old, while her husband was almost thrice that. Never mind, too, that she was already infected with two STDs, that she was 'single' when we first contacted her only a few weeks prior, and that her husband (following the lead of her father) is also her pimp, having already sold her sexually to a visiting sailor and long-time drinking mate. Her father sees increased betel-nut sales at the compound when such drinking mates of his new son-in-law arrive, so he doesn't seem to mind, and it was the partial bride-price payment that purchased the betel-nut in the first place. The husband will likely pressure her to pay the money back somehow ...

leadership to influence practices leading to a rapidly expanding epidemic – including unsafe sexual behaviour, and alcohol and gender-based violence – both physical and sexual. (IRG 2007: 15)

Nevertheless, I accept that others (maybe even most others) see things very differently. I accept that they think that abstinence is the way to go. I know that they believe strongly that all will be saved in marital fidelity. I hear those who say that more praying will dampen transmission. I have to acknowledge claims that the rhetorics of prevention are well-matched by activities. The NAC certainly looks busy, if the activities and stories covered in its *Bung Wantaim* newsletter are any clue. I must hope that leadership

> *'Where's our money?' they turned out to be saying. 'Her blood is a big thing, and how are you going to compensate us?' 'Her blood is our blood', they indicated, 'her body is our body'. I hope that I don't sound like a Magdalene Society relief worker filled with religiously fervent indignation in need of venting by a good smoting by saying so, but I confess to having imagined her as already spiralling downward into prostitution. We know too much already about the effects wrought in and on female bodies because of marriage. Their photographs and stories show evidence of beatings, rapes, dislocation, disturbed sleep and nutrition, and heightened chance of infection by boyfriend and husband, if not also by customer and pimp. Three days prior, when he found out why his new bride was in our truck, her new husband tried to pull her out through the window. It was seen as reasonable, however regrettable, by those around me. 'Em i marit pinis, ya!' Em i putim pe pinis, ya!' ('She's married already!' 'He already paid bride-price'). Indeed.*

forum attendance will somehow trickle down at the local level to effect positive behavioural change. So much of what is written about Papua New Guinea these days is negative, I know. Here comes yet another foreign researcher telling us of all the ways in which our social systems and customs are maladaptive, brutalising of women and girls and headed for certain ruin. Foreign(er) social scientific research in Papua New Guinea has often and many times rightly been accused of serving primarily foreign(er) ends to the exclusion of anything beneficial to the 'subjects,' often 'objects' of study. Every few days or weeks a new spate of articles circulates in the western press regarding yet another gruesome pack rape, yet more dead babies buried in mass graves, yet more millions of kina missing in theft and graft, and yet another highway holdup. The specter of AIDS is not improving the situation, either. It is feeding existing stereotypes regarding real and imagined sexuality, but without drawing westerners much closer in terms of intervention. In just the past several years, as I've tried my best to educate former students, family, friends, colleagues and acquaintances about AIDS in Papua New Guinea and

*We saw it happen on Daru, too, capital of Western Province.
Four young high school students raped a 15-year-old co-student
at knife-point while we conducted health awareness toksaves
close by. In the ensuing non-case, a corporate group of males
related to the young victim sought compensation through a
corporate group of policemen from a corporate group of male
kinsmen of the corporate group of male rapists. The K500 that
changed hands satisfied all four masculine corporations: the
police, because they wouldn't have to admit that the rapists
had already gone free; the rapists, for obvious reasons; the
kinsmen of the rapists, because the case could be hushed
up; and the kinsmen of the victim, because those K500 went
straight into beer. The crime and the victim had been erased,
and indeed she saw not one toea of 'her' compensation.*

about our *common* struggle, the response seems to have changed greatly. Whereas once the typical reply was along the lines of 'Oh, so they've got it, too, huh?; wow, it's everywhere', now it's 'yeah, I've heard it's really bad there, an African-style disaster; well, no wonder, I've heard those natives are really promiscuous. Is it really true that they're all gay'?

The reality of Papua New Guinea is of a truly magnificent country filled with incredibly interesting and memorable people who had no difficulty getting under my skin and into my heart. I have yet to meet more than two or three social scientists who do not feel that most Papua New Guineans are industrious, linguistically diverse, culturally rich, modern, emotionally giving and good-tempered. That stands for coastal Daruans as for highland coffee-growers, Papuan settlement-dwellers no less than border crossers in Vanimo. This is not always the received picture here in the West, of course. Historical and social scientific research has distorted Papua New Guinea communities and customs in a variety of ways. Bias consists variously of ethnocentrism, of remaining traces of social evolutionary ranking of world cultures, of racism pure and simple, of mere incomprehension, of paternalism, of the results of linguistic incompetence–and the list goes on. I do not want to contribute to this, nor am I here to tell Papua New Guineans what to do.

Nevertheless, Papua New Guinea, just like the contemporary US, is riddled with sexual and other double standards that spawn and justify a level and kind of sexual violence that appears to be 'acceptable' to most people. There is now on the part of powers-that-be an undeniable interest in AIDS and maybe even in women's plight, and partly by the degree to which females in particular have internalised their own oppression. Women *not* in this or that local sex industry have appeared to me over the years to be just as heavily invested in the denigration of those who are as were males who more directly use them sexually or otherwise profit from their exploitation, although there seems to be positive change in that regard. Sisterhood is, if not fully global, at least fully globalising.

I'd like to close by making a few suggestions regarding some of the ideas we've broached here, about what is likely going to begin being registered very soon in terms of the clinical presentations of AIDS. As a social scientist I'm very respectful of the legacy of the tenets of germ theory, which have undoubtedly helped to reduce disease and suffering. Nevertheless, I think that on another level it has dampened our ability to think about disease causation (and its corollary, normal immune system function) in other ways. Because we think so much in terms of viruses, bacteria, fungi and protozoa, heads bent, microscopes focused, clinical trials 'controlled', placebos at the ready, we seek cures first in highly technical, often highly expensive experimentation and pharmaceutical intervention. We're the first to tout the awesome power of antibiotics, but among the last to raise the issue of resistance, at least not without a lot of prodding. If we recognise the cultural and the social-structural at all, in terms of disease causation, it is usually to invoke them as obstacles to this or that biomedical finding or public health promotion, for example, when patients don't 'comply', when they remain 'naïve' to therapy. I accept Mark Boyd's point in the previous chapter that that's not what medical doctors mean when they use that term, and yet that's now what naïve means in the dictionary and in common usage and that there might be something more there. My point as a social scientist is that such language use, whether calculated or not, conscious or not, both hides the source of medical power to begin with and redoubles it anew. More pathology ensues, for now the non-compliance must be dealt with and naiveté reined in. Why do they fail? How often do they fail? Why is their culture stubborn? Why don't their bodies get wise?

Again, I'm not denying that such 'magic bullets' as Paul Ehrlich proclaimed when he tested his 606th arsenical compound and found one that worked (for awhile) against spirochetes can be profound achievements. Nevertheless, when the cause of disease isn't quite so singular, stable and

One bright, crisp morning in 2004, my adoptive mother came to pick me up, as we had planned to visit her older cousin to discuss the upcoming coffee season. Crying upon arrival, she said that she had spent all night tending to our relative, who had passed away after spending the last six weeks of her life in total agony. Her husband had been displeased with her and one night had poured out the contents of a kerosene bottle onto her, lit a book of matches, and set her aflame. Now, he may or may not stay in the jail cell, but we know the Daru rapists won't. Her people may or may not find solace in a compensation payment, but we suspect the pregnant girl in Porgera won't see a single toea, and it's too late for the beheaded woman and woman set aflame.

minute, but rather, protean and ever shape-shifting, multi-factorial and synergistic – as clearly is 'AIDS' – then hearts, minds and wallets must be opened to new approaches. We've talked about how iatrogenic antiretrovirals can be on the corporeal, bodily level. I don't think that we've yet grasped to what extent is this sickness one that inheres not just in but also between bodies and between those bodies and the chemicals and techniques that are supposed to make them well. This is a first intended meaning of sexually transmitted *dis*-ease, which a number of social and political theorists have called attention to over the past couple of decades.

I mean the phrase also to refer to the highly gendered double-standards of kinship and marriage, of labor and production, of post-marital residence patterns and sociality, and of sexual identity and expression, as I've talked about in previous chapters. Rape, for example, is said conservatively to occur in PNG to the tune of about 45 per 100,000 persons (Zimmer-Tamakoshi 2004), which is one of the highest frequencies in the world. Yet and still, rape doesn't just *occur*, like flash floods or hot weather. Rape is committed by and happens amidst soldiers, priests, 'intimate partners', policemen, teachers, family friends, family members, strangers and politicians. Because they are reported (much less successfully prosecuted) to an infinitesimally small degree, they leave behind traces on and in, but more to the point, between bodies. 'That's their business', some say, 'he already paid the bride-price', say others, and 'it's her fault, not his', say yet others. Of a 15-year-old girl pack-raped on Daru by her fellow students, for example, two of the 'investigating' policemen whom I questioned about their less than vigorous approach replied: 'well, she's already had sex, anyway' (author's fieldnotes, Daru, 2003). A top government lawyer in PNG, meanwhile, was convicted (but whose appeal was successful) for possessing 'pornographic materials' that consisted of videotaped sexual activities between himself, his wife and another man (Anonymous 2005b). Carol Jenkins and colleagues found that in the *week* prior to their being interviewed by researchers, 10% of the policemen and 11% of the security guards had engaged in *lainap* sex or serial copulation, almost always without the consent of the woman (and never with the consent of the *girl*) in question (Jenkins 2000). Think of the rates they might have generated had they inquired of the previous *year*! Helen Epstein (2007) investigated the prominence in rural South Africa of what was called 'streamlining'; again, the root cause is men's punishment of women but in a homosocial way. All five members of a focus group interview I conducted in Lae with young women in prostitution told of policemen and/ or jail warders who had raped them or their best friends as a condition of their captivity and/or eventual release. One said that the police usually told them that (translated from the Tok Pisin) 'you're the ones who have done wrong, and now you've come inside the jail, inside the police station, and we're here and we're the ones who can release you. You're gonna have to give us your vaginas to go free' (author's field-notes, Lae, 30 April 2004). That's what I mean by the term in a second way.

If I can really stand up on my soapbox now, I'd say that to imagine non-microbial sexually transmitted *dis*-ease is, third, to attend to the embodied nature of genital and reproductive traumas, not just to the discharge, but also to the girl around it; not just to the penile sore, but to the cognitive outlook, too, that guided the man's preceding sexual activity; not just to the HIVab test result *per se*, but also to the fear and shame and stigma that follow in its wake and that may have prevented its occurrence until now. I think that too much attention is paid to the properties *in vivo* of this or that anti-retroviral, but just as Mark Boyd said in the previous chapter, not enough to their propensity also to reveal other bodily signs and symptoms, many of which become new reference points of stigma and discrimination, for example, the gluteal muscle wasting he mentioned. Women suffer vaginal discharges not just because their bodies were exposed to and became infected with the gonococcus, but also because they were beaten and abused by their so-called 'intimate partners'. Young girls get cervical cancers not just because they have been infected with HPV, but also because they have reached coitarche too soon and too often against their will – it means too often that their cervixes have been bludgeoned. If you don't believe me, ask any nurse, ask any family counsellor, ask any police-woman (and not a few policemen). This fact is neatly camouflaged by use of the term, 'sexual debut', as if there has occurred a ballyhooed Hollywood opening, implying a degree of agency in coitarcheal females (whether 8 or 12 or 16) that even some grown-up women don't have. Not just because their blood has antibodies to HIV in it, but because they are beaten, pimped out or raped by the ones who are supposed to love, cherish and protect them, some girls and women literally weep through and because of their sex in the form of cervical and vaginal tearing, dampened desires, depressed immune response, and vaginas that both don't express enough (in dryness) and that express too much (in the form of discharges). It would be ironic if it weren't so sad that sexual molestation and wife-beating is euphemised as 'domestic violence', as if violence is being done to a kitchen cabinet or an ideological construction.

Without vaginas, many women would simply not be allowed to live. Just as bodies incorporate signs of sickness in the form of sores, discharge, tears and cancers, so do communities surround bodies rendered ill by sorcery accusations, harmful contraceptive devices and unwanted pregnancies. In similar fashion, economic systems and political relations surround those sickened communities by way of resource extraction, warfare, systemic corruption and crippling debt structure. What I'm calling for is for both biomedical practitioners and social scientists to work together more closely and imagine disease causation more broadly and with the same degree of complexity as are most social relations and processes.

Although I neither deserve nor desire any special credit, I do wish to conclude by saying that I consider the contents of this book to represent my special responsibilities in the world, and I hope that it is not the last thing I'll ever say. I have tried my best to speak Truth as clearly as I can to Power and to have joined others who are trying to make the world safer for all, especially for its most vulnerable residents. Inattention to matters of social-structure and gender relations will doom any national response. So will inattention to the significant condom disinformation throughout the country. I hope that my analyses will enable health officials, politicians, policy-makers and ordinary citizens to recognise their special responsibilities in taking on-board more critical and self-reflexive approaches to what promises otherwise to be the mutual destruction of many Pacific island countries and cultures.

In the interest of furthering this important dialogue, I want to close with a passage from Barry Lopez's *Arctic Dreams*, so that my friends and colleagues in Papua New Guinea may intuitively understand and appreciate what they are up against:

> No culture has yet solved the dilemma each has faced with the growth of a conscious mind: how to live a moral and compassionate existence when one is fully aware of the blood, the horror inherent in all life, when one finds darkness not only in one's own culture but within oneself. If there is a stage at which an individual life becomes truly adult, it must be when one grasps the irony in its unfolding and accepts responsibility for a life lived in the midst of such paradox. (Lopez 1986: 413)

Bibliography

Abbott, T.K. 1962. 'Minute – Venereal Disease, Pt. Moresby, Oct. 4th'. N.A. Public Health Registry Files, Accession 23, Box 8599, File 15-18-1, 'Venereal Disease Control (Pt. 1), 1959–1970'.

Aderinto, S. 2006. 'Mines'. In M. Ditmore (ed.), *Encyclopedia of Prostitution and Sex Work*, pp. 315–7. Westport, Connecticut: Greenwood Press.

Adlersberg, J. 2006. 'Do Condoms Protect Against HPV?' Available on-line (accessed 6 August 2007) at: http://abclocal.go.com/wabc/story?section=health&id=4291805 .

Agenzia Fides. 2008. '"We need to keep the youth from contracting AIDS, not lead them into promiscuity": the Bishop of Vanimo shares his concerns with Agenzia Fides'. Available on-line (accessed 28 July) at: http://www.fides.org/aree/news/newsdet.php?idnews=16450&lan=eng .

Aggleton, P. 2007. '"Just a Snip"?: a social history of male circumcision'. *Reproductive Health Matters* 15(29): 15–21.

AIDWATCH. 2005. 'Boomerang AID: not good enough Minister'! Available on-line (accessed 6 August 2007) at: http://aidwatch.org.au/assets/aw00728/Boomerang%20aid%20final%20jun%2005.pdf .

Ali, S. 2006. 'Violence Against the Girl Child in the Pacific Islands Region'. Florence, Italy: UNICEF.

Allen, B. 1997. 'HIV/AIDS in Rural Melanesia and South-East Asia: divination or description?' In G. Linge and D. Porter (eds) *No Place for Borders: the HIV/AIDS epidemic and development in Asia and the Pacific*, pp. 114–23. New York: St. Martin's Press.

Allen, M. 1993[1984]. 'Homosexuality, Male Power, and Political Organization'. In G. Herdt (ed.) *Ritualized Homosexuality in Melanesia*, new, revised edition, pp. 83–126. Berkeley: University of California Press.

Allen, J. and P. Corris (eds). 1977. *The Journal of John Sweatman*. St. Lucia: University of Queensland Press.

Alpers, P. 2005. *Gun-Running in Papua New Guinea: from arrows to assault weapons in the Southern Highlands Province*. Special Publication 5. Geneva, Switzerland: Small Arms Survey.

AMFAR (American Federation of AIDS Research). 2005. 'The Effectiveness of Condoms in Preventing HIV Transmission'. Issue Policy Brief 1.

Amnesty International. 2006. *Papua New Guinea: Violence Against Women – Not Inevitable, Never Acceptable*.

Amstel, H. Van and S. van der Geest. 2004. 'Doctors and Retribution: the hospitalization of compensation claims in the highlands of Papua New Guinea'. *Social Science and Medicine* 59: 2089–94.

Anglican Board of Missions (ABM). 2005. 'For Goodness Sake!: Asia-Pacific faith-based organizations battle HIV/AIDS'. Available on-line (accessed 7 August 2007) at: http://www.hivpolicy.org/Library/HPP000987.pdf .

Anonymous. 2005a. 'Church Supports Condoms'. *Post-Courier*, 20 January.

Anonymous. 2005b. 'Top Lawyer in Porno Claims'. *The National*, 17 January.

Anonymous. 2006. 'HIV/AIDS Awareness Lags at Unis'. *Post-Courier*, 12 April.

Anti MSM. 2003. 'It is Moral to Discriminate'. *Post-Courier*, 22 September.

Arek, M. 2008. 'PNG Unlikely to Meet HIV/AIDS Goals: UN'. *The National*, 17 September.

Armstrong, W. 1996. 'Providing Sexual and Reproductive Health Services in a Developing Country: a challenge to a Eurocentric Model'. In M. Spongberg, J. Larbalestier and M. Winn (eds), *Women Sexuality Culture*, pp. 58–63. Sydney: University of Sydney Women's Studies Centre.

Arno, P. and K. Feiden. 1992. *Against the Odds: the story of AIDS drug development, politics and profits*. New York: HarperCollins.

Aruwafu-Buchanan, H. 2007. 'Youth Vulnerability to HIV in the Pacific'. In C. Jenkins and H. Aruwafu-Buchanan, *Cultures and Contexts Matter: understanding and preventing HIV in the Pacific*, pp. 71–130. Manila: Asian Development Bank.

Ashley-Montagu, M.F. 1937. 'The Origin of Subincision in Australia'. *Oceania* 8: 193–207.

—— 1968. 'Has Chastity a Chance in College?' In *Man Observed*, pp. 121–32. New York: G.P. Putnam's.

Asian Development Bank (ADB) 2006. 'HIV/AIDS Prevention and Control in Rural Development Enclaves Project'. Available on-line (accessed 7 August 2007) at: http://www.adb.org/Documents/Legal-Agreements/PNG/39033/39033-PNG-GRJ.pdf .

Australian Agency for International Development (AusAID). 2004. *Meeting the Challenge: Australia's International HIV/AIDS Strategy*. Canberra: Australian Agency for International Development.

—— 2005a. *Evaluation of the PNG National HIV/AIDS Support Project*. Evaluation and Review Series 38. Canberra: Australian Agency for International Development.

—— 2005b. *Evaluation of the PNG National HIV/AIDS Support Project, Appendices*. Evaluation and Review Series 38. Canberra: Australian Agency for International Development.

Australian Nursing Journal. 2007. 'PNG on Verge of AIDS Epidemic'. October, p. 16.

Baal, J. Van. 1966. *Dema*. The Hague: Martinus Nijhoff.

—— 1993[1984]. 'The Dialectics of Sex Among the Marind-anim'. In G. Herdt (ed.) *Ritualized Homosexuality in Melanesia*, new, revised edition, pp. 128–66. Berkeley: University of California Press.

Babona, D. and G. Nurse. 1988. 'HTLV-I Antibodies in Papua New Guinea'. *The Lancet* ii (8620): 1148.

Babona, D., G. Slama and E. Puiahi. 1996. 'Laboratory Diagnosis of HIV Infection in Papua New Guinea'. *Papua New Guinea Medical Journal* 39: 200–4.

Bailey, B. and D. Farber. 1992. *The First Strange Place: race and sex in WWII Hawaii*. New York: Free Press.

Ballard, J. and C. Malau. 2002. 'Policy-Making on AIDS in PNG to 2000'. Draft Paper for Workshop on Policy-Making in PNG, 1980–2000. Canberra and Port Moresby.

Barber, K. 2003. 'The Bugiau Community at Eight Mile: an urban community in Port Moresby, Papua New Guinea'. *Oceania* 73: 287–97.

Barham, A., M. Rowland and G. Hitchcock. 2004. 'Torres Straits Bepotaim: an overview of archaeological and ethnoarchaeological investigations and research'. *Memoirs of the Queensland Museum*, Cultural Heritage Series 3(1): 1–72.

Barnett Report, The. 1990. *A Summary of the Report of the Commission of Inquiry into Aspects of the Timber Industry in Papua New Guinea*. Hobart, Tasmania: Asia-Pacific Action Group.

Barter, P. 2007. 'Foreword' to 'The 2007 Estimation Report on the HIV Epidemic in Papua New Guinea'. Port Moresby: National AIDS Council.

Basedow, R. 1927. 'Subincision and Kindred Rites of the Australian Aboriginal'. *Journal of the Royal Anthropological Institute* 57: 123–56.

Beardmore, E. 1890. 'The Natives of Mowat, Daudai, New Guinea'. *Journal of the Royal Anthropological Institute of Great Britain and Ireland* 19: 459–68.

Bearman, P. and H. Brückner. 2001. 'Promising the Future: virginity pledges and first intercourse'. *American Journal of Sociology* 106 (4): 859–912.

Beaver, W. 1912. 'Western Division'. In *Annual Report for the Territory of Papua*, for the year ended June 30th. Port Moresby: National Archives.

—— 1920. *Unexplored New Guinea*. London: Seeley and Service.

Beer, B. 2008. 'Buying Betel and Selling Sex: contested boundaries, risk milieus, and discourses about HIV/AIDS in the Markham Valley, Papua New Guinea'. In L. Butt and R. Eves (eds) *Making Sense of AIDS: culture, sexuality, and power in Melanesia*, pp. 97–115. Honolulu: University of Hawai'i Press.

Bellamy, R.L. 1913. 'Special Report from Losuia, July 1st'. In *Annual Report for the Territory of Papua*, 1914. Port Moresby: National Archives.

Bennett, L. 2007. *Women, Islam and Modernity: single women, sexuality and reproductive health in contemporary Indonesia*. New York: Routledge.

Bennett, S. 2008. 'Condoms "Promote Sin" in Papua New Guinea as AIDS, Faith Cross'. Available on-line (accessed 22 August 2008) at: http://www.bloomberg.com/apps/news?pid=20601087&sid=acEj93SR3hsw&refer=home .

Benton, K.W. 2008. 'Saints and Sinners: training Papua New Guinean (PNG) Christian clergy to respond to HIV and AIDS using a model of care'. *Journal of Religion and Health*. Online First! Publication, no pagination available.

Berer, M. 2007a. Taking on the Opposition, Male Circumcision and Other Themes. *Reproductive Health Matters* 15(29): 6–8.

—— 2007b. 'Male Circumcision for HIV Prevention: perspectives on gender and sexuality'. *Reproductive Health Matters* 15(29): 45–8.

Berreman, G. 1962. *Behind Many Masks*. Ithaca: The Society for Applied Anthropology.

Berry, J. and G. Renner. 2004. *Vows of Silence: abuses of power in the papacy of John Paul II*. New York: Free Press.

Bettelheim, B. 1971[1954]. *Symbolic Wounds: puberty rites and the envious male*, new revised ed. New York: Collier Books.

Bevan, T. 1890. *Toil, Travel, and Discovery in British New Guinea*. London: Kegan Paul, Trench, Trubner, and Co.

Biehl, J. 2007. *Will to Live: AIDS therapies and the politics of survival*. Princeton: Princeton University Press.

Black, R.H. 1957. 'Dr Bellamy of Papua'. *Medical Journal of Australia* ii: 189 97, 232 8, 279–84.

Bladon, M. 1983. *Tidal Waves on the Bamu*. Bundeena, Australia: Mabel Anne Bladon Books and Tapes.

—— 1984. *The Song of the Bamu*. Sydney: Mabel Anne Bladon Books and Tapes.

Bleeker M.C., J. Berkhof, C.J. Hogewoning, F.J. Voorhorst, A.J. van den Brule, T.M. Starink, P.J. Snijders and C.J. Meijer. 2005. 'HPV Type Concordance in Sexual Couples Determines the Effect of Condoms on Regression of Flat Penile Lesions'. *British Journal of Cancer* 92(8): 1388–92.

Bonivento, C. 2001a. 'Do Condoms Stop or Spread AIDS?' Goroka: Family Life Apostolate.

—— 2001b. 'AIDS and Condoms: the teachings of the Church'. Vanimo: Pastoral Letter.

—— 2003. 'John Paul II and Oceania'. Available on-line (accessed 7 August 2007) at: http://www.fides.org/aree/news/newsdet.php?idnews=916&lan=eng .

—— 2005a. 'Dr. Mola is to Give Right Information'. *The National*, 14 February.

—— 2005b. 'Pastoral Letter Bilong Bishop Bilong Vanimo Long Laikim na Helpim Ol Bratasusa Bilong Mipela I sik long HIV-AIDS'.

—— 2006. 'Everyone Has a Right to Speak on Condoms'. *The National*, 17 January.

—— 2008. 'On the HIV/AIDS Awareness in the Schools'. Vanimo: Pastoral Letter.

Boone, P. 1997. *In a Heavy Metal Mood: no more Mr. Nice-Guy*. Hip-O Records. HIPD 40025.

Boone, S. 1972. *One Woman's Liberation*. Carol Stream, Illinois: Creation Press.

Borrey, A. 1992. *Ol Kalabus Meri: a study of female prisoners in Papua New Guinea*. Port Moresby: Papua New Guinea Law Reform Commission.

Borthwick, P. 1999. 'Developing Culturally Appropriate HIV/AIDS Education Programs in Northern Thailand'. In P. Jackson, N. Cook (eds), *Genders & Sexualities in Modern Thailand*, pp. 206–25. Chiang Mai, Thailand: Silkworm Books.

Bouten, M. 1996. 'Sex Education to Grade Seven Students in Papua New Guinea, Yes or No?' *Papua New Guinea Medical Journal* 39: 225–27.

Bowtell, B. 2007. 'HIV/AIDS: the looming Asia Pacific pandemic'. Policy Brief. Sydney: Lowy Institute for International Policy.

Boyd, M. 2007. 'Using HIV-Protease Inhibitors in Resource-Poor Settings'. PowerPoint presentation delivered to the Bangkok Symposium on HIV Medicine.

Boyd, M. and D. Cooper. 2007. 'Second-Line Combination Antiretroviral Therapy in Resource-Limited Settings: facing the challenges through clinical research'. *AIDS* 21 (Supplement 4): S55–S63.

Boyd, M., N. Dixit, U. Siangphoe, N. Buss, M. Salgo, J. Lange, P. Phanuphak, D. Cooper, A. Perelson and K. Ruxrungtham. 2006. 'Viral Decay Dynamics in HIV-Infected Patients Receiving Ritonavir-Boosted Saquinavir and Efavirenz With or Without Enfuvirtide: a randomized, controlled trial (HIV-NAT 012)'. *Journal of Infectious Diseases* 194: 1319–22.

Bradley, C. 1998. 'Changing a "Bad Old Tradition": wife-beating and the work of the Papua New Guinea Law Reform Commission'. In L. Zimmer-Tamakoshi (ed.) *Modern Papua New Guinea*, pp. 351–63. Kirksville, Missouri: Thomas Jefferson University Press.

—— 2000. 'Family and Sexual Violence in PNG: an integrated long term strategy'. Port Moresby: Institute of National Affairs.

Bradshaw, S. 2003. 'Vatican – condoms don't stop HIV'. BBC News. Available on-line (accessed 23 August 2007) at: http://news.bbc.co.uk/2/hi/programmes/panorama/3180236.stm .

Brown, D. 2006. 'Africa Gives "ABC" Mixed Grades: AIDS abstinence plan raises awareness but has small effect on behavior'. *Washington Post*, 15 August.

Brown, D., J. Edwards and R. Moore. 1988. *The Penis Inserts of Southeast Asia: an annotated bibliography with an overview and comparative perspectives*. Center for South and Southeast Asia Studies Occasional Paper 15. Berkeley: University of California.

Brückner, H. and P. Bearman. 2005. 'After the Promise: the STD consequences of adolescent virginity pledges'. *Journal of Adolescent Health* 36(4): 271–8.

Buchanan-Aruwafu, H. and R. Maebiru. 2008. 'Smoke From Fire: desire and secrecy in Auki, Solomon Islands'. In L. Butt and R. Eves (eds) *Making Sense of AIDS: culture, sexuality, and power in Melanesia*, pp. 168–86. Honolulu: University of Hawai'i Press.

Buhrich, E.N. 1983. 'The Association of Erotic Piercing with Homosexuality, Sadomasochism, Bondage, Fetishism, and Tattoos'. *Archives of Sexual Behavior* 12: 167–171.

BW (Bung Wantaim, a newsletter). 2008a. April.

—— 2008b. July.

—— 2008c. May.

Burchill, E. 1972. *Thursday Island Nurse*. Adelaide: Rigby.

Burslem, F., O. Laohapensang, J. Sauvarin, M. Young and A. Larson. 1998. 'Naked Wire and Naked Truths: reproductive health risks faced by teenage girls in Honiara, Solomon Islands'. *Pacific Health Dialog* 5(1): 8–15.

Butcher, B. 1964. *My Friends, the New Guinea Headhunters*. Garden City: Doubleday and Company.

Butcher, K. 2007. 'HIV Mainstreaming in Papua New Guinea, and its Role in Supporting Good Governance'. *Pacific Economic Bulletin* 22(1): 158–64.

Butt, L. 1998. *The Social and Political Lives of Infants*. Ph.D. dissertation. McGill University.

—— 1999. 'Medicine, Morality and the Politics of "Normal" Infant Growth'. *Journal of Medical Humanities* 20(2): 81–100.

—— 2002. 'The Suffering Stranger: medical anthropology and international morality'. *Medical Anthropology* 21(1): 1–24.

—— 2005. '"Lipstick Girls" and "Fallen Women": AIDS and conspiratorial thinking in Papua, Indonesia. *Cultural Anthropology* 20(3): 412–42.

—— 2008. 'Silence Speaks Volumes: elite responses to AIDS in Highlands Papua'. In L. Butt and R. Eves (eds) *Making Sense of AIDS: culture, sexuality, and power in Melanesia*, pp. 116–32. Honolulu: University of Hawai'i Press.

Butt, L. and R. Eves (eds). 2008. *Making Sense of AIDS: culture, sexuality, and power in Melanesia*. Honolulu: University of Hawai'i Press.

Butt, L. and J. Munro. 2007. 'Rebel Girls?: unplanned pregnancy and colonialism in highlands Papua, Indonesia'. *Culture, Health & Sexuality* 9(6): 585–98.

Butt, L., J. Munro and J. Wong. 2004. 'Border Testimonials: patterns of AIDS awareness across the island of New Guinea'. *Papua New Guinea Medical Journal* 47 (1–2): 65–76.

Butt, L., G. Numbery and J. Morin. 2002a. 'The Smokescreen of Culture: AIDS and the indigenous in Papua, Indonesia'. *Pacific Health Dialog* 9(2): 283–9.

—— 2002b. *Preventing AIDS in Papua: revised research report*.

Bynum, C. 1987. *Holy Feast and Holy Fast: the religious significance of food to medieval women*. Berkeley: University of California Press.

Caldwell, J. 2000. 'AIDS in Melanesia', Special AusAID Seminar: 'It's Everyone's Problem: HIV/AIDS and Development in Asia and the Pacific'. Canberra: Australian Agency for International Development.

Caldwell, J. and G. Isaac-Toua. 2002. 'AIDS in Papua New Guinea: situation in the Pacific'. *Journal of Health, Population, and Nutrition* 20(2): 104–11.

Caldwell, M. 1994. 'Blessed With Resistance'. *Discover*, January.

Callinan, R. 2004. 'A Price Too High To Pay'. *The Weekend Australian Magazine*, 9–10 October: 18–9, 21.

Calov, W.L. and M.B. Webb. 1925. 'Gonorrhoea in Natives of New Guinea: a record of twelve months' work in a venereal disease campaign in Rabaul'. *Medical Journal of Australia* ii: 720–4.

Cameron, E. 2005. *Witness to AIDS*. I.B. Taurin. New York: Palgrave/McMillan.

Carey, R.F. 1994. 'Letter in response to "Condom safety and HIV"'. *Sexually Transmitted Disease* 21: 60.

Carey, R.F., W.A. Herman, S.M. Retta, J.E. Rinaldi, B.A. Herman and T.W. Athey. 1992. 'Effectiveness of Latex Condoms as a Barrier to Human Immunodeficiency Virus-sized Particles Under Conditions of Simulated Use'. *Sexually Transmitted Diseases* 19: 230–4.

Carney, M. 2006. 'Sick No Good'. ABC Four Corners. Available on-line (accessed 7 August 2007) at: http://www.abc.net.au/4corners/content/2006/s1711584. htm .

Carpenter, L.M., A. Kamali, A. Ruberantwari, S.S. Malamba and J.A. Whitworth. 1999. 'Rates of HIV-1 Transmission Within Marriage in Rural Uganda in Relation to the HIV Sero- Status of the Partners'. *AIDS* 13(9): 1083–9.

Casey, S. 2007. 'Papua New Guinea - epicenter of HIV in the Asian Pacific region'. Available on-line (7 August 2007) at: on-line at: http://www.afao.org.au/ view_articles.asp?pxa=ve&pxs=103&pxsc= 27&pxsgc=138&id=607 .

Cassell, J. 1991. *Expected Miracles: surgeons at work*. Philadelphia: Temple University Press.

Cawte, J. 1978. 'Gross Stress in Small Islands: a study in macropsychiatry'. In C. Laughlin and I. Brady (eds), *Extinction and Survival in Human Populations*, pp. 95–121. New York: Columbia University Press.

Center for International Economics (CIE). 2002. *Potential Impacts of an HIV/AIDS Epidemic in PNG*. Canberra: Australian Agency for International Development.

Centers for Disease Control (CDC). 1990. 'Catholic Bishop Says Condom Distribution Helps Spread AIDS'. *AIDS Weekly*. 5 November, p. 11.

Chappell, D. 1992. 'Shipboard Relations Between Pacific Islander Women and Euroamerican Men, 1767–1887'. *Journal of Pacific History* 27(2): 131–49.

Chung, M. 2000. 'Summary of Research Findings on Adolescent Sexuality & Men's Attitudes to Family Planning in Pacific Island Countries'. Suva: Secretariat of the Pacific Community.

Clark, J. 1991. 'Pearlshell Symbolism in Highlands Papua New Guinea, with Particular Reference to the Wiru People of Southern Highlands Province'. *Oceania* 61: 309–39.

—— 1997. 'State of Desire: transformations in Huli sexuality'. In L. Manderson and M. Jolly (eds) *Sites of Desire/Economies of Pleasure: sexualities in Asia and the Pacific*, pp. 191–211. Chicago: University of Chicago Press.

Clark, J. and J. Hughes. 1995. 'A History of Gender and Sexuality in Tari'. In A. Biersack (ed.) *Papuan Borderlands*, pp. 315–40. Ann Arbor: University of Michigan Press.

Clune, F. 1943. *Prowling Through Papua*. London: Angus and Robertson.

Coates, T., O. Grinstead, S. Gregorich, D. Heilbron, W. Wolf, K-H. Choi, J. Schacter, P. Scheirer and A. van der Straten. 2000. 'The Voluntary HIV-1 Counseling and Testing Efficacy Study: a randomized controlled trial in three developing countries'. *Science to Community*. Prevention 1. Available on-line (accessed 30 July 2007) at: http://caps.ucsf.edu/pubs/reports/pdf/VCTS2C.pdf .

Cohen, J. 2005. 'ABC in Uganda: success or subterfuge'. *HIV/AIDS Policy and Law Review* 10(2): 23–4.

Cohen, S. 2004. 'Beyond Slogans: lessons from Uganda's experience with ABC and HIV/AIDS'. *Reproductive Health Matters* 12(23): 132–5.

—— 2007. 'Promoting the "B" in "ABC": its value and limitations in fostering reproductive Health'. *The Guttmacher Report on Public Policy* 7(4): 11–3.

Conant, M.A., D.W. Spicer and C.D. Smith. 1984. 'Herpes Simplex Virus Transmission: condom studies'. *Sexually Transmitted Diseases* 11: 94–5.

Copeland, B. 2007. 'AIDS Holistics'. Available on-line (accessed 30 July 2007) at: http://www.geocities.com/aids_holisticspng/ .

Courier, The. 2001. 'Finding the Right Approach'. September–October: 52–3.

Couriermail. 2007. 'Drug Bust Could Unravel Pacific Ring'. Available on-line (accessed 9 October 2007) at: http://www.news.com.au/couriermail/story/0,23739,22210508-5003402,00.html .

Crawford, A.L. 1981. *Aida: life and ceremony of the Gogodala*. Bathhurst: The National Cultural Council of Papua New Guinea, in association with Robert Brown and Associates.

Crittenden, S. 2006. 'Catholics and Condoms'. *The Religion Report*, 3 May.

Crockett, S. 2000. 'The Future State and Predictions of HIV/AIDS in Papua New Guinea'. *Pacific AIDS Alert Bulletin* 20: 12–5.

Cronau, P. 2006. 'Catastrophe on Our Doorstep'. Available on-line (accessed 30 July 2007) at: http://www.eurekastreet.com.au/article.aspx?aeid=1826 .

Cullen, T. 2000. *HIV/AIDS Press Coverage in the South Pacific*. Ph.D. Thesis. Department of Journalism, University of Queensland.

—— 2003a. 'Press Coverage of HIV/AIDS in the South Pacific: short-term view of a long-term problem'. *Pacific Journalism Review* 9(1): 139–48.

—— 2003b. 'HIV/AIDS: 20 years of press coverage'. *Australian Studies in Journalism* 12: 64–82.

—— 2006. 'HIV/AIDS in Papua New Guinea: a reality check'. *Pacific Journalism Review* 12(1): 153–65.

Cummings, M. 2008. 'The Trouble With Trousers: gossip, *kastom* and sexual culture in Vanuatu'. In L. Butt and R. Eves (eds) *Making Sense of AIDS: culture, sexuality, and power in Melanesia*, pp. 133–49. Honolulu: University of Hawai'i Press.

Currie, B., S. Naraqi, D. Babona, T. Pyakalyia, S. Webb and W. Maskill. 1988. 'Human Immunodeficiency Virus Infection in Papua New Guinea'. *The Medical Journal of Australia* 148: 100–1.

—— 1989. 'Acquired Immunodeficiency Syndrome in Papua New Guinea'. *The Medical Journal of Australia* 150: 541.

Curry, C., P. Bunungan, C. Annerud and D. Babona. 2005. 'HIV Antibody Seroprevalence in the Emergency Department at Port Moresby General Hospital, Papua New Guinea'. *Emergency Medicine Australasia* 17: 359–62.

Daia-Bore, J. 2006. 'Send Parents of Girl to Jail: WIP leader'. *The National*, 31 March.

Darius, M. 2004. 'Women, Young Girls Helpless Against Virus'. *The National*, 2 December.

Dateline. 2001. 'Dateline'. SBS TV Programme, aired on 2 May 2001. Available on-line (accessed 7 August 2007) at: http://www.pomcci.org.pg/SBSTV2001.html .

Dawson, J., R. Fitzpatrick, J. McLean, G. Hart and M. Boulton. 1991. 'The HIV Test and Sexual Behavior in a Sample of Homosexually Active Men'. *Social Science and Medicine* 32(6): 683–8.

Department for Community Development. 2004. Progress Report on the Status of Implementation of the East Asia Pacific (EAP) Regional Commitment and Action Plan Against Commercial Sexual Exploitation of Children (CSEC). Port Moresby.

Department of Education. 2006a. *HIV & AIDS and Reproductive Health: lecturer's guide*. Port Moresby: Department of Education.

—— 2006b. *HIV & AIDS and Reproductive Health: student teacher course book*. Port Moresby: Department of Education.

Deschamps, M-M., J.W. Pape, A. Hafner and W.D. Johnson. 1996. 'Heterosexual Transmission of HIV in Haiti'. *Annals of Internal Medicine* 125: 324–30.

Diamond, M. 1990. 'Selected Cross-Generational Sexual Behavior in Traditional Hawai'i: a sexological ethnography'. In J.R. Feierman (ed.) *Pedophilia: biosocial dimensions*, pp. 422–43. New York: Springer-Verlag.

Dilger, H. 2007. 'Healing the Wounds of Modernity: salvation, community and care in a neo-Pentecostal church in Dar Es Salaam, Tanzania'. *Journal of Religion in Africa* 37: 59–83.

Ditmore, M. (ed.). 2006. *Encyclopedia of Prostitution and Sex Work*, in two volumes. Westport, Connecticut: Greenwood Press.

Donald, A. 2007. 'AIDS Epidemic Threatens Papua New Guinea'. Available on-line (accessed on 21 September 2007) at: http://www.pinknews.co.uk/news/competitions/2005-5289.html .

Donaldson, B. 2003. 'Usage of Queensland Health Torres Strait Primary Health Care Facilities in the Torres Strait Treaty Area by Papua New Guinea Nationals'. Unpublished Report. Thursday Island: Thursday Island Hospital, Queensland Health.

Dore, G., J. Kaldor, K. Ungchusak and T. Mertens. 1996. 'Epidemiology of HIV and AIDS in the Asia-Pacific Region'. *Medical Journal of Australia* 165: 494–8.

Dorney, S. 2005. 'Papua New Guinea – What Can Australia Do (successfully)?'. Australian Security in the 21st Century Seminar Series. Radio Australia, 3 November.

Dowsett, G. and M. Couch. 2007. 'Male Circumcision and HIV Prevention: is there really enough of the right kind of evidence?' *Reproductive Health Matters* 15(29): 33–44.

Draus, P., H. Siegal, R. Carlson, R. Falck and J. Wang. 2005. 'Cracking the Cornfields: recruiting illicit stimulant drug users in Rural Ohio'. *The Sociological Quarterly* 46: 165–89).

Drysdale, R. 2007. 'In the Face of Gender Inequality, Married Women are Among Most Vulnerable to HIV'. Press Release posted to AIDSTOK, 26 August.

Dufour, P. [Paul Lecroix] 1926. *History of Prostitution, Volume Three: "The Christian Era."* Chicago: Pascal Covici.

Duncombe, C., S.J. Kerr, K. Ruxrungtham, G.J. Dore, M.G. Law, S. Emery, J.P. Lange, D.A. Cooper and P. Phanuphak. 2005. 'HIV Disease Progression: a patient cohort treated via a clinical research network in a resource limited setting'. *AIDS* 19(2): 169–78.

Dundon, A. 2002. 'Mining and Monsters: a dialogue on development in Western Province, Papua New Guinea'. *The Australian Journal of Anthropology* 13(2): 139–54.

—— 2007. 'Warrior Women, the Holy Spirit and HIV/AIDS in Rural Papua New Guinea'. *Oceania* 77(1): 29–42.

Dundon, A. and C. Wilde. 2007. 'Introduction: HIV and AIDS in rural Papua New Guinea'. *Oceania* 77(1): 1–11.

Dureau, C. 2001. 'Mutual Goals: Family Planning on Simbo, Solomon Islands'. In M. Jolly and K. Ram (eds), *Borders of Being: citizenship, fertility, and sexuality in Asia and the Pacific*, pp. 232–261. Ann Arbor: University of Michigan Press.

Economic and Social Commission for Asia and the Pacific (ESCAP). 2005. 'Gender and HIV/AIDS in the Asia and Pacific Region'. Gender and Development Discussion Paper 18. United Nations.

Economist, The. 2006. 'Asia: help thy neighbour; Australia and AIDS'. 379(8471): 56.

Edgerton, R. 1992. *Sick Societies: challenging the myth of primitive harmony*. New York: Free Press.

Edwards, J.H.D. 1964. 'Foreword' to Mabel Anne Bladon, *Song of the Bamu*, pp. iii. Lawson, N.S.W.: Mission Publications of Australia.

Elias, I., J. Gillett, B. Karlin, T. Pyakalyia and D. Turner. 1990. 'Sexually Transmitted Diseases in PNG'. *Point* 14: 179–90.

Epigee Women's Health (EWH). 2007. 'Safe Sex vs. Safer Sex'. Available on-line (accessed 7 August 2007) at: http://www.epigee.org/guide/risks.html .

Epstein, H. 2005. 'The Lost Children of AIDS'. *New York Review of Books*, 3 November.
—— 2007. *The Invisible Cure: Africa, the West and the fight against AIDS*. New York: Farrar, Strauss & Giroux.
Eric. 2005. 'Make Condoms an Illegal Product'. *Post-Courier*, 26 January.
Ernst, T. 1978. 'Myth, Ritual, and Population Among the Marind-anim'. *Social Analysis* 1: 34–53.
Errington, F. 1974. *Karavar: masks and power in a Melanesian ritual*. Ithaca: Cornell University Press.
Esso Highlands Limited (EHL). 2005. 'Sociocultural Impacts and Mitigation Measures'. PNG Gas Project and Environmental Impact Statement, Chapter 15.
Etkin, N. 1992. 'Side Effects': cultural constructions and reinterpretations of Western pharmaceuticals. Medical Anthropology Quarterly 6(2): 99–113.
Eves, R. 2003a. 'AIDS and Apocalypticism: interpretations of the epidemic from Papua New Guinea'. *Culture, Health & Sexuality* 5(3): 249–64.
—— 2003b. 'Mayhem and the Beast: narratives of the world's end from New Ireland (Papua New Guinea)'. *Journal of the Royal Anthropological Institute* 9: 527–47.
—— 2008. 'Moral Reform and Miraculous Cures: Christian healing and AIDS in New Ireland, Papua New Guinea'. In L. Butt and R. Eves (eds) *Making Sense of AIDS: culture, power, and sexuality in Melanesia*, pp. 206–23. Honolulu: University of Hawai'i Press.
Eves, R. and L. Butt. 2008. 'Introduction: making sense of AIDS'. In L. Butt and R. Eves (eds) *Making Sense of AIDS: culture, power, and sexuality in Melanesia*, pp. 29–69. Honolulu: University of Hawai'i Press.
Fabrega, H. and D. Silver. 1973. *Illness and Shamanistic Curing in Zinacantan: an ethnomedical analysis*. Stanford: Stanford University Press.
Fadiman, A. 1998. *The Spirit Catches You and You Fall Down*. New York: Farrar, Strauss & Giroux.
Fanon, F. 1967. *Black Skins, White Masks*, translated by Charles Lam Markmann. New York: Grove Press.
Farmer, E. 1996. 'AIDS and the Community'. *Papua New Guinea Medical Journal* 39: 214–7.
Farmer, P. 2004. 'An Anthropology of Structural Violence'. *Current Anthropology* 45(3): 305–25.
Festinger, L., H. Riecken and S. Schacter. 1956. *When Prophecy Fails: a social and psychological study of a modern group that predicted the destruction of the world*. New York: Harper Torchbooks.
FHI (Family Health International). 2007. *IMPACT: Implementing AIDS Prevention and Care Project, Final Report*. Arlington, Virginia: FHI.
Fink, S. 2006. 'Papua New Guinea: no escaping the virus'. Available on-line (accessed 7 August 2007) at: http://www.pbs.org/frontlineworld/blog/2006/06/papua_new_guine.html .
Fiti-Sinclair, R. 1996, 'Female Prostitutes in Port Moresby, Papua New Guinea: STDs & HIV/AIDS knowledge, attitudes, beliefs and practices'. In M. Spongberg, J. Larbalestier and M. Winn (eds) *Women Sexuality Culture*, pp. 116–23. Sydney: University of Sydney Women's Studies Centre.
Fitzpatrick R, G. Hart, M. Boulton J. McLean and J. Dawson. 1989. 'Heterosexual Sexual Behaviour in a Sample of Homosexually Active Men'. *Genitourinary Medicine* 65: 259–262.
Flaws, B. 2006. 'The Church in Papua New Guinea: a blessing or a curse?' Available on-line (accessed 7 August 2007) at: http://www.dev-zone.org/downloads/jc6bonnie.pdf .
Flint, L.A. 1919. 'Muguru at Torobina, Bamu River'. *Man* 19: 38–9.

Fordham, G. 2005. *A New Look at Thai Aids: perspectives from the margin*. New York: Berghahn Books.

Fowke, J. 2006. 'Getting it Wrong in Papua New Guinea'. *Quadrant* 50(12): 28–31.

Fox, P. 2006. 'A Condom Might Save Another Life'. *The National*, 10 January.

Frank, D. and T. Duke. 2000. 'Congenital Syphilis at Goroka Base Hospital'. *Papua New Guinea Medical Journal* 43(1–2): 121–6.

Franklin, K. 2006. 'The HIV/AIDS Situation in PNG'. Media Release. Wycliffe Australia.

Frontline. 2005. 'Interview: Randall Tobias'. Available on-line (accessed on 24 September 2007) at: http://www.pbs.org/wgbh/pages/frontline/aids/interviews/tobias.html .

Gamson, J. 1990. 'Rubber Wars: struggles over the condom in the United States'. *Journal of the History of Sexuality* 1: 262–82.

Gare, J. T. Lupiwa, D. Suarkia, M. Paniu, A. Wahasoka, H. Nivia, J. Kono, W. Yeka, J. Reeder and C. Mgone. 2005. 'High Prevalence of Sexually Transmitted Infections Among Female Sex Workers in the Eastern Highlands Province of Papua New Guinea'. *Sexually Transmitted Diseases* 32(8): 466–73.

Garg, S., P. Bhalla, N. Sharma, R. Sahay, A. Puri, R. Saha, P. Sodhani, N. Murthy and M. Mehra. 2001. 'Comparison of Self-reported Symptoms of Gynaecological Morbidity with Clinical and Laboratory Diagnosis in a New Delhi Slum'. *Asia-Pacific Population Journal* 16(2): 75–92.

Gauri, V and E. Lieberman. 2006. 'Boundary Institutions and HIV/AIDS Policy in Brazil and South Africa'. *Studies in Comparative International Development* 41(3): 47–73.

Gege, A. 2003. 'Current Situation of HIV/AIDS in Papua New Guinea and its Implications'. Presented at the Women in Mining Conference, 3–6 August.

Gellner, E. 1986. 'Original Sin'. *Times Higher Education Supplement*. 10 October, p. 13.

Gerawa, M. 2003. 'Papua New Guinea: AIDS "reporting" to see increase'. *Post-Courier*, 11 April.

—— 2005. 'Catholics Tackle HIV Issues'. *Post-Courier*, 15 February.

—— 2006. 'Commentary: PNG Is Diverse – Let It Be'. *Pacific Magazine*, 16 March. Available on-line (accessed 30 July 2007) at:http://www.pacificmagazine.net/news/2006/03/16/commentary-png-is-diverse--let-it-be .

—— 2008. 'Condom Talk Angers Church Pastors'. *Post-Courier*, 25 June.

Geyle, A. 1998. 'Bamu Patrol'. Originally published in *Una Voce*, p. 18. Available on-line (accessed 30 July 2007) at: http://www.pngaa.net/Articles/articles_bamu_patrol.htm .

Gibson, J. 2006. 'AIDS Alert for Promiscuous Pacific'. *Sydney Morning Herald*, 11 July.

Gill, I. 2007. 'New Condom Campaign to Combat HIV/AIDS'. Asian Development Bank.

Glick, L. 1977 [1967] 'Medicine as an Ethnographic Category: the Gimi of the New Guinea Highlands'. In D. Landy (ed.) *Culture, Disease, and Healing: studies in medical anthropology*, pp. 58–70. New York: Macmillan.

Goinau, W. 1995. 'The Impact of Wawoi Guavi Logging in the Bamu Area of The Western Province'. The Department of Anthropology and Sociology, Social Work Programme. Port Moresby: University of Papua New Guinea.

Goldman, E. 1970[1917]. *The Traffic in Women, and other essays*, A.K. Shulman (ed.). New York: Times Change Press.

Goldman, R. and S. Papson. 1993. *Sign Wars: the cluttered landscape of advertising*. New York: The Guilford Press.

Government of Papua New Guinea. (GoPNG). 1998. 'National HIV/AIDS Medium Term Plan, 1998–2002'. Port Moresby.

—— 2003. 'HIV/AIDS Management and Prevention Act 2003'.

—— 2006. 'First National Summit on HIV Prevention: Full Report and Recommendations, April'.

Green, E. and A. Ruark. 2008. 'AIDS and the Churches: getting the story right'. *First Things: the Journal of Religion, Culture and Public Life*. April, 22–26.

Greer, A. 2006. 'Papua New Guinea's HIV Crisis'. Available on-line (accessed 30 July 2007) at: http://www.wo-magazine.com/website/stories/hiv.html .

Gregg, J. 2003. *Virtually Virgins: sexual strategies and cervical cancer in Recife, Brazil.* Stanford: Stanford University Press.

Gregory, C. 1982. *Gifts and Commodities*. New York: Academic Press.

Griffin, J., H. Nelson and S. Firth. 1979. *Papua New Guinea: a political history*. Victoria: Heineman Education Australia.

Grimwade, G. 2004. 'Japanese Pearlers' Bathhouses, Thursday Island, Torres Strait'. *Memoirs of the Queensland Museum*, Cultural Heritage Series 3(1): 379–86.

Gross, M. & S. Manning. 2005. 'Time Runs Out on Pacific HIV/AIDS Crisis'. *Scoop*. Available on-line (accessed 30 July 2007) at: http://www.scoop.co.nz/stories/HL0506/S00001.htm .

Gumuno, J. 2008. 'AusAID Team Checks on Its HIV/AIDS Projects'. *The National*, 6 April.

Gunther, J. 1990. 'Post-War Medical Services in Papua New Guinea: a personal view'. In B.G. Burton-Bradley (ed.) *A History of Medicine in Papua New Guinea: vignettes from an earlier period*, pp. 47–76. Kingsgrove, New South Wales: Australasian Medical Publishing Company, Limited.

Guss, S. 2008. '"C" is Change in Attitude, Not Condom'. *The National*, 7 April.

Haddon, A.C. 1890. 'Ethnography of the Western Tribe of Torres Straits'. *Journal of the Royal Anthropological Institute* 19: 297–422.

—— 1914. 'The Outrigger Canoes of Torres Straits and North Queensland'. In E.C. Quiggin (ed.), *Essays and Studies Presented to William Ridgeway on his 60th Birthday, 6th August 1913*, pp. 609–34. Cambridge University Press: Cambridge.

—— 1920. *Migrations of Cultures in British New Guinea*. Huxley Memorial Lecture for 1920.

Haley, N. 2008. 'When There's No Accessing Basic Health Care: local politics and responses to HIV/AIDS at Lake Kopiago, Papua New Guinea'. L. Butt and R. Eves (eds) *Making Sense of AIDS: culture, sexuality, and power in Melanesia*, pp. 24–40. Honolulu: University of Hawai'i Press.

Hammar, L. n.d. 'From Gift to Commodity … and Back Again: form and fluidity of sexual networking in Papua New Guinea'. Forthcoming in V. Luker, S. Dinnen and A. Patience (eds) *Law, Order and HIV/AIDS in PNG*. Canberra: Australian National University.

—— 1989. 'Gender and Class on the Fringe: a feminist analysis of ethnographic theory and data in Papua New Guinea'. Working Paper 189 in the Michigan State University Series, Women in International Development, R. Gallin (ed.).

—— 1992. 'Sexual Transactions in Daru: with some observations on the ethnographic enterprise'. *Research in Melanesia* 16: 21–54.

—— 1993a. 'AIDS Issue in the Open'. *Research in Melanesia* 17: 187–8.

—— 1993b. 'AIDS Won't Discriminate'. *Research in Melanesia* 17: 189–90.

—— 1996a. 'Brothels, Bamu, and *Tu Kina Bus* in South Coast New Guinea: human rights issues and global responsibilities'. *Anthropology and Humanism* 21(2): 140–58.

—— 1996b. 'Bad Canoes and *Bafalo*: the political economy of sex on Daru island, Western Province, Papua New Guinea'. *Genders* 23: 212–43.

—— 1997. 'The Dark Side to Donovanosis: color and climate, race and racism in American South Venereology'. *Journal of Medical Humanities* 18(1): 29–58.

—— 1998a. 'AIDS, STDs, and Sex Work in Papua New Guinea'. In L. Zimmer-Tamakoshi (ed.) *Modern Papua New Guinea*, pp. 257–96. Kirksville, Missouri: Thomas Jefferson University Press.

—— 1998b. 'Music, Drugs, and Sex in the South Fly: a brief look at music styles, narcotics, and the sex industry on Daru Island, Western Province, Papua New Guinea'. In A. Kaeppler and J. Wainwright Love III (eds) *The Garland Encyclopedia of World Music*, Oceania volume, pp. 178–80. New York: Garland.

—— 1998c. 'Sex Industries and Sexual Networks: complicated risks and public health implications'. *Pacific Health Dialog* 5(3): 47–53.

—— 1999a. 'Caught Between Structure and Agency: gendered violence and prostitution in Papua New Guinea'. *Transforming Anthropology* 8(1–2): 77–96.

—— 1999b. 'To Be Young, Female and Normal: the health risks of absent sexual citizenship'. *Journal of Medical Humanities* 20(2): 133–52.

—— 2003. 'Confessions of a (Somewhat) Reluctant Consultant: or, what happens when academic dreams go "poof"'. *The Qualitative Report* 8(2): 286–305.

—— 2004a. 'Sexual Health, Sexual Networking, and Sexually Transmitted Disease in (Papua) New Guinea'. *Papua New Guinea Medical Journal* 47(1–2): 1–12.

—— 2004b. '4,275 and Counting: telling stories about sexually transmitted diseases on Daru island, Western Province'. *Papua New Guinea Medical Journal* 47(1–2): 88–113.

—— 2004c. 'Bodies and Methods in Motion'. *Practicing Anthropology* 26(4): 8–12.

—— 2006a. 'Incest'. In M. Ditmore (ed.) *Encyclopedia of Prostitution and Sex Work*, two volumes, pp. 224–5. Westport, Connecticut: Greenwood Press.

—— 2006b. '"It's in Every Corner Now": a nationwide study of HIV, AIDS and STDs'. Submitted to the NHASP, the Burnet Institute and to AusAID.

—— 2006c. 'Sex, Drugs and Rock and Roll: summary findings from Vanimo'. Submitted to the NHASP, the Burnet Institute and to AusAID.

—— 2007b. 'Epilogue: Homegrown in PNG – rural responses to HIV and AIDS'. *Oceania* 77(1): 72–94.

—— 2007c. 'The Many Sexes of Risk'. *Reviews in Anthropology* 36(4): 335–56.

—— 2008b. 'Fear and Loathing in Papua New Guinea: sexual behaviour and sexual health in a nation under siege'. In L. Butt and R. Eves (eds) *Making Sense of AIDS: culture, sexuality, and power in Melanesia*, pp. 60–79. Honolulu: University of Hawai'i Press.

Hammel, E. and D. Friou 1994. 'Anthropology and Demography: marriage, liaison or encounter'? Available on-line (accessed 30 July 2007) at: http://www.demog.berkeley.edu/~gene/brown.94.rev.2.html .

Hankins, C. 2007. 'Male Circumcision: implications for women as sexual partners and parents'. *Reproductive Health Matters* 15(29): 62–7.

Harder, B. 2005. 'Death Can Outdo ABCs of Prevention'. *Science News*, 167(11): 173.

Harrison, A. 2008. 'Hidden Love: sexual ideologies and relationship ideals among rural South African adolescents in the context of HIV/AIDS'. *Culture, Health & Sexuality* 10(2): 175–89.

Hart, C. 2007. 'PM Blasted Over HIV Comments'. *The Australian*, 14 April.

Hauck, V., A. Mandi-Filer and J. Bolger. 2005. 'Ringing the Church Bell: the role of churches in governance and public performances in Papua New Guinea'. Discussion Paper 57E. Canberra: Australian Agency for International Development.

Hayes, G. 2007. The Demographic Impact of the HIV/AIDS Epidemic in Papua New Guinea, 1990–2030. *Asia-Pacific Population Journal* 22(3): 11–30.

Heider, K. 1976a. 'Dani Sexuality: a low energy system'. *Man* 11:188–211.

—— 1976b. *Grand Valley Dani: peaceful warriors*. New York: Holt, Rinehart & Winston.

Help Resources. 2005. 'A Situational Analysis of Child Sexual Abuse & the Commercial Sexual Exploitation of Children in Papua New Guinea'. Draft manuscript.

Henry, J. 1965. *Pathways to Madness*. New York: Random House.

Herbert, T. 2007. 'Commercial Sexual Exploitation of Children in the Solomon Islands: a report focusing on the presence of the logging industry in a remote region'. The Solomon Islands: Christian Care Centre.

Herdt, G. (ed.). 1993a[1984]. *Ritualized Homosexuality in Melanesia*, new, revised edition. Berkeley: University of California Press.

—— 1993b[1984]. 'Introduction to the Paperback Edition'. In G. Herdt (ed.) *Ritualized Homosexuality in Melanesia*, new, revised edition, pp. vii–xliv. Berkeley: University of California Press.

Hermkens, A.-K. 2007. 'The Power of Mary in Papua New Guinea'. *Anthropology Today* 23(2): 4–8.

Hewat, S. 2008. 'Love as Sacrifice: the romantic underground and beliefs about HIV/ AIDS in Manokwari, Papua'. In L. Butt and R. Eves (eds) *Making Sense of AIDS: culture, sexuality, and power in Melanesia*, pp. 150–67. Honolulu: University of Hawai'i Press.

Hides, J. 1936. *Papuan Wonderland*. Glasgow: Blackie and Son.

Higgins, D.L., C. Galavotti, K.R. O'Reilly, D.J. Schnell, M. Moore, D.L. Rugg and R. Johnson. 1991. 'Evidence of the Effects of HIV Antibody Counseling and Testing on Risk Behaviors'. *Journal of the American Medical Association* 266(17): 2419–29.

Hilder, B. 1980. *The Voyage of Torres*. Brisbane: University of Queensland Press.

Hira, S.K., P.J. Feldblum, J. Kamanga, G. Mukelabai, S.S. Weir and J.C. Weir. 1997. 'Condom and Nonoxynol-9 Use and the Incidence of HIV infection in Serodiscordant Couples in Zambia'. *International Journal of STD & AIDS* 8(4): 243–50.

Hirsch, J. 2007. 'The Inevitability of Infidelity: sexual reputation, social geographies, and marital HIV risk in Rural Mexico'. *American Journal of Public Health* 97(6): 986–996.

Hirsch, J. and H. Wardlow (eds). 2006. *Modern Loves: the anthropology of romantic courtship and companionate marriage*. Ann Arbor: University of Michigan Press.

Hitchcock, G. 2004. *Wildlife is Our Gold: political ecology of the Torassi River Borderland, Southwestern New Guinea*. Ph.D. Dissertation. University of Queensland.

Hoffman, A. 2007. 'Diocese Settles Abuse Claims for $198M'. Available on-line (accessed on 7 September 2007) at: http://www.comcast.net/news/index.jsp?cat=GENERAL&fn=/2007/09/07/757978.html .

Hofman, R. 2007. 'A Positive Papua New Guinean Speaks Out Against Stigma'. *AIDSmeds & Poz*. Available on-line (accessed 22 August 2007) at: http://www.aidsmeds.com/articles/stigma_hiv_maura_2021_12665.shtml .

Hogbin, I. 1970. *The Island of Menstruating Men: religion in Wogeo, New Guinea*. Scranton, Pennsylvania: Chandler Publishing.

Holmes, J.H. 1924. *In Primitive New Guinea*. London: Seeley and Service.

Hooper, E. 1999. *The River: a journey to the source of HIV and AIDS*. Boston: Little, Brown.

Hotchin, P., P. Tapelu, V. Chetty, R. Hakwa and D. Phillips. 1996. 'Knowledge, Attitudes and Behaviour of Reinfected Patients – Suva STD clinic, Fiji 1994/5'. *Pacific Health Dialog* 2(2): 45–7.

Huang, J. S. Harrity, D. Lee, K. Becerra, R. Santos and W. C. Mathews. 2006. 'Body Image in Women with HIV: a cross-sectional evaluation'. *AIDS Research and Therapy* 3(17): 1–7.

Hughes, J. 1991. 'Impurity and Danger: the need for new barriers and bridges in the prevention of sexually-transmitted disease in the Tari Basin, Papua New Guinea'. *Health Transition Review* 1(2): 131–40.

—— 1997. 'A History of Sexually Transmitted Diseases in Papua New Guinea'. In M. Lewis, S. Bamber and M. Waugh (eds) *Sex, Disease, and Society: a comparative history of sexually transmitted diseases and HIV/AIDS in Asia and the Pacific*, pp. 231–48. Westport, Connecticut: Greenwood Press.

—— 2002. 'Sexually Transmitted Infections: a medical anthropological study from the Tari Research Unit 1990–1991'. *Papua New Guinea Medical Journal* 45(1–2): 128–33.

Hull, T. and M. Budiharsana. 2001a. 'Putting Men in the Picture: problems of male reproductive health in Southeast Asia'. IUSSP XXIV Congress, Salvador, Brazil, 18–24 August.

Hull, T. and M. Budiharsana. 2001b. 'Male Circumcision and Penis Enhancement in Southeast Asia: matters of pain and pleasure'. *Reproductive Health Matters* 9(18): 60–7.

Human Rights Watch (HRW). 2005. '"Making Their Own Rules": police abuses and HIV/AIDS'. Available on-line (accessed 7 August 2007) at: http://hrw.org/reports/2005/png0905/7.htm .

Ickovics, J.R., A.C. Morrill, S.E. Beren, U. Walsh and J. Rodin. 1994. 'Limited Effects of HIV Counseling and Testing for Women'. *Journal of the American Medical Association* 272(6): 443–8.

Inglis, A. 1974. *Not a White Woman Safe: sexual anxiety and politics in Port Moresby*. Canberra: Australian National University Press.

International HIV/AIDS Alliance (IHAA). 2006. 'Civil Society and the "Three Ones"'. Discussion Paper.

Iqbal, S., T. Ball, J. Kimani, P. Kiama, P. Thottingal, J. Embree, K. Fowke and F. Plummer. 2005. 'Elevated T Cell Counts and RANTES Expression in the Genital Mucosa of HIV-1–Resistant Kenyan Commercial Sex Workers'. *Journal of Infectious Diseases* 192: 728–38.

IRG (Independent Review Group). 2007. 'Independent Review Group on HIV/AIDS'. Authored by P. Aggleton, S. Bharat, A. Coutinho, R. Drew and S. Wignall. Used by permission of the first author.

Irumai, A., E. Bruce and J. Nonwo. 2004. 'Qualitative Assessment and Response Report on HIV/AIDS/STI Situation Among Sex Workers and Their Clients in Port Moresby, Papua New Guinea'. Unpublished report. Port Moresby: World Vision.

Islands Business International. 2006. 'No Deal on Condoms'. Available on-line (accessed 25 August 2007) at: http://www.islandsbusiness.com .

—— 2007. 'Poor Condom Usage in the Islands'. Available on-line (accessed 7 August 2007) at: http://www.islandsbusiness.com .

Ivarature, H. 1998. 'Introduction and Development of Family Planning in Tonga 1958–1990'. In D. Carr, N. Gunson and J. Terrell (eds) *Echoes of Pacific War*, pp. 99–109. Canberra: Target Oceania.

—— 2000. 'The Institutionalization and "Medicalization" of Family Planning in Tonga'. *Asia-Pacific Population Journal* 15(2): 35–52.

Jackson, R. 1976. 'An Introduction to the Urban Geography of Papua New Guinea'. University of Papua New Guinea, Department of Geography, Occasional Papers 13. Port Moresby: University of Papua New Guinea.

Jakarta Post, The. 2007a. 'Impact of High-Risk Sexual Behavior Knocks on the Doors of Nation's Families'. 5 May.

—— 2007b. 'Half in Indonesia's Remote Papua Province Unaware of HIV/AIDS'. 21 June.

Janzen, J. 1978. *The Quest for Therapy in Lower Zaire*. Berkeley: University of California Press.

Jenkins, C. 1996. 'Editorial: AIDS in Papua New Guinea'. *Papua New Guinea Medical Journal* 39(3): 164–5.

—— 1997. *Youth in Danger: AIDS and STDs among young people in Papua New Guinea*. Port Moresby: Papua New Guinea Institute of Medical Research and United Nations Population Fund.

—— 2000. 'Female Sex Worker HIV Prevention Projects: lessons learnt from Papua New Guinea, India and Bangladesh'. UNAIDS Case Study.

—— 2002. 'Situation Analysis of HIV/AIDS in Papua New Guinea'. Unpublished review.

—— 2004. 'HIV/AIDS and Culture: implications for policy'. In V. Rao and M. Walton (eds) *Culture and Public Action: a cross-disciplinary dialogue on development policy*, pp. 260–81. Stanford: Stanford University Press.

—— 2006. 'Male Sexuality and HIV: the case of male-to-male sex'. A background paper produced for Risks and Responsibilities: Male Sexual Health and HIV in Asia and the Pacific. International Consultation held in New Delhi, India, 23–6 September.

—— 2007. 'HIV/AIDS, Culture and Sexuality in Papua New Guinea'. In C. Jenkins and H. Buchanan-Aruwafu, *Cultures and Contexts Matter: understanding and preventing HIV in the Pacific*, pp. 1–69. Manila: Asian Development Bank.

Jenkins, R. 2001. 'Riddle Women'. *TAGLine* 8(9): 1–5.

Jenkins, C. and M. Alpers. 1996. 'Urbanization, Youth and Sexuality: insights for an AIDS campaign for youth in Papua New Guinea'. *Papua New Guinea Medical Journal* 39: 248–51.

Jenkins, C. and M. Passey. 1998. 'Papua New Guinea'. In T. Brown, R. Chan, D. Mugrditchian, B. Mulhall, D. Plummer, R. Sarda and W. Sittitrai (eds), *Sexually Transmitted Diseases in Asia and the Pacific*, pp. 230–54. Armidale: Venereology Publishing.

Jenkins, C. and K. Pataki-Schweitzer. 1993. 'Knowledge of AIDS in Papua New Guinea'. *Papua New Guinea Medical Journal* 36(3): 192–204.

Jiear, A.H. 1903. 'Annual Report 1902–03, Daru Western Division, British New Guinea, July 1st'. In *Annual Report of British New Guinea*, 1903, British New Guinea and Papua, Government Secretary, Files of Correspondence, Journals and Patrol Reports from Out-Stations. Commonwealth Record Series, Box 6522, Folder 181.

John, M. 2003. 'DPM: Gays promoting sex hatred'. *Post-Courier*, 28 August.

Joku, H. 2008. 'Sex Scandal'. *The National*, 7 April.

Jolly, M. 1997. 'From Point Venus to Bali Ha'i: eroticism and exoticism in representations of the Pacific'. In L. Manderson and M. Jolly (eds). *Sites of Desire/Economies of Pleasure*, pp. 99–122. Chicago: University of Chicago Press.

Jolly, M. and L. Manderson. 1997. 'Sites of Desire/Economies of Pleasure in Asia and the Pacific'. In L. Manderson and M. Jolly (eds) *Sites of Desire/Economies of Pleasure: sexualities in Asia and the Pacific*, pp. 1–26. Chicago: University of Chicago.

Jorgenson, D. 2006. 'Hinterland History: the Ok Tedi mine and its cultural consequences in Telefolmin'. *The Contemporary Pacific* 18(2): 233–63.

Kaitani, M. 2003. 'Young Men and Sexual Risk Behaviour in Fiji'. *Development Bulletin* 62: 188–208, 123–5.

Kaldor, J., P. Effler, R. Sarda, G. Petersen, D. Gertig and J. Narain. 1994. 'HIV and AIDS in Asia and the Pacific: an epidemiological overview'. *AIDS 1994* 8 (Supplement 1): S165–S172.

Kampen, J. van. 2006. 'The ABC Disaster'. *The Drum Beat* (345). Available on-line (accessed 7 August 2007) at: http://www.comminit.com/drum_beat_345. html .

Kanu, Z. 2008. 'HIV/AIDS Rate Very High in PNG'. *The National*, April14.

Karel, H. 1995. 'The Knowledge of AIDS in Morobe Province, Papua New Guinea'. *Pacific Health Dialog* 2(2): 20–4.

Katz, A. 2002. 'AIDS, Individual Behaviour and the Unexplained Remaining Variation'. *African Journal of AIDS Research* 1: 125–42.

Kaul, R., F. Plummer, J. Kimani, T. Dong, P. Kiama, T. Rostron, E. Njagi, K.S. MacDonald, J.J. Bwayo, A.J. McMichael and S.L. Rowland-Jones. 2000. 'HIV-1-Specific Mucosal CD8+Lymphocyte Responses in the Cervix of HIV-1-Resistant Prostitutes in Nairobi'. *Journal of Immunology* 164: 1602–11.

Keck, V. 2007. 'Knowledge, Morality and "Kastom": SikAIDS among young Yupno people, Finisterre Range, Papua New Guinea'. *Oceania* 77(1): 43–57.

Kelly, R. 1980. *Etoro Social Structure*. Ann Arbor: University of Michigan Press.

Kelo, Y. 2005. 'Skul Meri Kilim Em Yet ... Bikos famili pusim em long marit'. *Wantok*, Jenuari 20–6.

Kempf, W. 2002. 'The Politics of Incorporation: masculinity, spatiality and modernity among the Ngaing of Papua New Guinea'. *Oceania* 73(1): 56–77.

Kenyon, M. and J. Power. n.d. 'Family Planning in the Pacific Region: getting the basics right'. Australian Reproductive Health Alliance.

Kewa, C. 2003. 'Military Deemed as HIV High Risk'. *Post-Courier*, 5 September.

Kewande, J. 2008. 'Don't Preach on Condoms'. *Post-Courier*, 26 June.

Kidu, C. 2003. 'Last Say: action against violence'. *Post-Courier*, 18 September.

King, D. 1994. 'Interim Findings for 1994'. Ok-Fly Social Monitoring Project Report 8. Available on-line (accessed 30 July 2007) at: http://rspas.anu.edu. au/rmap/projects/Ok-Fly_social_monitoring/Ofsmp08-Burton1994- interim-findings-1994.pdf .

Kippax, S. 2006. 'A Public Health Dilemma: a testing question'. *AIDS Care* 18(3): 230–5.

Kirsch, S. 2001. 'Lost Worlds: environmental disaster, "culture loss" and the law'. *Current Anthropology* 42(2): 167–98.

——— 2006. *Reverse Anthropology: indigenous analysis of social and environmental relations in New Guinea*. Stanford: Stanford University Press.

Kish, L.S., J.T. McMahon and W.F. Bergfeld. 1983. 'An Ancient Method and a Modern Scourge: the condom as a barrier against herpes (Letter)'. *Journal of the American Academy of Dermatologists* 9: 769–70.

Kituai, A.I.K. 1998. *My Gun, My Brother: the world of the Papua New Guinea colonial police, 1920–1960*. Honolulu: University of Hawai'i Press.

Kleinman, A. 1995. *Writing at the Margin*. Berkeley: University of California Press.

Knauft, B. 1990. 'The Question of Homosexuality Among the Kiwai of South New Guinea'. *Journal of Pacific History* 25: 188–210.

——— 1993. *South Coast New Guinea Cultures: history, comparison, dialectic*. Cambridge: Cambridge University Press.

——— 1994. 'Foucault Meets South New Guinea: knowledge, power, sexuality'. *Ethos* 22(4): 391–438.

——— 2003. 'What Ever Happened to Ritualized Homosexuality?: modern sexual subjects in Melanesia and elsewhere'. *Annual Review of Sex Research* 14:137–59.

Koczberski, G. 2000. 'The Sociocultural and Economic Context of HIV/AIDS in Papua New Guinea'. *Development Bulletin* 52: 61–3.

Krakauer, J. 2003. *Under the Banner of Heaven: a story of violent faith*. New York: Doubleday.

Kramer, P. 1993. *Listening to Prozac*. New York: Penguin.

Kramer, P.B. 1995. 'Knowledge About AIDS and Follow-up Compliance in Patients Attending a Sexually Transmitted Disease Clinic in the Highlands of Papua New Guinea'. *Papua New Guinea Medical Journal* 38(3): 178–90.

Kroeger, K. 2003. 'AIDS Rumors, Imaginary Enemies, and the Body Politic in Indonesia'. *American Ethnologist* 30(2): 243–57.

Laade, W. 1971. *Oral Traditions and Written Documents on the History and Ethnography of the Northern Torres Strait Islands, Saibai-Dauan-Boigu*, Volume 1. Wiesbaden: Franz Steiner Verlag GMBH.

Lafitani, S. 1998. 'New Behaviours and Migration Since WWII'. In D. Carr, N. Gunson and J. Terrell (eds) *Echoes of Pacific War*, pp. 76–86. Canberra: Target Oceania.

Landtman, G. 1927. *The Kiwai Papuans of British New Guinea*. London: Macmillan and Co.

—— 1917 *The Folk-tales of the Kiwai Papuans*. Helsingfors: Acta Societatis Scientiarum Fennicae.

—— 1954 'Initiation Ceremonies of the Kiwai Papuans'. In M. Mead and N. Calas (eds), *Primitive Heritage*, pp. 179–86. New York: Random House.

Langmore, D. 1989. *Missionary Lives: Papua, 1874–1914*. Honolulu: University of Hawai'i Press.

Langness, L.L. 1969. 'Marriage Among the Bena Bena'. In R. Glasse and M. Meggitt (eds), *Pigs, Pearlshells and Women: marriage in the New Guinea highlands*, pp. 38–55. Englewood Cliffs, New Jersey: Prentice-Hall.

Lattas, A. 1996. 'Humanitarianism and Australian Nationalism in Colonial Papua: Hubert Murray and the project of caring for the self of the coloniser and colonised'. *The Australian Journal of Anthropology* 7: 141–64.

Lavu, E., N. Kutson, C. Connie, G. Tau and P. Sims. 2004. 'Total Lymphocyte Counts in Adult HIV/AIDS Patients in Port Moresby General Hospital'. *Papua New Guinea Medical Journal* 47(1–2): 31–8.

Lawrence, D. 1989a. *The Material Culture of Customary Exchange in the Torres Strait and Fly Estuary Region*. Ph.D. Thesis. James Cook University.

—— 1989b. 'From the Other Side: recently collected oral evidence of contacts between the Torres Strait Islanders and the Papua peoples of the southwestern coast'. *Aboriginal History* 13(2): 95–123.

—— 1990a. '"Canoe Traffic" of the Torres Strait and Fly Estuary'. In J. Siikala (ed.) *Culture and History in the Pacific*, pp. 184–201. Helsinki: Suomen Anthropologinen Seura.

—— 1990b. 'Sustainable Development for Traditional Inhabitants of the Torres Strait Region: the Torres Strait Baseline Study'. Sustainable Development for Traditional Inhabitants of the Torres Strait Region. Workshop Series 16. D. Lawrence and T. Cansfield-Smith (eds), pp. 481–92. Cairns: Great Barrier Reef Marine Park Authority.

—— 1991. 'Re-evaluating Interpretations of Customary Exchange in the Torres Strait'. *Australian Aboriginal Studies* (2): 2–12.

—— 1994. 'Customary Exchange Across Torres Strait'. *Memoirs of the Queensland Museum* 34(2): 214–446.

—— 1995. '"You Can't Buy Another Life From a Store": Lower Fly Area Study'. Ok-Fly Social Monitoring Programme Report No. 9. National Capital District: Unisearch PNG Party Ltd.

—— 1998. 'Customary Exchange in the Torres Strait'. *Australian Aboriginal Studies* 2: 13–25.

Layard, J. 1942. *Stone Men of Malekula*. London: Chatto and Windus.

Leach, T., S.L. Gooey, M. Elaripe. 2006. 'The Involvement of People with HIV in PNG's HIV Response'. Final Report to Oxfam Australia.

Lee, R. 2006. 'Filipino Experience of Ritual Male Circumcision: knowledge and insights for anti-circumcision advocacy'. *Culture, Health & Sexuality* 8(3): 225–34.

Lee, R., L. Norella, B. Ragas, R. Rola, M. Sibbaluca and C. Tena. 2002. *Between the Thighs: penile circumcision, implants and sexual gadgets*. Jakarta: the Ford Foundation.

Lemeki, M., M. Passey and P. Setel. 1996. 'Ethnographic Results of a Community STD Study in the Eastern Highlands Province'. *Papua New Guinea Medical Journal* 39: 239–42.

Lennox, S. 2000. 'Impact of Logging on the Bamu River'. Available on-line (accessed 23 April 2005) at: http://www.ozgreen.org.au/Web%20Files/Newsletter%20 Articles/PNGNov99No2.htm .

Lepani, K. 2004. 'HIV/AIDS High Risk Settings Strategy: focal point project analysis'.

———2007a. 'Sovasova and the Problem of Sameness: converging interpretative frameworks for making sense of HIV and AIDS in the Trobriand Islands'. *Oceania* 77(1): 12–28.

———2007b. *In the Process of Knowing: making sense of HIV and AIDS in the Trobriand Islands of Papua New Guinea*. Ph.D. dissertation. Australian National University.

———2008a. 'Fitting Condoms on Culture: rethinking approaches to HIV prevention in the Trobriand Islands, Papua New Guinea'. In L. Butt and R. Eves (eds) *Making Sense of AIDS: culture, sexuality, and power in Melanesia*, pp. 246–66. Honolulu: University of Hawai'i Press.

———2008b. 'Mobility, Violence, and the Gendering of HIV in Papua New Guinea'. *The Australian Journal of Anthropology* 19(2): 150–64.

Leslie, H.Y. 2002. 'Producing *What* in the Transition?: health messaging and cultural constructions of health in Tonga'. *Pacific Health Dialog* 9(2): 296–302.

Lett, L. 1942. *The Papuan Achievement*. Melbourne: Oxford University Press.

Levi-Strauss, C. 1963. 'The Sorcerer and His Magic'. In *Structural Anthropology*, pp. 167–85. Garden City: Doubleday.

Levy, C. 2005. 'Attitudes and Behaviours Toward HIV and AIDS and Persons Living with AIDS'. Madang: VSO Tokaut AIDS Baseline Report.

———2006. 'Research and Evaluation on the Impact of the Awareness Community Theatre Program In Raikos and Jimi Districts'. Madang: VSO Tokaut AIDS Project.

Lewis, G. 1975. *Knowledge of Illness in a Sepik River Society*. London: Athlone.

——— 1980. *Day of Shining Red: an essay on understanding ritual*. Cambridge: Cambridge University Press.

Lifeline. 2004. *The National*, 29 August.

Lima, V.D., P. Kretz, A. Palepu, S. Bonner, T. Kerr, D. Moore, M. Daniel, J. Montaner and R. Hogg. 2006. 'Aboriginal Status is a Prognostic Factor for Mortality Among Antiretroviral Naïve HIV-Positive Individuals First Initiating HAART'. *AIDS Research and Therapy* 3(14): 1–9.

Limpakarnjanarat, K. 2000. 'Improving the Surveillance, Monitoring and Evaluation of the National Program'. Appended to C. Jenkins (2002).

Lindenbaum, S. 1972. 'Sorcerers, Ghosts and Polluting Women: an analysis of religious belief and population control'. *Ethnology* 11: 241–53.

——— 1979. *Kuru Sorcery: disease and danger in the New Guinea Highlands*. Palo Alto: Mayfield.

——— 2008. 'Foreword'. In L. Butt and R. Eves (eds) *Making Sense of AIDS: culture, sexuality, and power in Melanesia*, pp. vii–xiv. Honolulu: University of Hawai'i Press.

Lopez, B. 1986. *Arctic Dreams*. New York: Scribners.

Lovelock, J.E. 1987 [1979]. *Gaia*. New York: Oxford University Press.

Luker, V. 2004. 'Civil Society, Social Capital and the Churches: HIV/AIDS in Papua New Guinea'. State, Society and Governance in Melanesia Project Working Paper 2004/1.

Luluaki, J. 2003. 'Sexual Crimes Against and Exploitation of Children and the Law in Papua New Guinea'. *International Journal of Law, Policy and the Family* 17: 275–307.

Lush, L., G. Walt and J. Ogden. 2003. 'Transferring Policies for Treating Sexually Transmitted Infections: what's wrong with global guidelines?' *Health Policy and Planning* 18(1): 18–30.

Lyons, A.P. 1914. 'Daru, Western Division, Patrol Reports, 1913–1914'. CRS G91, Item 194.

—— 1926. 'Notes on the Gogodara Tribe of Western Papua'. *Journal of the Royal Anthropological Institute of Great Britain and Ireland* 56: 329–59.

Macintyre, M. 2008. 'Police and Thieves, Gunmen and Drunks: problems with men and problems with society in Papua New Guinea'. *Australian Journal of Anthropology* 19: 179–93.

Maddocks, I. 1967. 'Donovanosis in Papua'. *Papua and New Guinea Medical Journal* 10: 49–53.

—— 1975. 'Medicine and Colonialism'. *The Australian and New Zealand Journal of Sociology* 11(3): 27–33.

Maddocks, I., E.M. Anders and E. Dennis. 1976. 'Donovanosis in Papua New Guinea'. *British Journal of Venereal Disease* 52: 190–6.

Magaña, R. 1991. 'Sex, Drugs and HIV: an ethnographic approach'. *Social Science and Medicine* 33(1): 5–9.

Mageo, J. 1991. 'Inhibitions and Compensations: a study of the effects of negative sanctions in three Pacific cultures'. *Pacific Studies* 14(3): 1–40.

—— 1998. *Theorizing the Self in Samoa: emotions, genders, and sexualities*. Ann Arbor: University of Michigan Press.

Maher, R.F. 1961. *New Men of Papua: a study of culture change*. Madison: University of Wisconsin Press.

Makoae, M. and K. Jubber 2008. 'Confidentiality or Continuity?: family caregivers experiences with care for HIV/AIDS patients in home-based care in Lesotho'. *Journal of Social Aspects of HIV/AIDS* 5(1): 36–46.

Malau, C. and S. Crockett. 2000. 'HIV and Development, the Papua New Guinea Way'. *Development Bulletin* 52: 58–60.

Malau, C., M. O'Leary, C. Jenkins and N. Faraclas 1994. 'HIV/AIDS Prevention and Control in Papua New Guinea'. *AIDS 1994* 8 (Supplement 2): S117–S124.

Malinowski, B. 1929. *The Sexual Life of Savages*. New York: Harcourt, Brace & World.

Malins, I. 1987. *Christian Marriage and Family Life*. Wewak: Christian Books, Melanesia.

Mallett, S. 2003. *Conceiving Cultures: reproducing people and places on Nuakata, Papua New Guinea*. Ann Arbor: University of Michigan Press.

Mamu, M. 2006. 'Rise of STI, a Threat to SI'. *Nation*, 28 March.

Manderson, L. 1997. 'Parables of Imperialism and Fantasies of the Exotic: western representations of Thailand – Place and Sex'. In L. Manderson and M. Jolly (eds) *Sites of Desire/Economies of Pleasure: sexualities in Asia and the Pacific*, pp. 123–44. Chicago: University of Chicago Press.

Manderson, L. and M. Jolly (eds). 1997. *Sites of Desire/Economies of Pleasure: sexualities in Asia and the Pacific*. Chicago: University of Chicago Press.

Marksbury, R. (ed.). 1993. *The Business of Marriage: transformations in Oceanic matrimony*. Pittsburgh: University of Pittsburgh Press.

Massey-Baker, G.W. 1911. 'Patrol Reports, Western Division, 1911'. Commonwealth Archives, C.R.S. G91, Item 192.

Matane, P. 1992. 'Research Tarnishes Our Image'. *Post-Courier*, September.

Matit, P. 2005. 'Papua New Guinea: the impact of Ok Tedi Mine on indigenous women along the Fly River'. Available on-line (accessed 23 April 2005) at: http://www.mmpindia.org/womenandminigreport.pdf .

McBride, W. 2005. 'HIV/AIDS in Papua New Guinea: an unfolding disaster?' *Emergency Medicine Australasia* 17: 304–6.

McBride, J. and D. Bradford. 2004. 'Antiretroviral Therapy for HIV-infected People in Papua New Guinea: challenges and opportunities'. *Papua New Guinea Medical Journal* 47(1–2): 22–30.

McCarthy, J. 1970. *New Guinea Journeys*. Adelaide: Rigby.

McKellar-James, G. 2004. 'Review of *Missionaries, Headhunters & Colonial Officials*, by Peter Maiden'. Available on-line (accessed 24 April 2005) at: http://www.asopa.com.au/archives/mh&co_review.htm .

McNiven, I., F. von Gnielinski and M. Quinell. 2004. 'Torres Strait and the Origin of Large Stone Axes From Kiwai Island, Fly River Estuary (Papua New Guinea)'. *Memoirs of the Queensland Museum*, Cultural Heritage Series 3(1): 271–89.

McPherson, Naomi. 2008. 'SikAIDS: deconstructing the awareness campaign in rural West New Britain, Papua New Guinea'. In L. Butt and R. Eves (eds) *Making Sense of AIDS: culture, sexuality, and power in Melanesia*, pp. 224–45. Honolulu: University of Hawai'i Press.

Mead, M. 1963. *Sex and Temperament in Three Primitive Societies*. New York: Morrow-Quill.

Meggitt, M. 1964. 'Male-Female Relationships in the Highlands of Australian New Guinea'. *American Anthropologist* 66(4, Pt. 2): 204–24.

—— 1969. 'Introduction'. In R.M. Glasse and M.J. Meggitt (eds), *Pigs, Pearlshells, and Women: marriage in the New Guinea Highlands*, pp. 1–15. Englewood Cliffs, New Jersey: Prentice-Hall.

Melrose, D. 2002. *Tropical Public Health Studies in Papua New Guinea With Emphasis on Filariasis and Other Parasitic Diseases*. Thesis for Doctor of Public Health, James Cook University.

Mgone, C., M. Passey, J. Anang, W. Peter, T. Lupiwa, D. Russell and M. Alpers. 2002. 'Human Immunodeficiency Virus and Other Sexually Transmitted Infections Among Female Sex Workers in Two Major Cities in Papua New Guinea'. *Sexually Transmitted Diseases* 29: 265–70.

Middleton, J. 2006a. 'Violence Against Women the Norm in Papua New Guinea'. *New Zealand Herald*, 23 May.

—— 2006b. 'Papua New Guinea's Sex Disease Time Bomb Ticks Away'. *New Zealand Herald*, 15 May.

Miller, L. and M. Gur. 2002. 'Religiousness and Sexual Responsibility in Adolescent Girls'. *Journal of Adolescent Health* 31: 401–6.

Mishra, V. 2007. 'Why Do So Many HIV-Discordant Couples in Sub-Saharan Africa Have Female Partners Infected, Not Male Partners?' Available on-line (accessed 27 July 2008) at: http://hivimplementers.org/agenda/pdf/U3/U3-Mishra%20Abstract%201717.ppt.pdf .

Mola, G. 2005. 'Caring for Pregnant Women with Donovanosis or HIV in the Low-Resource Setting of Papua New Guinea'. *O&G* 7(3): 22–4.

—— 2006. 'The Fight Against HIV/AIDS in Papua New Guinea'. Originally published in the *Post-Courier*, 4 December.

—— 2008. 'Pastors Sounded More Like the Pharisees'. *Post-Courier*, 8 July.

Mond, L. 1999. Press Statement, 'On the Current Status of HIV/AIDS in Papua New Guinea – May 13'. Available on-line (accessed 7 August 2007) at: http://portmoresby.anglican.org/org/ais.html .

Mondia, P. 1990. 'Editorial: The Impact of Acquired Immunodeficiency Syndrome (AIDS) on Tuberculosis Control in Papua New Guinea'. *Papua New Guinea Medical Journal* 33: 81–3.

Mondia, P. and J. Perera. 1990. 'A Limited Serosurveillance of HIV Infection Among Tuberculosis Patients Attending a Tuberculosis Clinic: a preliminary report'. Paper presented to the 26th Annual Medical Symposium. Draft Manuscript.

Moral and Social Issues Council (MSIC). 2006. 'Discussion Paper on Homosexuality and the Salvation Army'. Available on-line (accessed 2 August 2007) at: http://www.salvationarmy.org.nz/SITE_Default/SITE_about/x-files/18431.pdf .

Morin, J. 2008. '"It's Mutual Attraction": transvestites and the risk of HIV transmission in urban Papua'. In L. Butt and R. Eves (eds) *Making Sense of AIDS: culture, sexuality, and power in Melanesia*, pp. 41–59. Honolulu: University of Hawai'i Press.

Morobean Observer. 2008. 'Scrutiny into Health Dept Lauded'. *The National*, 7 March.

Mulhern, P. 2001. 'Medical Care for Prisoners in Papua New Guinea—2001'. Available on-line (accessed 30 September 2007) at: http://www.pfi.org/programmes/global_assistance_ programme/PNG%202001%20Reportpdf .

Mullings, L. 1984. *Therapy, Ideology, and Social Change*. Berkeley: University of California.

Murdoch, D., W. Venter, A. Van Rie and C. Feldman. 2007. 'Immune Reconstitution Inflammatory Syndrome (IRIS): review of common infectious manifestations and treatment options'. *AIDS Research and Therapy* 4(9): 1–10.

Murray, A. 2001. *Pink Fits: sex, subcultures and discourses in the Asia-Pacific*. Victoria: Monash University Press.

Murray, C.G. 1902. 'Report of the Resident Magistrate, Western Division, on a Visit to the Bamu Estates'. In Appendix B in *Annual Report on British New Guinea*, for the years 1900–01: 85–7.

Murray, J.H.P. 1927. *Annual Report for the Territory of Papua*, for the years 1926–27. Port Moresby: National Archives.

—— 1933. 'Head Hunting in Theory and Practice'. In *Annual Report for the Territory of Papua*, for the years 1931–32. Port Moresby: National Archives.

Mydans, S. 1997. 'A Bartered Bride's "No" Stuns Papua New Guinea: rejection of tribal customs is a sign of changing times'. *New York Times*, 7 May.

Myers, J. 1992. 'Nonmainstream Body Modification: genital piercing, branding, burning and cutting'. *Journal of Contemporary Ethnography* 21(3): 267–306.

Nadel, S.F. 1954. *Nupe Religion*. London: Oxford University Press.

Nagata, Y. 2004. 'The Japanese in Torres Strait'. In A. Shnukal, G. Ramsay and Y. Nagata (eds), *Navigating Boundaries: the Asian Diaspora in Torres Strait*, pp. 138–59. Canberra: Pandanus Books.

Nalu, M. 2004. 'AIDS Could Wipe Out PNG'. *Post-Courier*, 24 January.

Nash, J. 1981. 'Sex, Money, and the Status of Women in Aboriginal South Bougainville'. *American Anthropologist* 8(1): 107–26.

—— 1987. 'Gender Attributes and Equality: men's strength and women's talk among the Nagovisi'. In M. Strathern (ed.) *Dealing With Inequality: analyzing gender relations in Melanesia and beyond*, pp. 150–73. Cambridge: Cambridge University Press.

National, The. 2004. 'Sports Withdraw Makoma Visas'. 6 September.

—— 2005. 'The Settlement Issue'. 28 December.

—— 2006. 'Doctor Against Use of Condoms'. 12 July.

—— 2007. 'More Than 40,000 Living With HIV in PNG'. 9 August.

—— 2008. 'New HIV/AIDS Study to Focus on Attitudes'. 16 April.

National AIDS Council (NAC). 2006. *National Gender Policy and Plan on HIV and AIDS, 2006–2010*. Port Moresby: National AIDS Council.

—— 2007. *National Strategic Plan on HIV/AIDS, 2004–2008*. Port Moresby: National AIDS Council.

National AIDS Council Secretariat (NACS). 2002. (with Department of Health) 'HIV/AIDS Quarterly Report, September'. Port Moresby.

—— 2003. (with Department of Health) 'HIV/AIDS Quarterly Report, December'. Port Moresby.

—— 2005. (with Department of Health) 'HIV/AIDS Quarterly Report, March'. Port Moresby.

—— 2006a. 'Monitoring the Declaration of Commitment on HIV/AIDS, 2004–2005'. United Nations General Assembly Special Session on HIV/AIDS.

—— 2006b. 'HIV/AIDS Quarterly Report, December'. Port Moresby.

—— 2007. (with Department of Health) 'The 2007 Estimation Report on the HIV Epidemic in Papua New Guinea'. Port Moresby.—2008. (with partners). 'UNGASS 2008 Country Progress Report'. Port Moresby.

National Court of Justice. 2007. 'Regular Civil Motions'. 6 April, Judge J. Davani presiding.

National HIV and AIDS Support Project (NHASP). 2001. 'Clinical Research Priorities'. Milestone 13.

—— 2002a. 'An Overview of HIV'. Unpublished report.

—— 2002b. 'HIV Serum Surveillance Indonesia – PNG Border'. Unpublished report.

—— 2002c. 'Serum Surveillance Report'. Unpublished report.

—— 2003a. 'Social Science Research Priorities'. Milestone 44.

—— 2003b. 'Counselling Report: review of final counseling curricula, materials and training'. Milestone 45.

—— 2004a. 'Strategic Planning for HIV/AIDS and STI'. Milestone 66.

—— 2004b. 'Capacity-Building Status Report – Baseline'. Milestone 38.

—— 2005a. 'The Introduction of Antiretroviral Therapy in Papua New Guinea'. Milestone 58.

—— 2005b. 'Gender Impact Evaluation of the National HIV/AIDS Support Project in Papua New Guinea'. Milestone 95.

—— 2005c. 'Situational Analysis for Strategic Planning at the District Level: Western Province'.

—— 2005d. 'District Health Workers Competency in Syndromic Management of STIs'.

—— 2005e. '2004 National HIV/AIDS Consensus Workshop: key findings summary and analysis'. Milestone 82.

—— 2005f. 'Annual Monitoring & Evaluation Report For Year 4'. Milestone 74.

—— 2005g. 'Summary Report: Social Mapping of 19 Provinces in Papua New Guinea'.

—— 2005h. 'Annual Monitoring and Evaluation Report For Year 5'. Milestone 92.

—— 2005i. 'Situational Analysis for Strategic Planning at the District Level: Gulf Province'.

—— 2005j. 'Situational Analysis for Strategic Planning at the District Level: West New Britain Province'.

—— 2005k. 'Training Impact Assessment and Evaluation Report'. Milestone 78 – Parts 1 and 2.

—— 2005l. 'Situational Analysis for Strategic Planning at the District Level: Morobe Province'.

—— 2006a. 'Review of Coverage and Quality of VCT Services in PNG'.

—— 2006b. 'Evaluation of HIV and AIDS Community Theatre'.

—— 2006c. 'Review of Church Engagement and Future Directions'. Milestone 107.

—— 2006d. 'Review of the Papua New Guinea Provincial HIV Program'. Milestone 104.

—— 2006e. 'High Risk Settings Strategy Report: moving beyond awareness'. Milestone 90.

—— 2006f. 'Annual Plan, January 2006 – December 2006'. Milestone 96.

—— 2006g. 'Grant Scheme Impact Assessment'. Milestone 91.

—— 2006h. 'Social Marketing Evaluation Review'. Milestone 100.

—— 2006i. 'Annual Monitoring and Evaluation Report for Year 6'. Milestone 108.

National Sex and Reproduction Research Team (NSRRT) and C. Jenkins. 1994. *National Study of Sexual and Reproductive Knowledge and Behaviour in Papua New Guinea*. Papua New Guinea Institute of Medical Research Monograph No 10. Goroka: Papua New Guinea Institute of Medical Research.

Newman, P. and D. Boyd. 1982. 'The Making of Men: ritual and meaning in Awa male initiation'. In G. Herdt (ed.) *Rituals of Manhood: male initiation in Papua New Guinea*, pp. 239–85. Berkeley: University of California Press.

New Zealand Herald. 2007. 'Pacific Told It Can't Ignore Threat of AIDS'. 12 April.

New Zealand Parliamentarians' Group on Population and Development (NZPGPD). 2006. 'Study Tour to Papua New Guinea: raising awareness of the Millennial Development Goals in the Pacific'. Auckland: NZPPD Secretariat.

Nomelea, F. 1986. 'Western Province'. In *Marriage in Papua New Guinea*, pp. 7–9. Port Moresby: Law Reform Commission.

Nyanzi, S., B. Nyanzi, B. Kalina and R. Pool. 2007[2004]. 'Mobility, Sexual Networks and Exchange Among *bodabodamen* in Southwest Uganda'. In R. Parker, P. Aggleton (eds) *Culture, Society and Sexuality: a reader*, pp. 411–23. London: Routledge.

O'Brien, E. 2007. 'Papua New Guinea's AIDS Crisis May Mirror Africa's, says UN Official'. Available on-line (accessed on 4 September 2007) at: http://www.bloomberg.com/apps/news?pid=20601081&sid=ag58R85zpjE0&refer=australia .

O'Callaghan, M. 1995. 'The Battle to Stop Papua New Guinea Dying of Ignorance'. *The Health Worker* 1: 3.

—— 1999. 'PNG-Positive'. *The Australian Magazine*, 13–14 November.

Oelrichs, R. 2004. 'The Subtypes of Human Immunodeficiency Virus in Australia and Asia'. *Sexual Health* 1: 1–11.

O'Farrell, N. 2001. 'Enhanced Efficiency of Female-to-Male HIV Transmission in Core Groups in Developing Countries'. *Sexually Transmitted Diseases* 28(2): 84–91.

Ohtsuka, R. 1983. *Oriomo Papuans: ecology of sago-eaters in Lowland Papua*. Tokyo: University of Tokyo Press.

O'Keeffe, A., J. Godwin and R. Moodie. 2005. *HIV/AIDS in the Asia Pacific Region. Analytical Report for the White Paper on Australia's Aid Program*. Canberra.

Okuonzi, S. and H. Epstein. 2005. 'Editorial: Pragmatic Safe Sex, Not Abstinence or Faithfulness, Was Key in Uganda's HIV Decline'. *Health Policy and Development* 3(1): ii–iii.

O'Leary, M. 2001[1993]. 'Editorial: Mandatory Testing for HIV – no solution at all'. Reprinted in *Pacific AIDS Alert Bulletin* 22: 28–9.

O'Leary, M., W. van der Meijden, C. Malau, O. Delamare and T. Pyakalyia. 1993. 'HIV Serosurveillance in Papua New Guinea'. *Papua New Guinea Medical Journal* 36(3): 187–91.

Olivier-Miller, S. 2004. 'Papua New Guinea'. In R. Francoeur and R. Noonan (eds) *Continuum Complete International Encyclopedia of Sexuality*, Updated, with More Countries, pp. 813–23. New York: Continuum.

O'Neal, J. 1979. *Up From South: a prospector in New Guinea, 1931–1937*. Sydney: Oxford University Press.

Ostroff, S. 1998. 'Emerging Infectious Diseases: the Pacific at the crossroads'. *Pacific Health Dialog* 5(1): 167–70.

PAC Beat. 2007. 'PNG: HIV/AIDS Numbers Still Rising'. Radio broadcast. Available on-line (accessed (25 July 2007) at: http://www.radioaustralia.net.au/pacbeat/stories/s1882301.htm .

Pach, A., F.G. Cerbone and D.R. Gerstein. 2003. 'A Qualitative Investigation of Antiretroviral Therapy Among Injection Drug Users'. *AIDS and Behavior* 7(1): 87–100.

Pacific AIDS Alert Bulletin. 2007. 'Universal Access to HIV Treatment Achieved in Small Pacific Island Countries'. November, pp. 8–9.

Pacific Islands Monthly. 1950. 'Dr. Vernon Remembered at the Mission in the Mud'. February: 23–4.

—— 1953. 'Mission in the Mud Conducts a Travelling School'. October: 35.

—— 1975. 'Deadly Drink'. March: 22.

Pac News. 2005. 'Government Doctor Arrested with Australian in Small Arms Smuggling'. Available on-line (accessed 21 July 2007) at: http://www.gunpolicy.org/Articles/2005/270105.html .

Paiva, V. 2007[2004]. 'Gendered Scripts and the Sexual Scene: promoting sexual subjects among Brazilian teenagers'. In R. Parker, P. Aggleton (eds) *Culture, Society and Sexuality: a reader*, pp. 427–42. London: Routledge.

Pamba, K. 2005. 'Societal Norms and HIV/AIDS'. The Notebook, *The National*, 5 January.

—— 2008. 'No Sex Till Marriage: HIV virus carrier'. *The National*, 28 March.

Pantumari, J. 2003. 'Papua New Guinea HIV/AIDS Situation Analysis'. Women and Mining Conference, 3–6 August.

Paradi, N. 2002. 'HIV-AIDS Trip'. Unpublished manuscript.

Pareti, S. 2001. 'UNGASS: walking the talk in the Pacific'. *Pacific AIDS Alert Bulletin* 22: 4–5.

Parikh, S. 2007. 'The Political Economy of Marriage and HIV: the ABC approach, "safe" infidelity, and managing moral risk in Uganda'. *American Journal of Public Health* 97(7): 1198–1208.

Parliament of the Commonwealth of Australia. 1916. 'Pearl-Shelling Industry: report and recommendations of the Royal Commission'. Canberra: Government of Australia.

Passey, M. 1996. 'Issues in the Management of Sexually Transmitted Diseases in Papua New Guinea'. *Papua New Guinea Medical Journal* 39: 252–60.

Passey, M., C. Mgone, S. Lupiwa, N. Suve, S. Tiwara, T. Lupiwa, A. Clegg and M. Alpers. 1998a. 'Community Based Study of Sexually Transmitted Diseases in Rural Women in the Highlands of Papua New Guinea: prevalence and risk factors'. *Sexually Transmitted Infections* 74: 120–7.

Passey, M. C. Mgone, S. Lupiwa, S. Tiwara, S. Lupiwa and M. Alpers. 1998b. 'Screening for Sexually Transmitted Diseases in Rural Women in Papua New Guinea: are WHO therapeutic algorithms appropriate for case detection?' *Bulletin of the World Health Organization* 76(4): 401–11.

Pathanapornpandh, N. 2005. 'Establishment of Pilot HIV/AIDS Care Centers'. Technical Consultants Report prepared for the Asian Development Bank. Bangkok, Thailand.

People and Planet. 2006. 'AIDS Epidemic Taking Hold in Papua New Guinea'. Available on-line (accessed 30 July 2007) at: http://www.peopleandplanet.net .

Per, Z. 2006. 'AIDS Cases Rise to Over 11,800 in Q1'. *The National*, 4 April.

Persson, A. 2004. 'Incorporating *Pharmakon*: HIV, medicine, and body shape change'. *Body & Society* 10(4): 45–67.

Peseta, N. 2007. 'Second Generation Surveillance Surveys of Sexual Risk Behavior Among Youth in Tokelau'. Tokelau: Council for the Ongoing Government of Tokelau.

Peter, A. 2006. 'Doctor Against Use of Condoms'. *The National*, 12 July.

Pigg, S. 2001. 'Languages of Sex and AIDS in Nepal: notes on the social production of commensurability'. *Cultural Anthropology* 16(4): 481–541.

Pilkington, E. 2007. '$1bn "Don't Have Sex" Campaign a Flop as Research Shows Teenagers Ignore Lessons'. *The Guardian*, 16 April. Available on-line (accessed 23 April 2007) at: http://education.guardian.co.uk/schoolsworldwide/story/0,,2058181,00.html .

Pincock, S. 2006. 'Papua New Guinea Struggles to Reverse Health Care Decline'. *The Lancet* 368: 107–8.

Pirie, P. 2000. 'Untangling the Myths and Realities of Fertility and Mortality in the Pacific Islands'. *Asia-Pacific Population Journal* 15(2): 5–20.

Pitt-Rivers, G.H.L. 1927. 'The Effect on Native Races of Contact with European Civilisation'. *Man* 27: 2–10.

Pitts, M. 2001. 'Crime and Corruption – does Papua New Guinea have the capacity to control it'? *Pacific Economic Bulletin* 16(2): 127–34.

Plummer, D. and D. Porter. 1997. 'The Use and Misuse of Epidemiological Categories'. In G. Linge and D. Porter (eds) *No Place For Borders: the HIV/AIDS epidemic and development in Asia and the Pacific*, pp. 41–50. New York: St. Martin's Press.

Population Action International. 2007. *Abstaining From Reality: US restrictions on HIV prevention*. Washington, D.C.: Population Action International.

Porter, D. 1997. 'A Plague on the Borders: HIV, development, and traveling identities in the Golden Triangle'. In L. Manderson and M. Jolly (eds) *Sites of Desire/ Economies of Pleasure: sexualities in Asia and the Pacific*, pp. 21–32. Chicago: University of Chicago Press.

Pospisil, L. 1963. *The Kapauku Papuans of West New Guinea*. New York: Holt, Rinehart and Winston.

Post-Courier, The. 2001. 'AIDS No Laughing Matter'. 5 December.

—— 2002. 'Deadly Binge'. 18 June.

—— 2004. 'Trust in God for Change'. 7 October.

—— 2005. 'Provide Condoms!' 29 November.

—— 2006. 'Poverty is the Key Issue in the Fight Against HIV/AIDS'. 8 March.

—— 2007. 'Condoms Not Safe'. 26 February.

—— 2008a. 'Asian Sex Racket'. 20 March.

—— 2008b. 'Boy Raped by Women'. 4 April.

—— 2008c. 'More Mothers, Students HIV Positive in Morobe'. 6 June.

—— 2008d. 'Floating Brothels'. 26 September.

Powdermaker, H. 1971[1933]. *Life in Lesu: the study of a Melanesian society in New Ireland*. New York: W.W. Norton & Co.

Prior, J.M. 2001. 'Of Mud and Militias: Pentecost Thoughts from Papua New Guinea'. Available on-line (accessed 25 June 2007) at: http://eapi.admu.edu.ph/eapr001/prior1.htm .

Qalo, S. 2007. 'Police Humiliated Me: AIDS victim'. *The Fiji Times Online*. Available on-line (accessed on 22 August 2007) at: http://www.fijitimes.com.fj/story.aspx?id=68981 .

Radio Australia. 2007. 'PNG: HIV/AIDS numbers still rising'. Available on-line (accessed 25 July 2007) at: http://www.radioaustralia.net.au/pacbeat/stories/s1882301.htm .

Ralston, C. 1988. '"Polyandry," "Pollution," "Prostitution": the problems of eurocentrism and androcentrism in Polynesian studies'. In B. Caine, E.A. Grocz and M. de Lepervanche (eds), *Crossing Boundaries*, pp. 71–80. Sydney: Allen and Unwin.

—— 1992 'Dialogue: the study of women in the Pacific'. *The Contemporary Pacific* (Spring): 162–75.

Raynes, P. and G. Maibani. 2006. 'The Challenges to Scaling Up Antiretroviral Therapy in Papua New Guinea'. *Papua New Guinea Medical Journal* 49(1–2): 32–42.

Reed, A. 1997. 'Contested Images and Common Strategies: early colonial sexual politics in the Massim'. In L. Manderson and M. Jolly (eds) *Sites of Desire/ Economies of Pleasure: sexualities in Asia and the Pacific*, pp. 48–71. Chicago: University of Chicago Press.

—— 2003. *Papua New Guinea's Last Place: experiences of constraint in a postcolonial prison*. Oxford: Berghahn Books.

Reed, S. W. 1943. *The Making of Modern New Guinea, with special reference to Culture Contact in the Mandated Territory*. Philadelphia: The American Philosophical Society.

Rei, H. 2007. 'OTML Employees Take Part in Health Workshop'. *The National*, 7 June.

Re/Search. 1989. *Modern Primitives*. San Francisco: Re/Search Publications.

Reynolds, M. 2007. 'The Abstinence Gluttons'. *The Nation*, 18 June.

Rheeney, A. 2008. 'PNG Government's HIV Response in Crisis'. *Pacific Magazine*. Available on-line (accessed 22 August 2008) at: http://www.pacificmagazine. net/news/2008/03/12/png-governments-hiv-response-in-crisis .

Richards, S. 2004. 'God's Curse and Hysteria: women's narratives of AIDS, Manokwari, West Papua'. *Papua New Guinea Medical Journal* 47(1–2): 77–87.

Riley, E.B. 1925. *Among Papuan Headhunters*. Philadelphia: J.B. Lippincott.

Riley, I. 2000. 'Lessons from Sexually Transmitted Epidemics', Special AusAID Seminar: 'It's Everyone's Problem: HIV/AIDS and Development in Asia and the Pacific'. Canberra: Australian Agency for International Development.

Robbins, J. 2004. *Becoming Sinners: Christianity and moral torment in Papua New Guinea*. Berkeley: University of California Press.

Roheim, G. 1940. 'Professional Beauties of Normanby Island'. *American Anthropologist* 42: 657–61.

—— 1946. 'Ceremonial Prostitution in Duau (Normanby Island)'. *Journal of Clinical Psychopathology and Psychotherapy* 7: 753–64.

Ronayne-Ford, J. 2006. 'Prevention'. Available on-line (accessed 30 September 2006) at: http://www.aids.net.au/aids-global-png20060411a.htm .

Rosenhan, D. 1973. 'On Being Sane in Insane Places'. *Science* 179: 250–8.

Rubin, G. 1975. 'The Traffic in Women: notes on the "political economy" of sex'. In R. Reiter (ed.) *Toward an Anthropology of Women*, pp. 157–210. New York: Monthly Review.

Rupali, P., R. Condon, S. Roberts, L. Wilkinson, L. Voss and M.G. Thomas. 2007. 'Prevention of Mother to Child Transmission of HIV infection in Pacific Island Countries'. *Internal Medicine Journal* 37: 216–23.

Ryan, F. 1999. *Virus X: tracking the new killer plagues out of the present and into the future*. Boston: Little, Brown and Company.

Salamon, C and C. Hamelin. 2008. 'Why are Kanak Women More Vulnerable than Others to HIV?: ethnographic and statistical insights from New Caledonia'. In L. Butt and R. Eves (eds) *Making Sense of AIDS: culture, sexuality, and power in Melanesia*, pp. 80–96. Honolulu: University of Hawai'i Press.

Saracco, A., M. Musicco and A. Nicolosi. 1993. 'Man-to-Woman Sexual Transmission of HIV: longitudinal study of 343 steady partners of infected men'. *Journal of Acquired Immune Deficiency Syndromes* 6: 497–502.

Sarda, R. and J. Gallwey. 1995. 'STD Services in the Pacific: report of a survey'. *Pacific Health Dialog* 2(2): 37–44.

Satoro, L. 2008. 'PNG Tops STI Cases in Asia Pacific Region'. *The National*, 23 May.

Scheper-Hughes, N. 1994. 'AIDS and the Social Body'. *Social Science and Medicine* 39(7): 991–1003.

Schieffelin, E. 1976. *The Sorrow of the Lonely and the Burning of the Dancers*. New York: St. Martin's Press.

Schneebaum, T. 1989. *Where the Spirits Dwell: an odyssey in the jungle of New Guinea*. New York: Grove Press.

Schoeffel, P. 1994. 'Social Change'. In K.R. Howe, R.C. Kiste and B.V. Lal (eds) *Tides of History: the Pacific islands in the twentieth century*, pp. 350–80. Honolulu: University of Hawai'i Press.

Schoepf, B.G. 2003. 'Uganda: lessons for AIDS control in Africa'. *Review of African Political Economy* 30(98): 377–96.

—— 2004a. 'AIDS, History, and Struggles Over Meaning'. In E. Kalipeni, S. Craddock, J. Oppong and J. Ghosh (eds) *HIV and AIDS in Africa: beyond epidemiology*. pp. 15–28. Oxford: Blackwell.

—— 2004b. 'AIDS in Africa: structure, agency and risk'. In E. Kalipeni, S. Craddock, J. Oppong and J. Ghosh (eds) *HIV and AIDS in Africa: beyond epidemiology*. pp. 121–32. Oxford: Blackwell.

Schug, D. 1995. 'The Marine Realm and the Papua New Guinean Inhabitants of the Torres Strait'. *SPC Traditional Marine Resource Management and Knowledge Information Bulletin* 5: 16–23.

Seaton, B., J. Wembri, P. Armstrong, J. Ombiga, S. Naraqi and I. Kevau. 1996. 'Symptomatic Human Immunodeficiency Virus (HIV) Infection in Papua New Guinea'. *Australia and New Zealand Journal of Medicine* 26(6): 783–8.

Second Strategic Planning Workshop (SSPW). 2000. 'A Strategic Plan For Responding to HIV/AIDS and STIs in the Kingdom of Tonga, 2001–2005'. Tongatapu, Tonga: Australian Agency for International Development.

Serpenti, L. 1977. *Cultivators in the Swamps*. Assen, the Netherlands: Van Gorcum.

—— 1993[1984] 'Ritual Homosexuality and Pedophilia Among Kimam-Papuans'. In G. Herdt (ed.) *Ritualized Homosexuality in Melanesia*, revised, paperback edition, pp. 292–317. Berkeley: University of California Press.

Setel, P. 1999. *A Plague of Paradoxes: AIDS, culture, and demography in Northern Tanzania*. Chicago: University of Chicago Press.

Shapiro, R. and S.H. Kapiga. 2002. 'Male Condoms and Circumcision'. In M. Essex, S. Mboup, P. Kanki, R. Marlink and S. Tlou (eds) *AIDS in Africa*, 2nd ed., pp. 490–505. New York: Kluwer.

Sharp, N. 1993. *The Stars of Tagai: the Torres Strait islanders*. Canberra: Aboriginal Studies Press.

Shelton, J. and N. Fuchs. 2004. 'Opportunities and Pitfalls in Integration of Family Planning and HIV Prevention Efforts in Developing Countries'. *Public Health Reports* 119: 12–5.

Shnukal, A. 2004. 'The Post-Contact Created Environment in the Torres Strait Central Islands'. *Memoirs of the Queensland Museum*, Cultural Heritage Series 3(1): 317–46.

Sidibe, M., I. Ramiah and K. Buse. 2006. 'Alignment, Harmonisation and Accountability in HIV/AIDS'. *The Lancet* 368: 1853–4.

Siebers, R. and M. Lynch. 1998. 'HIV and AIDS Knowledge Among Medical Laboratory Technologists in the Pacific'. *Pacific Health Dialog* 5(1): 22–5.

Silverman, E. 2004. 'Anthropology and Circumcision'. *Annual Review of Anthropology* 33: 419–45.

Sims, P. 2003. 'Papua New Guinea Needs Law and Order Above All'. *BMJ* 326(7381): 165.

Singe, J. 1989. *The Torres Strait: people and history*. Townsville: University of Queensland.

Singer, P. and D.E. DeSole. 1967. 'The Australian Subincision Ceremony Reconsidered: vaginal envy or kangaroo bifid penis envy'. *American Anthropologist* 69: 355–8.

Singh, S., J. Darroch and A. Bankole. 2004. 'A, B and C in Uganda: the roles of abstinence, monogamy and condom use in HIV decline'. *Reproductive Health Matters* 12(23): 129–31.

Siriratmongkhon, W.I.-e.K. 2002. 'Gender and pleasure: exploration of sex gadgets, penile implants and related beliefs in Thailand'. Nakornprathom, Thailand: Institute for Population and Social Research.

Sissons, D.C.S. 1976. 'Karayuki-San: Japanese prostitutes in Australia, 1887–1916, pt. I'. *Historical Studies* 17(68): 323–41.

—— 1977. 'Karayuki-San: Japanese Prostitutes in Australia, 1887–1916, pt. II'. *Historical Studies* 17(69): 474–88.

Skrobanok, S., N. Boonpakdi and C. Janthakeero. 1997. *The Traffic in Women: human realities of the international sex trade*. London: Zed Books.

Sladden, T. 2005. 'Twenty Years of HIV Surveillance in the Pacific: what do the data tell us and what do we still need to know?' *Pacific Health Surveillance and Response* 12(2): 22–37.

Sloan, N., B. Winikoff, N. Haberland, C. Coggins and C. Elias. 2000. 'Screening and Syndromic Approaches to Identify Gonorrhea and Chlamydial Infection Among Women'. *Studies in Family Planning* 31: 55–68.

SMART Study Group. 2006. 'CD4+ Count: guided interruption of antiretroviral treatment'. *New England Journal of Medicine* 355(22): 2283–96.

Smith, D.J. 2004. 'Youth, Sin and Sex in Nigeria: Christianity and HIV/AIDS-related beliefs and behaviour among rural-urban migrants'. *Culture, Health & Sexuality* 6(5): 425–37.

Smith, G., S. Kippax, P. Aggleton and P. Tyrer. 2003. 'HIV/AIDS School-based Education in Selected Asia-Pacific Countries'. *Sex Education* 3(1): 3–21.

Snow, P. and S. Waine. 1979. *People From the Horizon: an illustrated history of the Europeans Among the South Sea Islanders*. Oxford: Phaidon Press.

Specht, J. and F. Fields. 1984. *Frank Hurley in Papua: photographs of the 1920–1923 Expeditions*. Bathurst: Robert Brown and Associates.

Spiller, P. 2006. 'Tackling PNG's Aids Epidemic'. BBC News, 28 September. Available on-line (accessed 24 July 2007) at: http://news.bbc.co.uk/2/hi/asia-pacific/5385436.stm .

Staff Writer. 1961. 'Quarter Century With the Mission in the Mud'. *Pacific Islands Monthly* 31(11): 45–7.

STD Nius. 1996. 'Health Minister Launches Sexual Health Prevention & Care Project'. April.

Steingraber, S. 1997. *Living Downstream: an ecologist looks at cancer and the environment*. New York: Addison-Wesley.

Steinberg, J. 2008. *Sizwe's Test: a young man's journey through Africa's AIDS epidemic*. New York: Simon and Schuster.

Stewart, C. 2004. 'Towards a Climate of Tolerance and Respect: legislating for HIV/AIDS and human rights in Papua New Guinea'. *Journal of South Pacific Law* 8(1). Available online (accessed on 20 August 2008) at: http://www.paclii.org/journals/fJSPL/vol08no1/2.shtml

—— 2006. 'Prostitution and Homosexuality in Papua New Guinea: legal, ethical and human rights issues'. Gender Relations Centre. Canberra: Australian National University.

—— 2008. 'Men Behaving Badly: sodomy cases in the Colonial Courts of Papua New Guinea'. *Journal of Pacific History* 43(1): 77–93.

Suaudeau, P. 2007. 'Safe Sex'. Available on-line (accessed 1 August 2007) at: http://www.hli.org/safe_sex.pdf .

Sullivan, N. 2007. 'God's Brideprice: laissez faire religion, and the fear of being left behind in PNG'. *Contemporary PNG Studies: DWU Research Journal* 6: 63–91.

Sullivan, N., T. Warr, J. Rainbubu, J. Kunoko, F. Akuane, M. Angasa and Y. Wenda. 2003. 'Tinpis Maror: a social impact study of proposed RD Tuna cannery in Vidar Wharf, Madang'. Madang: Nancy Sullivan and Associates.

Suzuki, K., Y. Motohashi, Y. Kaneko. 2006. 'Factors Associated With the Reproductive Health Risk Behavior of High School Students in the Republic of the Marshall Islands'. *Journal of School Health* 76(4): 138–44.

Sydney Morning Herald. 2005a. 'Ties are fraying with PNG'. Editorial, 18 May.

—— 2005b. 'Aussie Jailed in PNG for Gun Smuggling'. 27 January.

—— 2007a. 'Sorcery Murders Linked to AIDS Ignorance'. 30 January.

—— 2007b. 'HIV Stigma Made Worse'. 29 May.

—— 2007c. 'PM Endorses Strict HIV Screening'. 14 April.

Taime, M. 2006. 'Use Condoms to Fight Virus'. *Post-Courier*, 21 August.

Tau, G. 2007. 'Neuro AIDS in Papua New Guinea'. PowerPoint presentation to Pacific Neuro AIDS Meeting, Sydney, 20 July.

The Australian. 2008. 'Report Finds Australian Businessmen Contracting HIV in PNG'. Available on-line (accessed 21 September 2008) at: http://www.theaustralian. news.com.au/story/0,25197,24354594-5013404,00.html .

The Health Worker. 1995. 'HIV-Infection in PNG Hits the Highest in Mid-1995'. October.

Thierfelder, M.U. 1928. 'The Control of Granuloma Venereum Among the Marindinese in Dutch South-New-Guinea'. *Mededeelingen van den Dienst der Volksgzondheit in Nederlansch-Indie* 17: 393–423.

Tiwara, S., M. Passey, A. Clegg, C. Mgone, S. Lupiwa, N. Suve and T. Lupiwa. 1996. 'High Prevalence of Trichomonal Vaginitis and Chlamydial Cervicitis Among a Rural Population in the Highlands of Papua New Guinea'. *Papua New Guinea Medical Journal* 39: 234–8.

Tobia, B. 1998. 'The ILO Urges Govts to Recognise Booming Sex Industry'. *Pacific Islands Monthly*, November, p. 31.

Tobias, M. 2007. 'The HIV/AIDS Crisis in Papua New Guinea'. *Issue Analysis* 81: 1–20.

Toliman, P., T. Lupiwa, G. Law, J. Reeder and P. Siba. 2006. 'Gonococcal Drug Sensitivities, Gonorrhoea, Chlamydia, Trichomoniasis and High Risk Behaviours Among STI Clinic Attendees from Goroka, Lae, Mt Hagen and Port Moresby'. Goroka: Papua New Guinea Institute of Medical Research.

Tonny, M. 2008. 'Safe Sex, Whose Responsibility'. *The National*, 4 February.

Townsend, I. 2002. 'AIDS Epidemic Sweeps Across Papua New Guinea'. *The World Today*. Available on-line (accessed 7 August 2007) at: http://www.abc.net.au/ worldtoday/stories/s597683.htm .

Tozer, R.A. 1996. 'Papua New Guinea Red Cross Blood Transfusion Service: present status and future considerations'. *Papua New Guinea Medical Journal* 39(1): 38–42.

Treat Asia. 2007. 'Site Profile'. Available on-line (accessed 7 August 2007) at: http:// www.amfar.org/cgi-bin/iowa/asia/news/index.html?record=114 .

Trenholm, C., B. Devaney, K. Fortson, L. Quay, J. Wheeler and M. Clark. 2007. 'Impacts of Four Title V, Section 510 Abstinence Only Education Programs'. Available on-line (accessed 30 July 2007) at: http://www.mathematica-mpr. com/publications/PDFs/impactabstinence.pdf .

Tuzin, D. 1980. *The Voice of the Tambaran: truth and illusion in Ilahita Arapesh religion.* Berkeley: University of California Press.

—— 1982. 'Ritual Violence Among Ilahita Arapesh: the dynamics of moral and religious uncertainty'. In G. Herdt (ed.) *Rituals of Manhood: male initiation in Papua New Guinea*, pp. 321–56. Berkeley: University of California Press.

Underhill, K., P. Montgomery and D. Operario. 2007. 'Sexual Abstinence Only Programmes to Prevent HIV Infection in High Income Countries: systematic review'. BMJ 335(7613): 248–59.

UNICEF East Asia and Pacific Regional Office. 2006. *Pacific: Children and HIV/AIDS – a call to action.* Bangkok: UNICEF.

UNICEF, UNESCAP and ECPAT. 2006. *Commercial Sexual Exploitation of Children (CSEC) and Child Sexual Abuse (CSA) in the Pacific: A Regional Report.* Suva, Fiji: UNICEF Pacific.

United Nations. 1996. *Time to Act: The Pacific Response to HIV and AIDS.* Suva, Fiji: United Nations.

—— 2001. 'Papua New Guinea Common Country Assessment'.

United Nations Programme on HIV/AIDS, Australian Agency for International Development and National AIDS Council (UNAIDS-AusAID-NAC). 2004. *HIV/AIDS Stakeholder Mapping in Papua New Guinea.*

United Nations Programme on HIV/AIDS, United Nations Children's Fund and the World Health Organization (UNAIDS-UNICEF-WHO). 2004. 'Epidemiological Fact Sheets: Papua New Guinea'.

United States Conference of Catholics Bishops (USCCB). 2004. 'The Nature and the Scope of the Problem of Sexual Abuse of Minors by Catholic Priests and Deacons in the United States'.

Van der Geest, S. and S. Sarkodie. 1998. 'The Fake Patient: a research experiment in a Ghanaian hospital'. *Social Science and Medicine* 47(9): 1373–81.

Vanderwal, R. 2004. 'Early Historical Sources for the Top Western Islands in the Western Torres Strait Exchange Network'. *Memoirs of the Queensland Museum, Cultural Heritage Series* 3(1): 257–70.

de Vincenzi, I. and the European Study Group on Heterosexual Transmission of HIV. 1994. 'A Longitudinal Study of Human Immunodeficiency Virus Transmission by Heterosexual Partners'. *New England Journal of Medicine* 331: 341–6.

Vinit, T. 2004. 'HIV/AIDS Control: the PNG way'. Mass e-mailed PowerPoint presentation.

—— 2008. 'We Need a Tougher Adultery Act'. *The National*, 16 April.

Visnegarwala, F., S. Raghavan, C. Mullin, G. Bartsch, J. Wang, D. Kotler, C. Gibert, J. Shlay, C. Grunfeld, A. Carr and W. El-Sadr. 2005. 'Sex Differences in the Associations of HIV Disease Characteristics and Body Composition in Antiretroviral-Naive Persons'. *American Journal of Clinical Nutrition* 82(4): 850–6.

Vogel, L.C., with J. Richens. 1989. 'Donovanosis in Dutch South New Guinea: history, evolution of the epidemic and control'. *Papua New Guinea Medical Journal* 32: 203–18.

Vulum, S. 2001. 'Worry 1: HIV/aids on the increase'. *Pacific Magazine.* 1 December. Available on-line (accessed 7 August 2007) at: http://www.pacificmagazine. net/issue/2001/12/01/worry-1-hivaids-on-the-increase .

Vunisea, A. 2005. 'HIV Risks Through the Tuna Industry'. SPC Women in Fisheries Bulletin 15, April: 8–9.

Waiut, S. 2005. 'Skate Spells Out "Three Evils"'. *Post-Courier,* 2 December.

De Walque, D. 2006. 'Discordant Couples: HIV Infection Among Couples in Burkina Faso, Cameroon, Ghana, Kenya, and Tanzania'. World Bank Policy Research Working Paper No. 3956.

Wardlow, H. 2002a. 'Headless Ghosts and Roving Women: specters of modernity in Papua New Guinea'. *American Ethnologist* 29: 5–32.

—— 2002b. '"Giving Birth to *Gonolia*": "culture" and sexually transmitted disease among the Huli of Papua New Guinea'. *Medical Anthropology Quarterly* 16: 151–75.

—— 2002c. 'Public Health, Personal Beliefs: battling HIV and AIDS in Papua New Guinea'. *Cultural Survival Quarterly* 26(3): 29–32.

—— 2004. 'Anger, Economy and Female Agency: problematizing "prostitution" and "sex work" among the Huli of Papua New Guinea'. *Signs* 29(4): 1017–40.

—— 2006a. *Wayward Women: sexuality and agency in a New Guinea society*. Berkeley: University of California Press.

—— 2006b. 'All's Fair When Love is War: romantic passion and companionate marriage among the Huli of Papua New Guinea. In J. Hirsch and H. Wardlow (eds) *Modern Loves: the anthropology of romantic courtship & companionate marriage*, pp. 51–77. Ann Arbor: University of Michigan.

—— 2007. 'Men's Extramarital Sexuality in Rural Papua New Guinea'. *American Journal of Public Health* 97: 1006–14.

—— 2008. '"You Have to Understand: Some of Us are Glad AIDS has Arrived": Christianity and condoms among the Huli, Papua New Guinea'. In L. Butt and R. Eves (eds), *Making Sense of AIDS: culture, sexuality, and power in Melanesia*, pp. 187–205. Honolulu: University of Hawa'i Press.

Washington, H. 2007. *Medical Apartheid: the dark history of medical experimentation on Black Americans from colonial times to the present*. New York: Random House.

World Association for Sexual Health (WAS). 2007. 'Declaration of Human Sexual Rights'. Available on-line (accessed 23 July 2007) at: http://www.worldsexology. org/about_sexualrights.asp .

W.D. 1940. 'Papua's Western Division: it is not all mud'. *Pacific Islands Monthly*, 15 June, pp. 44–5.

Weed, S., I. Erickson, A. Lewis, G. Grant and K. Wibberly. 2008. 'An Abstinence Program's Impact on Cognitive Mediators and Sexual Initiation'. *American Journal of Health Behavior* 32(1): 60–73.

Westaway, J. 1989. 'Marshall Islands Employs Education to Reduce High Birthrate'. *Development* (Wellington) September: 4–13.

White, M. 2000. 'Australia's Contribution to Family Planning, Reproductive Health and Population Programs in the Pacific Islands and Papua New Guinea'. Australian Reproductive Health Alliance. Occasional Paper 1(1).

Whiteman, J. 1973. 'Chimbu Family Relationships in Port Moresby'. New Guinea Research Bulletin 52. Port Moresby and Canberra: Australian National University.

Widi-Wirski, R., S. Berkly and R. Downing. 1988. 'Evaluation of the WHO Clinical Case Definition for AIDS in Uganda'. *Journal of the American Medical Association* 260: 3286–9.

Wiebel, W. and Safika. 2001. 'Migration Patterns of Sex Workers in Irian Jaya, Indonesia'. Jakarta: Program for Appropriate Technology in Health.

Wilde, C. 2003. *Men at Work: masculinity, mutability, and mimesis among the Gogodala of Papua New Guinea*. Ph.D. dissertation. University of Sydney.

—— 2004. 'Acts of Faith: muscular Christianity and masculinity among the Gogodala of Papua New Guinea'. *Oceania* 75(1): 32–48.

—— 2007. '"Turning Sex into a Game": Gogodala men's response to the AIDS epidemic and condom promotion in rural Papua New Guinea'. *Oceania* 77(1): 58–71.

Wilkinson, D. and G. Dore. 2000. 'An Unbridgeable Gap?: comparing the HIV/AIDS epidemics in Australia and sub-Saharan Africa'. *Australian and New Zealand Journal of Public Health* 24(3): 276–80.

Williams, F.E. 1924. *The Natives of the Purari Delta*. Port Moresby: Government Printer.

—— 1969[1936]. *Papuans of the Trans-Fly*. Oxford: Clarendon Press.

Willis, I. 1974. *Lae: village and city*. Melbourne: Melbourne University Press.

Wilson, A. 2004. *The Intimate Economies of Bangkok: tomboys, tycoons, and Avon ladies in the global city*. Berkeley: University of California Press.

Windybank, C. and M. Manning. 2003. 'Papua New Guinea On the Brink'. *Issue Analysis* 30: 1–16.

Winn, M. and D. Lucas. 1993. 'Language, Videos and Family Planning in the South Pacific'. *Asia-Pacific Population Journal* 8(4): 19–38. Available on-line (accessed 29 July 2007) at: http://www.unescap.org/esid/psis/population/journal/1993/v08n4a2.htm .

Wood, M. 1987. 'Brideservice Societies and the Kamula'. *Canberra Anthropology* 10: 1–23.

—— 1996. 'Rimbunan Hijau's Wawoi-Guavi Timber Concession Exposed'. Available on-line (accessed 6 April 2005) at: http://forests.org/archived_site/today/recent/1996/wgtc.htm .

—— 1998. 'Logging, Women and Submarines: some changes in Kamula men's access to transformative power'. *Oceania* 68(4): 228–48.

Workman, R., A. Hill and T. Pinhey. 2001. 'Promoting HIV Testing Among Guam Sex Workers'. *Research for Sex Work* 4. Available on-line (accessed 23 August 2007) at: http://hcc.med.vu.nl/artikelen/workman.htm .

World Bank, Asian Development Bank and Australian Agency for International Development (WB-ADB-AusAID). 2006. 'Papua New Guinea Human Development Strategy'. Draft.

World Council of Churches. 2004. 'The *Nadi* Declaration: a statement of the World Council of Churches' Pacific Member Churches on HIV/AIDS'. Available on-line (accessed 4 September 2007) at: http://www.bloomberg.com/apps/news?pid=20601081&sid=ag58R85zpjE0&refer=australia .

World Health Organization (WHO). 2001a. 'HIV/AIDS in Asia and the Pacific Region'.

—— 2001b. 'STI/HIV: the condom situation assessment in 11 Asian and Western Pacific countries'.

—— 2005. 'WHO Multi-Country Study on Women's Health and Domestic Violence Against Women, Factsheet on Samoa'.

—— 2006. 'WHO Country Cooperation Strategy: Papua New Guinea – 2005–2009'.

World Health Organization, the National AIDS Council Secretariat and the National Department of Health (WHO-NACS-NDoH). 2000. 'STI/HIV 2000 Consensus Report'. Port Moresby: The Government of Papua New Guinea.

World Health Organization and the Secretariat of the South Pacific (WHOSSP). 2004. 'HIV/AIDS and Sexually Transmitted Infections'. Suva, Fiji.

—— 2006. 'Second Generation Surveillance Surveys of HIV, other STIs and Risk Behaviors in 6 Pacific Island Countries (2004–2005)'. Suva, Fiji.

World Health Organization, United Nations Agency for International Development and the United Nations Children's Fund (WHO-UNAID-UNICEF). 2008. *Towards Universal Access: scaling up priority HIV/AIDS interventions in the health sector*. Geneva: WHO.

World Health Organization Regional Office (WHORO) for the Western Pacific. 2005. 'HIV/AIDS and Sexually Transmitted Infections'. Manila: World Health Organization.

Wright, H. 1959. *New Zealand, 1769–1840: early years of Western contact*. Cambridge: Harvard University Press.

Yakaipoko, W. 2002. *The Blue Logic*. Port Moresby: University of Papua New Guinea Press.

Yamada, S. 1998. 'Prostitution in CNMI: political and economic aspects of emerging infectious diseases'. *Pacific Health Dialog* 5(1): 76–8.

Yeka, W., G. Maibani-Michie, D. Prybylski and D. Colby, 2006. 'Application of Respondent Driven Sampling to Collect Baseline Data on FSWs and MSM for HIV Risk Reduction Interventions in Two Urban Centres in Papua New Guinea'. *Journal of Urban Health* 83 (Supplement 7): 60–72.

Zenner, D. and S. Russell. 2005. 'Sexually Transmitted Diseases and HIV/AIDS in Vanuatu: a cause for concern and action'. *The New Zealand Medical Journal* 118 (1220). Available on-line (accessed 7 August 2007) at: http://www.nzma.org.nz/journal/118-1220/1610/content.pdf .

Zigas, V. 1971. 'A Donovanosis Project in Goilala (1951–54)'. *Papua and New Guinea Medical Journal* 14(4): 148–9.

Zimmer-Tamakoshi, L. 1993a. 'Nationalism and Sexuality in Papua New Guinea'. *Pacific Studies* 16(4): 61–98.

—— 1993b. 'Bachelors, Spinsters, and *Pamuk Meris*'. In R. Marksbury (ed.) *The Business of Marriage: transformations in Oceanic matrimony*, pp. 83–104. Pittsburgh: University of Pittsburgh Press.

—— 1997. '"Wild pigs and dog men": rape and domestic violence as "women's issues" in Papua New Guinea'. In C. Brettell and C. Sargent (eds) *Gender in Cross-Cultural Perspective*, 2nd ed, pp. 538–53. Englewood Cliffs, New Jersey: Prentice-Hall.

—— 2004. 'Rape and Other Sexual Aggression'. In C. Ember and M. Ember(eds) *The Encyclopedia of Sex and Gender*, Volume One, pp. 230–43. Amsterdam: Kluwer

Index

ABC (Abstain, Be faithful, use Condoms)   xi, 1–8 *passim*, 22–7 *passim*, 32, 37–8, 41, 48, 133, 137, 138, 143–4, 174, 180, 189, 192–4, 199, 203, 204, 214–18 *passim*, 227, 235, 247–8, 262–4, 276, 300, 302, 314, 320, 326–34n3 *passim*
abortion   41, 78, 208
Africa, relevance of HIV and AIDS prevalence there to Papua New Guinea   2, 8-9, 16, 32, 46, 55, 58, 119, 143, 146, 152, 157, 159, 172, 190, 199, 214, 220, 227–8, 248, 326, 337, 341, 344, 351, 355–6, 363–4, 374, 386
alcohol   65, 66, 70–1, 80, 95–6, 100–1, 104, 110, 158, 170, 202, 204, 220, 239, 248, 266, 298, 301, 305, 323, 380, 383
Asmat   82–3, 89

Bamu
    traditional sexual networking   60–98 *passim*
    centrality in trade throughout south coast New Guinea   63–8 *passim*, 76–8, 84–8, 95
    sagapari/tu kina bus   62, 70–2, 76, 78–9, 88, 93–4, 97n13
Bernard, Sister Rose   23, 44
Bonivento, Bishop Cesare   10, 22–3, 44, 48, 56–7, 135, 137, 192, 207–9, 212, 215–34, 242–4
Boyd, Mark   5, 29, 58, 269, 337–68 *passim*
Bush, George   48, 222–3, 245n2, 331, 351
bush medicine   15–16, 24, 40, 52, 192, 358–9
Butt, Leslie   3, 16, 19, 32, 55, 58, 139, 190–1, 274, 277, 281, 286, 288, 291, 300, 310

canoes, canoe-hulls, and their manufacture and trade   63–9, 76–8, 84–91 *passim*
Central Province   96, 126, 158, 172
Central Public Health Laboratory   114, 118, 129, 184
Christian, policies and doctrines of relevance to HIV, AIDS, STDs, sexuality and condoms   1–4, 8–32 *passim*, 38–55 *passim*, 61, 72, 80, 96, 121–4, 134–40 *passim*, 160–6, 170, 174, 181–2, 194–296 *passim*, 249–50, 255, 261–6, 272, 274–82 *passim*, 286, 297, 300, 307, 311, 314, 319–23, 324–34 *passim*, 360, 373
Churches, Christian
    Anglican   11, 30, 44, 175, 181, 233–5, 329
    Baptist   97n6, 198, 234, 238, 329–30
    Catholic   11, 20–3 *passim*, 44, 48, 54, 61, 79, 81, 111, 135, 183, 195–9 *passim*, 207, 211, 215, 217, 222–44 *passim*, 254, 289, 300, 329–30
    evangelical   29, 50, 58n1, 121, 126, 138, 182, 195, 198, 209, 214, 217, 234, 237–40, 311, 323
    faith healings, alleged   8, 16, 24, 38, 52, 261, 358
    Lutheran   177, 237, 254

www.ingramcontent.com/pod-product-compliance
Lightning Source LLC
Chambersburg PA
CBHW050520190326
41458CB00005B/1604